Bipolar
Psychopharmacotherapy

Bipolar Psychopharmacotherapy
Caring for the Patient
Second Edition

Edited by

Hagop S. Akiskal

University of California, San Diego, CA, USA

and

Mauricio Tohen

Department of Psychiatry,
University of Texas Health Science Centre, San Antonio, TX, USA
International Society for Bipolar Disorders

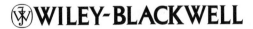
A John Wiley & Sons, Ltd., Publication

Library of Congress Cataloging-in-Publication Data

Bipolar psychopharmacotherapy : caring for the patient / edited by Hagop Akiskal and Mauricio Tohen. – 2nd ed.
       p. ; cm.
  Includes bibliographical references and index.
  ISBN 978-0-470-74721-6 (cloth)
  1. Manic-depressive illness–Chemotherapy. 2. Lithium–Therapeutic use. 3. Antipsychotic drugs.
4. Psychopharmacology. I.   Akiskal, Hagop S. II.   Tohen, Mauricio.
  [DNLM: 1.   Bipolar Disorder–drug therapy. 2.   Anticonvulsants–therapeutic use.
3.   Antimanic Agents–therapeutic use. 4.   Antipsychotic Agents–therapeutic use.
5.   Bipolar Disorder–prevention & control. WM 207]
  RC516.B529 2011
  616.89′5–dc22

                                                                                      2010046388

A catalogue record for this book is available from the British Library.

This book is published in the following electronic formats: ePDF: 9780470975107; Wiley Online Library: 9780470975114; ePub: 9780470976982

Set in 10/12pt Times Roman by Laserwords Private Limited, Chennai, India
Printed in Singapore by Ho Printing Singapore Pte Ltd

First Impression 2011

*This book is dedicated to patients with bipolar disorder
and their families for the privilege
of caring for them.*

*We also dedicate it to Pierre Deniker and Mogens Schou
for their pioneering research which made such caring possible.*

"To my wife Dianne" – Mauricio Tohen

Contents

Contents _____ ix

Contents ———————————————————————— xiii

List of Contributors

Hagop S. Akiskal, International Mood Center, University of California at San Diego, 9500 Gilman Drive, La Jolla, CA 92093-0603, USA

Kareen K. Akiskal, International Mood Center, University of California at San Diego, 9500 Gilman Drive, La Jolla, CA 92093-0603, USA; French Depressive and Manic-Depressive Association, Rennes, France

Lori L. Altshuler, Department of Psychiatry and Behavioral Sciences, Veterans Affairs Greater Los Angeles Healthcare System, The David Geffen School of Medicine at UCLA, Los Angeles, CA, USA

Lesley M. Arnold, Department of Psychiatry and Behavioral Neuroscience, Women's Health Research Program, University of Cincinnati College of Medicine, 231 Albert Sabin Way, Cincinnati, OH 45267, USA

Jean-Michel Azorin, Department of Psychiatry, Ste Marguerite Hospital, 13274 Marseille Cedex 9, France

Jacqueline Baumann, Experimental Therapeutics and Pathophysiology Branch, Intramural Research Program, National Institute of Mental Health, National Institutes of Health, Bethesda, MD, USA

Joris Berwaerts, Johnson & Johnson Pharmaceutical Research & Development, LIC Beerse, Belgium; JB Titusville, NJ, USA

Charles L. Bowden, Department of Psychiatry, University of Texas Health Science Center at San Antonio, 7703 Floyd Curl Drive, San Antonio TX 78229-3900, USA

L. Ivo Caers, Johnson & Johnson Pharmaceutical Research & Development, LIC Beerse, Belgium; JB Titusville, NJ, USA

Joseph R. Calabrese, School of Medicine, Case Western Reserve University and University Hospitals of Cleveland, Cleveland, OH 44106, USA

Giedra Campbell, Scientific Communications, Lilly Research Laboratories, Lilly Corporate Center, Indianapolis, IN 46285, USA

Francesc Colom, Head of Psychoeducation and Psychological Treatments Area, Barcelona Bipolar Disorders Program, IDIBAPS, Institute of Neurosciences, Hospital Clinic, Villarroel 170, 08036 Barcelona, Spain

John Cookson, The Royal London Hospital, Burdett House, Mile End Hospital, Bancroft Road, London E1 4DG, UK

V.E. Cosgrove, Stanford School of Medicine, Stanford University Medical Center, 300 Pasteur Drive, Stanford, CA 94305, USA

Robert L. Findling, Division of Child and Adolescent Psychiatry, University Hospitals Case Medical Center, 10524 Euclid Avenue, Cleveland, OH 44106, USA

Juan-Carlos Gómez, Psychosis Global Development Team, Lilly Research Laboratories, Lilly Corporate Center, Indianapolis, IN 46285, USA

Paul Grof, Mood Disorders Center of Ottawa, Smyth Medical Building, 1929 Russell Road, Ottawa, ON K1G 4G3, Canada

Heinz Grunze, Academic Psychiatry, Newcastle General Hospital, Westgate Road, Newcastle upon Tyne NE46BE, UK

Ioline Henter, Experimental Therapeutics and Pathophysiology Branch, Intramural Research Program, National Institute of Mental Health, National Institutes of Health, Bethesda, MD, USA

Nathan Herrmann, Department of Psychiatry, Faculty of Medicine, Sunnybrook Health Sciences Center, University of Toronto, 2075 Bayview Avenue, Toronto, ON M4N 3M5, Canada

Onur N. Karayal, Pfizer Inc., 235 East 42nd Street, New York, NY 10017, USA

A.E. Koukopoulos, Azienda Ospedaliera Sant'Andrea, Università La Sapienza Roma, Rome, Italy

Athanasios Koukopoulos, Centro Lucio Bini Roma, 42, Via Crescenzio, 00193 Rome, Italy

Mauricio Kunz, Department of Psychiatry, Mood Disorders Centre, University of British Columbia, Vancouver, Canada

David Latov, Experimental Therapeutics and Pathophysiology Branch, Intramural Research Program, National Institute of Mental Health, National Institutes of Health, Bethesda, MD, USA

Rodrigo Machado-Vieira, Experimental Therapeutics and Pathophysiology Branch, Intramural Research Program, National Institute of Mental Health, National Institutes of Health, Bethesda, MD, USA

Susan L. McElroy, Lindner Center of HOPE, Mason and Department of Psychiatry, and Behavioral Neuroscience University of Cincinnati College of Medicine, 231 Albert Sabin Way, Cincinnati, OH 45267, USA

Roger S. McIntyre, Departments of Psychiatry and Pharmacology and Institute of Medical Science, University of Toronto; Mood Disorders Psychopharmacology Unit, University Health Network, 399 Bathurst Street, Toronto M5T 2S8, Canada

Andrea Murru, Barcelona Bipolar Disorders Program, IDIBAPS, Institute of Neurosciences, Hospital Clinic, 08036 Barcelona, Spain

David J. Muzina, Department of Psychiatry and Psychology, The Cleveland Clinic Foundation, Cleveland, OH 44195, USA

Alessandra Nivoli, Bipolar Disorders Program, Clinical Institute of Neuroscience, Hospital Clinic, University of Barcelona, IDIBAPS-CIBERSAM, Villarroel 170, Barcelona 08036 Catalonia, Spain

Willem A. Nolen, Department of Psychiatry, University Medical Center Groningen, University of Groningen, Groningen, The Netherlands

Svante Nyberg, Neuroscience TA, AstraZeneca R&D, Södertälje, Sweden

Elizabeth Pappadopulos, Department of Psychiatry Research, Zucker Hillside Hospital, Glen Oaks, NY 11004, USA

Robert M. Post, The George Washington University, 5415 West Cedar Lane, Suite 201B, Bethesda, MD 20814, USA

Zoltán Rihmer,, Department of Clinical and Theoretical Mental Health, and Department of Psychiatry and Psychotherapy, Semmelweis University, Faculty of Medicine, Budapest, Hungary.

Martha Sajatovic, Department of Psychiatry, Case Western Reserve University School of Medicine and University Hospitals Case Medical Center, 10524 Euclid Avenue, Cleveland, OH 44106, USA

G. Sani, Azienda Ospedaliera Sant'Andrea, Università La Sapienza Roma, Rome, Italy

Mogens Schou, Deceased prior to the publishing of the 2nd edition of this book

Thomas L. Schwartz, Treatment Resistant Depression and Anxiety Disorders Program, SUNY Upstate Medical University, Syracuse NY 13210, USA

Kenneth I. Shulman, Department of Psychiatry, Faculty of Medicine, Sunnybrook Health Sciences Center, University of Toronto, 2075 Bayview Avenue, Toronto, ON M4N 3M5, Canada

J.S. Seo, Stanford School of Medicine, Stanford University Medical Center, 291 Campus Drive MC 5216, Stanford, CA 94305-5101, CA, USA

G. Serra, Azienda Ospedaliera Sant' Andrea, Università La Sapienza Roma, Rome, Italy

Vivek Singh, Department of Psychiatry, University of Texas Health Science Center at San Antonio, 7703 Floyd Curl Drive, San Antonio TX 78229-3900, USA

Stephen M. Stahl, Department of Psychiatry, University of California San Diego, 9500 Gilman Drive # 9116-A, La Jolla, CA 92093-9116-A, USA; Department of Psychiatry, University of Cambridge, Cambridge, UK

Trisha Suppes, VA Palo Alto Health Care System, Palo Alto; Stanford University Medical Centre, Stanford School of Medicine, 300 Pasteur Drive, Stanford, CA 94305, USA

Alan C. Swann, Department of Psychiatry and Behavioral Sciences, The University of Texas Health Science Center at Houston, 1300 Moursund Street, Houston TX 77030, USA

Tiffany Thomas, Division of Child and Adolescent Psychiatry, University Hospitals Case Medical Center, 10524 Euclid Avenue, Cleveland, OH 44106, USA

Mauricio Tohen, Department of Psychiatry, Division of Mood and Anxiety Disorders, University of Texas Health Science Centre at San Antonio, 7730 Floyd Curl Drive, San Antonio, TX 78229, USA

Marc L.M. van der Loos, Department of Psychiatry, Isala Klinieken, Location Sophia, Zwolle, The Netherlands

Eduard Vieta, Bipolar Disorders Program, Clinical Institute of Neuroscience, Hospital Clinic, University of Barcelona, IDIBAPS-CIBERSAM, Villarroel 170, Barcelona 08036, Catalonia, Spain

Cristina Wheeler-Castillo, Experimental Therapeutics and Pathophysiology Branch, Intramural Research Program, National Institute of Mental Health, National Institutes of Health, Bethesda, MD, USA

H. Yang, Stanford School of Medicine, Stanford University Medical Center, 300 Pasteur Drive, Stanford, CA 94305, USA

Lakshmi N. Yatham, UBC Department of Psychiatry, UBC Hospital, The University of British Columbia, 2255 Wesbrook Mall, Vancouver BC V6T2AI, Canada

Boghos I. Yerevanian, Department of Psychiatry and Biobehavioral Sciences, David Geffen School of Medicine, University of California, Los Angeles, CA, USA

Carlos A. Zarate, Experimental Therapeutics and Pathophysiology Branch, Intramural Research Program, National Institute of Mental Health, National Institutes of Health, Bethesda, Maryland, USA

F. Zazzara, Centro Lucio Bini Roma, 42, Via Crescenzio, 00193 Rome, Italy

Preface to the Second Edition

Although few new drugs have been introduced since the first edition of this book five years ago, the field of bipolar pharmacotherapy has grown sober and hopefully wiser. With the FDA approval of new indications for existing agents, we actually have an embarrassment of riches.

The generation of the senior editor, who started practicing in the early 1970s, had only lithium, the sole agent approved by the FDA specifically for the treatment of what was then called manic-depressive illness. And in a sense we were lucky because we had many years to learn how best to use this agent for the prophylaxis of the disruptive mood episodes of patients with this devastating condition. There was great enthusiasm, even though there were then very few clinical centers in North America where lithium was prescribed. The enthusiasm was due to the fact that lithium was – and still is – a very special agent, at that time unlike any other in our field. We had to follow strict protocols for its use and limit it largely to those who had the 'classical' presentations of the illness. Lithium helped 'medicalize' psychiatry because one had to be a well-trained physician to use it properly. Although some patients who were misinformed about the dangers of lithium shunned this product (just like some psychiatrists), many more wanted to have a therapeutic trial. Thus, it became a sign of prestige to be offered a trial with this 'miraculous' agent. Part of the mystique was that it was not a drug – it was a natural product. Unfortunately, it is not free of risk: despite proper work-up and expert follow-up, 25 years later a very small minority of patients may develop kidney or thyroid dysfunction. We, nonetheless, continue to believe that even with the availability of newer agents every bipolar patient, properly screened, needs to be evaluated for the benefits of a properly conducted lithium trial. With the publication of systematic long-term data from the BALANCE study in the UK (*Lancet* 375:385–395,2010), sceptics have been reminded of the benefits of lithium.

The anticonvulsant agents that are psychoactive with 'mood stabilizing' properties have been widely studied and were the first agents to provide an alternative to lithium, either as monotherapy or in combination with lithium. Although 'polypharmacy' has gained a bad reputation, it has become the standard in the treatment of many diseases such as hypertension and epilepsy: these conditions have indeed served as a model for combination therapy in psychiatry. Combination therapy has actually raised bipolar psychopharmacotherapy into an art form in the hands of experts, and we have therefore devoted a chapter to extensive coverage of its proper application. Mood and bipolar clinics nowadays depend on such experts to supervise the work of young psychiatrists. One can say that bipolar clinics have helped to make bipolarity a psychiatric subspecialty – almost. Such clinics conduct research not only on pharmaceutical aspects, but also on biomarkers of clinical response, as well as long-term observational studies of patient cohorts, and the development of psychoeducational and innovative psychotherapies specifically geared for bipolar disorder.

Enter the atypical antipsychotics, the main class of agents introduced in the last decade for bipolar disorder. Classical neuroleptics were very effective for acute mania, in fact they were the first pharmacological agents used in the treatment of bipolar mania over 60 years ago, but extrapyramidal, endocrine as well as depressive side effects limited their use. They can, however, still be used in selected patients, especially for acute treatment and in the elderly. That is why atypical antipsychotics have been welcomed in clinical practice, even though they are not entirely free of the limitations of the neuroleptics – and most bring their own liabilities in terms of metabolic side effects.

This edition builds on the comprehensive scope of the first edition in that we cover different classes of agents as well as different populations, namely children, women, and older patients. In view of major recent advances in atypical agents, each (including Clozapine) is now covered in a separate chapter, and the newer agents (including Asenapine) have been added to our coverage in separate chapters. A unique feature of this edition is the two chapters devoted to the pharmacological treatment of mixed states and rapid cycling, the forms of bipolar disorder which are all too common in current practice and often challenging for the patient, family, and psychiatrist. Although the use of antidepressants remains controversial in bipolar disorder, and certainly antidepressant monotherapy in bipolar illness is generally contra-indicated, in practice they are not infrequently combined with mood-stabilizing agents; for this reason a chapter meticulously summarizing the pros and cons of antidepressant use in bipolar disorder graces this new edition. We are also pleased that a team of clinical scientists from the National Institute of Mental Health, Bethesda, brings to this edition the latest expertise in novel and experimental approaches to the treatment of bipolarity.

As in the first edition – which also appeared in Spanish (2007) and Turkish (2009) – our monograph devoted to bipolar pharmacotherapy opens with a chapter on the scope of bipolar disorders from clinical and epidemiologic–public health perspectives. Suicide prevention, the major evidence for which comes from Hungary which has pioneered this field, is also described from such a dual perspective. We conclude with an expanded and extensively revised chapter on the principals of caring for bipolar patients and their families in a mood (bipolar) clinic; this chapter extends beyond the chapter on psychoeducation to weave, in association with the individual pharmacotherapy chapters, an even broader integrative philosophy of care for bipolar patients than in the first edition. The substantive advances in bipolar psychopharmacotherapy in the last five years have caused the book to grow from 19 to 25 chapters, which cover essentially all efficacious treatments for bipolar disorder with the exception of electroconvulsive and stimulation-modulation therapies.

We thank the staff at Wiley-Blackwell, in particular, Joan Marsh, who closely worked with the editors and the authors to achieve these goals. Nearly all authors represent pioneers, from both industry and academia, in the development of the individual drugs or therapeutic topics or modalities covered in this book. We sorely miss the late Mogens Schou who opened, with his ground-breaking research, one of the most glorious pages in the history of psychopharmacotherapy with his extensive research on lithium. For this reason the new edition has a dedication to him and the late Professor Pierre Deniker (who, with Jean Delay), led the introduction of Chlorpromazine, the first neuroleptic, into psychiatry.

We believe that the best weapon against the stigma of mental illness is research and the development of efficacious treatments for which this book stands as witness. We believe that drug development can improve further with synergistic efforts of scientists from industry and academia. Allies in this battle are the patients themselves, their families, and the clinical professionals privileged to care for them. This book is dedicated to them as well.

Hagop Akiskal
Mauricio Tohen

1

The Scope of Bipolar Disorders

Hagop S. Akiskal

University of California at San Diego, CA, USA

1.1   DIAGNOSTIC AND PUBLIC HEALTH ASPECTS

Recent advances in the epidemiology, psychopathology, and pharmacotherapy of bipolar disorders have led to a greater recognition of this illness in all of its varieties (Akiskal *et al.*, 2000; Maj *et al.*, 2002; Goodwin and Jamison, 2007). The lifetime risk for bipolar conditions is about 1% for the core (bipolar I) phenotype, making it at least equal in prevalence to schizophrenia. A higher percentage of acute psychiatric hospital admissions is now being assigned to the category of mania, and recognition of clinically attenuated outpatient forms of the illness (soft bipolar spectrum) is increasing. The latter (Bipolar II and beyond) is now estimated to be at least three to four times more prevalent than bipolar I (Angst *et al.*, 2003; Judd and Akiskal, 2003; Hirschfeld *et al.*, 2003); the current US prevalence of bipolar spectrum disorders, including bipolar I, is estimated at 4–5% (Merikangas *et al.*, 2007).

Reasons for the current focus on the entire diagnosable range of bipolar conditions are several. Predominant among these is the tendency of diagnostic practice to follow the availability of effective treatment modalities (Lehmann, 1969). After the discovery of chlorpromazine, North American psychiatrists were tacitly encouraged to elicit subtle degrees of formal thought disorder from their patients so as to bring them the benefits of this new class of drugs. By the early 1970s, schizophrenia had become more or less synonymous with psychosis. With the advent of lithium carbonate treatment and its well-documented efficacy for bipolar disorders, this trend became reversed in favor of bipolar disorders. Beginning with DSM-III (American Psychiatric Association, 1980), the concept of schizophrenia has been largely restricted to a core group of deteriorating psychotic disorders, while mood disorders have been broadened to include even those with mood-incongruent psychotic features that may or may not coincide with affective episodes. This diagnostic approach reflects more than just therapeutic fashion; it is supported by familial aggregation, course, and outcome (Akiskal, 2002). Available evidence indicates that mood disorders are often recurrent and, especially in bipolar conditions, can lead to considerable impairment in developmental, conjugal, and social spheres. The public health significance of bipolar disorder is summarized in Table 1.1. The most important of these is suicide, seen in as many as 20% of those who receive inadequate or no

Bipolar Psychopharmacotherapy: Caring for the patient, Second Edition. Edited by Hagop S. Akiskal and Mauricio Tohen.
© 2011 John Wiley & Sons, Ltd. Published 2011 by John Wiley & Sons, Ltd.

Table 1.1 Public health aspects of bipolar disorder.

Lifelong cyclical illness
1.0–1.5% of population
Peak onset 15–30 years
5–10 year delay in correct diagnosis
Frequent hospitalization
Repeated hospitalization
Repeated conjugal disruption: promiscuity
Repeated job change/loss
Financial disasters
Alcohol/substance abuse
50% nonadherence to medication
Increased cardiovascular mortality
Suicide (highest within 10 years of illness onset)

treatment, and must be considered a *preventable* complication (Khuri and Akiskal, 1983; Akiskal, 2007). It now appears that bipolar II may account for a disproportionately large portion of suicidal morbidity and mortality among bipolar disorders (Rihmer *et al.*, 1990; Rihmer and Pestality, 1999; Akiskal, 2007), emphasizing the importance of early and accurate diagnosis.

At the "softest" end of the spectrum, milder degrees of bipolar disorder – subsumed under the rubrics of cyclothymic disorder (Akiskal *et al.*, 1977) and bipolar disorder not otherwise specified – are now categorized as mood disorders rather than being grouped with neurotic or personality disorders. Although these seemingly attenuated and "atypical" variants may not be easily distinguishable from nonaffective personality disorders, the clinician is advised to err on the side of affective diagnosis because of treatment implications, including their potential to engage in suicidal acts (Azorin *et al.*, 2010).

External validating strategies – such as family history, course, and inter-episodic temperamental features – are often necessary to confirm the diagnosis of the bipolar spectrum (Akiskal, 2003). The most established of bipolarity beyond classic mania and bipolar I (Akiskal, 1999) is the bipolar II type, so-named originally by Dunner, Gershon, and Goodwin (1976). Like diabetes type II, its onset is often insidious, but its ravages no less devastating than that of the psychotic forms of the illness. This is particularly true for cyclothymic depression, a variant of bipolar II we have termed bipolar II$^1/_2$ (Akiskal *et al.*, 2006), arising from a cyclothymic temperament, it pursues an unstable course; and is likely to be misdiagnosed as axis II cluster B (Akiskal, 2004). These patients represent the "dark side" of bipolarity (Akiskal, Hantouche, and Lancrenon, 2003; Hantouche, Angst, and Akiskal, 2003).

The American Psychiatric Association Diagnostic Manual of Mental Disorders, even in its last published edition (DSM-IV, 2000), does not recognize hypomanic or manic switches occurring during pharmacotherapy, electroconvulsive therapy, phototherapy, and sleep deprivation as indicators of bipolar disorder. These patients are obviously not unipolar MDD, nor are they classified under bipolar NOS. Therefore, this common clinical phenomenon is voted by the DSM Committee out of existence. Since at least 1983, there has been good evidence that such switching of antidepressants requires bipolar family history (Akiskal *et al.*, 2000; Akiskal, Hantouche, and Lancrenon, 2003). They are best regarded as less penetrant forms of bipolar disorder (bipolar III). Diagnostic studies of depressive states with mood swings in the setting of multiple drug abuse, particularly that of stimulants, is controversial, but we contend that many of these individuals belong to a provisional bipolar type III-$^1/_2$ (Akiskal and Pinto, 1999; Maremmani *et al.*, 2003; Camacho and Akiskal, 2005). This is relevant in a book on advances in bipolar disorder, because many of these patients respond favorably to anticonvulsant mood stabilizers. Finally, I would like to mention bipolar type IV, which refers to individuals who develop depression later in life from a lifelong background of hyperthymic temperament (hypomanic traits without clear cut episodes); their bipolar status might be inferred from familial bipolarity (Cassano *et al.*, 1992). It is uncertain how DSM-V in progress will deliberate on the status of bipolar spectrum disorders. Suffice it to say that their public health significance (that is,, early diagnosis and treatment) warrants a more appropriate nosological designation than the inglorious dumping ground of "bipolar NOS."

In a French national study (see Table 1.2), 65% of all major depressions belonged to the bipolar spectrum, of which the most prevalent were the bipolar II and II$^1/_2$ phenotypes (Akiskal *et al.*, 2005b, 2006). These considerations are important, because nearly all pharmacologic treatments covered in this book – certainly those approved by regulatory bodies – pertain to bipolar I. Thus, there is a wide gap between the psychopharmacology of bipolar disorder and the public health significance of the phenotypes observed in the community and the clinic.

Lithium was the first specific agent for bipolar disorder for clinical use. This was four decades ago. Many other agents have been approved since then, almost all of them in the last decade. They are all covered in this book. Lithium medicalized psychiatry in bringing significant attention to the course of bipolar disorder. Its importance should not be overshadowed by these new developments. Many patients, especially those in the "core" classic form of the illness (mania-depression free interval type, (Koukopoulos *et al.*, 1995; Goodwin and Jamison, 2007)), do respond to lithium. Its judicious use, often in combination with other agents in rational polypharmacy, requires intimate knowledge of its physiological and medical characteristics. Regrettably, young psychiatrists are not

Table 1.2 Bipolar spectrum subtypes in the French EPIDEP study (n = 493): validation by bipolar family history.

	N	%
Bipolar I	41	8.4
Bipolar II	61	12.4
Bipolar II-$^1/_2$	164	33.5
Bipolar III	28	5.7
Bipolar IV	22	4.5
Total	319	64.5

Akiskal *et al.*, *J Affect Disord*, 2005b.

having adequate experience with this agent. A summary of the medical workup of patients in preparation of lithium use (see Akiskal, 1999) is given in Appendix 1.A.

1.2 PSYCHOLOGICAL AND SOCIAL ASPECTS

The long term, essentially life-long, nature of bipolar disorder, and its vicissitudes dictate continuity of treatment and long-term caring. To solve practical problems in the patients' lives requires caring that goes beyond medications and psychotherapy, to include the family, significant others, and the community.

Bipolar disorder continues to be poorly understood by both the public and doctors. More often than not, a bipolar child is classified as having conduct disorder or ADHD (Dilsaver, Henderson-Fuller, and Akiskal, 2003). A teenager's suicide attempt is mis-attributed to problems of the heart, adolescent crisis, or substance abuse; promiscuous behavior is blamed on early "sexual abuse." Bipolar patients from time to time describe their parents as "monsters" or "emotionally-abusive," which some psychotherapists accept on blind faith without ever talking to the parents or significant others. Bipolar II patients are often diagnosed as unipolar and/or borderline personality (Akiskal, 2004), treated with antidepressant without mood stabilizers, resulting in tragic aggravation of the course of the illness (Akiskal and Mallya, 1987; Akiskal et al., 2005a). Excessive spending or squandering of one's economic resources and pathological generosity may lead to financial ruin before bipolarity is considered.

Polls of members of the Depressive and Manic-Depressive Association in the U.S. have shown a latency of 10 years from the onset of symptoms until the correct diagnosis of bipolar disorder (Hirschfeld, Lewis, and Vornik, 2003). Early diagnosis is critical, because suicide in bipolar patients often occurs within this early period. The comfort, support, destigmatization, information, and advocacy provided by such a conglomeration of patients, families, and community leaders (many of whom are themselves bipolar) represents a novel approach in the rehabilitation of the bipolar patient into society. This is a humane and just cause.

Given that a proportion of bipolar individuals have artistic and leadership talents (Akiskal and Akiskal, 1988), sophisticated clinical management of bipolarity can poten-tially safeguard the adaptive capacity and contributions that gifted bipolar people provide to society. Although psychotically ill (bipolar) patients are represented in the media as being creative, this is a destigmatization campaign at best and glamorizing madness at worst. Achievement and creativity are attributes of the "softer" spectrum represented in the attenuated temperamental expressions of bipolarity often involving and extending into bipolar II (Akiskal and Akiskal, 1988, 2005).

To what extent cognitive dysfunction in bipolar illness precedes clinical onset is not entirely settled. Nor is it known how it specifically impacts functioning and creativ-ity. These are new vistas of scientific investigation (Torres et al., 2010; Frangou, 2009; Germana et al., 2010; Giakoumaki et al., 2010). Goodwin and Jamison (2007), based on animal studies, raise the possibility that early treatment with certain agents used in bipolar disorder might increase neuronal growth and thereby contribute to better cognitive functions. This is an open field of investigation for the next generation of neuroscientists and psychopharmacologists in this area (Burdick *et al.*, 2007; Goldberg and Chengappa, 2009).

Spanning from temperament to psychosis, bipolar disorder is a fascinating yet tragic human condition. Mental health professionals who treat these individuals must use pharmacotherapy and psychosocial interventions compassionately, judiciously, and rigorously, – only rarely "aggressively." Severe bipolar illness is not just an ordinary illness to be medicated to "mediocrity." The temperament of these individuals deserves all our consideration and respect. While most *psychotic* bipolar patients are neither leaders nor creators, they are the reservoir of the genes, which in dilute form, might be the seeds of genius (Akiskal *et al.*, 2000).

APPENDIX 1.A: LABORATORY CONSIDERATIONS IN THE CLINICAL USE OF LITHIUM

More than any other development, the introduction of lithium has emphasized the role of physicianship in psychiatry. The scientific literature and clinical wisdom on the therapeutic aspects of this salt have been well summarized in a monograph by Jefferson *et al.* (1983). The success of lithium treatment is dependent on the thoroughness of the initial workup, on dosage titration procedures, and on appropriate monitoring throughout therapy.

The type of workup depends on the age of the patient and concurrent medical conditions (Table 1.3). In young (less than 40 years), physically healthy subjects, preparation for lithium therapy should include medical history (especially focused on neurologic, renal, cardiac, gastrointestinal, endocrine, and cutaneous systems), physical examination, and laboratory evaluation focusing on electrolytes and thyroid. In older patients or those with a history of cardiac disease, a baseline electrocardiogram (EKG) should be obtained and an electroencephalogram (EEG) performed if brain disease is suspected; if there is a history of renal disease, thorough evaluation of baseline kidney function is mandatory. Given rigorous indications for lithium, major medical illness, and abnormalities in laboratory indices do not necessarily contraindicate its use; they do dictate, however, greater medical vigilance, including frequent determination of blood levels and use of lower doses.

Table 1.3 Recommended laboratory workup of patients considered for lithium therapy.

Healthy <40 years	All others
Weight	EKG
CBC	EEG
T4/TSH	TRH test
FBS/serum electrolytes	24-h urine volume
Urinalysis	Urine concentration test
BUN/creatinine	Creatinine clearance

A short-term lithium trial in the controlled environment of a hospital is relatively easy to administer and is recommended for acutely manic, medically ill, or elderly subjects. In outpatient practice, the physician must make sure that the patient and significant others understand the importance of adherence to periodic laboratory procedures and monitoring of side effects.

Lithium is rapidly and completely absorbed from the gastrointestinal tract and peaks in the serum in about 1.5–2.0 (standard preparation) or 4.0–4.5 hours (slow release preparation), depending on age. Its half-life varies from 24 to 36 hours; steady state is reached in about four days. Lithium is not protein-bound and is excreted unchanged almost entirely through the kidneys. It can be safely combined with most classes of drugs except diuretics and nonsteroidal anti-inflammatory agents (other than aspirin), which tend to increase the serum lithium level.

Acutely manic- and possibly bipolar depressive-patients have a high tolerance for lithium and preferentially retain it during the first 10 days while excreting sodium; a regular diet is recommended. Postpubertal bipolar patients, who typically have excellent glomerular function, require higher doses to achieve the same level of equilibrium in the serum. The reverse is true in the geriatric age group. Elderly subjects with adequate glomerular function can benefit considerably from judicious lithium use. However, greater medical vigilance is required for this group; initial doses should be low (150–300 mg/day), with frequent clinical and laboratory monitoring to maintain blood levels in the lower range (0.3–0.8 mEq/l). Special attention must be paid to signs of sinus node dysfunction (bradycardia) or neurotoxicity; the latter is particularly likely in patients with concurrent neurologic disease or sedative and alcohol abuse.

In healthy subjects who achieve good episode prevention, quarterly serum levels (12 hours after the last dose) and serum creatinine are generally sufficient; thyroid indices must be obtained at least once a year. For elderly or medically compromised patients, laboratory tests should be repeated as dictated by the medical condition, with frequent serum lithium levels; the dosage should be kept at the lowest possible level compatible with prophylaxis.

References

Akiskal, H.S. (ed.) (1999) *Bipolarity: Beyond Classic Mania. Psychiatric Clinics of North America*, WB Saunders, September 1999.

Akiskal, H.S. (2002) Classification, diagnosis and boundaries of bipolar disorders, in *Bipolar Disorder* (eds M. Maj, H.S. Akiskal, J.J. Lopez-Ibor, and N. Sartorius), John Wiley & Sons, Ltd, London, pp. 1–52.

Akiskal, H.S. (2003) Validating "hard" and "soft" phenotypes within the bipolar spectrum: continuity or discontinuity? *J. Affect. Disord.*, **73**, 1–5.

Akiskal, H.S. (2004) Demystifying borderline personality: critique of the concept and unorthodox reflections on its natural kinship with the bipolar spectrum. *Acta Psychiatr. Scand.*, **110**, 401–407.

Akiskal, H. (2007) Targeting suicide prevention to modifiable risk factors: has bipolar II been overlooked? *Acta Psychiatr. Scand.*, **116**, 395–402.

Akiskal, H.S. and Akiskal, K.K. (1988) Re-assessing the prevalence of bipolar disorders: Clinical significance and artistic creativity. *Psychiatr. Psychobiol.*, **3**, 29s–36s.

Akiskal, K. and Akiskal, H.S. (2005) The theoretical underpinnings of affective temperaments: implications for evolutionary foundations of bipolarity and human nature. *J. Affect. Disord.*, **85**, 231–239.

Akiskal, H.S., Akiskal, K.K., Lancrenon, S., and Hantouche, E. (2006) Validating the soft bipolar spectrum in the French National EPIDEP Study: the prominence of BP-II1/2. *J. Affect. Disord.*, **96**, 207–213.

Akiskal, H.S., Benazzi, F., Perugi, G., and Rihmer, Z. (2005a) Agitated "unipolar" depression re-conceptualized as a depressive mixed state: implications for the antidepressant-suicide controversy. *J. Affect. Disord.*, **85**, 245–258.

Akiskal, H.S., Hantouche, E.G., Allilaire, J.F., and Akiskal, K.K. (2005b) Validating the bipolar spectrum: overview of the phenomenology and relative prevalence of clinical subtypes in the French national EPIDEP study. *J. Affect. Disord.*, **85**, 29–36.

Akiskal, H.S., Bourgeois, M.L., Angst, J. *et al.* (2000) Re-evaluating the prevalence of and diagnostic composition within the broad clinical spectrum of bipolar disorders. *J. Affect. Disord.*, **59** (Suppl. 1), 5s–30s.

Akiskal, H.S., Djenderedjian, A.H., Rosenthal, R.H., and Khani, M.K. (1977) Cyclothymic disorder: validating criteria for inclusion in the bipolar affective group. *Am. J. Psychiatry*, **134**, 1227–1233.

Akiskal, H., Hantouche, E.G., Allilaire, J.F. *et al.* (2003) Validating antidepressant-associated hypomania (bipolar III): a systematic comparison with spontaneous hypomania (bipolar II). *J. Affect. Disord.*, **73**, 65–74.

Akiskal, H.S., Hantouche, E.G., and Lancrenon, S. (2003) Bipolar II with and without cyclothymic temperament: "dark" and "sunny" expressions of soft bipolarity. *J. Affect. Disord.*, **73**, 49–57.

Akiskal, H.S. and Mallya, G. (1987) Criteria for the "soft" bipolar spectrum: treatment implications. *Psychopharmacol. Bull.*, **23**, 68–73.

Akiskal, H.S. and Pinto, O. (1999) The evolving bipolar spectrum: prototypes I, II, III, IV. *Psychiatr. Clin. N. Am.*, **22**, 517–534.

American Psychiatric Association (1980) *DSM-III. Diagnostic and Statistical Manual of Mental Disorders*, American Psychiatric Press, Washington, DC.

American Psychiatric Association (2000) *DSM-IV. Diagnostic and Statistical Manual of Mental Disorders*, American Psychiatric Press, Washington, DC.

Angst, J., Gamma, A., Benazzi, F. *et al.* (2003) Toward a re-definition of subthreshold bipolarity: epidemiology and proposed criteria for bipolar-II, minor bipolar disorders and hypomania. *J. Affect. Disord.*, **73**, 133–146.

Azorin, J.M., Kaladjian, A., Besnier, N. *et al.* (2010) Suicidal behavior in a French Cohort of major depressive patients: characteristics of attempters and nonattempters. *J. Affect. Disord.*, **123**, 87–94.

Burdick, K.E., Braga, R.J., Goldberg, J.F., and Malhotra, A.K. (2007) Cognitive dysfunction in bipolar disorder: future place of pharmacotherapy. *CNS Drugs*, **21**, 971–981.

Camacho, A. and Akiskal, H.S. (2005) Proposal for a bipolar-stimulant spectrum: temperament, diagnostic validation and therapeutic outcomes with mood stabilizers. *J. Affect. Disord.*, **85**, 217–230.

Cassano, G.B., Akiskal, H.S., Savino, M. *et al.* (1992) Proposed subtypes of bipolar II and related disorders: with hypomanic episodes (or cyclothymia) and with hyperthymic temperament. *J. Affective. Disord.*, **26**, 127–140.

Dilsaver, S.C., Henderson-Fuller, S., and Akiskal, H.S. (2003) Occult mood disorders in 104 consecutively presenting children referred for the treatment of attention-deficit/hyperactivity disorder in a community mental health clinic. *J. Clin. Psychiatry*, **64**, 1170–1176.

Dunner, D.L., Gershon, E.S., and Goodwin, F.K. (1976) Heritable factors in the severity of affective illness. *Biol. Psychiatry*, **11**, 31–42.

Frangou, S. (2009) Risk and resilience in bipolar disorder: rationale and design of the Vulnerability to Bipolar Disorders Study (VIBES). *Biochem. Soc. Trans.*, **37** (Pt 5), 1085–1089.

Germana, C., Kempton, M.J., Sarnicola, A. *et al.* (2010) The effects of lithium and anticonvulsants on brain structure in bipolar disorder. *Acta Psychiatr. Scand.*, **122**, 481–487.

Giakoumaki, S.G., Bitsiois, P., Frangou, S. *et al.* (2010) Low baseline startle and deficient affective startle modulation in remitted bipolar disorder patients and their unaffected siblings. *Psychophysiology*, **47**, 659–668.

Goldberg, J.F. and Chengappa, K.N. (2009) Identifying and treating cognitive impairment in bipolar disorder. *Bipolar Disord.*, **11**, 123–137.

Goodwin, F.K. and Jamison, K.R. (2007) *Manic-Depressive Illness: Bipolar Disorders and Recurrent Depression*, Oxford University Press, New York.

Hantouche, E.G., Angst, J., and Akiskal, H.S. (2003) Factor Structure of hypomania: interrelationships with cyclothymia and the soft bipolar spectrum. *J. Affect. Disord.*, **73**, 39–47.

Hirschfeld, R.M., Holzer, C., Calabrese, J.R. *et al.* (2003) Validity of the mood disorder questionnaire: a general population study. *Am. J. Psychiatry*, **160**, 178–180.

Hirschfeld, R.M., Lewis, L., and Vornik, L.A. (2003) Perceptions and impact of bipolar disorder: how far have we really come? Results of the national depressive and manic-depressive association 2000 survey of individuals with bipolar disorder. *J. Clin. Psychiatry*, **64**, 161–174.

Jefferson, J., Jefferson, J.W., Greist, J.H. and Ackerman, D.L. (1983) *Lithium Encyclopedia*, American Psychiatric Press, Washington, DC.

Judd, L.L. and Akiskal, H.S. (2003) The prevalence and disability of bipolar spectrum disorders in the U.S. population: Re-analysis of the ECA database taking into account subthreshold cases. *J. Affect. Disord.*, **73**, 123–131.

Khuri, R. and Akiskal, H.S. (1983) Suicide prevention: the necessity of treating contributory psychiatric disorders. *Psychiatr. Clin. N. Am.*, **6**, 193–207.

Koukopoulos, A., Reginaldi, D., Minnai, G. *et al.* (1995) The long term prophylaxis of affective disorders. *Adv. Biochem. Psychopharmacol.*, **49**, 127–147.

Lehmann, H.E. (1969) The impact of the therapeutic revolution on nosology, in *Problematique de la Psychose* (eds P. Doucet and C. Laurin), Excerpta Medica Foundation, New York, pp. 136–153.

Maj, M., Akiskal, H.S., Lopez-Ibor, J.J., and Sartorius, N. (2002) *Bipolar Disorder*, John Wiley & Sons, Ltd, Chichester.

Maremmani, I., Pacini, M., Lubrano, S. *et al.* (2003) Dual diagnosis heroin addicts. The clinical and therapeutic aspects. *Heroin Add. Rel. Clin. Probl.*, **5**, 7–98.

Merikangas, K.R., Akiskal, H.S., Angst, J. *et al.* (2007) Lifetime and 12-month prevalence of bipolar spectrum disorder in the National Comorbidity Survey replication. *Arch. Gen. Psychiatry.*, **64**, 543–552.

Rihmer, Z., Barsi, J., Arato, M., and Demeter, E. (1990) Suicide in subtypes of primary major depression. *J. Affect. Disord.*, **18**, 221–225.

Rihmer, Z. and Pestality, P. (1999) Bipolar II disorder and suicidal behavior. *Psychiatr. Clin. N. Am.*, **22**, 667–673.

Torres, I.J., Defreitas, V.G., Defreitas, C.M. *et al.* (2010) Neurocognitive functioning in patients with bipolar I disorder recently recovered from a first manic episode. *J. Clin. Psychiatry*, **71**, 234–242.

Lithium Treatment: Focus on Long-Term Prophylaxis

Paul Grof and Mogens Schou[*]

Mood Disorders Center of Ottawa, Ontario, Canada

2.1 INTRODUCTION

Long-term treatment with lithium has had a rather stormy past, tainted with misunderstandings and misinterpretations. But appreciating its past is helpful for the appropriate use of lithium in the present, and we will therefore briefly summarize the history.

How long lithium prophylaxis has been used for mood disorders is difficult to say exactly. In the 1880s lithium was used for the treatment and prevention of recurrent depressions (Lange, 1886; Schioldann, 2001), but statistics and controlled trials were not known at that time, and the observations remained clinical impressions. In the 1950s lithium treatment for mania became evidence-based (Schou *et al.*, 1954), and between 1967 and 1970 prophylactic lithium treatment achieved the same (Baastrup and Schou, 1967; Baastrup *et al.*, 1970).

There is nevertheless good reason to count the age of lithium treatment from 1949, when Cade (1949) published his paper "Lithium salts in the treatment of psychotic excitement," for lithium has remained in psychiatric use since then. Why is lithium treatment still being used after 60 years? A systematic, chronological exposition of the history of lithium treatment in psychiatry has been done in other publications to which the reader is referred, for example, Johnson (1984), Schou (1992), and Healy (1997). We will attempt, however, to answer this question by recounting and commenting selected relevant events.

Methodological problems will be given more attention than the presentation of data because they have caused most misunderstandings about lithium. The main ones will be addressed in this chapter. Since lithium is used primarily for the prevention of recurrences, this review, reflecting on particular previous work by Schou (1993b, 1998c, 2001), deals primarily with prophylactic treatment of "typical" or "classical" bipolar disorders; and disregards treatment of single manic and depressive episodes and touches

---

[*] Deceased prior to the publishing of the second edition of this book.

Bipolar Psychopharmacotherapy: Caring for the patient, Second Edition. Edited by Hagop S. Akiskal and Mauricio Tohen.
© 2011 John Wiley & Sons, Ltd. Published 2011 by John Wiley & Sons, Ltd.

only peripherally on atypical cases. We focus on the more recent challenges in the long-term treatment.

2.2 CADE'S PIONEERING STUDY

It has often been claimed that the so-called "psychopharmacological era" started with the introduction of chlorpromazine in 1952. The era actually began when Cade introduced lithium as an antimanic drug in 1949. When the word "serendipity" was used about his discovery, Cade became annoyed and pointed out that it was based on a specific hypothesis and experimental observations. The hypothesis was that mental illnesses are caused by intoxication with an unknown compound, and that this toxic agent can be found in the patients' urine. His hypothesis led him to inject lithium urate, the only soluble salt of uric acid, into guinea pigs, and when he saw that they became docile and lethargic, he started treating psychiatric patients with lithium carbonate after having tried it on himself without ill effects.

Whereas schizophrenic and depressed patients did not show positive changes, all 10 manic patients showed abatement or cessation of their symptoms. Later attempts to induce lethargy in guinea pigs with lithium showed, however, that this was possible only with high doses. Some of Cade's animals were presumably intoxicated rather than merely lethargic. To make therapeutic discoveries on the basis of misinterpreted experiments requires curiosity, daring, luck, and compassion for patients!

2.3 DISCOVERY OF THE PROPHYLACTIC ACTION OF LITHIUM

By 1964 Schou (1956), Hartigan (1963), and Baastrup (1964) had independently of each other made observations on small groups of patients that seemed to indicate that prolonged treatment with lithium might ameliorate or prevent not only manic but also depressive recurrences. This was a new and unexpected observation, and it called for closer examination.

2.3.1 NON-BLIND MIRROR TRIAL

A confirmation of the original observations came from a large, open study. A nonblind trial lasting six years and involving 88 bipolar and unipolar patients who had suffered at least two episodes within two years provided the first systematically collected evidence of a prophylactic action of lithium against both manic and depressive episodes of classical manic-depressive illness (Baastrup and Schou, 1967). The average number of episodes per year decreased by 87% from the time before lithium treatment to the time during lithium treatment ($p < 0.001$). A Swiss–Czech–Danish collaborative trial confirmed the findings (Angst et $al.$, 1970). Psychiatrists in other countries then initiated lithium treatment and confirmed the observation of depressive as well as manic recurrences diminishing in intensity and frequency.

However, Blackwell and Shepherd (1968) expressed sharp skepticism. They never tried treating patients with lithium; so their disbelief was purely speculative. Yet, they contested the validity of the evidence. They felt that bias and the suggestive power of the psychiatrists accounted for the observations, and that patients selected because they had suffered frequent episodes during recent years could be expected to have fewer episodes during the following years.

In their reply Baastrup and Schou (1968) pointed out that most of the patients were discharged soon after starting lithium treatment. General practitioners, who were unaware of the ongoing trial and therefore unbiased, determined when a recurrence had taken place. Moreover, rather than decrease, the frequency of episodes may be expected to increase. At that time a frequency increase in time was considered characteristic of recurrent affective disorders (Angst and Weis, 1969; Grof *et al.*, 1970a). Blackwell and Shepherd chose to overlook these findings. The discussions between Blackwell and Shepherd, and Baastrup and Schou went on for some time and created uncertainty among British and American psychiatrists, who hesitated to start prophylactic lithium treatment. Baastrup and Schou felt that double-blind observations were required to terminate this dispute.

2.3.2   DOUBLE-BLIND DISCONTINUATION TRIAL

Baastrup *et al.* and their associates (1970) therefore carried out a double-blind discontinuation trial. Bipolar and unipolar patients who had been given lithium for at least a year were allocated randomly to either placebo or continued lithium treatment. Within six months the difference between the groups had reached a pre-determined significance level ($p < 0.01$), and sequential analysis terminated the trial. While 21 of 39 placebo-treated patients had relapsed, none of the 45 lithium-treated patients had done so. The final analysis revealed a statistical difference of $p < 0.001$. Later randomized, placebo-controlled trials of both discontinuation design and prospective design confirmed the findings, for example, Melia (1970), Coppen *et al.* (1971), Cundall, Brooks, and Murray (1972), Hullin, McDonald, and Allsopp (1972), Prien, Caffey, and Klett (1973), and Stallone *et al.* (1973). The evidence was now so strong that lithium became approved for prophylactic treatment of bipolar disorder by the FDA (in 1974) and by regulatory agencies in many countries.

2.3.3   OBSERVER BIAS, DISEASE COURSE

There are few psychiatric treatments that have been debated as hotly as prophylactic treatment with lithium. Most of the disagreements had methodological roots, in particular different attitudes toward clinical trials. Shepherd was convinced that valid evidence could be obtained only with randomized, placebo-controlled trials; any other evidence had to be rejected. The 1967 trial by Baastrup and Schou was not randomized and placebo controlled, the reason being that it had started more or less on an exploratory basis and then had gradually grown. The authors felt, however, that data collected in an open prophylactic study of mirror-design need not necessarily be disregarded. The marked and long-lasting change produced by lithium in the course of disease was unlikely to have been fortuitous. Schou, Thomsen, and Baastrup (1970) tested the assumptions on which Blackwell and Shepherd had based their criticism. The effect of observer bias and psychological factors on the recording of recurrences was investigated by comparing the disease course of a group of patients in whom lithium treatment was switched double-blind to placebo, and another group who stopped taking lithium on their own initiative. When lithium is discontinued during a double-blind study, observer bias and suggestion continue to work at full force; when lithium is discontinued openly, their psychological effect ends. The percentage of patients who suffered relapse each month was the same in the two groups.

The calculations showed that in manic-depressive patients neither observer bias nor placebo effects were strong enough to exert significant influence on the recorded recurrence rate. A survival analysis of the same data revealed that the low frequency of episodes during lithium treatment was accordingly not a result of "regression toward the mean" as Blackwell and Shepherd had suggested.

2.3.4   FURTHER DOUBTS ABOUT THE EFFICACY OF LITHIUM TREATMENT

Lithium prophylaxis became widely used during the following years, but occasionally doubts about its efficacy were still expressed. For example, Dickson and Kendell (1986) found that even though long-term lithium treatment was being increasingly administered in Edinburgh during the period 1970–1981, admission rates for mania and depression were on the rise; the authors felt that this cast doubts on the efficacy of lithium treatment.

In response, Schou (1986) pointed out that drawing conclusions about the efficacy of a treatment administered to a limited number of patients from the admission rates of a much larger number is a dubious procedure. Prophylactic lithium treatment is given only to manic-depressive patients with frequent recurrences, so even if lithium treatment were 100% effective, it could only be expected to prevent a small fraction of re-admissions. Grof (1987) drew attention to the many other factors that could have led to a rise in the number of admissions, for example, a broadening in diagnostic practice. In other hospitals rises in admissions for comparable reasons were observed.

Moncrieff (1995) claimed that a prophylactic action of lithium treatment was never satisfactorily demonstrated. She felt that development of side effects had probably compromised the blindness of the prophylactic lithium trials, but she presented no evidence in support of that notion. But the available evidence shows that the blindness had not been invalidated (Schou, 1998a). Basing her arguments again purely on speculation, Moncrieff claimed that the rise in frequency of manic recurrences after discontinuation of lithium was not caused by the removal of an active prophylactic drug. The cause was instead, she insisted, rebound recurrences precipitated by withdrawal of lithium. But even if a discontinuation design with rebound manias might inflate the size of lithium's effect, this in itself shows that lithium is not without effect (Goodwin, 1995).

Moncrieff also referred to a study by Suppes *et al.* (1993) that reported rapid development of predominantly manic recurrences after abrupt discontinuation of lithium. These observations were impressive, but they were made in patients who differed diagnostically from those in whom lithium was originally shown to be prophylactically effective in 1967–1970. During the last decades the expanded use of bipolar diagnoses and of the DSM approach has led to a substantial widening of the indications for lithium use (Grof, 1998). In the early prophylactic trials the patients were diagnosed according to ICD criteria and had classical manic-depressive illness, and in these patients discontinuation of lithium did not produce rebound. It led to re-emergence of recurrences at a rate that did not exceed their experiences before they started lithium treatment (Grof, Cakuls, and Dostal, 1970b; Schou, Thomsen, and Baastrup, 1970; Rifkin, Quitkin, and Howard, 1975; Fyrö and Petterson, 1977; Sashidharan and McGuire, 1983; Mendlewicz, 1984; Berghöfer, Kossman, and Müller-Oerlinghausen, 1996). Moncrieff's principal argument failed.

2.3.5 "NATURALISTIC" TRIALS

In some "naturalistic" or "outpatient" or "clinical practice" trials the prophylactic effectiveness of lithium has been found to be lower than it was in the early trials. The explanations of this discrepancy between efficacy and effectiveness are most likely treatment adherence and patient selection.

In naturalistic trials the patients are usually not sufficiently supervised to ensure sufficient compliance (Schou, 1993a). Poor compliance is the major cause of the difference between efficacy, the potential of a treatment and effectiveness – the result obtained under clinical conditions (Guscott and Taylor, 1994). Efforts should be made to improve compliance and increase effectiveness also when lithium treatment is given under naturalistic or outpatient or clinical practice conditions (Schou, 1997).

In some of the naturalistic trials lithium treatment was been given to patients with atypical features and comorbid psychopathology and to patients who previously had been found refractory to lithium (Schou, 1998a). The indications for lithium treatment had been influenced by the introduction of new diagnostic criteria (Gershon and Soares, 1997; Gitlin and Altshuler, 1997). The effectiveness of lithium prophylaxis in clinical practice should be assessed during carefully monitored lithium treatment given on indications where it has been shown to be efficacious.

2.4 PRACTICAL ISSUES

2.4.1 EFFECT OF THE SERUM LITHIUM CONCENTRATION

The frequency and severity of side effects depends primarily on the serum lithium concentration being kept low and competently tailored to each patient. At the psychiatric hospital in Risskov, Denmark, the range of serum lithium concentrations was lowered from 0.8–1.0 to 0.5–0.8 mmol/l (Schou, 1988; Vestergaard and Schou, 1988; Schou and Vestergaard, 1988; Vestergaard, Poulstrup, and Schou, 1988). The average serum lithium concentration decreased by about 30%, and the proportion of patients not having side effects rose markedly. Lithium-induced tremor and diarrhea were strikingly less pronounced during treatment with low serum concentrations than with high; so were lithium-induced increase of urine volume and reduction of renal concentrating ability. In Europe the recommended serum lithium range has for several years been 0.4–0.8 mmol/l, to be exceeded at each end in particularly sensitive and particularly resistant patients respectively (Birch *et al.*, 1993).

The claims of many and severe side effects of lithium are made primarily in the United States where relatively higher lithium levels have been used. In 1989 a group from Boston (Gelenberg *et al.*, 1989) compared doses leading to what they called "standard" serum lithium levels, 0.8–1.0 mmol/l, with doses leading to low levels, 0.4–0.6 mmol/l. The trial showed that the former levels were not only more effective but also associated with a higher incidence of side effects than the latter. There was more noncompliance in the high level group; the authors nevertheless chose to recommend the high levels. They did not examine effects and side effects of the levels in between 0.6 and 0.8 mmol/l. Later a recalculation of the data showed that more recurrences on a lower lithium level were due primarily to observations in patients who were switched from higher to lower levels.

In another American study by Gitlin (1993), using serum lithium concentrations between 0.6 and 1.2 mmol/l, 3 out of 82 patients showed gradual rises of the serum creatinine concentration. We found only a single American author who has recommended lower serum lithium concentrations, between 0.3 and 0.8 mmol/l (Akiskal, 1999).

2.4.2 PREVENTION OF LITHIUM INTOXICATION

Patients undergoing lithium treatment rarely commit suicide by taking overdoses of lithium, but lithium intoxications can develop under various unfortunate circumstances. Intoxication does not develop randomly. The mechanisms governing the excretion of lithium by the kidney have by now been unraveled through animal experiments and clinical experiences over many years. This knowledge has led to precautionary guidelines (Thomsen and Schou, 1999). Situations to be avoided during lithium treatment include overdose, kidney disease, dehydration, sodium deficiency, and interaction with various drugs. It is useful for physicians and patients to keep such conditions in mind.

2.4.3 USE DURING PREGNANCY

Early experiments on primitive aquatic animals had shown that exposure to high concentrations of lithium in the surrounding fluid led to malformations of the offspring. In 1949, a "Register of Lithium Babies" was established (Schou, 1969) in order to reveal whether malformed children would be born to mothers having been in lithium treatment during pregnancy. The register was based on voluntary reports, and it indicated an increased frequency of congenital malformations of the heart. However, these findings exaggerated the risk because congenitally malformed babies were more likely to be reported than normal babies, and the retrospective register was closed in 1990 (Schou, 1990). When the lithium baby register was started, psychiatrists were not used to thinking along teratogenic lines, and the register's estimate of *maximum* teratogenic risk was taken as a measure of the *true* teratogenic effect of lithium. That gave lithium a "bad press."

Later investigations without the bias of the register have given more reassuring results and could not demonstrate a relationship between malformations and lithium given during pregnancy. The risk of fetal changes in more recent studies was minimal (Jacobson *et al.*, 1992; Schou, 1998b). Lithium can be given safely during the last six months of pregnancy. If the risk of recurrence is high and the illness severe, lithium can also be given during the first three months; but the patient and her partner should be fully involved in such a decision and made aware that it was not possible to obtain relevant experimental data.

2.4.4   BREASTFEEDING DURING LITHIUM TREATMENT

Small but variable amounts of lithium pass from the mother's blood to her milk and hence to the nursing child. However, breastfeeding plays an important role for both mother and child, physically and psychologically. Fortunately, one can today measure the lithium concentration in the mothers' milk and relate it to her blood level. Thus it has become doubtful that it is advisable to abstain from breastfeeding during lithium treatment, as long as the concentration remains low (for example,, stays below 15%).

2.4.5   LITHIUM AND KIDNEY FUNCTION

Newer observations on patients who have been on lithium for many years indicate that in long-term treatment it is very important to pay special attention to the patients' kidney function. Earlier, mostly negative studies included patients who had been treated with lithium up to 15 years; more recent investigations of patients with longer treatment duration show that a proportion of patients develops chronic lithium nephropathy (Grof *et al.*, 1980; Schou and Vestergaard, 1988; Povlsen *et al.*, 1992; Bendz, Sjödin, and Aurell, 1996; Schou and Kampf, 2006). In most patients the glomerular filtration rate remains stable during long-term lithium administration and the primary manifestation of this condition is impaired urinary concentration, usually but not always accompanied by polyuria. By itself, mild polyuria is of minimal clinical importance, but patients with severe polyuria may be at a greater risk of lithium intoxication as a result of dehydration and fluctuation of sodium levels. Thus, the renal adverse effects of lithium primarily affect the tubuli and interstitium.

It is very important, particularly when reading the literature, to make a careful distinction between the effects of properly supervised lithium therapy and lithium intoxication. Many reports have failed to differentiate between the two conditions. Lithium intoxication, particularly a repeated one, can lead to a drop in the glomerular filtration rate and, ultimately, to acute oligoanuric renal failure.

A rare adverse effect of lithium prophylaxis is nephrotic syndrome. Morphologically it may present as a minimal lesion or as focal segmental glomerular sclerosis. Stopping lithium treatment tends to result in full remission of the minimal lesion, but restarting lithium therapy usually leads to a rapid relapse. In isolated cases, lithium has been shown to impair renal tubular acidification by way of incomplete distal renal tubular acidosis.

However, this impairment is not accompanied by systemic acidosis and thus has no clinical relevance.

Most adverse effects of chronic lithium treatment appear to be due to chronic, uninterrupted administration. In patients with classic, episodic bipolar disorder the potential adverse effect on the kidney function can be avoided by carefully planned, intermittent treatment with lithium given only during high risk periods determined by serial dexamethasone suppression tests. This helpful but experimental approach should be left to specialized lithium clinics.

In clinical practice it is essential to obtain renal baseline information before lithium treatment, to maintain each patient on the lowest effective lithium concentration, to monitor the patient and the kidney function regularly and to refer to a nephrologist if the kidney function shows signs of deterioration.

2.5 ARE NEW AND BETTER PROPHYLACTIC AGENTS ABOUT TO OUST LITHIUM?

During the recent decades, new medications have been introduced for long-term treatment of bipolar disorder. Lithium treatment has side effects, and it would be welcome if something better were forthcoming and its advantages convincingly demonstrated (Schou, 1998a). For some time lithium and other mood stabilizers appeared to be in direct competition, especially for the market share. The question in the title of this section reflects that reality and was particularly opportune at the time of the first edition of this book.

However, with the increasing recognition of the heterogeneity of bipolar disorders the query is shifting from finding the single best drug to selecting the correct mood stabilizer for the given patient – the patient who is likely to respond to it. There is now extensive evidence for stabilizing ability of lithium, quetiapine, olanzapine, lamotrigine, and carbamazepine. But who are the patients for whom lithium works best and who gets more benefit from atypical neuroleptics or antiepileptics? And who will require combinations?

When the new, putative mood stabilizers have compared with lithium, experience from recent decennia has shown it important to distinguish between typical and atypical bipolar disorder (Schou, 1998a). Patients with typical, classical bipolar disorder have a fully episodic course, often present with mood-congruent symptoms and family history positive for episodic depressive or bipolar disorder and are rarely accompanied by psychiatric comorbidity. Patients with atypical bipolar disorder have a nonepisodic, incompletely remitting course with residual psychopathology, often including mood-incongruent symptoms, ultrarapid cycling, dysphoric mania, and comorbidity, and have a family history of chronic or protracted psychiatric disorders. Likely to respond well to lithium are patients with typical bipolar disorders, likely to benefit from atypical neuroleptics and selected anticonvulsants are patients with atypical presentations.

Accumulated evidence now supports this approach. For example, in two prospective randomized double-blind studies (Placidi et al., 1986; Greil et al., 1997, 1998; Greil and Kleindienst, 1999) the prophylactic efficacies of lithium and carbamazepine were compared. Whereas lithium was consistently superior to carbamazepine in patients with typical bipolar disorder, carbamazepine had the same efficacy as lithium or showed an edge to be better in patients with atypical bipolar disorder. Furthermore, studies by researchers from Ottawa and Halifax compared lithium, lamotrigine, and olanzapine and were primarily patient-oriented rather than drug-oriented. Passmore *et al.* (2003) studied 164 subjects from 21 families of bipolar probands, 14 responders to lithium and 7 responders to lamotrigine. There were differences between the drugs with respect to clinical course (episodic in the lithium group, rapid cycling in the lamotrigine group) and comorbidity (panic attacks and substance abuse in the lamotrigine group). The relatives of lithium responders had significantly higher risk of bipolar disorder, and the relatives of lamotrigine responders had higher prevalence of schizoaffective disorder, major depression, and panic attacks. Grof (2003) discussed in more detail the principles and the execution of selective long-term monotherapy with the individual agents in bipolar patients.

A current, widespread practice is to add further mood stabilizers already when the first mood stabilizer has been given for only a short time. It has, however, been found in the above studies that many patients can be successfully stabilized on one main mood stabilizer if the drug is initially selected according to the patients' clinical characteristics.

2.6 COMBINATION TREATMENT

There are many clinical observations that in patients who do not tolerate lithium or patients who are refractory to long-term lithium, the addition of an antiepileptic or of atypical neuroleptics may be of use (for example, Yatham, Calabrese, and Kusumakar, 2003; Grof, 2003). There has, however, been a scarcity of controlled trials exploring efficacy of the combination over either drug given alone. Such studies are described elsewhere in this book in Chapters 3, 6, 7, and 10. It is noteworthy that in nearly all of them lithium is considered the gold standard to be augmented. While giving two drugs together might achieve better results by reaching two subgroups of bipolar patients in a heterogeneous population, the real question that needs to be answered is whether such a side effect-prone combination works better than the tailoring of each drug to appropriately selected patients. During unsatisfactory maintenance treatment for recurrent major depressions with antidepressant drugs, augmentation with lithium is frequently useful. In patients who respond to antidepressants plus augmentation with lithium it may be worth trying to discontinue the antidepressant after some time. The patients may then remain stabilized on long-term lithium alone.

2.7 PROPHYLAXIS IN RECURRENT DEPRESSIVE DISORDER

There is substantial evidence that, in patients with the classical type of bipolar disorder, long-term lithium treatment exerts a recurrence-preventive action not only in bipolar disorder but also in depressive disorder (Baastrup and Schou, 1967; Angst *et al.*, 1970; Baastrup *et al.*, 1970). This observation has not had any noticeable effect on the prophylactic treatment for depressive disorder. The antidepressant drugs had been introduced in the late 1950s, and they have later dominated both the acute and the prophylactic treatments for this disorder.

It should, however, be noted that many patients are treated with antidepressants who according to present-day international classifications have, or must be suspected of having, bipolar disorder. They are, for example, patients with bipolarity in the family, patients whose depressive disorder started in puberty, patients in whom there is information about at least one episode with hypomanic symptoms and patients with antidepressant-induced hypomania (Akiskal *et al.*, 2003; Chun and Dunner, 2004). Such patients with recurrent depressions may with advantage be treated with lithium instead of with antidepressants. These observations are in good agreement with the conclusion of recent extensive epidemiological studies indicating that many patients with recurrent depressive disorders may in fact have bipolar propensity (Angst *et al.*, 2003; Judd and Akiskal, 2003).

Such patients are prevalent in clinical practice and if the bipolar nature of their disorder is not recognized, their clinical management represents a formidable challenge.

2.8 THE EFFECT OF LITHIUM ON THE PATIENTS' SUICIDAL BEHAVIOR

In the 1980s clinical observations on both side of the Atlantic pointed out to a possible beneficial effect of lithium on suicidal behavior (Hanus and Zapletalek, 1984; Jamison, 1986). For example, Jamison noted that among about 9000 lithium-treated patients in three major mood disorder clinics in the United States the frequency of suicides was conspicuously low. In the 1990s systematic investigations on very large groups of patients from clinical settings revealed that the frequencies of suicides and of suicide attempts were about 10–15 times lower in patients given prophylactic lithium treatment than in patients not given such treatment (Coppen *et al.*, 1991; Müller-Oerlinghausen *et al.*, 1992; Tondo, Jamison, and Baldessarini, 1997; Kallner *et al.*, 2000; Schou, 2000; Baldessarini, Tondo, and Hennen, 2001; Goodwin *et al.*, 2003). Reviews by Akiskal *et al.* (2000) and Akiskal (2002).

However, an antisuicidal effect of lithium cannot be definitively proven through a randomized, double-blind methodology. This is in principle not possible for any kind of antisuicidal intervention because there won't be any matching patient control group to compare with. One cannot, after all, keep suicide-threatened patients on placebo or deprived of psychological and social support merely to observe if and when they will commit suicide. Nor can one determine by throwing a dice when and in whom an ongoing and possibly effective intervention should be discontinued. But the studies reviewed are highly significant and fully *compatible* with the assumption that lithium has a striking antisuicidal effect. As scientists we must concede that the investigations strongly indicate such a possibility. As responsible clinicians we owe it to patients and relatives alike to make appropriate use of that probability.

2.9 BENEFITS OF PROPHYLACTIC LITHIUM TREATMENT

The discovery and implementation of prophylactic lithium treatment have had far-reaching results.

1. The efficacy of lithium therapy and prophylaxis has established recurrent mood disorders to be treatable conditions and has contributed to recognizing psychiatry as a medical discipline.
2. Lithium was the first psychotropic drug for which a recurrence-preventive action in mood disorders was demonstrated. This paved the way for other medications to be studied on this indication. Lithium prevents recurrences not only in bipolar disorder but also in related recurrent unipolar depressions.
3. During the last 60 years lithium has stimulated research in numerous fields, for example, clinical, pharmacological, physiological, biochemical, and genetic.
4. Mood disorders place a heavy burden on the economy of individuals, the health system and society at large (Wyatt and Henter, 1995). Since lithium treatment is effective and inexpensive, its widespread use has reduced such costs substantially (Reifman and Wyatt, 1980).
5. Last but not least, prophylactic lithium treatment has changed the lives of millions of people with recurrent mood disorders for the better. After years in the shadow of fear it may be difficult to hope again, but gradually patients and family experience how the course of the disease has been altered, and how fear loses its grip. Patients feel that life once more becomes predictable, and that normal friendships can be established or re-established. Prophylactic lithium treatment can improve the quality of life significantly for patients whose existence was dominated by frequent and severe recurrences.

    (See further discussion in Chapter 19.)

2.10 CONCLUSION

Prophylactic lithium treatment for mood disorders was introduced over 50 years ago, and in spite of being an inexpensive drug, unsupported by powerful pharmaceutical industries, lithium is still used all over the world. Lithium is, with the exception of the U.S.A., the prophylactic agent most widely used in bipolar disorder. This substance produces the most dramatic benefits of any medication used in psychiatry if it is used correctly. It is the treatment of choice for patients who suffer from recurrent "classic" bipolar disorder, effectively preventing both the manic and the depressed phases of the disorder.

Few psychiatric treatments have been debated so hotly. Misunderstandings and mis-statements about lithium have abounded, and this chapter attempts to rectify the common ones. Competition from pharmaceutical companies trying to replace lithium with new prophylactic medications has been fierce. All this foresaw a short life for lithium. But prophylactic lithium treatment is still widely in use and effective in recurrent episodic bipolar and depressive disorders; it is waiting for something indisputably better to replace it, or parallel its benefits in other types of bipolar spectrum.

References

Akiskal, H.S. (1999) Affective disorders, in *Merck Manual of Diagnosis and Therapy*, 14th edn (ed. R. Berkow), Merck, Sharp and Dohme Research Laboratories, New Jersey, pp. 1525–1544.

Akiskal, H.S. (2002) The bipolar spectrum – the shaping of a new paradigm in psychiatry. *Curr. Psychiatry Rep.*, **4** (1), 1–3.

Akiskal, H.S., Bourgeois, M.L., Angst, J. *et al.* (2000) Reevaluating the prevalence of and diagnostic composition within the broad clinical spectrum of bipolar disorders. *J. Affect. Disord.*, **59** (Suppl. 1), 5s–30s.

Akiskal, H.S., Hantouche, E.G., Allilaire, J.F. *et al.* (2003) Validating antidepressant-associated hypomania (bipolar III): a systematic comparison with spontaneous hypomania (bipolar II). *J. Affect. Disord.*, **73**, 65–74.

Angst, J., Gamma, A., Benazzi, F. *et al.* (2003) Toward a re-definition of subthreshold bipolarity: epidemiology and proposed criteria for bipolar-II, minor bipolar disorders and hypomania. *J. Affect. Disord.*, **23**, 133–146.

Angst, J. and Weis, P. (1969) Zum Verlauf depressiver Psychosen. In W. Schulte and W. Mende (Eds.), *Melancholie in Forschung, Klinik und Behandlung*, pp. 2–9. Stuttgart: Georg Thieme.

Angst, J., Weis, P., Grof, P. *et al.* (1970) Lithium prophylaxis in recurrent affective disorders. *Br. J. Psychiatry*, **116**, 604–614.

Baastrup, P.C. (1964) The use of lithium in manic-depressive psychosis. *Compr. Psychiatry*, **5**, 396–408.

Baastrup, P.C., Poulsen, J.C., Schou, M. *et al.* (1970) Prophylactic lithium: double-blind discontinuation in manic-depressive disorders. *Lancet*, **II**, 326–330.

Baastrup, P.C. and Schou, M. (1967) Lithium as a prophylactic agent: its effect against recurrent depressions and manic-depressive psychosis. *Arch. Gen. Psychiatry*, **16**, 162–172.

Baastrup, P.C. and Schou, M. (1968) Prophylactic lithium. *Lancet*, **I**, 1419–1422.

Baldessarini, R.J., Tondo, L., and Hennen, J. (2001) Treating the suicidal patient with bipolar disorder. Reducing suicide risk with lithium. *Ann. N. Y. Acad. Sci.*, **932**, 24–38.

Bendz, H., Sjödin, I., and Aurell, M. (1996) Renal function on and off lithium in patients treated with lithium for 15 years or more: a controlled, prospective lithium withdrawal study. *Nephrol. Dial. Transplant.*, **11**, 457–460.

Berghöfer, A., Kossman, A.B., and Müller-Oerlinghausen, B. (1996) Course of illness and pattern of recurrences in patients with affective disorders during long-term lithium prophylaxis: a retrospective analysis over 15 years. *Acta Psychiatr. Scand.*, **93**, 349–354.

Birch, N.J., Grof, P., Hullin, R.P. *et al.* (1993) Lithium prophylaxis: proposed guidelines for good clinical practice. *Lithium*, **4**, 225–230.

Blackwell, B. and Shepherd, M. (1968) Prophylactic lithium: another therapeutic myth? An examination of the evidence to date. *Lancet*, **I**, 968–971.

Cade, J.F.J. (1949) Lithium salts in the treatment of psychotic excitement. *Med. J. Aust.*, **36**, 349–352.

Coppen, A., Noguera, R., Bailey, J. *et al.* (1971) Prophylactic lithium in affective disorders: controlled trial. *Lancet*, **II**, 275–279.

Coppen, A., Standish-Barry, H., Bailey, J. *et al.* (1991) Does lithium reduce the mortality of recurrent mood disorders? *J. Affect. Disord.*, **23**, 1–7.

Chun, B.J.D.H. and Dunner, L.D. (2004) A review of antidepressant-induced hypomania in major depression: suggestions for DSM-V. *Bipolar Disord.*, **6**, 32–42.

Cundall, R.L., Brooks, P.W., and Murray, L.G. (1972) A controlled evaluation of lithium prophylaxis in affective disorders. *Psychol. Med.*, **2**, 308–311.

Dickson, W.E. and Kendell, R.E. (1986) Does maintenance lithium therapy prevent recurrences of mania under ordinary clinical conditions? *Psychol. Med*, **16**, 521–530.

Fyrö, B. and Petterson, U. (1977) A double blind study of the prophylactic effect of lithium in manic-depressive illness. *Acta Psychiatr. Scand.*, **269**, 17–22.

Gelenberg, A.J., Kane, J.M., Keller, M.B. *et al.* (1989) Comparison of standard and low serum levels of lithium for maintenance treatment of bipolar disorder. *N. Engl. J. Med.*, **321**, 1489–1493.

Gershon, S. and Soares, J.C. (1997) Current therapeutic profile of lithium. *Arch. Gen. Psychiatry*, **54**, 16–20.

Gitlin, M.J. (1993) Lithium-induced renal insufficiency. *J. Clin. Psychopharmacol.*, **13**, 276–279.

Gitlin, M.J. and Altshuler, L.L. (1997) Unanswered questions, unknown future for one of our oldest medications. *Arch. Gen. Psychiatry*, **54**, 21–23.

Goodwin, G.M. (1995) Lithum revisited. A reply. *Br. J. Psychiatry*, **167**, 573–574.

Goodwin, F.K., Fireman, B., Simon, G.E. *et al.* (2003) Suicide risk in bipolar disorder during treatment with lithium and divalproex. *J. Am. Med. Assoc.*, **290**, 1467–1473.

Greil, W. and Kleindienst, N. (1999) Lithium versus carbamazepine in the maintenance treatment of bipolar II disorder and bipolar disorder not otherwise specified. *Int. Clin. Psychopharmacol.*, **14**, 283–285.

Greil, W., Kleindienst, N., Erazo, N., and Müller-Oerlinghausen, B. (1998) Differential response to lithium and carbamazepine in the prophylaxis of bipolar disorder. *J. Clin. Psychopharmacol.*, **18**, 455–460.

Greil, W., Ludwig-Mayerhofer, W., Erazo, N. *et al.* (1997) Lithium vs carbamazepine in the maintenance treatment of schizoaffective disorder: a randomised study. *Eur. Arch. Psychiatry Clin. Neurosci.*, **247**, 42–50.

Grof, P. (1987) Admission rates and lithium therapy. *Br. J. Psychiatry*, **150**, 264–265.

Grof, P. (1998) Has the effectiveness of lithium changed? Impact of the variety of lithium's effects. *Neuropsychopharmacology*, **19**, 183–188.

Grof, P. (2003) Selecting effective long-term treatment for bipolar patients: monotherapy and combination therapy. *J. Clin. Psychiatry*, **64** (Suppl. 5), 53–61.

Grof, P., MacCrimmon, D., Smith, E.K.M. *et al.* (1980) Long-term lithium treatment and the kidney. *Can. J. Psychiatry*, **25**, 535–544.

Grof, P., Schou, M., Angst, J. *et al.* (1970a) Methodological problems of prophylactic trials in recurrent affective disorders. *Br. J. Psychiatry*, **116**, 599–603.

Grof, P., Cakuls, P., and Dostal, T. (1970b) Lithium drop-outs: a follow-up study of patients who discontinued prophylactic treatment. *Int. Pharmacopsychiatry*, **5**, 162–169.

Guscott, R. and Taylor, L. (1994) Lithium prophylaxis in recurrent affective illness: efficacy, effectiveness and efficiency. *Br. J. Psychiatry*, **164**, 741–764.

Hanus, K. and Zapletalek, M. (1984) Suicidal activity of patients with affective disorders during the preventive use of lithium. *Cesk. Psychiatr.*, **80**, 97–100.

Hartigan, G.P. (1963) The use of lithium salts in affective disorders. *Br. J. Psychiatry*, **109**, 810–814.

Healy, D. (ed.) (1997) Lithium. Interview with Mogens Schou, *The Psychopharmacologists II*, Chapman & Hall, London, pp. 259–284.

Hullin, R.P., McDonald, R., and Allsopp, M.N.E. (1972) Prophylactic lithium in recurrent affective disorders. *Lancet*, **1**, 1044–1046.

Jacobson, S.J., Jones, K., Johnson, K. *et al.* (1992) Prospective multicentre study of pregnancy outcome after lithium exposure during first trimester. *Lancet*, **339**, 530–533.

Jamison, K.R. (1986) Suicide and bipolar disorders. *Ann. N. Y. Acad. Sci.*, **487**, 301–315.

Johnson, F.N. (1984) *The History of Lithium Treatment*, Mcmillan, London.

Judd, L.L. and Akiskal, H.S. (2003) The prevalence and disability of bipolar spectrum disorders in the US population: re-analysis of the ECA database taking into account subthreshold cases. *J. Affect. Disord.*, **73**, 123–131.

Kallner, G., Lindelius, R., Petterson, U. *et al.* (2000) Mortality in 497 patients with affective disorders attending a lithium clinic or after having left it. *Pharmacopsychiatry*, **33**, 8–13.

Lange, C. (1886) Bidrag til urinsyrediatesens klinik. *Hospitalstidende*, **5**, 1–15, 21–38, 45–63, 69–83.

Melia, P.I. (1970) Prophylactic lithium: a double-blind trial in recurrent affective illness. *Br. J. Psychiatry*, **116**, 621–624.

Mendlewicz, J. (1984) Lithium discontinuation in bipolar Illness: a double-blind prospective controlled study, in *Current Trends in Lithium and Rubidium Therapy* (ed. G.U. Corsini), MTP Press, Stuttgart, pp. 125–141.

Moncrieff, J. (1995) Lithium revisited: a re-examination of the placebo-controlled trials of lithium prophylaxis in manic-depressive disorder. *Br. J. Psychiatry*, **167**, 569–574.

Müller-Oerlinghausen, B., Ahrens, B., Grof, E. *et al.* (1992) The effect of long-term lithium treatment on the mortality of patients with manic-depressive or schizo-affective illness. *Acta Psychiatr. Scand.*, **86**, 218–222.

Passmore, M.J., Garnham, J., Duffy, A. *et al.* (2003) Phenotypic spectra of bipolar disorder in responders to lithium versus lamotrigine. *Bipolar Disord.*, **5**, 110–114.

Placidi, G.F., Lenzi, A., Lazzerini, F. *et al.* (1986) The comparative efficacy and safety of carbamazepine versus lithium: a randomized, double-blind, 3-year trial in 83 patients. *J. Clin. Psychiatry*, **47**, 490–494.

Povlsen, U.J., Hetmar, O., Ladefoged, J., and Bolwig, T.B. (1992) Kidney functioning during lithium treatment: a prospective study of patients treated with lithium for up to ten years. *Acta Psychiatr. Scand.*, **85**, 56–60.

Prien, R.F., Caffey, E.M., and Klett, C.J. (1973) Prophylactic efficacy of lithium carbonate in manic-depressive illness. *Arch. Gen. Psychiatry*, **28**, 337–341.

Reifman, A. and Wyatt, R.J. (1980) Lithium: a brake in the rising cost of mental illness. *Arch. Gen. Psychiatry*, **37**, 355–388.

Rifkin, A.F., Quitkin, F., and Howard, A. (1975) A study of abrupt lithium withdrawal. *Psychopharmacology*, **44**, 157–158.

Sashidharan, S.P. and McGuire, R.J. (1983) Recurrence of affective illness after withdrawal of long-term lithium treatment. *Acta Psychiatr. Scand.*, **68**, 126–133.

Schioldann, J. (2001) *In Commemoration of the Century of the Death of Carl Lange. The Lange Theory of 'Periodical Depressions'. A Landmark in the History of Lithium Therapy*, Adelaide Academic Press.

Schou, M. (1956) Lithiumterapi ved mani: praktiske retningslinier. *Nord. Med.*, **55**, 790–794.

Schou, M. (1969) The 'Scandinavian register of lithium babies', in *Lithium in Psychiatry*, Acta Psychitr. Scand. Suppl., Vol. 207 (eds N. Diding, J.O. Ottosson, and M. Schou), p. 97.

Schou, M. (1986) Admission rates and lithium therapy. *Br. J. Psychiatry*, **149**, 798–799.

Schou, M. (1988) Effects of long-term lithium treatment on kidney function: an overview. *J. Psychiatr. Res.*, **22**, 287–296.

Schou, M. (1990) Lithium treatment during pregnancy, delivery, and lactation. An update. *J. Clin. Psychiatry*, **51**, 410–413.

Schou, M. (1992) Phases in the development of lithium treatment in psychiatry, in *The Neurosciences: Paths of Discovery*, vol. 2 (eds F. Samson and G. Adelman), Birkhäuser, Boston, pp. 147–166.

Schou, M. (1993a) Lithium prophylaxis: about 'naturalistic' or 'clinical practice' studies. *Lithium*, **4**, 77–81.

Schou, M. (1993b) *Lithium Treatment of Manic-Depressive Illness: A Practical Guide*, 5th edn, Karger, Freiburg, London, New York.

Schou, M. (1997) The combat of non-compliance during prophylactic lithium treatment. *Acta Psychiatr. Scand.*, **95**, 361–363.

Schou, M. (1998a) Has the time come to abandon prophylactic lithium treatment? A review for clinicians. *Pharmacopsychiatry*, **31**, 210–215.

Schou, M. (1998b) Treating recurrent affective disorders during and after pregnancy: what can be taken safely? *Drug Saf.*, **18**, 143–152.

Schou, M. (1998c) The effect of prophylactic lithium treatment on mortality and suicidal behavior: a review for clinicians. *J. Affect. Disord.*, **50**, 253–259.

Schou, M. (2000) Suicidal behavior and prophylactic lithium treatment of major mood disorders: a review for clinicians. *Suicide Life Threat. Behav.*, **30**, 289–293.

Schou, M. (2001) Lithium treatment at 52. *J. Affect. Disord.*, **67**, 21–23.

Schou, M. and Kampf, D. (2006) Lithium and the kidneys, in *Lithium in Neuropsychiatry* (eds M. Bauer, P. Grof, and B., Müller-Oerlinghausen), Informa, London, pp. 251–259.

Schou, M., Juel-Nielsen, N., Strömgren, E., and Voldby, H. (1954) The treatment of manic psychoses by the administration of lithium salts. *J. Neurol. Neurosurg. Psychiatry*, **17**, 250–260.

Schou, M., Thomsen, K., and Baastrup, P.C. (1970) Studies on the course of recurrent endogenous affective disorders. *Int. Pharmacopsychiatry*, **5**, 100–106.

Schou, M. and Vestergaard, P. (1988) Prospective studies on a lithium cohort. 2. Renal function. Water and electrolyte metabolism. *Acta Psychiatr. Scand.*, **78**, 427–433.

Stallone, F., Shelley, E., Mendlewicz, J., and Fieve, R.R. (1973) The use of lithium in affective disorders, III. A double-blind study of prophylaxis in bipolar illness. *Am. J. Psychiatry*, **130**, 1006–1010.

Suppes, T., Baldessarini, R.J., Faedda, G.I. *et al.* (1993) Discontinuation of maintenance treatment of bipolar disorder: risks and implications. *Harv. Rev. Psychiatry*, **1**, 131–144.

Thomsen, K. and Schou, M. (1999) Avoidance of lithium intoxications: advice based on knowledge about the renal lithium clearance under various circumstances. *Pharmacopsychiatry*, **32**, 83–86.

Tondo, L., Jamison, K.R., and Baldessarini, R.J. (1997) Effect of lithium maintenance on suicidal behavior in major mood disorders. *Ann. N. Y. Acad. Sci.*, **836**, 339–351.

Vestergaard, P., Poulstrup, I., and Schou, M. (1988) Prospective studies on a lithium cohort. 3. Tremor, weight gain, diarrhea, psychological complaints. *Acta Psychiatr. Scand.*, **78**, 343–441.

Vestergaard, P. and Schou, M. (1988) Prospective studies on a lithium cohort. 1. General features. *Acta Psychiatr. Scand.*, **78**, 434–441.

Wyatt, R.J. and Henter, I. (1995) An economic evaluation of manic-depressive illness. *Soc. Psychiatry Psychiatr. Epidemiol.*, **30**, 213–219.

Yatham, L.N., Calabrese, J.R., and Kusumakar, V. (2003) Bipolar depression: criteria for treatment selection, definition of refractoriness, and treatment options. *Bipolar Disord.*, **5**, 85–97.

Valproate: Clinical Pharmacological Profile

Charles L. Bowden and Vivek Singh

The University of Texas Health Science Center at San Antonio, TX, USA

3.1 HISTORICAL BACKGROUND

Valproic acid (valproate), synthesized by Burton in the United States in 1882, was initially used as an organic solvent for other compounds. It was during its use as a solvent for a series of compounds being tested for anti-seizure activity that Meuiner serendipitously discovered that valproate inherently possessed anti-seizure properties. He observed that compounds which did not appear to possess anti-seizure qualities, when administered alone, inhibited seizure activity when valproiate was employed as the delivery solvent. With this observation, he concluded that valproate, rather than the test compounds possessed anti-seizure effects (Meunier *et al.*, 1975; Fariello and Smith, 1989; Bowden and McElroy, 1995). Interest in valproate as a putative mood stabilizing agent began following the first observational report of its efficacy in bipolar disorder (Lambert *et al.*, 1966). Divalproex sodium, an enteric and delayed release formulation of valproate was introduced in the U.S. in 1983 and received U.S. Food and Drug Administration (FDA) approval in 1995 for the treatment of acute mania associated with bipolar I disorder. An extended-release formulation of divalproex was approved by the FDA for migraine in 2001 and acute mania and mixed mania associated with bipolar I disorder in 2006. Valproate, either as divalproex or other formulations, is now an approved and widely used treatment option for acute mania and maintenance therapy for bipolar disorder worldwide.

3.2 STRUCTURE–ACTIVITY RELATIONSHIPS

Valproate (dipropylacetic acid) is an eight-carbon, branched-chain carboxylic acid, that is, structurally different from the other antiepileptic and psychotropic compounds (Bocci and Beretta, 1976; Levy *et al.*, 2002). Branched-chain carboxylic acids effectively antagonize pentylenetetrazole-induced seizures while straight-chain acids have little or no antiepileptic activity.

Bipolar Psychopharmacotherapy: Caring for the patient, Second Edition. Edited by Hagop S. Akiskal and Mauricio Tohen.
© 2011 John Wiley & Sons, Ltd. Published 2011 by John Wiley & Sons, Ltd.

3.3 PHARMACODYNAMIC PROPERTIES

Over the past decade, studies of valproate and lithium indicate converging, additive mechanisms for the drugs. These results provide heuristic evidence that other molecules with similar mechanisms could be effective in bipolar disorder and several other CNS disorders. Since many effective anticonvulsants are ineffective in bipolar disorder, anti-seizure properties are not fundamental to bipolar mechanisms. For several of these biological systems, functional actions of the system are at least partially understood. Treatment of cultured cortical neurons with therapeutic concentrations of valproate or lithium increased the levels of brain derived neurotrophic factor (BDNF) mRNA. The primary actions of the two drugs on BDNF neuroprotection reside upstream from the calcium-responsive elements, involving GSK-3 inhibition by lithium and valproate and histone deacetylase (HDAC) inhibition by valproate, hypothesized to be fundamental to the action of valproate in bipolar disorders (Leng *et al.*, 2008; Wu *et al.*, 2008; Yasuda *et al.*, 2009). Through its HDAC inhibition, valproate increases activity of heat shock protein-7 mRNA levels and thereby provides neuroprotection against glutamate induced excitotoxicity (Marinova *et al.*, 2009; Geddes *et al.*, 2010). Studies in cortical neurons suggest that other mechanisms common to lithium and valproate include calcium signaling, extracellular signal-regulated kinase (ERK) cascade, inhibition of phospholipase A-2 and of inositol biosynthesis, Akt signaling, and PKC inhibition (Einat *et al.*, 2003). Both lithium and valproate lengthen the period of circadian rhythms and increase arrhythmicity in Drosophila, which may explain a portion of their efficacy in bipolar illness (Dokucu, Yu, and Taghert, 2005). Inhibition of HDAC was associated with antidepressant-like effects in a mouse model for behavioral despair (Leng *et al.*, 2008). These studies, limited in that nonhuman systems were investigated, nevertheless consistently indicate synergistic neuroprotective effects of lithium via glycogen synthase kinase-3 inhibition and valrpoate via HDAC inhibition. The results, consistent with implications of a recent randomized trial in which bipolar patients treated with both valproate and lithium had superior maintenance results compared with those treated with either drug alone, suggest that the combined use of valproate and lithium in the treatment of bipolar disorder warrants further study (Geddes *et al.*, 2010). Additionally, combined use of both drugs to treat glutamate-related neurodegenerative diseases, for example, multiple sclerosis, appears to be a promising area of investigation (Gray *et al.*, 2003). Valproate and lithium also have other overlapping effects on neuronal systems involved in maintaining mood stability and alertness that have not been observed in studies of similar system with carbamazepine or second generation antipsychotics (Harwood and Agam, 2003).

Several additional neurochemical systems have been identified as impacted by valproate. However, at least some of these effects appear consequent to HDAC inhibition. Briefly, these systems include stimulation of the ERK pathway in the rat hippocampus and frontal cortex (Einat *et al.*, 2003; Yuan *et al.*, 2001) implicated in the mediation of antimanic effects of mood stabilizers (Gould and Manji, 2002) and increased expression of the cytoprotective protein B-cell lymphoma/leukemia-2 gene (Bcl-2) in the CNS in vivo and in cells of human neuronal origin. (Gray *et al.*, 2003) Valproate activates **two** prominent substrates for PKC in the brain, myristoylated alanine-rich C kinase substrate (MARCKS), and GAP-43, which have been implicated in actin-membrane plasticity and neurite outgrowth during neuronal differentiation, respectively, and are essential to normal brain development and may play a role in the long term efficacy of mood stabilizers (Watson, Watterson, and Lenox, 1998; Hasegawa *et al.*, 2003). Valproate reduced corticotrophin releasing factor (CRF) mRNA expression and CRF1 receptor binding, damping the tone in this pathway, that is, associated with stress linked psychopathology, including mixed mania (Watterson *et al.*, 2002).

3.4 PHARMACOKINETICS AND METABOLIC CLEARANCE

Valproate is available in five different formulations: (i) divalproex sodium, an enteric-coated, compound containing valproic acid and sodium valproate in equal proportions; (ii) valproic acid; (iii) sodium valproate; (iv) divalproex sodium sprinkle capsules containing enteric-coated particles of divalproex sodium that can be administered orally or be sprinkled on food; and (v) an extended- release form of divalproex, to be dosed once a day, with a much lower differential between the peak-to-trough serum levels. Sodium valproate can be delivered intravenously and is associated with amelioration of manic symptoms within one day or less (Grunze *et al.*, 1999). Valproate is also available in suppository form for rectal administration.

The valproate moiety, common to all formulations, is rapidly absorbed, except in its formulation as divlaproex sodium, and is 100% bioavailable with all preparations (Levy *et al.*, 2002; Penry and Dean, 1989; Wilder, 1992). The absorption of valproate is delayed with food, which may mitigate side effects. Valproate and sodium valproate attain their peak serum concentrations within 2 hours while divalproex sodium reaches its peak serum concentration within 3–8 hours of oral intake. The extended release (ER) formulation of divalproex has an earlier onset of absorption than divalproex sodium regular-release tablets and about a 20% lesser difference in trough-peak serum concentrations compared to the regular-release divalproex sodium.

Valproate demonstrates high binding affinity for serum proteins, especially for serum albumin. However, lower level of serum proteins, seen particularly in the elderly and women, does not affect the steady state concentration of the drug as there is a higher level of the unbound fraction of the drug and thus enhanced rate of clearance of the drug. Since only the unbound fraction of valproate is bioactive and crosses the blood brain barrier, valproate's pharmacological activity is solely determined by the unbound fraction of the drug. Enhanced valproate activity, and hence higher incidence of adverse events, may also be seen following its displacement from serum protein binding sites when administered with drugs with greater binding affinity for serum proteins, despite unaltered total valproate serum concentrations.

Conjugation, through glucoronidation in the liver, is the predominant mode of metabolic clearance of valproate. Oxidative pathways lead to the production of metabolite that are bioactive and toxic (4-en- and 2,4-en metabolites) (Bocci and Beretta, 1976; Levy *et al.*, 2002; Wilder, 1992; Schatzberg, 1998). Valproate's elimination half-life, typically 5–20 hours, can be affected by agents that induce or inhibit the mitochondrial and/or microsomal enzymes systems involved in its clearance.

3.5   SERUM CONCENTRATION AND EFFICACY

The antimanic efficacy of valproate is most pronounced at serum concentration of 45–125 µg/ml (Bowden *et al.*, 1996). At serum levels greater than 110 µg/ml, advantages of higher efficacy may be offset by greater incidence of adverse effects and poor tolerability (Allen *et al.*, 2006). Valproate, at lower serums concentrations, may be efficacious in patients with bipolar II disorder or cyclothymia (Jacobsen, 1993). Long term outcomes are also related to serum concentrations with intervention for a developing mood episode significantly longer with maintenance of serum valproate concentrations between 75 and 100 µg/ml compared to patients with serum levels either lower or higher than this range (Calabrese and Shelton, 2002). Clinicians should take into consideration both the response and the side effects of valproate in determining the daily dose of valproate. Adverse events such as increased appetite, sedation, leukopenia, and thrombocytopenia are a direct function of the valproate serum concentration (Bowden *et al.*, 2000). Treatment with valproate is initiated at 15 mg/kg body weight and the daily dosage titrated upwards till the desired response is achieved or adverse effects are seen.

3.6   EFFICACY AND INDICATIONS

Valproate has gained FDA indications for the treatment of manic or mixed episodes associated with bipolar disorder I, with or without psychotic features; as a monotherapeutic or adjunctive agent in the treatment of simple and complex absence seizures; for adjunctive therapy in multiple seizure types, including absence seizures; and as a prophylactic agent in migraine. Large, placebo-controlled clinical trials have demonstrated valproate's efficacy in prophylaxis from mania (Bowden *et al.*, 2000; Tohen, Ketter, and Zarate, 2003) and in prolonging time to recurrence of depression in bipolar disorder (Gyulai *et al.*, 2003). Controlled studies additionally indicate that valproate is effective in generalized epilepsies, including generalized tonic-clonic and myoclonic seizures, as well as in secondarily generalized tonic-clonic seizures, infantile spasms, photosensitive epilepsy, and febrile seizures (Rimmer and Richens, 1985).

3.7   EFFICACY IN BIPOLAR DISORDER

3.7.1   ACUTE MANIA AND MIXED MANIA

Valproate has proven to be an effective treatment for mania and mixed mania based on several open label and controlled studies (five placebo-controlled, one haloperidol-controlled, one lithium controlled, and one placebo-and lithium-controlled) (McElroy *et al.*, 1993; Bowden *et al.*, 1994). In the controlled trials, valproate demonstrated significant superiority to placebo and was comparable to lithium and haloperidol in the acute treatment of mania associated with bipolar I disorder (Emirch, Doae, and von Zerssen, 1985; Pope *et al.*, 1991; Freeman *et al.*, 1992; Bowden *et al.*, 1994; McElroy *et al.*, 1996;

Bowden *et al.*, 2006). In the most recently concluded placebo-controlled study in acute mania, response to valproate was directly related to the severity of manic symptoms with patients with greater severity of manic symptoms experiencing greater benefits with valproate compared to placebo than those with lesser severity of manic symptoms (Bowden *et al.*, 2006). These studies also showed the onset of antimanic response with valproate as early as day 5.

The response latency to valproate is reduced following "oral loading" dosages with valproate. Following an oral loading strategy with valproate, 20 mg/kg body weight, in an open label, rater-blinded study of patients with acute mania, ≥50% of the patients had significant response within five days. Valproate was well tolerated and patients experienced minimal adverse events (Keck *et al.*, 1993). Hirschfield *et al.* also demonstrated the safety and efficacy of an accelerated loading strategy, 30 mg/kg/day on days 1 and 2 and then 20 mg/kg/day on days 3–10 (Hirschfeld *et al.*, 1999). The dosing strategy aimed to expedite attainment of trough serum concentrations of valproate ≥50 mg/l in patients meeting DSM-IV diagnostic criteria for a manic episode. Patients were randomly assigned to a loading group (N = 20), nonloading group (N = 20) with divalproex started at 250 mg t.i.d. on day 1 followed by standard titration between days 3–10; or lithium (N = 19) started at 300 mg t.i.d. followed by standard dose titrations between days 3–10. Significantly greater number of patients in the loading group than in the nonloading group (84% vs. 30%) attained a valproate concentration of ≥50 mg/l by day 3 with no differentiation between the three groups in the frequency or type of adverse events. In a double-blind study (Oluboka *et al.*, 2002) comparing the efficacy and tolerability of oral loading (N = 5), 20 mg/kg/day, and slower titration (n = 6), 10 mg/kg/day, regimens of valproate in acutely manic patients, the mean serum valproate concentration in the loading group compared to the titration group was significantly higher at day 1 (72.1 vs. 34.6, $p < 0.05$). The loading group continued to have a higher valproate serum concentration at day 3, (71.7 vs. 59), though the differential diminished. Reduction in manic symptoms was significantly greater in the loading group than in the titration group at day 3 with comparable tolerability in the two groups, with the loading group more likely to experience sedation.

Valproate was comparable to haloperidol in the reduction of manic and psychotic symptoms in patients with acute mania, when administered at 20 mg/kg/day (McElroy *et al.*, 1996). Valproate demonstrated superiority in the reduction of manic symptoms, shorter response latency and lower rates of adverse events when compared to carbamazepine in a small (*n* = 30) blinded randomized study in acute mania (Vasudev, Goswami, and Kohli, 2000).

These studies of the past two decades provide firm evidence for the role of valproate in the treatment of acute mania. The studies also demonstrate the wide spectrum of efficacy of valproate and the breadth of circumstances in which it can be effectively employed. There continues to be a paucity of data on the efficacy of valproate, as well as of other antimanic agents, in the treatment of hypomania and cyclothymia (Jacobsen, 1993). Sample sizes were consistently small in the loading dosage and comparative effectiveness studies summarized above, therefore limiting the strength of the results.

3.8   COMBINATION STRATEGY IN ACUTE MANIA

Valproate, when used as an adjunct to antipsychotics (haloperidol, risperidone, olan-zapine, quetipaine) in the treatment of acute mania, is associated with approximately 20% higher rates of antimanic response than with treatment with either antipsychotics or valproate alone (Muller-Oerlinghausen *et al.*, 2000; Sachs *et al.*, 2002; Tohen *et al.*, 2002; Yatham *et al.*, 2003; Yatham, 2005). The Sachs *et al.* study allowed patients whose manic symptoms had failed to respond to monotherapy with either valproate or lithium at an adequate dose for ≥2 weeks or longer to receive either risperidone or haloperidol (add-on therapy), or patients who were manic without treatment, in which case both risperidone and either lithium or valproate were started concurrently (co-therapy). The study reported no advantage for the combination treatment in the cotherapy group when compared to monotherapy, but in the group of patients who had failed to respond to monotherapy with valproate or lithium an advantage for the add-on therapy compared to the monotherapy was seen. All of the other adjunctive studies required some unre-sponsiveness to monotherapy treatment therefore strongly indicating that a combination treatment regimen is more likely to have additional benefits when used in situations where monotherapy has been ineffective.

3.9   PROPHYLAXIS IN BIPOLAR DISORDER

In a large, double-blind, placebo controlled monotherapy study (Geddes *et al.*, 2010), patients who fulfilled recovery criteria within three months of an index manic episode after open label treatment with either lithium or valproate (n = 372) were randomized to receive treatment with divalproex, lithium, or placebo in a 2 : 1 : 1 assignment for 52 weeks. The primary outcome measure was time to any mood episode; secondary mea-sures were time to a manic episode, time to a depressive episode, average change from baseline in Schedule for Affective Disorders and Schizophrenia-Change Version subscale scores for depression and mania, and Global Assessment of Function (GAF) scores. Nei-ther valproate nor lithium demonstrated significant superiority to placebo in time to any mood episode (p = 0.06), in part due to the substantially lower rates of relapse into mania in the placebo group than had occurred in early lithium studies which may have been consequent to lithium withdrawal induced rebound episodes. Significantly lower rates of discontinuation for either a recurrent mood or depressive episode were seen in the val-proate group than the placebo group (Bowden, 2004). Valproate proved more efficacious than lithium in longer duration of successful prophylaxis, less deterioration in depres-sive symptoms, and GAF scores. Patients who were treated with valproate during the open phase and were randomized to receive valproate had wider advantages compared to placebo for time to mania or depression (P = 0.05), time to depression (P = 0.03) pro-portion of patients who completed the trial and did not have either a manic or depressive episode (McElroy *et al.*, 2008). Among patients who were treated with lithium in the open phase, there was no significant advantage among those subsequently randomized to lithium compared to those randomized to receive either placebo or valproate. A post hoc secondary analysis demonstrated that valproate treatment was associated with lower rates of discontinuation for a mood episode compared to those who received lithium (relative risk (RR) = 0.63, 95% confidence interval (CI) = 0.44–0.90) (Macritchie *et al.*, 2000). Another post hoc analysis showed that valproate was superior to lithium ($P > 0.004$) for time to a mood episode or early discontinuation for any reason, a measure of effectiveness that has been incorporated in recent maintenance studies in bipolar disorder (Bowden, 2003).

Valproate and olanzapine did not differentiate from each other in a 12-week randomized blinded comparison in patients with mania (Zajecka *et al.*, 2002). Valproate and olanzapine, in a 47-week study, showed equivalent efficacy but were both associated with high rates of study discontinuation (85% vs. 84%). Patients who attained remission at the end of three weeks were more likely to complete the entire duration of the study than those who were not remitted (divalproex: 26.2% vs. 11.1%; olanzapine: 20.3% vs. 10.6%, $P = 0.001$) indicating a greater probability of long term effectiveness of either olanzapine or valproate amongst patients who demonstrate an acute response to the same medication during a manic episode. Valproate was better tolerated and was associated with significantly lesser weight gain and reduction in cholesterol, while olanzapine caused increase in cholesterol in both the studies (Zajecka *et al.*, 2002; Tohen, Ketter, and Zarate, 2003).

A randomized, blinded comparative study of lithium and valproate in patients with rapid-cycling bipolar disorder did not differentiate between the two groups with only 25% of patients meeting criteria for a bimodal response. Patients who demonstrated a bimodal response were randomized to a 20-month maintenance phase. Less than one-quarter of acute responders randomized to either lithium or valproate maintained benefits without developing a new mood episode in either of the two treatment arms (Calabrese *et al.*, 2005). In a combination study of valproate and lithium, patients on the combination regimen were less likely to relapse over a course of 12 months but more likely to experience side effects than those treated with lithium alone (Solomon *et al.*, 1997). In a pragmatic trial utilizing practicing clinicians which allowed clinician choice of acute medication, patients randomized to valproate plus lithium had generally more favorable continuation outcomes than those randomized to treatment with valproate or lithium alone (Geddes *et al.*, 2010)

3.10 TREATMENT OF BIPOLAR DEPRESSION

A recent meta-analysis has been published of the four small, randomized blinded single center trials that have compared valproate semisodium with placebo in a total of 142 participants (Davis, Bartolucci, and Petty, 2005; Sachs, 2001; Muzina, Ganocy, and Khalife, 2008). The dosing strategy varied between studies with valproate dosed to achieve mean serum levels between 61.5 and 83 µg/ml. The extended release (ER) formulation of divalproex was used in two studies (Muzina, Ganocy, and Khalife, 2008; Ghaemi, Gilmer, and Goldberg, 2007), participants were adults with a mean age from 35 to 41 years old with bipolar I and II disorder with or without rapid cycling course based on DSM-IV criteria, and were moderately to severely depressed. Results were reported for follow-up at six weeks (Muzina, Ganocy, and Khalife, 2008; Ghaemi, Gilmer, and Goldberg, 2007) and eight weeks (Davis, Bartolucci, and Petty, 2005; Sachs, 2001). In three of the studies

(140 participants) depression as measured by depression rating scale scores was significantly lower with valproate compared with placebo at study endpoint. The random effects meta-analysis showed significant reduction in depression symptoms; standardized mean difference (SMD): -0.35 (-0.69, -0.02; $p = 0.04$) with no heterogeneity detected (Smith et al., 2010). In the one study that reported results for participants by bipolar subtype, statistically significant improvement in MADRS scores was shown in the bipolar I, but not in the bipolar II group (Muzina, Ganocy, and Khalife, 2008). However, the difference in effect size between the subgroups was not reported, and the number of participants in each subgroup was small so this result should be interpreted with caution. Proportions of patients meeting similar response criteria were also calculated. In each study, participants treated with valproate semisodium were more likely to respond by the end of the trial compared with those on placebo. The pooled treatment effect using a random effects model was statistically significant (RR 2.00 [95% CI: 1.13, 3.53; $p = 0.02$]) with no heterogeneity detected $I^2 = 0\%$. The absolute risk difference was 0.22% (0.07, 0.36; $p = 0.003$; $I^2 = 0\%$) or 22% generating a number needed to treat (NNT) of 5 (Smith et al., 2010).

3.11 VALPROATE IN TREATMENT OF BIPOLAR DISORDER IN CHILDREN AND ADOLESCENTS

In a double-blind four-week (N = 150) comparison of divalproex ER to placebo in patients 10–17 years old with mania or mixed mania, valproate was non superior to placebo on change in YMRS score (divalproex ER -8.8 (n = 74); placebo -7.9 (n = 70)), the primary efficacy measure or on secondary measures. There was no difference between the two groups on the incidence of adverse effects (Wagner et al., 2009). Valproate and quetiapine did not differ in efficacy or adverse effects in a randomized double-blind four week study of 50 patients aged 12–18 years with acute mania or mixed mania (DelBello et al., 2006). In an open, randomized six-week study, (n = 42) (Kowatch et al., 2000) patients aged 9–18 years with mania, received either valproate, or lithium, or carbamazepine. No significant differences across the three different groups were noted but the effect size for improvement was greatest for the valproate group compared to that for either lithium or carbamazepine groups (valproate = 1.63; lithium = 1.06, carbamazepine = 1.00) (Kowatch et al., 2000). Mixed mania, a common manifestation of bipolar disorder in adolescents, responded well to open six-month treatment with valproate, with high rates of patients who completed the entire duration of the study (Pavuluri et al., 2005).

Valproate did not differ from lithium in either time to development of symptoms indicative of relapse or time to discontinuation for any reason in patients, aged 5–17 years with bipolar disorder I and II, who had been previously stabilized on combination of valproate and lithium (n = 60) (Findling et al., 2005). Several of these studies in children and adolescents acknowledge the methodological difficulties of conduct of studies in this age group and the difficulty in achieving all of the aims that are desired to provide effectiveness data to guide psychiatrists in practice. Small sample sizes, difficulties in recruitment, and uncertainties about ascertainment of diagnosis of bipolar disorder are among the methodological limitations that leave us with inadequate information for treatments for bipolar disorder in adolescents and children.

3.12   USE IN BIPOLAR ILLNESS COMORBID WITH ALCOHOLISM

Bipolar disorder is highly comorbid with substance use disorders, with alcohol use disorder being the most common. In the largest prospective, blinded, placebo controlled study, 59 bipolar I patients with alcohol dependence were treated with lithium carbonate and psychosocial interventions for 24 weeks, with half randomized to receive valproate additionally. Patients assigned to the valproate group had significantly fewer heavy drinking days and fewer drinks per heavy drinking day, and lower levels of gamma-glutamyl transpeptidase (GGT) compared with the placebo group. Higher serum valproate concentrations were associated with improved alcohol use outcomes. The decline in heavy drinking was exclusive of the improvement in the manic and depressive symptoms, which improved equivalently in both the groups (Salloum et al., 2005).

3.12.1   RELAPSE PREVENTION

Valproate was associated with a significantly smaller percentage of individuals relapsing to heavy drinking in another, double-blind, placebo-controlled trial but there were no significant differences in other alcohol-related outcomes. The valproate group demonstrated greater decreases in irritability and a trend toward greater decreases on measures of lability and verbal assault. There were no significant variations between group differences on measures of impulsivity (Brady et al., 1995). Valproate, in a small randomized study (n = 16), demonstrated safety and faster and greater consistency in symptom reduction compared to benzodiazepine (Longo, Campbell, and Hubatch, 2002).

3.12.2   ALCOHOL WITHDRAWAL

Reoux et al., conducted a randomized, double-blind, placebo-controlled trial of valproate in 36 hospitalized patients experiencing moderate alcohol withdrawal. All subjects received a baseline dose of oxazepam and had additional oxazepam available as a rescue medication in accordance with a standard, symptom-triggered detoxification protocol. Valproate demonstrated a significantly positive affected on alcohol withdrawal course and reduced the use of oxazepam (p < 0.033) (Reoux et al., 2001).

3.13   BIPOLAR DISORDER COMORBID WITH ADHD

Attention deficit hyperactivity disorder (ADHD) is often comorbid in patients with bipolar disorder. Scheffer et al. conducted a study to determine whether adjunctive use of a psychostimulant was safe and efficacious for treatment of symptoms of ADHD in 40 pediatric outpatients with bipolar I or II disorder and concurrent ADHD who had their manic symptoms stabilized through open label treatment with valproate for eight weeks. Thirty of the stabilized patients were then treated in a four-week randomized, double-blind, placebo-controlled crossover trial during which valproate was continued.

Psychostimulants combined with valproate were significantly more efficacious than valproate plus placebo for the ADHD symptoms with no evidence of worsening of manic symptoms (Scheffer et al., 2005). This practical study indicates that psychostimulants can be used concomitantly with valproate to treat concurrent ADHD with bipolar disorder without increasing the risk of relapse to mania.

3.14 BIPOLAR DISORDER COMORBID WITH BORDERLINE PERSONALITY DISORDER

In a six month placebo controlled double-blind study of valproate of 30 women ages 18–40 years with borderline personality disorder and bipolar II disorder, divalproex was significantly superior to placebo in diminishing interpersonal sensitivity and anger/hostility as well as overall aggression (Frankenburg and Zanarini, 2002).

3.15 ADVERSE EFFECTS

There is a great deal of understanding of the adverse effect profile of valproate given experience with its usage for the past five decades (DeVane, 2003; Prevey et al., 1996). The adverse effects associated with valproate are seen at higher frequency in patients treated for epilepsy than in patients with bipolar disorder. This is most likely related to higher doses of valproate as well as concomitant use of other antiepileptics in the treatment of epilepsy than in those with bipolar disorder (DeVane, 2003).

3.16 COMPARATIVE ADVERSE EFFECTS

Valproate has been compared with other drugs employed in treatment of bipolar disorder. In general, adverse effects have been relatively favorable compared with lithium (Bowden et al., 2000), carbamazepine (Vasudev, Goswami, and Kohli, 2000), and olanzapine (Tohen, Ketter, and Zarate, 2003; Zajecka et al., 2002). Rates of early discontinuation for side effects or other reasons have generally been lower for valproate than for these three comparator drugs. One post hoc analysis conducted in the one-year maintenance study comparing valproate, lithium, and placebo added early (Bowden et al., 2000) discontinuation for any reason to the primary planned outcome of time to a full episode of mania or depression. In the post hoc effectiveness analysis, incorporating tolerability by assessing time to discontinuation for any reason, valproate was significantly superior to lithium, even applying Bonferroni correction for multiple comparisons ($p = 0.004$) (Bowden, 2004).

3.17 ADVERSE EFFECTS IN COMBINATION THERAPY, COMPARED WITH MONOTHERAPY

Several studies have compared valproate alone vs valproate plus other drugs (olanzapine, risperidone, quetiapine) (Tohen, Ketter, and Zarate, 2003; Sachs et al., 2002). Conclusions from these studies are limited because about half the patients were receiving lithium in lieu of valproate, making the sample size insufficient for analyzing the difference between lithium and valproate.

3.18 ADVERSE EFFECTS BY BODILY SYSTEM

Valproate has been extensively used over several decades and is generally well tolerated, based on evidence from several controlled studies (DeVane, 2003; Prevey *et al.*, 1996). Epilepsy patients on valproate are more likely to experience adverse events than patients being treated for migraine or bipolar disorder, again a consequence of lower dosage for migraine than for epilepsy (DeVane, 2003). In a large one year controlled study in bipolar disorder, tremor, and reported weight were the only adverse effects more commonly seen with valproate than placebo (Prevey *et al.*, 1996).

3.18.1 GASTROINTESTINAL EFFECTS

Gastrointestinal side effects, directly related to the peak serum concentration of valproate, manifest most commonly as nausea, vomiting, diarrhea, dyspepsia, and anorexia (DeVane, 2003). These can be minimized by the use of extended or delayed release formulations of valproate or by lowering the dose (Horne, 2003; Zarate *et al.*, 2000).

3.18.2 TREMORS

Since the incidence of tremors (9–22%) is related to the serum concentration of valproate, its more likely to occur in patients with epilepsy than bipolar disorder (DeVane, 2003). Tremors associated with valproate resemble benign essential tremors and may respond to a lowering of the dose or the use of delayed release or ER formulations (Zarate *et al.*, 2000).

3.18.3 SEDATION

Sedation (20–25%), dose, and peak serum concentration associated, usually occurs during the initiation of treatment and can be minimized by initiating treatment with lower doses and a more gradual titration, reduction of dose, use of extended or delayed release formulations, or by administering the medication at bedtime (DeVane, 2003).

3.18.4 COGNITIVE IMPAIRMENT

Valproate has minimal negative effects on cognitive functioning and may even improve cognition (DeVane, 2003; Aldenkamp *et al.*, 2000). Open reports findings suggest valproate may slow cognitive decline in patients with dementia, which are intriguing in light of the indirect but strong evidence for neuroprotective effects of valproate

(Tariot, Schneider, and Mintzer, 2001). A multicenter, 20-week, randomized, observer-blinded, parallel group trial showed that addition of valproate (target dose 1800 mg/day) to carbamazepine, led to improvement on a test measuring short-term verbal memory (Aldenkamp et al., 2000). Several studies have shown that valproate does not negatively impact motor speed and coordination, memory, concentration, and mental flexibility (Prevey et al., 1996; Craig, 1994).

3.18.5   PANCREATITIS

In 34 clinical trials involving 3007 patients, only two cases of pancreatitis (0.07%), both nonfatal, were thought to be related to valproate (Bowden, 2003). In studies of patients with migraine, the rates of elevation of amylase were similar between the valproate and the placebo groups (5.9 and 6.1%) (Pellock, 2002). Since pancreatitis is an infrequent and idiosyncratic adverse effect of valproate, monitoring amylase levels will provide little benefit in predicting pancreatitis.

3.18.6   HEMATOLOGICAL

Hematological adverse effects, most commonly manifested as leukopenia (0.4%) and thrombocytopenia (1–32%), are a direct function of serum valproate concentration, usually emerging at concentrations ≥ 100 μg/ml (Bowden, 2003). Thrombocytopenia associated with valproate is usually mild and rarely associated with bleeding complications (Acharya and Bussel, 1996) and can be reversed with dose reduction. As higher serum levels are more likely to cause thrombocytopenia, platelet counts should be monitored following dose escalation (Acharya and Bussel, 1996).

3.18.7   ALOPECIA

Chelation of essential trace elements such as selenium and zinc and its effect on HDAC are postulated as the etiology for hair loss associated with valproate. Reducing the dose of valproate may prove beneficial in reducing the risk of this side effect. Use of vitamin preparations containing zinc, selenium, folate, and biotin may also help reverse this adverse event. Care should be taken to space the administration of valproate and the vitamin preparations to avoid chelating of these elements by valproate (Bowden, 2003; Hurd et al., 1984).

3.18.8   HEPATOTOXICITY

The overall risk of hepatotoxicity associated with valproate is 1/20 000 but may be as high as 1/600–800 in patients younger than two years receiving concomitant anticonvulsants given the relative immaturity of their hepatic system (Perucca, 2002). In two long term studies in bipolar disorder (Bowden *et al.*, 2000; Tohen, Ketter, and Zarate, 2003) no hepatotoxicity was reported with valproate. In fact, hepatic function measures tended to improve with long term valproate treatment.(Bowden *et al.*, 2000) Taken in the aggregate, the risk of hepatoxicity from valproate appears to be real, but limited to infants with immature hepatic systems exposed to treatment with concurrent anticovulsants. Such age groups are potentially candidates for treatment with valproate for epilepsy, but not for treatment for bipolar disorder.

3.18.9   BIRTH DEFECTS

Valproate is associated with an increased incidence of birth defects, including neural tube defects, craniofacial anomalies, limb abnormalities, and cardiovascular anomalies, if exposure to valproate occurs in the first 10 weeks of gestation (RR 4.9, 95% CI:1.4–67.3) (Samren *et al.*, 1997; Kinrys *et al.*, 2003). Neural tube defects, the most serious of the congenital anomalies occur in 1–4% of infants with exposure to valproate (Bowden, 2003). Exposure to valproate during the first trimester, prior to the closure of the neural tube, leads to spina bifida in 1–2% of infants, a rate 10–20 times greater than in the general population. The risk of malformations is increased with higher dosage and serum levels, concomitant use of other anticonvulsants, and may possibly be decreased with supplemental folic acid (Bowden, 2003).

3.18.10   WEIGHT GAIN

Valproate use is associated with weight gain ranging from 3 to 24 pounds in 3–20% of patients treated over 3–12 months (Bowden, 2003). Weight gain is more likely to occur at valproate serum levels greater than 125 μg/ml (Bowden, 2003). Hence, maintaining the dosage and serum level at the lowest effective level may help mitigate the effect of valproate on weight gain.

3.18.11   LIPID PROFILE

Studies have shown that valproate does not cause elevation of lipids (Tohen *et al.*, 1995; Geda, Caske, and Icagasioglu, 2002; Demirocioglu, Soylu, and Dirik, 2000). Additionally, several studies designed to provide more reliable assessments of lipid and glucose metabolism indicate that valproate is associated with reductions in total cholesterol, low-density lipoprotein (LDL) and high-density lipoprotein (HDL) cholesterol levels and protects against the adverse effects of some antipsychotic drugs on lipid profile (Bowden *et al.*, 2000, 2006; Tohen, Ketter, and Zarate, 2003; Zajecka *et al.*, 2002; Casey *et al.*, 2003).

3.18.12   POLYCYSTIC OVARIAN SYNDROME (PCOS)

Polycystic Ovarian Syndrome (PCOS), the leading cause of anovulatory infertility in women, occurs in 4–12% of women (Geddes *et al.*, 2010; Dunaif and Thomas, 2001). Menstrual disturbance is more commonly seen in bipolar patients than in the general population irrespective of the medication used, probably due to a dysfunction of the hypothalamic-pituitary-gonadal axis in this group of patients (Rasgon *et al.*, 2000). Valproate, as a component of treatment regimens prior to entry into the National Institute of Mental Health Systematic Treatment Enhancement Program for Bipolar Disorder (STEP-BD) program, was associated with new-onset menstrual cycle irregularities and hyperandrogenism in 10.5% of women (Joffe *et al.*, 2006). Findings from this study are limited by the cross sectional, retrospective design of the study. In a follow-up study of 14 women with PCOS, PCOS reproductive features remitted in three put of four women who discontinued and persisted in three patients who continued treatment with valproate (Joffe *et al.*, 2006). No changes in polycystic ovarian morphology were associated with valproate in either study.

High frequency of menstrual dysfunction was observed in women with bipolar disorder who were treated with lithium, valproate, or carbamazepine exclusive of the medication. Ultrasound identified an increased number of ovarian follicles in one of the lithium-treated patients but no increase in any valproate-treated patient. Hormonal assessment of estrone, luteinizing hormone, follicle-stimulating hormone, testosterone, and dehydroepiandrosterone (DHEA) yielded no abnormal values in any patient (Rasgon *et al.*, 2000).

3.19   SUMMARY

Valproate has established a broad and fundamental role for itself in the acute and prophylactic treatment of bipolar disorder throughout the world due to its generally good tolerability and broad spectrum of efficacy. However, some side effects, particularly weight gain, limit effectiveness in long term management. Valproate, as well as other agents employed in the treatment of bipolar disorder, is increasingly used in some form of combination therapy. Recent studies consistently support the safety, efficacy, and generally good tolerability of valproate in combination with the following drugs: lithium, olanzapine, risperidone, quetiapine, haloperidol, ziprasidone and, most recently, lamotrigine. Valproate, as is the case with an increasing proportion of primary medications utilized in treatment of bipolar disorder, is no longer patent protected. Therefore, the likelihood of future large scale studies to advance or keep up to date clinical knowledge about the drug is much diminished. Practicing psychiatrists and other physicians and prescribers of such medications will therefore do well to seek updated review articles on individual drugs, drug classes, and treatment guideline updates to incorporate into their knowledge base and pharmaceutical management.

The exciting recent development of evidence for overlapping intracellular neuronal signaling system effects of valproate and lithium, may lead both to improved understanding of the biochemical pathophysiology of the disorder, as well as clarification of the mechanisms of both valproate and lithium, and also provide insights into the development of additional treatments for bipolar disorders.

References

Acharya, S., Bussel, J.B. (1996) Hematologic toxicity of sodium valproate. *J. Pediatr. Neurol.*, **14**, 303–307.

Aldenkamp, A.P., Baker, G., Mulder, O.G. *et al.* (2000) A multicenter, randomized clinical study to evaluate the effect on cognitive function of topiramate compared with valproate as add-on therapy to carbamazepine in patients with partial-onset seizures. *Epilepsia*, **41** (9), 1167–1178.

Allen, M.H., Hirschfeld, R.M., Wozniak, P.J. *et al.* (2006) Linear relationship of valproate serum concentration to response and optimal serum levels for acute mania. *Am. J. Psychiatry*, **163** (2), 272–275.

Bocci, U. and Beretta, G. (1976) Esperienze sugli alcoolisti e tossicomania con dipropilacetate di sodio. *Lav. Neuropsichiatr.*, **58**, 51–61.

Bowden, C.L. (2003) Valproate. *Bipolar Disord.*, **5**, 189–202.

Bowden, C.L. (2004) The effectiveness of divalproate in all forms of mania and the broader bipolar spectrum: many questions, few answers. *J. Affect. Disord.*, **79**, S9–S14.

Bowden, C.L., Brugger, A.M., Swann, A.C. *et al.* (1994) Efficacy of divalproex vs lithium and placebo in the treatment of mania. *J. Am. Assoc.*, **271**, 918–924.

Bowden, C.L., Calabrese, J.R., McElroy, S.L. *et al.* (2000) A randomized, placebo-controlled 12-month trial of divalproex and lithium in treatment of outpatients with bipolar I disorder. *Arch. Gen. Psychiatry*, **57**, 481–489.

Bowden, C.L., Calabrese, J.R., Swann, A.C. *et al.* (2006) Divalproex sodium extended-release versus placebo in the treatment of acute mania. Presented at the Annual Meeting of the American Psychiatric Association in Toronto, Canada, May, 22, 2006.

Bowden, C.L., Janicak, P.G., Orsulak, P. *et al.* (1996) Relation of serum valproate concentration to response in mania. *Am. J. Psychiatry*, **153**, 765–770.

Bowden, C.L. and McElroy, S.L. (1995) History of the development of valproate for treatment of bipolar disorder. *J. Clin. Psychiatry*, **56** (S3), 3–5.

Brady, K.T., Myrick, H., Henderson, S. *et al.* (2002) The use of divalproex in alcohol relapse prevention: a pilot study. *Drug Alcohol Depend.*, **67** (3), 323–330.

Calabrese, J.R. and Shelton, M.D. (2002) Long term treatment of bipolar disorder with lamotrigine. *J. Clin. Psychiatry*, **63** (S10), 18–22.

Calabrese, J.R., Shelton, M.D., Rapport, D.J. *et al.* (2005) A 20-month, double-blind, maintenance trial of lithium versus divalproex in rapid-cycling bipolar disorder. *Am. J. Psychiatry*, **162** (11), 2152–2161.

Casey, D.E., Daniel, D.G., Wassef, A.A. *et al.* (2003) Effect of divalproex combined wth olanzapine or risperidone in patients with an acute exacerbation of schizophrenia. *Neuropsychopharm*, **28**, 182–192.

Craig, I. and Tallis, R. (1994) Impact of valproate and phenytoin on cognitive function in elderly patients: results of a single-blind randomized comparative study. *Epilepsia*, **35** (2), 381–390.

Davis, L.L., Bartolucci, A., and Petty, F. (2005) Divalproex in the treatment of bipolar depression: a placebo-controlled study. *J. Affect. Disord.*, **85** (3), 259–266.

DelBello, M.P., Kowatch, R.A., Adler, C.M. *et al.* (2006) A double-blind randomized pilot study comparing quetiapine and divalproex for adolescent mania. *J. Am. Acad. Child. Adolesc. Psychiatry*, **45** (3), 305–313.

Demirocioglu, S., Soylu, A., and Dirik, E. (2000) Carbamazepine and valproic acid: effects on serum lipids and liver function tests. *Pediatr. Neurol.*, **23** (2), 142–146.

DeVane, C.L. (2003) Pharmacokinetics, drug interactions, and tolerability of valproate. *Psychopharm. Bull.*, **37** (S2), 25–42.

Dokucu, M.E., Yu, L., and Taghert, P.H. (2005) Lithium- and valproate-induced alterations in circadian locomotor behavior in Drosophila. *Neuropsychopharmacology*, **30** (12), 2216–2224.

Dunaif, A. and Thomas, A. (2001) Current concepts in the polycystic ovary syndrome. *Ann. Rev. Med.*, **52**, 401–419.

Einat, H., Yuan, P., Gould, T.D. *et al.* (2003) The role of the extracellular signal-regulated kinase signaling pathway in mood modulation. *J. Neurosci.*, **23** (19), 7311–7316.

Emirch, H.M., Dose, M., and von Zerssen, D. (1985) The use of sodium valproate, carbamazepine and oxcarbazepine in patients with affective disorders. *J. Affect. Disord.*, **8** (3), 243–250.

Fariello, R. and Smith, M.C. (1989) *Valproate: Mechanisms of Action, in Antiepileptic Drugs*, 3rd edn, vol. 3, Raven, New York, pp. 567–575.

Findling, R.L., McNamara, N.K., Youngstrom, E.A. *et al.* (2005) Double-blind 18-month trial of lithium versus divalproex maintenance treatment in pediatric bipolar disorder. *J. Am. Acad. Child Adolesc. Psychiatry*, **44** (5), 409–417.

Frankenburg, F.R. and Zanarini, M.C. (2002) Divalproex sodium treatment of women with borderline personality disorder and bipolar II disorder: a double-blind placebo-controlled pilot study. *J. Clin. Psychiatry*, **63** (5), 442–446.

Freeman, T.W., Clothier, J.L., Pazzaglia, P. *et al.* (1992) A double-blind comparison of valproate and lithium in the treatment of acute mania. *Am. J. Psychiatry*, **149**, 108–111.

Geda, G., Casken, H., and Icagasioglu, D. (2002) Serum Lipids, vit B-12 and folic acid levels in children receiving long term valproate therapy. *Acta Neurol. Belg.*, **102** (3), 122–126.

Geddes, J.R., Goodwin, G.M., Rendell, J. *et al.* (2010) Lithium plus valproate combination therapy versus monotherapy for relapse prevention in bipolar I disorder (BALANCE): a randomized open-label trial. *Lancet*, **375** (9712), 385–395.

Ghaemi, N.S., Gilmer, W.S., and Goldberg, J.F. (2007) Divalproex in the treatment of acute bipolar depression: A preliminary double-blind, randomized, placebo-controlled pilot study. *J. Clin. Psychiatr.*, **68** (12), 1839–1840.

Gould, T.D. and Manji, H.K. (2002) The Wnt signaling pathway in bipolar disorder. *Neuroscientist*, **8** (5), 497–511.

Gray, N.A., Zhou, R., Du, J. *et al.* (2003) The use of mood stabilizers as plasticity enhancers in the treatment of neuropsychiatric disorders. *J. Clin. Psychiatry*, **64S** (5), 3–17.

Grunze, H., Erfurth, A., Amann, B. *et al.* (1999) Intravenous valproate loading in acutely manic and depressed bipolar I patients. *Clin. Psychopharmacol.*, **19** (4), 303–309.

Gyulai, L., Bowden, C.L., McElroy, S.L. *et al.* (2003) Maintenance efficacy of divalproex in the prevention of bipolar depression. *Neuropsychopharmacology*, **28** (7), 1374–1382.

Harwood, A.J. and Agam, G. (2003) Search for a common mechanism of mood stabilizers. *Biochem. Pharmacol.*, **66** (2), 179–189.

Hasegawa, H., Osada, K., Misonoo, A. *et al.* (2003) Chronic carbamazepine treatment increases myristoylated alanine-rich C kinase substrate phosphorylation in the rat cerebral cortex via down-regulation of calcineurin A alpha. *Brain Res.*, **994** (1), 19–26.

Hirschfeld, R.M., Allen, M.H., McEvoy, J.P. *et al.* (1999) Safety and tolerability of oral loading divalproex sodium in acutely manic bipolar patients. *J. Clin. Psychiatry*, **60** (12), 815–818.

Horne, R.L. and Cunenan, C. (2003) Safety and efficacy of switching psychiatric patients from a delayed-release to an extended-release formulation of divalproex sodium. *Clin. Psychopharmacol.*, **23** (2), 176–181.

Hurd, R.W., Van Rinsvelt, H.A., Wilder, B.J. *et al.* (1984) Selenium, zinc, and copper changes with valproic acid: possible relation to drug side effects. *Neurology*, **34** (10), 1393–1395.

Jacobsen, F.M. (1993) Low dose valproate: a new treatment for cyclothymia, mild rapid cycling disorders, and premenstrual syndrome. *J. Clin. Psychiatry*, **54**, 229–234.

Joffe, H., Cohen, L.S., Suppes, T. *et al.* (2006) Valproate is associated with new-onset oligoamenorrhea with hyperandrogenism in women with bipolar disorder. *Biol. Psychiatry*, **59** (11), 1078–1086.

Keck, P.E. Jr., McElroy, S.L., Tugrul, K.C. *et al.* (1993) Valproate oral loading in the treatment of acute mania. *J. Clin. Psychiatry*, **54** (8), 305–308.

Kinrys, G., Pollack, M.H., Simon, N.M. *et al.* (2003) Valproic acid for the treatment of social anxiety disorder. *Int. Clin. Psychopharmacol.*, **18** (3), 169–172.

Kowatch, R.A., Suppes, T., Carmody, T.J. *et al.* (2000) Effect size of lithium, divalproex sodium, and carbamazepine in children and adolescents with bipolar disorder. *J. Am. Acad. Child Adolesc. Psychiatry*, **39** (6), 713–720.

Lambert, P.A., Cavaz, G., Borselli, S. *et al.* (1966) Action neuropsychotrope d'un nouvel antiepileptique: le depamide. *Ann. Med. Psychol.*, **1**, 707–710.

Leng, Y., Liang, M.H., Marinova, Z. *et al.* (2008) Synergistic neuroprotective effects of lithium and valproic acid or other histone deacetylase inhibitors in neurons: roles of glycogen synthesis kinase-3 inhibition. *J. Neurosci.*, **28** (5), 2576–2588.

Levy, R.H., Mattson, R.H., Meldrum, B.S. *et al.* (2002) *Antiepileptic Drugs*, 5th edn, Lippincott Williams & Wilkins, New York.

Longo, L.P., Campbell, T., and Hubatch, S. (2002) Divalproex sodium (Depakote) for alcohol withdrawal and relapse prevention. *J. Addict. Dis.*, **21** (2), 55–64.

Macritchie, K.A., Geddes, J.R., Scott, J. *et al.* (2000) Valproic acid, valproate and divalproex in the maintenance treatment of bipolar disorder. *Psychiatr. Serv.*, **51** (9), 1179–1181.

Marinova, Z., Ren, M., Wendland, J.R. *et al.* (2009) Valproic acid induces functional heat-shock protein 70 via Class I histone deacetylase inhibition in cortical neurons: a potential role of Sp1 acetylation. *J. Neurochem.*, **111** (4), 976–987.

McElroy, S.L., Bowden, C.L., Collins, M.A. *et al.* (2008) Relationship of open acute mania treatment to blinded maintenance outcome in bipolar I disorder. *J. Affect. Disord.*, **107** (4), 127–133.

McElroy, S.L., Keck, P.E., Stanton, S.P. *et al.* (1996) A randomized comparison of divalproex oral loading versus haloperidol in the initial treatment of acute psychotic mania. *J. Clin. Psychiatry*, **57**, 142–146.

McElroy, S.L., Keck, P.E., Tugrul, K.C. *et al.* (1993) Valproate as a loading treatment in acute mania. *Neuropsychobiology*, **27**, 146–149.

Meunier, H., Carraz, G., Meunier, V. *et al.* (1975) Proprietes pharmacodynamiques de l'acide n-propylacetique. *Therapie*, **18**, 435–438.

Muller-Oerlinghausen, B., Retzow, A., and Henn, F.A. (2000) Valproate as an adjunct to neuroleptic medication for the treatment of acute episodes of mania: a prospective, randomized, double-blind, placebo-controlled, multicenter study. *J. Clin. Psychopharmacol.*, **20** (2), 195–203.

Muzina, D., Ganocy, S., and Khalife, S. (2008) A double-blind, placebo-controlled study of Divalproex extended-release in newly diagnosed mood stabilizer naive patients with acute bipolar I or II depression. Presented at the 48th NCDEU Meeting: New Approaches for Mental Health Interventions, Phoenix, AZ.

Oluboka, O.J., Bird, D.C., Kutcher, S. *et al.* (2002) A pilot study of loading versus titration of valproate in the treatment of acute mania. *Bipolar Disord.*, **4** (5), 341–345.

Pavuluri, M.N., Henry, D.B., Carbray, J.A. *et al.* (2005) Divalproex sodium for pediatric mixed mania: a 6-month prospective trial. *Bipolar Disord.*, **7** (3), 266–273.

Pellock, J.M. (2002) Treatment considerations: traditional antiepileptic drugs. *Epilepsy Behav.*, **2** (6S1), 18–23.

Penry, J.K. and Dean, J.C. (1989) The scope and use of valproate in epilepsy. *J. Clin. Psychiatry*, **40**, 17S–22S.

Perucca, E. (2002) Pharmacological and therapeutic properties of valproate: a summary after 35 years of clinical experience. *CNS Drugs*, **16** (10), 695–714.

Pope, H.G. Jr., McElroy, S.L., Keck, P.E. Jr. *et al.* (1991) Valproate in the treatment of acute mania: a placebo-controlled study. *Arch. Gen. Psychiatry*, **48**, 62–68.

Prevey, M.L., Cattanach, L., Collins, J.F. *et al.*, The Department of Veterans Affairs Epilepsy Cooperative Study 264 Group (1996) Effect of valproate on cognitive functioning. Comparison with carbamazepine. *Arch. Neurol.*, **53** (10), 1008–1016.

Rasgon, N.L., Altshuler, L.L., Gudeman, D. *et al.* (2000) Medication status and polycystic ovary syndrome in women with bipolar disorder: a preliminary report. *J. Clin. Psychiatry*, **61** (3), 173–178.

Reoux, J.P., Saxon, A.J., Malte, C.A. *et al.* (2001) Divalproex sodium in alcohol withdrawal: a randomized double-blind placebo-controlled clinical trial. *Alcohol Clin. Exp. Res.*, **25** (9), 1324–1329.

Rimmer, E. and Richens, A. (1985) An update on sodium valproate. *Pharmacotherapy*, **5**, 171–184.

Sachs, G. (2001) Design and promise of multicenter effectiveness trials. 4th International Conference on Bipolar Disorder, Pittsburgh.

Sachs, G.S., Grossman, F., Ghaemi, S.N. *et al.* (2002) Combination of a mood stabilizer with risperidone or haloperidol for treatment of actue mania: a double -blind, placebo-controlled comparison of efficacy and safety. *Am. J. Psychiatry*, **159**, 1146–1154.

Salloum, I.M., Cornelius, J.R., Daley, D.C. *et al.* (2005) Efficacy of valproate maintenance in patients with bipolar disorder and alcoholism: a double-blind placebo-controlled study. *Arch. Gen. Psychiatry*, **62** (1), 37–45.

Samren, E.B., Van Duijn, C.M., Koch, S. *et al.* (1997) Maternal use of antiepileptic drugs and the risk of major congenital malformations: a joint European prospective study of human teratogenesis associated with maternal epilepsy. *Epilepsia*, **38** (9), 981–990.

Schatzberg, A.F. (1998) Bipolar disorder: recent issues in diagnosis and classification. *J. Clin. Psychiatry*, **59** (Suppl. 6), 35–36.

Scheffer, R.E., Kowatch, R.A., Carmody, T. *et al.* (2005) Randomized, placebo-controlled trial of mixed amphetamine salts for symptoms of comorbid ADHD in pediatric bipolar disorder after mood stabilization with divalproex sodium. *Am. J. Psychiatry.*, **162** (1), 58–64.

Smith L.A., Cornelius V.R., Azorin J.M. *et al.* (2010) Valproate for the treatment of acute bipolar depression: Systematic review and meta-analysis. *J. Affect. Disorders*, **122**, 1–9.

Solomon, D.A., Ryan, C.E., Keitner, G.I. *et al.* (1997) A pilot study of lithium carbonate plus divalproex sodium for the continuation and maintenance treatment of patients with bipolar I disorder. *J. Clin. Psychiatry*, **58** (3), 95–99.

Tariot, P.N., Schneider, L.S., and Mintzer, J.E. (2001) Safety and tolerability of divalproex sodium in the treatment of signs and symptoms of mania in elderly patients with dementia: results of a double-blind, placebo-controlled trial. *Curr. Ther. Res.*, **62** (1), 51–67.

Tohen, M., Castillo, J., Baldessarini, R.J. *et al.* (1995) Blood dyscrasias with carbamazepine and valproate: a pharmacoepidemiological study of 2,228 patients at risk. *Am. J. Psychiatry*, **152** (3), 413–418.

Tohen, M., Chengappa, K.N.R., Suppes, T. *et al.* (2002) Efficacy of olanzapine in combination with valproate or lithium in the treatment of mania in patients partially nonresponsive to valproate or lithium monotherapy. *Arch. Gen. Psychiatry*, **59**, 62–69.

Tohen, M., Ketter, T.A., and Zarate, C.A. (2003) Olanzapine versus divalproex sodium for the treatment of acute mania and maintenance of remission: a 47-week study. *Am. J. Psychiatry*, **160**, 1263–1271.

Vasudev, K., Goswami, U., and Kohli, K. (2000) Carbamazepine and valproate monotherapy: feasibility, relative safety and efficacy, and therapeutic drug monitoring in manic disorder. *Psychopharmacology*, **150**, 15–23.

Wagner, K.D., Redden, L., Kowatch, R.A. *et al.* (2009) A double-blind, randomized, placebo-controlled trial of divalproex extended-release in the treatment of bipolar disorder in children and adolescents. *J. Am. Acad. Child Adolesc. Psychiatry*, **48** (5), 519–532.

Watson, D.G., Watterson, J.M., and Lenox, R.H. (1998) Sodium valproate down-regulates the myristoylated alanine-rich C kinase substrate (MARCKS) in immortalized hippocampal cells: a property of protein kinase C-mediated mood stabilizers. *J. Pharmacol. Exp. Ther.*, **285** (1), 307–316.

Watterson, J.M., Watson, D.G., Meyer, E.M. *et al.* (2002) A role for protein kinase C and its substrates in the action of valproic acid in the brain: implications for neural plasticity. *Brain Res.*, **934** (1), 69–80.

Wilder, B.J. (1992) Pharmacokinetics of valproate and carbamazepine. *J. Clin. Psychopharmacol.*, **12**, 64S–68S.

Wu, X., Chen, P.S., Dallas, S. *et al.* (2008) Histone deacetylase inhibitors up-regulate astrocyte GDNF and BDNF gene transcription and protect dopaminergic neurons. *Int. J. Neuropsychopharmacol.*, **11** (8), 1123–1134.

Yasuda, S., Liang, M.H., Marinova, Z. *et al.* (2009) The mood stabilizers lithium and valproate selectively activate the promoter IV of brain-derived neurotrophic factor in neurons. *Mol. Psychiatry*, **14** (1), 51–59.

Yatham, L.N. (2005) Atypical antipsychotics for bipolar disorder. *Psychiatr. Clin. North Am.*, **28** (2), 325–347.

Yatham, L.N., Davis, K.H., Khan, A. *et al.* (2003) Effect of lamotrigine on neurocognitive measures in patients with bipolar I disorder. *J. Eur. Coll. Neuropsychopharmacol.*, **13** (S4), S227.

Yuan, P.X., Huang, L.D., Jiang, Y.M. *et al.* (2001) The mood stabilizer valproic acid activates mitogen-activated protein kinases and promotes neurite growth. *J. Biol. Chem.*, **276** (34), 31674–31683.

Zajecka, J., Weisler, R., Sachs, G. *et al.* (2002) A comparison of the efficacy, safety and tolerability of divalproex sodium and olanzapine in the treatment of bipolar disorder. *J. Clin. Psychiatry*, **63**, 1148–1155.

Zarate, C.A. Jr., Tohen, M., Narendran, R. *et al.* (2000) The adverse effect profile and efficacy of divalproex sodium compared with valproic acid: a pharmacoepidemiology study. *J. Clin. Psychiatry*, **60** (4), 232–236.

4

Pharmacological Profile and Clinical Utility of Lamotrigine in Mood Disorders

Marc L.M. van der Loos[1], Joseph R. Calabrese[2], Willem A. Nolen[3] and David J. Muzina[4]

[1]Department of Psychiatry, Isala Klinieken, Zwolle, The Netherlands
[2]School of Medicine, Case Western Reserve University and University Hospitals of Cleveland, OH, USA
[3]Department of Psychiatry, University Medical Center Groningen, University of Groningen, The Netherlands
[4]Department of Psychiatry and Psychology, Cleveland Clinic Foundation, OH, USA

4.1 INTRODUCTION

There remains a pressing need for additional treatment options for mood disorders, particularly those refractory or difficult to treat disorders such as bipolar disorder. Estimates of the prevalence of bipolar I disorder across diverse cultures and ethnic groups are consistent, ranging between 0.4 and 1.6% in adults (Weissman *et al.*, 1996; Regeer *et al.*, 2004). Recent estimates of the overall prevalence of bipolar disorder (types I and II as well as NOS) suggest that 4–5% suffers from this debilitating mental disorder (Hirschfeld *et al.*, 2003; Regeer *et al.*, 2004). Bipolar disorders carry a high burden, negatively affecting lives in many areas, most notably the performance of work-related, leisure, and interpersonal activities (Calabrese *et al.*, 2003b). The greatest need exists in the treatment of depressive episodes associated with bipolar disorders as symptoms of depression are much more commonly experienced and more difficult to treat than manic symptoms (Post, Denicoff, and Leverich, 2002; Judd *et al.*, 2002; Kupka *et al.*, 2005).

Reports of lamotrigine's beneficial effects on mood in epilepsy patients led to its use and study in affective disorders. Studies involving bipolar patients suggested that lamotrigine possessed a broad spectrum of therapeutic activity in bipolar disorder, with later descriptions of greater efficacy for depressive than for manic symptoms. Given the significant burden, prevalence, and recurrent nature of bipolar disorder – especially

Bipolar Psychopharmacotherapy: Caring for the patient, Second Edition. Edited by Hagop S. Akiskal and Mauricio Tohen.
© 2011 John Wiley & Sons, Ltd. Published 2011 by John Wiley & Sons, Ltd.

bipolar depression – lamotrigine appears to begin to address an area of serious unmet public health need (Calabrese *et al.*, 2003b).

4.2 CLINICAL PHARMACOLOGY OF LAMOTRIGINE

4.2.1 PHARMACODYNAMICS

Lamotrigine is an antiepileptic drug of the phenyltriazine class that has demonstrated efficacy as an add-on treatment of partial seizures (Mikati *et al.*, 1989; Matsuo *et al.*, 1993) and as maintenance treatment of bipolar I disorder to delay the time of occurrence of mood episodes (Bowden, 2003; Calabrese *et al.*, 2003a). Although its mechanism of therapeutic action in humans is not definitively understood, lamotrigine is thought to possess modulatory and protective effects on neurotransmission and intracellular signal transduction processes.

Structurally distinct from other antiepileptic drugs, lamotrigine interacts preferentially on the slow inactivated state of presynaptic neuronal sodium and calcium channels to prolong inactivation of the neuron and promote stabilization of the neuronal membrane (Xie and Hagan, 1998). This effect is augmented by a use-dependent action in which further inhibition by the drug develops during rapid, repetitive stimulation (that is, epileptiform bursts). Consequently, the release of the excitatory amino acid glutamate is antagonized (Fitton and Goa, 1995; Li, Ketter, and Frye, 2002). Lamotrigine has also been observed to inhibit cortical and amygdaloid kindling (Gilman, 1995; Leach, Marden, and Miller, 1986; Xie *et al.*, 1995).

Lamotrigine has no substantial *in vitro* affinity for adenosine, adrenergic, dopaminergic, muscarinic, and opioid receptors at clinically applicable concentrations and binds only weakly to inhibit serotonin 5HT3 receptors (Leach, Baxter, and Critchley, 1991). Lamotrigine lacks clinically meaningful activity at the 5HT1A receptor, where changes in 5HT1A receptor-mediated cyclic adenosine monophosphate pathway have been implicated in affective disorders (Shiah *et al.*, 1998; Vinod and Subhash, 2002).

In early epilepsy studies with lamotrigine it was noted that many patients reported improvement in mood and psychological well-being independent from reduction in seizure frequency, which led to its investigation for use in affective disorders (Smith *et al.*, 1993a, 1993b). Significantly, lamotrigine has minimal negative effects on cognitive, memory, or psychomotor function and is not associated with sedative effects or weight gain (Goa, Ross, and Chrisp, 1993, Cohen *et al.*, 1985; Ginsberg, Sachs, and Ketter, 2003).

4.2.2 PHARMACOKINETICS

Lamotrigine is extensively absorbed demonstrating linear kinetics, resulting in 98% bioavailability (Garnett, 1997). Peak plasma concentrations are attained after 1–3 hours with mean plasma protein binding of 55–68% (Cohen *et al.*, 1987, Ramsay *et al.*, 1991; Rambeck and Wolf, 1993). Lamotrigine readily crosses the placental barrier causing fetal blood concentrations similar to maternal levels and passes into breast milk reaching

40–80% of the maternal lamotrigine concentration (Ohman, Vitols, and Tomson, 2000; Pennell, 2003).

The rate-limiting step in the elimination of lamotrigine is N-glucoronidation by the liver with a plasma elimination half-life of 25 ± 10 hours (Cohen *et al.*, 1987). Autoinduction of its own metabolism does not occur and there are no active metabolites. Pregnancy increases lamotrigine clearance by more than 50% early during pregnancy and reverts quickly after delivery (Tran *et al.*, 2002). Clearance may be reduced in the elderly and in patients with moderate to severe hepatic dysfunction.

4.2.3 DRUG INTERACTIONS

Lamotrigine administration hardly affects the serum concentrations of other drugs. However, enzyme-inhibiting drugs such as divalproex sodium increase lamotrigine concentrations by significantly competing for metabolism through glucoronidation effectively increasing the mean half-life of lamotrigine to about 70 hours (Yuen *et al.*, 1992; Anderson *et al.*, 1996). Enzyme-inducing drugs, such as phenytoin, carbamazepine, and phenobarbital, reduce the lamotrigine's mean elimination half-life to about 12 hours and decrease lamotrigine concentrations (Hachad, Ragueneau-Majlessi, and Levy, 2002). There are pharmacokinetic interactions between lamotrigine and anti-conceptive medication (Sidhu *et al.*, 2006). The clearance of levonogestrel is increased with a possible decrease of the anti-conceptive reliability (Sidhu *et al.*, 2006). On the other hand is the clearance of lamotrigine enhanced by anti-conceptive medication, with a lowering of lamotrigine plasma levels (Sidhu *et al.*, 2006).

Lamotrigine does not significantly affect the pharmacokinetics of lithium (Chen, Veronese, and Yin, 2000). Table 4.1 summarizes lamotrigine drug interaction information.

4.3 LAMOTRIGINE AND MOOD DISORDERS

The observations of Smith and Colleagues (1993a, 1993b) that patients treated with add-on lamotrigine for partial seizures experienced improved mood apart from effects on epilepsy stimulated investigations of lamotrigine's efficacy to treat mood disorders.

Table 4.1 Lamotrigine drug interactions.

Lamotrigine has no known effects on levels of:	Lithium Carbamazepine Divalproex	Phenytoin Phenobarbital Mesuximide	Antidepressants Benzodiazepines Antipsychotics
Increased levels of lamotrigine caused by: (estimated % increase LTG)	**Divalproex/valproate** (~100%)		
Decreased levels of lamotrigine caused by: (estimated % decrease LTG)	**Carbamazepine** (40%) **Phenytoin** (50%)	**Phenobarbital** (40%) Oxcarbazepine (30%)	

Bold indicates interaction with clinically significant importance.

Early case reports involving bipolar patients suggested that lamotrigine possessed a broad spectrum of therapeutic activity in bipolar disorder, including rapid cycling and mixed states (Weisler *et al.*, 1994; Calabrese, Fatemi, and Woyshville, 1996; Walden *et al.*, 1996). A subsequent open-label study provided preliminary data that lamotrigine was effective for patients with refractory bipolar disorder, with 68% of depressed patients and 84% of manic/hypomanic/mixed patients showing moderate to marked response (Calabrese *et al.*, 1999a).

4.3.1 ACUTE MOOD DISTURBANCES

4.3.1.1 Bipolar Depression

An open naturalistic study of 22 depressed bipolar patients who were refractory to treatment with a combination of divalproex sodium and another mood stabilizer or divalproex sodium and an antidepressant for six weeks were treated with add-on lamotrigine. Sixteen out of 22 (72%) responded by the end of week 4, suggesting that lamotrigine may be useful in bipolar depression (Kusumakar and Yatham, 1997). In a double-blind placebo-controlled study of lamotrigine monotherapy in outpatients with non rapid-cycling bipolar I depression, treatment with lamotrigine over seven weeks (50 or 200 mg/day) did not result in a significant difference versus placebo on the primary outcome measure (HAM-D), but did so on all several secondary outcome measures including the MADRS, particularly in the 200 mg group, compared with placebo (Calabrese *et al.*, 1999b). Improvements were observed as early as week 3. Figure 4.1 demonstrates the percentage of patients showing a response to treatment at endpoint.

After this first positive result for lamotrigine in a RCT, lamotrigine was tested against placebo in four other RCTs (Calabrese *et al.*, 2007; Goldsmith *et al.*, 2003). None of

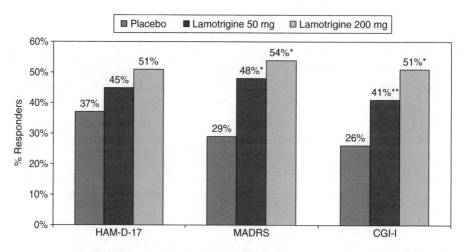

Figure 4.1 Lamotrigine vs placebo in bipolar 1 depression. *P < 0.05 vs placebo; **P < 0.1 placebo.

Calabrese, *J. Clin. Psychiarty.*, 1999; **60**: 79–88.

these RCTs discriminated significantly between lamotrigine and placebo on the primary outcome criteria. Part of this negative result was because of a high placebo response in all four studies. Nevertheless, a meta-analysis of all five studies showed a significant although modest benefit for lamotrigine (Geddes, Calabrese, and Goodwin, 2009).

Thirty-one patients with refractory bipolar and unipolar mood disorders participated in a double-blind, randomized, crossover study of three six-week monotherapy evaluations including lamotrigine, gabapentin, and placebo. Using the Clinical Global Impressions Scale for Bipolar Illness (CGI-BP) as the primary outcome variable, this study reported a 52% response rate (CGI-BP as much or very much improved) for lamotrigine, compared to 26% for gabapentin and 23% for placebo-treated patients (Frye *et al.*, 2000).

In a recent double-blind placebo-controlled study lamotrigine was tested as an adjunct to lithium during breakthrough depression. One hundred and twenty four bipolar I or II patients all on lithium (lithium serum levels 0.6–1.0 mmol/l) were randomized to addition of lamotrigine (up-titrated from 25 to 200 mg/day in six weeks) or placebo. During the study lithium serum levels were kept stable. After eight weeks the difference between lamotrigine addition to lithium and placebo addition to lithium on the change of MADRS score (primary outcome criterion) was significant (15.38 vs. 11.03 respectively, $p = 0.024$) (Figure 4.2). Also response according to a decrease of the MADRS >50% was significant (Van der Loos *et al.*, 2009). As a second step in this study paroxetine (open label 20 mg fixed dose) was added for another eight weeks in nonresponders to addition of lamotrigine or placebo. Lithium dosage and blind lamotrigine or placebo remained unaltered. Although the patients in the lithium-lamotrigine group (with or without paroxetine addition in nonresponders after eight weeks) improved further, the improvement in the lithium-placebo (with or without paroxetine addition in nonresponders after eight weeks) was even greater, resulting in a nonsignificant difference between both groups

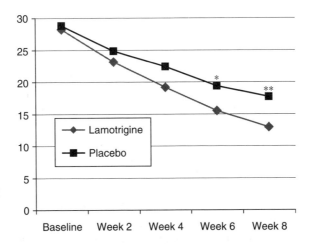

Figure 4.2 MADRS scores during eight weeks of treatment (MMRM). Lamotrigine versus Placebo. *p = 0.031, **P = 0.006.

Van der Loos, M.L. (2009) *J. Clin Psychiatry*, **70**, 223–231.

after 16 weeks (Van der Loos *et al.*, 2010). This study not only represents the first unequivocally positive double-blind, placebo controlled study of lamotrigine when used adjunctively, but was also the first time a large-scale double-blind, placebo controlled adjunctive bipolar depression study design has been successfully executed.

The final study (n = 410) compared lamotrigine (dose uptitrated to 200 mg/day) with olanzapine/fluoxetine (dose 6/25, 6/50, 12/25, or 12/50 mg/day) (Brown *et al.*, 2006) and showed a small but significant advantage (improvement on the MADRS after seven weeks of 14.91 vs 12.92 respectively p = 0.002) for the olanzapine/fluoxetine combination.

4.3.1.2 Unipolar Depression

A placebo-controlled, double-blind study of lamotrigine as adjunct to paroxetine in acute depression (unipolar) did not find a significant difference in HAM-D total score at the endpoint of the study for the paroxetine plus lamotrigine group when compared with paroxetine alone (Normann *et al.*, 2002). However, lamotrigine appeared to accelerate the onset of action of the antidepressant and improved core depressive symptoms as reflected by HAM-D items 1 (depressed mood), 2 (guilt feelings), and 7 (work and interest) and the CGI-Severity of Illness scale (p < 0.0001). Lamotrigine-treated patients had fewer days on treatment with benzodiazepines and fewer withdrawals for treatment failure.

A double-blind, randomized, placebo-controlled trial of augmentation with lamotrigine or placebo in patients concomitantly treated with fluoxetine for resistant major depressive episodes produced mixed results concerning lamotrigine's antidepressant efficacy (Barbosa, Berk, and Vorster, 2003). Twenty-three patients with a resistant major depressive episode (unipolar N = 15, bipolar II N = 8) were treated with fluoxetine 20 mg/day and concomitantly randomly assigned to receive either lamotrigine (N = 13) or placebo (N = 10) over six weeks. Lamotrigine was initiated at 25 mg/day and titrated to 100 mg/day. Although lamotrigine was statistically superior to placebo on the Clinical Global Impressions scale at endpoint (absolute score and responder analysis) for both unipolar and bipolar II patients, it failed to separate statistically from placebo on the Hamilton Rating Scale for Depression and Montgomery-Asberg Depression Rating Scale. The authors suggested that this negative study may have been the result of artifact from the small sample size used and the limited power of the study. The brief duration of the study (six weeks), the need to titrate lamotrigine slowly to minimize rash risk, and the use of relatively low dose lamotrigine (maximum of 100 mg/day) also contributed to the observed findings.

4.3.1.3 Mania/Mixed States

The 1999 open-label study by Calabrese and colleagues observed a robust response to lamotrigine (primarily as add-on therapy) in 84% of manic/hypomanic/mixed patients (Calabrese *et al.*, 1999a). In the first double-blind, randomized, controlled study of lamotrigine in acute mania lamotrigine titrated to 100 mg/day over three weeks was as effective as lithium 800 mg/day (mean blood level 0.77 mmol/l) in reducing manic symptoms (Ichim, Berk, and Brook, 2000). However, lamotrigine has not shown anti-manic activity in placebo-controlled studies (Bowden, 2003). Unpublished studies in patients with acute manic or mixed exacerbations of bipolar I disorder have found no significant difference from baseline in the 11-item Mania Rating Scale (MRS) between lamotrigine and placebo (Goldsmith *et al.*, 2003).

4.3.1.4   Prevention of Mood Disturbances: Maintenance Therapy

The initial lamotrigine maintenance study was a double-blind, placebo-controlled study in rapid cycling bipolar disorder (Calabrese *et al.*, 2000). Open label lamotrigine added to the treatment regimens of 324 patients meeting DSM-IV criteria for rapid cycling bipolar disorder resulted in 182 stabilized patients who were then randomly assigned to the double-blind maintenance phase after being stratified for bipolar I or II disorder. Other psychotropic agents were tapered and patients randomly assigned to either lamotrigine monotherapy or placebo in a 1 : 1 ratio for the six-month maintenance phase. Overall 49 placebo patients (56%) and 45 lamotrigine-treated patients (50%) required treatment of an emerging mood episode with additional pharmacotherapy. Although there was no statistical significance between these two treatment groups on the primary outcome measure of time to additional pharmacotherapy (median of 12 weeks for placebo versus 18 weeks for lamotrigine), lamotrigine was significantly more effective than placebo in the survival in study analysis (median of 8 weeks for placebo versus 14 weeks for lamotrigine). In the sub-analysis according to disease type, lamotrigine was significantly more effective than placebo in delaying time to additional pharmacotherapy for bipolar II patients than bipolar I patients. Forty-six percent of bipolar II patients on lamotrigine monotherapy were stable without relapse after six months compared to only 18% of placebo-treated bipolar II patients. These results were confirmed in a post hoc analysis of the same patient sample with the life chart method. Measured with the life chart at least once weekly patients taking lamotrigine were 1.8 times more likely to achieve euthymia than those taking placebo (Goldberg *et al.*, 2008). In an unpublished study, these findings were not replicated. However, significantly fewer lamotrigine treated rapid cyclers required intervention for a depressive episode. Collectively, these results suggest that lamotrigine may be a useful treatment for rapid cycling bipolar patients, especially for type II and for the prevention of depressive relapses.

Two 18-month maintenance studies (Bowden *et al.*, 2003; Calabrese *et al.*, 2003a) comparing lamotrigine, lithium, and placebo provided further support for the use of lamotrigine as a mood stabilizer and led to its approval by the US FDA in June 2003 as a maintenance treatment for bipolar I disorder. These complementary studies enrolled patients in a double-blind phase of maintenance therapy after a recent depressed, hypomanic, or manic episode remitted (CGI-S score of ≤3 for four consecutive weeks) during open-label stabilization during which lamotrigine was initiated as adjunctive or monotherapy and other psychotropics discontinued. In both studies, 50% of patients achieved stabilization criteria allowing for progression into double-blinded maintenance therapy with lamotrigine (50–400 mg/day), lithium (0.8–1.1 mEq/l), or placebo. The primary efficacy endpoint used was time to intervention for any mood episode.

In both of these studies, lamotrigine and lithium demonstrated effective prophylaxis against any emerging mood episode compared with placebo. There were statistically fewer relapsing mood episodes and longer median survival in lamotrigine and lithium treated patients compared with placebo. Median survival before intervention for any mood episode for lamotrigine-treated patients ranged from 118 to 256 days, significantly better than placebo (85–93 days). Lithium also outperformed placebo with a median survival of 170–292 days. However, there were important differences in the spectra of maintenance efficacy.

In both studies, lithium, but not lamotrigine was superior to placebo at delaying the time to intervention for a manic or hypomanic episode. In total for both studies 123 hypomanic/manic events emerged during maintenance, with 25% of placebo treated patients experiencing a hypomanic, manic, or mixed episode (47 of 188); 21% of the lamotrigine group relapsed (58 of 273), but only 11% of patients in the lithium-treatment arm had breakthrough mania or hypomania (18 of 164). Lithium was clearly more effective than placebo and lamotrigine in preventing manic and hypomanic relapse in recently symptomatic bipolar I patients.

In contrast, lamotrigine appears to be more effective than lithium in the prevention of depressive relapse in bipolar I patients. In both studies, lamotrigine but not lithium, was significantly better than placebo at prolonging time to intervention for a depressive mood episode. There were 209 depressive relapses in the patients observed in the two studies, with a higher rate of relapse in the placebo (68 of 188, or 36%) and lithium treatment groups (56 of 164, or 34%); lamotrigine was better at preventing recurrence of depression with a 31% rate of depressive relapse and a longer median survival before treatment of depression was necessary. The difference was particularly evident in the treatment of recently manic or hypomanic patients in whom only 14% of those receiving lamotrigine (8 of 58) needed intervention for emergent depression compared with 23% of patients receiving lithium (10 of 44) and 30% receiving placebo (21 of 69). In a post hoc analysis of the first six months of the bipolar I patients (index episode depression) there was no evidence for a greater risk for mood destabilization (emergent (hypo) manic symptoms) in the lamotrigine group versus the placebo group (Goldberg *et al.*, 2009).

4.4 SAFETY

4.4.1 RASH

Rashes requiring hospitalization and discontinuation of treatment have been reported with lamotrigine. The reported rash rate is 10% in adult patients with epilepsy treated with adjunctive lamotrigine and 7% in bipolar I adults treated with monotherapy; the placebo rate is 5% in both populations (lamotrigine package insert). Serious rash rates are considerably lower at 0.8% in pediatric epilepsy patients, 0.3% in epileptic adults as monotherapy, and 0.13% as adjunctive therapy. A retrospective analysis conducted of rates of lamotrigine-related rash in 12 multicenter studies of lamotrigine for mood disorders (n = 1955), including one open study, seven randomized controlled acute trials, and four randomized controlled maintenance trials from 1996 to 2001 reported serious rash in 0% with lamotrigine, 0.1% (N = 1) with placebo, and 0% with comparators (Calabrese *et al.*, 2002). Across all bipolar disorder studies with 2272 patients on lamotrigine, serious rash was observed in three patients for an overall rate of 0.1% (lamotrigine package insert). One of these three patients experienced a mild Stevens-Johnson syndrome (SGS) on adjunctive lamotrigine and did not require hospitalization.

In a randomized trial Usual Care Precautions were compared with Dermatologic Precautions (UCPs plus additional specific precautions intended to decrease the risk of rash) for 12 weeks (Ketter *et al.*, 2006). Lamotrigine was added (target dose 200 mg/day) to ongoing medication with a slow uptitration. UCPs were:

- not exceeding the initial dose or dose-escalation schedule
- if a rash developed during the study the patient contacted the investigator immediately
- lamotrigine was stopped in case of rash.

Patients in the Dermatologic Precautions group were, besides UCP, advised:

- not to take new medications or foods, use new cosmetics, deodorants, detergents, or fabric softeners
- stimulate the immune system through excessive sun exposure
- participate in activities that might lead to exposure to poison oak or poison ivy
- receive any immunizations.

Over 1175 patients were included. In both groups there were no reports of serious rash. The rate of non-serious rash was low for UCP as well as for DP (8.8 and 8.6% respectively, OR 0.99) which is comparable with rates of rash in previous studies. Clinical response was 50% with 29% remission over both groups (according to the Clinical Global Impressions Bipolar version).

A German registry that documents the incidences of serious rash has been in place since 1990 and ascertains hospitalized cases of SJS and toxic epidermal necrolysis (TEN) related to antiepileptic drug use (Rzany *et al.*, 1996). Reported cases are confirmed by a registry physician and reviewed by a dermatological expert committee ensuring high diagnostic accuracy. The incidence of serious rash rising to the level of SJS/TEN diagnosis in the German registry was 0.02% from 1993 to 2001 (Messenheimer, 2002).

Risk of rash is noted to be higher in pediatric patients and may be increased by co-administration of divalproex sodium or exceeding the recommended initial dose or dose escalation schedule for lamotrigine. Women may be at increased risk for rash compared with men, with a relative risk of 1.8 (Wong, Mawer, and Sander, 1999).

4.4.2 OTHER SIDE EFFECTS AND TOLERABILITY

Lamotrigine is known to be generally well tolerated in the treatment of epilepsy (Choi and Morrell, 2003). A great deal of data generated by the 18-month lamotrigine maintenance trials (Bowden *et al.*, 2003; Calabrese *et al.*, 2003a) confirms clinical experience and epilepsy management reports of lamotrigine's favorable side effect profile in the treatment of bipolar patients. In 280 patients on maintenance lamotrigine during double-blinded treatment in both trials combined, only 23 (8.2%) discontinued study participation prematurely due to an adverse event; 7.9% of placebo treated patients experienced adverse events that led to end of study (15 of 191). Over the 18 months randomized phase, lamotrigine treated patients exhibited a 4.9 pound mean decrease in

Table 4.2 Adverse events observed during randomized phase of lamotrigine maintenance studies (in percent)[a].

Event	Lamotrigine (n = 227)	Placebo (n = 190)
Nausean	14	11
Insomnia	10	6
Somnolence	9	7
Back pain	8	6
Fatigue	8	5
Rhinitis	7	4
Benign rash	7	5
Abdominal pain	6	3
Dry mouth	6	4
Constipation	5	2
Vomiting	5	2
Cough exacerbation	5	3
Pharyngitis	5	4

[a] Adverse events listed had incidence $\geq 5\%$ and were numerically greater than placebo. (Bowden, 2003; Calabrese *et al.*, 2003a).

body weight, compared to a 2.6 pound mean weight gain in the placebo group. In a combined analysis of both studies, the incidence of mania/hypomania/mixed episodes reported as adverse events was 5% for patients treated with lamotrigine, 4% for patients treated with lithium, and 7% for patients treated with placebo. In general, lamotrigine exhibits placebo level rates of treatment-emergent adverse events and is better tolerated than lithium (Calabrese *et al.*, 2003a). Table 4.2 lists treatment-emergent adverse events for the combined maintenance studies during the randomized phase.

4.5 CLINICAL APPLICATIONS FOR LAMOTRIGINE IN MOOD DISORDERS

4.5.1 ACUTE MOOD DISTURBANCES: DEPRESSION

With the wealth of available pharmacotherapies, especially antidepressants, for the treatment of unipolar major depressive disorder and the relative paucity of data to support its use for acute depression, lamotrigine remains a distant option in any medication algorithm to manage unipolar depressive disorder. However, there is sufficient available literature and clinical experience to suggest a possible adjunctive role for lamotrigine in some patients only partially responsive to traditional antidepressants or suffering with treatment refractory depression.

Patients experiencing ongoing depressive symptoms despite adequate antidepressant medication dosing may benefit from augmentation with lamotrigine titrated to 100–200 mg/day (Barbosa, Berk, and Vorster, 2003; Normann *et al.*, 2002). A minimum of six to nine weeks of adjunctive lamotrigine should be considered an adequate trial when used as an off-label add-on therapy in these cases.

Table 4.3 Recommended lamotrigine dosing schedule.

Concomitant medication?	Weeks 1 and 2	Weeks 3 and 4 (mg qd)	Week 5 (mg qd)	Week 6 (mg qd)	Week 7 (mg qd)
Not on divalproex or carbamazepine	25 mg qd	50	100	200	200
On divalproex	25 mg qod	25	50	100	100
On carbamazepine or phenytoin	50 mg qd	100	200	300	300

For the management of acute bipolar depression, the APA Practice Guidelines of 2002 recommended lamotrigine as a first-line option with moderate clinical confidence. Since then other options have become available, especially quetiapine en the combination of olanzapine plus fluoxetine. With the data that became available after the 2002 guideline, lamotrigine has a place in the treatment of acute bipolar depression, especially in patients experiencing a depressive episode despite adequate treatment with lithium. In these patients lamotrigine can be recommended as add-on therapy with substantial clinical confidence (Van der Loos et al., 2009).

Dosing should follow published titration schedules to minimize the risk of rash, with a minimum dose of 50 mg/day and a target dose of 200 mg/day for most patients (see Table 4.3). There is no pharmacokinetic interaction with lithium, however, in bipolar patients experiencing a breakthrough depression on carbamazepine or valproate, lamotrigine should be added while keeping in mind pharmacokinetic interactions that may affect dosing: double dose of lamotrigine in combination with carbamazepine, half the dose in combination with valproate.

4.5.2 ACUTE MOOD DISTURBANCES: MANIA/MIXED STATES

Lamotrigine monotherapy is not recommended for the acute management of mania or mixed states associated with bipolar I disorder. Despite limited case reports and early data suggesting that lamotrigine may possess anti-manic properties, further study has led to the conclusion that lamotrigine has only mild to moderate efficacy in mania and should not be reliably used as monotherapy in these urgent above baseline mood disturbances. The addition of lamotrigine to other first-line antimanic agents, such as lithium, divalproex, olanzapine, or quetiapine may hasten or complete recovery from acute manic or mixed states. Lamotrigine should definitely be considered as an initial adjunctive treatment for these bipolar I patients to address the need to prevent future mood episodes after recovery from the current manic or mixed episode. Again, dosing guidelines should be followed as indicated previously and in the package insert to avoid increased risk of rash.

In bipolar II patients experiencing acute hypomania, lamotrigine can be used as a monotherapy or in conjunction with another mood stabilizer such as lithium. One effective strategy is the prescription of lamotrigine plus a short-term atypical antipsychotic.

4.5.3 PREVENTION OF MOOD DISTURBANCES: MAINTENANCE THERAPY

Lamotrigine is indicated by the US FDA and the EMEA for the maintenance treatment of bipolar I disorder to delay the time to occurrence of mood episodes. It should therefore be considered in the treatment of all bipolar patients due to the inherent natural tendency for the illness to be chronic and recurrent.

Maintenance monotherapy with lamotrigine can be considered in those individuals with nonbipolar I illness, milder forms of bipolar II disorder with predominant depressive course, and in other bipolar spectrum disorders such as cyclothymic or hyperthymic personalities. In theory, lamotrigine monotherapy could also be considered as a maintenance therapy after successful ECT for either unipolar or bipolar depression. In most patients, lamotrigine should be part of a combined pharmacological strategy to prevent relapse. Although lamotrigine has been demonstrated an effective maintenance treatment for bipolar I disorder, its ability to prevent manic episodes was considerably less robust than its antidepressant ability. A comprehensive bipolar maintenance medication treatment plan must address prevention of depressive and manic phases, and lamotrigine is only moderately effective in the delay of manic episodes necessitating use of other mood stabilizers with a complementary efficacy profile, such as lithium, divalproex, or atypical antipsychotics.

4.5.4 LAMOTRIGINE USE IN WOMEN

There have been reports of lamotrigine serum concentrations decreasing in women after starting oral contraceptives and increasing after oral contraceptives were discontinued (Sidhu *et al.*, 2006). Dosage adjustments may have to be made in women taking lamotrigine during times of oral contraceptive initiation or termination, although no known link exists between blood levels and therapeutic effects for affective disorders.

Lamotrigine carries a Category C FDA warning for use during pregnancy. Pregnant women maintained on lamotrigine during pregnancy should have blood levels of lamotrigine checked monthly as its clearance increases significantly as pregnancy progresses. A preconception determination of lamotrigine blood level in a stable bipolar woman may provide a target dose range to maintain during pregnancy. Clearance of lamotrigine drops quickly after delivery, requiring dosage reduction in most postpartum patients. Breast-feeding is not recommended to nursing mothers on lamotrigine since significant levels of lamotrigine are present in breast milk and long term effects of exposure to neonates is unknown. Although there are some reports of an increased risk for isolated cleft palate or lip deformity after exposure to lamotrigine monotherapy during the first trimester of pregnancy (Holmes *et al.*, 2008) the overall risk for major birth defects appear to be similar to that of the general population (Cunnington and Tennis, 2005).

4.6 SUMMARY

The discovery of lamotrigine's positive effects on mood in epilepsy patients led to its investigations in and eventual approval for treating bipolar I disorder. Although the exact mood stabilizing mechanism of action for this novel anticonvulsant is unknown, it is thought to work by inhibiting voltage-sensitive sodium currents, in this manner stabilizing neuronal membranes and as a result modulating the presynaptic transmitter release of excitatory amino acids such as glutamate. Although there is some suggestion that lamotrigine may have some beneficial effect in the treatment of unipolar depression, available evidence points to a primary role in the treatment of bipolar depression. It is approved for maintenance treatment of bipolar disorder to prevent depressive episodes. In addition, it deserves a place in the treatment of acute bipolar depression, with the strongest evidence as add-on treatment to lithium. Lamotrigine is well tolerated, the major risk is a severe rash, and it requires careful dose monitoring.

References

Anderson, G.D., Yau, M.K., Gidal, B.E. *et al.* (1996) Bidirectional interaction of valproate and lamotrigine in healthy subjects. *Clin. Pharmacol. Ther.*, **60**, 145–156.

Barbosa, L., Berk, M., and Vorster, M. (2003) A double-blind, randomized, placebo-controlled trial of augmentation with lamotrigine or placebo in patients concomitantly treated with fluoxetine for resistant major depressive episodes. *J. Clin. Psychiatry*, **64**, 403–407.

Bowden, C.L. (2003) Acute and maintenance treatment with mood stabilizers. *Int. J. Neuropsychopharmacol.*, **6**, 269–275.

Bowden, C.L., Calabrese, J.R., Sachs, G. *et al.* (2003) A placebo-controlled 18-month trial of lamotrigine and lithium maintenance treatment in recently manic or hypomanic patients with bipolar I disorder. *Arch. Gen. Psychiatry*, **60**, 392–400.

Brown, E.B., McElroy, S.L., Keck, P.E. *et al.* (2006) Olanzapine/Fluoxetine Combination versus Lamotrigine in the treatment of bipolar I depression. *J. Clin. Psychiatry*, **67**, 1025–1033.

Calabrese, J.R., Bowden, C.L., McElroy, S.L. *et al.* (1999a) Spectrum of activity of lamotrigine in treatment-refractory bipolar disorder. *Am. J. Psychiatry*, **156**, 1019–1023.

Calabrese, J.R., Bowden, C.L., Sachs, G.S. *et al.* (1999b) A double-blind placebo-controlled study of lamotrigine monotherapy in outpatients with bipolar I depression. Lamictal 602 study group. *J. Clin. Psychiatry*, **60**, 79–88.

Calabrese, J.R., Bowden, C.L., Sachs, G. *et al.* (2003a) A placebo-controlled 18-month trial of lamotrigine and lithium maintenance treatment in recently depressed patients with bipolar I disorder. *J. Clin. Psychiatry*, **64**, 1013–1024.

Calabrese, J.R., Hirschfeld, R.M., Reed, M. *et al.* (2003b) Impact of bipolar disorder on a U.S. community sample. *J. Clin. Psychiatry*, **64**, 425–432.

Calabrese, J.R., Fatemi, S.H., and Woyshville, M.J. (1996) Antidepressant effects of lamotrigine in rapid cycling bipolar disorder. *Am. J. Psychiatry*, **153**, 1236.

Calabrese, J.R., Huffman, R.F., White, R.L. *et al.* (2007) Additional clinical trial data and a retrospective pooled analysis of response rates across all randomized trials conducted by GSK. *Bipolar Disord.*, **8** (Suppl. 1), 323–333.

Calabrese, J.R., Sullivan, J.R., Bowden, C.L. *et al.* (2002) Rash in multicenter trials of lamotrigine in mood disorders: clinical relevance and management. *J. Clin. Psychiatry*, **63**, 1012–1019.
Calabrese, J.R., Suppes, T., Bowden, C.L. *et al.*, Lamictal 614 Study Group (2000) A double-blind, placebo-controlled, prophylaxis study of lamotrigine in rapid-cycling bipolar disorder. *J. Clin. Psychiatry*, **61**, 841–850.
Calabrese, J.R., Vieta, E., and Shelton, M.D. (2003c) Latest maintenance data on lamotrigine in bipolar disorder. *Eur. Neuropsychopharmacol.*, **13** (Suppl. 2), S57–S66.
Chen, C., Veronese, L., and Yin, Y. (2000) The effects of lamotrigine on the pharmacokinetics of lithium. *Br. J. Clin. Pharmacol.*, **50**, 193–195.
Choi, H. and Morrell, M.J. (2003) Review of lamotrigine and its clinical applications in epilepsy. *Exp. Opin. Pharmacother.*, **4**, 243–251.
Cohen, A.F., Ashby, L., Crowley, D. *et al.* (1985) Lamotrigine (BW430C), a potential anticonvulsant. Effects on the central nervous system in comparison with phenytoin and diazepam. *Br. J. Clin. Pharmacol.*, **20**, 619–629.
Cohen, A.F., Land, G.S., Breimer, D.D. *et al.* (1987) Lamotrigine, a new anticonvulsant: pharmacokinetics in normal humans. *Clin. Pharmacol. Ther.*, **42**, 535–541.
Cunnington, M. and Tennis, P., The International Lamotrigine Pregnancy Registry Scientific Advisory Committee (2005) Lamotrigine and the risk of malformations in pregnancy. *Neurology*, **64**, 955–960.
Fitton, A. and Goa, K.L. (1995) Lamotrigine. An update of its pharmacology and therapeutic use in epilepsy. *Drugs*, **50**, 691–713.
Frye, M.A., Ketter, T.A., Kimbrell, T.A. *et al.* (2000) A placebo-controlled study of lamotrigine and gabapentin monotherapy in refractory mood disorders. *J. Clin. Psychopharmacol.*, **20**, 607–614.
Garnett, W.R. (1997) Lamotrigine: pharmacokinetics. *J. Child Neurol.*, **12** (Suppl. 1), S10–S15.
Geddes, J.R., Calabrese, J.R., and Goodwin, G.M. (2009) Lamotrigine for treatment of bipolar depression: independent meta-analysis and meta-regression of individual patient data from five randomised trials. *Br. J. Psychiatry*, **194**, 4–9.
Gilman, J.T. (1995) Lamotrigine: an antiepileptic agent for the treatment of partial seizures. *Ann. Pharmacother.*, **29**, 144–151.
Ginsberg, L., Sachs, G., and Ketter, T. (2003) Poster presented at the American Psychiatric Association 2003 Annual Meeting, San Francisco, CA, pp. 173–174.
Goa, K.L., Ross, S.R., and Chrisp, P. (1993) Lamotrigine. A review of its pharmacological properties and clinical efficacy in epilepsy. *Drugs*, **46**, 152–176.
Goldberg, J.F., Bowden, C.L., Calabrese, J.R. *et al.* (2008) Six-month prospective life charting of mood symptoms with lamotrigine monotherapy versus placebo in rapid cycling bipolar disorder. *Biol. Psychiatry*, **63**, 125–130.
Goldberg, J.F., Calabrese, J.R., Saville, B.R. *et al.* (2009) Mood stabilization and destabilization during acute and continuation phase treatment for bipolar I disorder with lamotrigine or placebo. *J. Clin. Psychiatry*, **70**, 1273–1280.
Goldsmith, D.R., Wagstaff, A.J., Ibbotson, T. *et al.* (2003) Lamotrigine: a review of its use in bipolar disorder. *Drugs*, **63**, 2029–2050.
Hachad, H., Ragueneau-Majlessi, I., and Levy, R.H. (2002) New antiepileptic drugs: review on drug interactions. *Ther. Drug Monit.*, **24**, 91–103.
Hirschfeld, R.M., Calabrese, J.R., Weissman, M.M. *et al.* (2003) Screening for bipolar disorder in the community. *J. Clin. Psychiatry*, **64**, 53–59.
Holmes, L.B., Baldwin, E.J., Smith, C.R. *et al.* (2008) Increased frequency of isolated cleft palate in infants exposed to lamotrigine during pregnancy. *Neurology*, **70**, 2152–2158.

Ichim, L., Berk, M., and Brook, S. (2000) Lamotrigine compared with lithium in mania: a double-blind randomized controlled trial. *Ann. Clin. Psychiatry*, **12**, 5–10.

Judd, L.L., Akiskal, H.S., Schettler, P.J. *et al.* (2002) The long-term natural history of the weekly symptomatic status of bipolar I disorder. *Arch. Gen. Psychiatry*, **59**, 530–537.

Kupka, R.W., Luckenbaugh, D.A., Post, R.M. *et al.* (2005) Comparison of rapid-cycling and non-rapid-cycling bipolar disorder based on prospective mood ratings in 539 outpatients. *Am. J. Psychiatry*, **162**, 1273–1280.

Ketter, T.A., Greist, J.H., Graham, J.A. *et al.* (2006) The effect of dermatologic precautions on the incidence of rash with addition of lamotrigine in the treatment of bipolar i disorder: a randomized trial. *J. Clin. Psychiatry*, **67**, 400–406.

Kusumakar, V. and Yatham, L.N. (1997) An open study of lamotrigine in refractory bipolar depression. *Psychiatry Res.*, **72**, 145–148.

Leach, M.J., Baxter, M.G., and Critchley, M.A. (1991) Neurochemical and behavioral aspects of lamotrigine. *Epilepsia*, **32** (Suppl. 2), S4–S8.

Leach, M.J., Marden, C.M., and Miller, A.A. (1986) Pharmacological studies on lamotrigine, a novel potential antiepileptic drug: II. Neurochemical studies on the mechanism of action. *Epilepsia*, **27**, 490–497.

Li, X., Ketter, T.A., and Frye, M.A. (2002) Synaptic, intracellular, and neuroprotective mechanisms of anticonvulsants: are they relevant for the treatment and course of bipolar disorders? *J. Affect. Disord.*, **69**, 1–14.

Matsuo, F., Bergen, D., Faught, E. *et al.*, U.S. Lamotrigine Protocol 0.5 Clinical Trial Group (1993) Placebo-controlled study of the efficacy and safety of lamotrigine in patients with partial seizures. *Neurology*, **43**, 2284–2291.

Messenheimer, J.A. (2002) Poster presented at the American Academy of Neurology Annual Meeting Denver, CO.

Mikati, M.A., Schachter, S.C., Schomer, D.L. *et al.* (1989) Long-term tolerability, pharmacokinetic and preliminary efficacy study of lamotrigine in patients with resistant partial seizures. *Clin. Neuropharmacol.*, **12**, 312–321.

Normann, C., Hummel, B., Scharer, L.O. *et al.* (2002) Lamotrigine as adjunct to paroxetine in acute depression: a placebo-controlled, double-blind study. *J. Clin. Psychiatry*, **63**, 337–344.

Ohman, I., Vitols, S., and Tomson, T. (2000) Lamotrigine in pregnancy: pharmacokinetics during delivery, in the neonate, and during lactation. *Epilepsia*, **41**, 709–713.

Pennell, P.B. (2003) Antiepileptic drug pharmacokinetics during pregnancy and lactation. *Neurology*, **61**, S35–S42.

Post, R.M., Denicoff, K.D., and Leverich, G.S. (2002) Presentations of depression in bipolar illness. *Clin. Neurosci. Res.*, **2**, 142–157.

Rambeck, B. and Wolf, P. (1993) Lamotrigine clinical pharmacokinetics. *Clin. Pharmacokinet.*, **25**, 433–443.

Ramsay, R.E., Pellock, J.M., Garnett, W.R. *et al.* (1991) Pharmacokinetics and safety of lamotrigine (Lamictal) in patients with epilepsy. *Epilepsy Res.*, **10**, 191–200.

Regeer, E.J., ten Have, M., Rosso, M.L. *et al.* (2004) Prevalence of bipolar disorder in the general population: a reappraisal study of the Netherlands mental health survey and incidence study. *Acta Psychiatr. Scand.*, **110**, 5374–5382.

Rzany, B., Mockenhaupt, M., Baur, S. *et al.* (1996) Epidemiology of erythema exsudativum multiforme majus, Stevens-Johnson syndrome, and toxic epidermal necrolysis in Germany (1990–1992): structure and results of a population-based registry. *J. Clin. Epidemiol.*, **49**, 769–773.

Shiah, I.S., Yatham, L.N., Lam, R.W. *et al.* (1998) Effects of lamotrigine on the 5-HT1A receptor function in healthy human males. *J. Affect. Disord.*, **49**, 157–162.

Sidhu, J., Job, S., Singh, S. *et al.* (2006) The pharmacokinetic and pharmacodynamic consequences of the co-administration of lamotrigine and a combined oral contraceptive in healthy female subjects. *Br. J. Clin. Pharmacol.*, **61**, 191–199.

Smith, D., Baker, G., Davies, G. *et al.* (1993a) Outcomes of add-on treatment with lamotrigine in partial epilepsy. *Epilepsia*, **34**, 312–322.

Smith, D., Chadwick, D., Baker, G. *et al.* (1993b) Seizure severity and the quality of life. *Epilepsia*, **34** (Suppl. 5), S31–S35.

Tran, T.A., Leppik, I.E., Blesi, K. *et al.* (2002) Lamotrigine clearance during pregnancy. *Neurology*, **59**, 251–255.

Van der Loos, M.L., Mulder, P.G., Hartong, E.G. *et al.* (2009) Efficacy and safety of lamotrigine as add-on treatment to lithium in bipolar depression: a multicenter, double-blind, placebo-controlled trial. *J. Clin. Psychiatry*, **70**, 223–231.

Van der Loos, M.L., Mulder, P., Hartong, E.G. *et al.* (2010 Sep.) Efficacy and safety of two treatment algorithms in bipolar depression: lithium plus lamotrigine versus lithium plus placebo both followed by addition of paroxetine in non-responders. *Acta Psychiatr. Scand.*, **122**(3), 246–254.

Vinod, K.Y. and Subhash, M.N. (2002) Lamotrigine induced selective changes in 5-HT(1A) receptor mediated response in rat brain. *Neurochem. Int.*, **40**, 315–319.

Walden, J., Hesslinger, B., van Calker, D. *et al.* (1996) Addition of lamotrigine to valproate may enhance efficacy in the treatment of bipolar affective disorder. *Pharmacopsychiatry*, **29**, 193–195.

Weisler, R., Risner, M., Ascher, J. *et al.* (1994) Poster presented at the American Psychiatric Association 1994 Annual Meeting, Philadelphia, PA.

Weissman, M.M., Bland, R.C., Canino, G.J. *et al.* (1996) Cross-national epidemiology of major depression and bipolar disorder. *J. Am. Med. Assoc.*, **276**, 293–299.

Wong, I.C., Mawer, G.E., and Sander, J.W. (1999) Factors influencing the incidence of lamotrigine-related skin rash. *Ann. Pharmacother.*, **33**, 1037–1042.

Xie, X. and Hagan, R.M. (1998) Cellular and molecular actions of lamotrigine: possible mechanisms of efficacy in bipolar disorder. *Neuropsychobiology*, **38**, 119–130.

Xie, X., Lancaster, B., Peakman, T. *et al.* (1995) Interaction of the antiepileptic drug lamotrigine with recombinant rat brain type IIA Na+ channels and with native Na+ channels in rat hippocampal neurones. *Pflugers Arch.*, **430**, 437–446.

Yuen, A.W., Land, G., Weatherley, B.C. *et al.* (1992) Sodium valproate acutely inhibits lamotrigine metabolism. *Br. J. Clin. Pharmacol.*, **33**, 511–513.

5

Carbamazepine and other Anticonvulsants

Heinz Grunze

Institute of Neuroscience, Academic Psychiatry, Newcastle University, Newcastle, UK

5.1 INTRODUCTION

Despite the fact that several well studied mood stabilizing agents, including some atypical antipsychotics, are nowadays promoted as monotherapy of bipolar disorder, a fair proportion of bipolar patients need treatment with additional drugs. As described in greater detail in a separate chapter, the concomitant use of different agents is rather the rule than the exception (Wolfsperger *et al.*, 2007). Whereas carbamazepine is often used in monotherapy or in combination with lithium, polypharmacy with three or more psychotropics regularly makes use of its off-spring, oxcarbazepine, other older anticonvulsants with so far limited scientific evidence or anticonvulsants which only became available recently. This chapter aims to summarize the scientific evidence supporting the use of these agents in bipolar disorder.

5.1.1 CARBAMAZEPINE

Starting with the first studies of Okuma *et al.* (1973) the efficacy of carbamazepine for the acute treatment of mania has first been demonstrated in several, mostly small studies, both by the group of Okuma and by other investigators (for example, Ballenger and Post, 1980; Emrich, Dose, and von Zerssen, 1985; Müller and Stoll, 1984; Post *et al.*, 1987).

Three more recent, double-blind, and placebo-controlled large studies, using an extended release formulation of carbamazepine, finally gave conclusive evidence for its antimanic efficacy (Weisler *et al.*, 2005; Weisler, Kalali, and Ketter, 2004; Zhang *et al.*, 2007b). Whereas the studies by Weisler *et al.* were short term 3 week studies, the study of Zhang also shows continuous antimanic efficacy over a 12 week study period. Post-hoc analysis of the Hamilton Depression Rating Scale (HAM-D) scores in the two studies by Weisler, Kalali, and Ketter (2004) and Weisler *et al.* (2005) also demonstrated significant improvement of depressive symptoms in patients with mixed mania. This is in line with the antidepressant effects observed in the study by Zhang *et al.* (2007a, 2007b) who also studied carbamazepine's efficacy in a sample of

Bipolar Psychopharmacotherapy: Caring for the patient, Second Edition. Edited by Hagop S. Akiskal and Mauricio Tohen.
© 2011 John Wiley & Sons, Ltd. Published 2011 by John Wiley & Sons, Ltd.

bipolar depressed patients. The main side effects that were higher than placebo in these controlled studies were dizziness, nausea, and somnolence; however, extended release carbamazepine still seems to be better tolerated than immediate release formulations, especially considering gastrointestinal side effects (El-Mallakh *et al.*, 2009). More detailed information on the tolerability and safety profile, including teratogenicity, of carbamazepine is also available in recent reviews (Fenn *et al.*, 2006; Gajwani *et al.*, 2005; Morrow *et al.*, 2006).

Comparative studies in mania have been conducted as well with conventional antipsychotics as with lithium and valproate (Brown, Silverstone, and Cookson, 1989; Klein *et al.*, 1984; Lerer *et al.*, 1987; Okuma *et al.*, 1979, 1990; Stoll *et al.*, 1986; Vasudev, Goswami, and Kohli, 2000). The general impression of these studies was that carbamazepine was overall equally effective as the comparators, with a probably slightly slower onset of response compared to antipsychotics and valproate, but still slightly faster acting than lithium (Small *et al.*, 1996).

Summarizing these trials, the short-term and intermediate antimanic efficacy of carbamazepine appears apparent, including patients with mixed mania.

For the depressed phase of bipolar disorder, the evidence for the usefulness of carbamazepine is less numerous. Only one randomized, placebo controlled study backs up antidepressant efficacy of carbamazepine (Zhang *et al.*, 2007a). In addition, small, mainly open, studies (reviewed by Brambilla, Barale, and Soares, 2001) suggest that carbamazepine may be useful in the treatment of both unipolar and bipolar depression.

First evidence for a prophylactic efficacy of carbamazepine in bipolar disorder was established by five randomized, controlled trials in the 1980s and early 1990s.

Four of these studies compared carbamazepine with lithium (Coxhead, Silverstone, and Cookson, 1992; Lusznat, Murphy, and Nunn, 1988; Placidi *et al.*, 1986; Watkins *et al.*, 1987) and one small study with placebo (Okuma *et al.*, 1981). A meta-analysis of the four lithium trials concluded that carbamazepine's efficacy as a prophylactic agent could not be established on the basis of these trials because of the heterogeneity in design, differences in statistical power and sensitivity of outcome measures (Dardennes *et al.*, 1995).

Probably more convincing evidence for prophylactic efficacy of carbamazepine is supplied by three additional maintenance studies. Denicoff *et al.* (1997) compared carbamazepine, lithium, and the combination of both in 52 bipolar I patients.

Patients were randomized either to carbamazepine or lithium treatment for the first year, then switched over to the alternative treatment for the second year and finally to combination treatment for the third year. Whereas the prophylactic efficacy of both monotherapies was disappointing, combination treatment with both lithium and carbamazepine was clearly superior to each monotherapy.

Greil *et al.* (1997b) and Greil and Kleindienst (1999a, 1999b) compared carbamazepine and lithium in an open-label, but randomized parallel group study, lasting for 2.5 years and involving 144 patients with bipolar I, II, and not otherwise specified bipolar disorders. No significant difference was observed between both treatments based on survival analysis with time to hospitalization or episode recurrence.

However, when combining different outcome-measures (recurrence and need for additional medication and/or adverse events) lithium was significantly better than carbamazepine. Additionally, less suicide attempts and completed suicides were observed in the lithium group (Thies-Flechtner *et al.*, 1996); this finding is also supported by a chart analysis by Yerevanian, Koek, and Mintz (2003) showing a trend toward better antisuicidal properties for both lithium and valproate compared to carbamazepine.

The impression that lithium may be overall more efficacious than carbamazepine in the prophylactic treatment for bipolar disorders is also backed up by a Dutch study (Hartong *et al.*, 2003) comparing 94 patients in a randomized, two-year double-blind design. Out of 44 patients on lithium, 12 patients developed a new episode compared with 21/50 on carbamazepine treatment. Although there was a clear trend, significant superiority for lithium was not shown in the total study population, but in those patients who were not previously treated with any other mood stabilizer. Interestingly, relapse with lithium occurred almost exclusively within the first three months of the trial while carbamazepine patients carried a constant risk of a new episode of about 40% per study year.

Looking across studies into specific sub-groups of patients where carbamazepine may be especially helpful, it seems indicated in patients with incomplete response to lithium in acute mania, rapid cycling (Denicoff *et al.*, 1997), patients with comorbid organic (neurological) disorders (Schneck, 2002), and schizoaffective patients (Elphick, 1985; Goncalves and Stoll, 1985; Greil *et al.*, 1997a).

However, in combination treatments, a major disadvantage of carbamazepine is the induction of different members of the cytochrome P 450 family (Spina, Pisani, and Perucca, 1996). This may cause an increased metabolism of different antidepressants and antipsychotics, including olanzapine (Tohen *et al.*, 2008) and risperidone (Yatham *et al.*, 2003) leading to reduced effectiveness. In addition, carbamazepine shows significant interactions both with valproate and lamotrigine.

In conclusion, carbamazepine appears to be an effective drug in bipolar disorder (Post *et al.*, 2007), especially in the treatment for acute mania, but not of special utility. There is evidence for antidepressant efficacy, and in long-term treatment the general impression is that it is less efficacious than lithium and lacks special antisuicidal properties. Additionally, induction of the cytochrome P 450 metabolism and competition for plasma protein binding complicates combination treatments both with other mood stabilizers and with several antipsychotics and antidepressants.

5.1.2   OXCARBAZEPINE

Oxcarbazepine is the 10-keto-analog of carbamazepine and uses a different pathway of metabolism. It avoids the formation of the 10,11-epoxide metabolite of carbamazepine which is thought to be responsible for the majority of neurological side effects. Instead, oxcarbazepine is reduced by a cytosolic reductase to its 10-mono-hydroxy derivative (MHD). Avoiding the metabolism by cytochrome P 450 3A4, oxcarbazepine does not induce its own metabolism and has less significant drug interactions than carbamazepine (Andreasen, Brosen, and Damkier, 2007). As a drawback, the scientific evidence for efficacy in bipolar disorder is considerably less than for carbamazepine (Hellewell, 2002; Hirschfeld and Kasper, 2004; Mazza *et al.*, 2007; Popova *et al.*, 2007; Pratoomsri *et al.*, 2006).

Most of the work on oxcarbazepine in bipolar disorder, especially in acute mania, was performed by Emrich *et al.* in the early 1980s (Emrich, 1994; Emrich, Dose, and von Zerssen, 1984). The antimanic effect of oxcarbazepine appeared comparable to the one of valproate in these early studies. In a double-blind comparative trial with haloperidol by Müller and Stoll (1984) no difference in efficacy was observed between oxcarbazepine and haloperidol. This impression was also supported by another study by Emrich (1990). With similar efficacy, the tolerability of oxcarbazepine was significantly better, with the incidence of side effects 3.5 times higher in the haloperidol group compared to the oxcarbazepine group. These studies are also comprehensively reviewed by Dietrich, Kropp, and Emrich (2001). More recently, a study by Hummel *et al.* (2002) supplied further supporting evidence for antimanic efficacy of oxcarbazepine, using an on–off–on design. Oxcarbazepine monotherapy appeared effective in patients with mild to moderate mania (Young Mania Rating Score < 25) but not in severely manic patients. Clearly, this makes it difficult to differentiate true efficacy from spontaneous remission. A single-blind study comparing oxcarbazepine and valproate in hypomania found similar improvement with both medications (Suppes *et al.*, 2007). The latest evidence comes from a double-blind, randomized, but not placebo-controlled study comparing valproate and oxcarbazepine in acute mania. Both treatments were effective, and no difference was observed between these treatment modalities in all reported outcomes (Kakkar *et al.*, 2009). On the other hand, there is conflicting evidence, as a large, placebo- controlled study in adolescent mania was negative for oxcarbazepine (Wagner *et al.*, 2006).

So far, no controlled studies are available for oxcarbazepine in bipolar depression. Retrospective chart reviews (Ghaemi, Ko, and Katzow, 2002; Pratoomsri *et al.*, 2005) suggest that oxcarbazepine may possess some efficacy in bipolar depressed patients. However, this impression has not been verified by controlled studies so far.

Considering prophylactic treatment, the available studies do not provide a recommendation (Vasudev *et al.*, 2008). In a study of Reinstein *et al.* (2003) 42 patients with bipolar or schizoaffective disorder were stabilized with valproate. Half of them were switched to oxcarbazepine after 10 weeks of treatment and followed up for another 10 weeks. Compared to patients remaining on valproate, mood stability was maintained to a similar degree. As a secondary outcome, it was noted that 47% of patients on valproate gained weight compared to only 26% of patients on oxcarbazepine, and a substantial proportion (70%) of patients lost weight after being switched from valproate to oxcarbazepine. Another open study in patients previously responsive to oxcarbazepine suggested reasonable prophylactic efficacy up to 12 months (Benedetti *et al.*, 2004). One underpowered double blind, randomized study looked into the efficacy of oxcarbazepine + lithium versus lithium + placebo. Although there was a trend toward better functionality and less depressive episodes with oxcarbazepine, the finding was not significant, most likely due to a lack of power (Vieta *et al.*, 2008).

A recent study compared carbamazepine and oxcarbazepine in the treatment of residual symptoms in patients on lithium prophylactic treatment. Although both substances lead to improvement, oxcarbazepine appeared more efficacious with a faster onset of full remission and less side effect burden (Juruena *et al.*, 2009).

In conclusion, there is some evidence for acute antimanic effects of oxcarbazepine, at least in mild to moderate manic patients, but probably not in severely ill patients. Data on the treatment for bipolar depression and prophylactic efficacy are sparse. However, oxcarbazepine remains a potential candidate drug for patients who previously responded well to carbamazepine, but had problems with tolerability or drug interactions in combination treatment.

The side effect profile of oxcarbazepine is largely similar to the one of carbamazepine, except with a lower incidence and severity. The exception is hyponatremia which might be more common with oxcarbazepine than with carbamazepine.

5.1.3 ESLICARBAZEPINE

Licarbazepine is the primary metabolite of oxcarbazepine. Two double-blind, placebo-controlled studies failed to separate between licarbazepine and placebo in acute mania; thus, it appears unlikely that this compound will be subject to more proof-of-concept studies in bipolar disorder. Eslicarbazepine (ESL) is the $S(+)$-enantiomer of licarbazepine. Similarly to oxcarbazepine, it is not metabolized to carbamazepine-10,11-epoxide, and is not susceptible to auto-induction or inhibition or induction of most Cytochrome P (CYP) isozymes (McCormack and Robinson, 2009). It is 90% excreted in urine either unchanged or as glucoronide. Recently, ESL has been examined for its antimanic properties in a randomized, controlled Phase II study. ESL was administered in two different dose regimens: Starting dose 600 mg/day with a maximum dose of 1800/day, or starting dose 800 mg/day with a maximum dose of 2400 mg/day. Although the higher dose range of ESL just missed significance in separating from placebo in the primary outcome (reduction of the Young Mania Rating Scale (YMRS) from baseline to endpoint), significantly more patients achieved remission with ESL (800–2400 mg/day) : YMRS reduction: -10.3 for Placebo, -14.2 for ESL 800–2400 mg/day, $p = 0.052$, Response: 50% for Placebo, 66.7 for ESL 800–2400 mg/day, $p = $ n.s., Remission: 27.5% for Placebo, 50.9% for ESL 800–2400 mg/day, $p = 0.02$ (all numbers baseline-endpoint Last Observation Carried Forward (LOCF) comparison). Thus, depending on further investigations ESL might become an emerging treatment option in bipolar disorder (Robertson _et al._, 2010).

5.1.4 PHENYTOIN

Although phenytoin has been a first choice treatment for epilepsies since the 1940s, it has never been studied until recently in a thorough way in bipolar disorder.

Mishory _et al._ (2000) were the first who published a placebo-controlled add-on trial with phenytoin in acute mania. Patients entering the study were started on haloperidol in a dose of the physician's discretion and then randomly assigned to receive either phenytoin or placebo as an add-on treatment. The improvement for the phenytoin group was significantly better starting from week 3 until the end of the study (week 5). In general, phenytoin was well tolerated, except for one patient developing tachycardia at 500 mg/day at week 4 and another patient developing dizziness at study initiation which responded to reduction of the dose. The same group also investigated the acute antimanic effect of fosphenytoin in a small open trial, observing no antimanic effects after one hour despite using doses which are effective in status epilepticus (Applebaum, Levine, and Belmaker, 2003).

Pilot studies with phenytoin exist for unipolar (Nemets, Bersudsky, and Belmaker, 2005), but not bipolar depression.

Finally, one study looked into prophylactic efficacy of phenytoin (Mishory, Winokur, and Bersudsky, 2003). Phenytoin or placebo were randomly added to ongoing and unchanged prophylactic treatment in stabilized bipolar patients. After six months patients who had not relapsed were crossed over to the other study agent without breaking the blind. There were only three patients (21.4%) who had a relapse on phenytoin, nine (56.3%) relapsed on placebo. This effect was significantly in favor of phenytoin. However, with the small sample size of the study, further conclusive trials have to be awaited before a more extensive use of phenytoin in bipolar disorder can be recommended.

5.1.5   CLONAZEPAM AND LORAZEPAM

These two benzodiazepam derivatives are quite frequently used in bipolar disorder. However, they are generally not considered as primarily mood stabilizing agents, but are used as add-on treatment to calm down the patient and relieve anxiety. This is especially true for lorazepam. Nevertheless, there are some studies supporting mood stabilizing effects of these two drugs. A Bayesian metaanalysis of published studies found statistically significant antimanic efficacy for clonazepam, but – at the time of the metaanalysis – not for Lorazepam (Curtin and Schulz, 2004).

Clonazepam is a high-potency 1,4-benzodiazepine derivative. Besides acting on the γ-amino butyric acid (GABA) A receptor (Haefely, 1983) clonazepam may also modulate the central serotonergic metabolism (Lima, 1991). Several open trials and case series support antimanic efficacy (Adler, 1986; Bottai *et al.*, 1995; Chouinard, 1985; Chouinard *et al.*, 1993; Chouinard, Young, and Annable, 1983; Morishita and Aoki, 1999; Pande, 1988).

For treating the depressed phase of the illness, evidence for efficacy of clonazepam appears less convincing. In a study of Kishimoto *et al.* (1988) 27 patients with major depression, among them 9 with bipolar depression, were treated openly with clonazepam. The authors report marked or moderate improvement to be obtained in 84% of the patients with a rapid onset of the antidepressive effect of clonazepam.

For maintenance treatment diverging results have been reported. Sachs (1990), Sachs, Rosenbaum, and Jones (1990) and Sachs, Weilburg, and Rosenbaum (1990) describe positive effects of add-on clonazepam for maintenance treatment. This is also in line with previous results of the study of Chouinard (1987) where clonazepam was administered as an adjunct to lithium or combined lithium/tryptophane treatment. However, the most recent study of Winkler *et al.* (2003) could not establish prophylactic efficacy for clonazepam in bipolar patients. Interestingly, however, they noticed a prophylactic efficacy of clonazepam in recurrent unipolar depression.

Summarizing these results most evidence points toward antimanic efficacy of clonazepam (Curtin and Schulz, 2004) whereas data for the treatment of bipolar depression and maintenance treatment are either missing or ambiguous.

As for lorazepam, it is often used as a standard rescue medication in controlled bipolar studies, but it may by itself influence the outcome of the trial when not applied in a controlled and restricted manner (see discussion on failed aripiprazole studies in bipolar depression, (Thase et al., 2008)). Several studies point toward an antimanic efficacy of lorazepam which may even be comparable to the one of haloperidol (Lenox et al., 1992).

Used as an add-on medication to haloperidol, lorazepam was less efficacious than lithium add-on treatment (Chou et al., 1999). In a double-blind randomized comparison with clonazepam, however, Lorazepam appeared more efficacious for treating acute mania (Bradwejn et al., 1990).

More recently, parenteral administration of lorazepam was also studied in comparison to olanzapine and placebo in 201 acutely manic patients. At endpoint after 24 hours, lorazepam injections were significantly superior to placebo in several outcome parameters measuring agitated behavior, although the study was not powered to show differences between lorazepam and placebo (Meehan et al., 2001). In another study, not only aripiprazole, but also i.m. Lorazepam (2 mg) was significantly better than placebo in reducing the Positive and Negative Syndrome Scale Excited Component score at 2 hours (Zimbroff et al., 2007). Thus, with these new studies, the outcome of the original metaanalysis of lorazepam's antimanic effects (Curtin and Schulz, 2004) might be different.

Due to the imminent danger of dependency, long-term use of lorazepam cannot be recommended. Thus, prophylactic efficacy has not been studied in a controlled manner so far.

5.1.6 LEVETIRACETAM

Levetiracetam is a pyrrolidine derivative which has been approved for add-on treatment of refractory partial epilepsy in adults. Its mechanisms of action appear different from those known from other classic antiepileptic drugs (Hovinga, 2001). In an animal model of mania, levetiracetam appeared efficacious (Lamberty, Margineanu, and Klitgaard, 2001). Case reports (Desarkar, Das, and Sinha, 2007; Goldberg and Burdick, 2002; Kaufman, 2004; Kyomen, 2006) and one open add-on study (Grunze et al., 2003) are supportive of antimanic efficacy, whereas another open trial could not show a benefit of levetiracetam as adjunctive medication to valproate in acute mania (Krüger et al., 2008). Double-blind randomized controlled trials which could clarify the antimanic properties of levetiracetam haven't been conducted to date. A case report suggests also efficacy in long-term mood stabilization in rapid cycling patients (Bräunig and Krüger, 2003). Further data on long-term maintenance treatment or on the treatment for bipolar depression are currently not available.

5.1.7 ZONISAMIDE

Zonisamide has been approved in several countries for the adjunctive treatment of refractory epilepsies. With classical antiepileptic drugs it shares several mechanisms of actions, such as sodium and T-type calcium channel blocker properties. Additionally, zonisamide also exerts effects on serotonin and dopamin turnover (Okada *et al.*, 1995, 1999; Oommen and Mathews, 1999). Zonisamide also binds to the GABA A receptor and inhibits carbonic anhydrase which, in turn, effects both extra- and intracellular pH-dependent neurotransmitter systems. In 1994, Kanba *et al.* (1994) presented evidence of antimanic effects of zonisamide in an open study with a responder rate of 80%. In bipolar depression, several prospective open studies suggest efficacy (Anand *et al.*, 2005; Ghaemi *et al.*, 2006; Wilson and Findling, 2007). These findings were also followed up in a study of the Stanley Foundation Bipolar Network where 63 bipolar outpatients received zonisamide adjunctive open treatment in mania, bipolar depression, or continuous cycling. In all phases of the illness, the addition of zonisamide appeared helpful (McElroy *et al.*, 2005). In addition, zonisamide seems to have a potentially beneficial side-effect profile in terms of weight loss (Leverich *et al.*, 2005; Wang *et al.*, 2008a). On the other hand, high drop out rates in some open studies due to nausea, vomiting, and sedation hint toward tolerability problems. With currently more controlled data lacking zonisamide may be a future choice as add-on treatment in patients who are not sufficiently responsive to standard therapy (Ghaemi *et al.*, 2008), especially, if weight gain constitutes an additional problem.

5.1.8   TOPIRAMATE

Several open studies and case reports favored topiramate as a potential antimanic agent (Calabrese *et al.*, 2001; Grunze *et al.*, 2001; Marcotte, 1998; Normann *et al.*, 1999) including adolescent mania (Lung *et al.*, 2009) and reporting also about beneficial weight loss properties (Ghaemi *et al.*, 2001; McElroy *et al.*, 2000). However, this positive first impression of antimanic efficacy could not hold true in five rigorous randomized, placebo-controlled trials with negative outcome (Kushner *et al.*, 2006; Roy Chengappa *et al.*, 2006).

For the depressed phase of the illness, an open trial with adjunctive topiramate by McElroy *et al.* (2000) showed no improvement. However, McIntyre *et al.* (2002) found in an eight week, single-blind, randomized comparator trial with bupropion similar efficacy of topiramate in patients with bipolar I or II depression.

As far as long term treatment is concerned, we rely only on open data (Vieta *et al.*, 2004; Wang *et al.*, 2008b). Clearly, more controlled data are needed, not only for bipolar depressed patients but also for long-term treatment in order to make any statement on topiramate's efficacy in bipolar disorder.

As far as its usefulness is concerned, several studies reported on significant weight loss which might make it an attractive add-on medication to counteract weight gain induced by some atypical antipsychotics (Vieta *et al.*, 2004) in the absence of significant drug-drug interactions (Migliardi *et al.*, 2007). However, tolerability might be a problem as studies repeatedly report on higher rates of neurological side effects such as paresthesia, sedation, word-finding difficulty, sleepiness, and forgetfulness compared to placebo. Transient hemiparesis with topiramate has also been reported in rare cases (Stephen, Maxwell, and Brodie, 1999).

5.1.9   GABAPENTIN

Although several open trials have favored gabapentin treatment in acute mania, the two double-blind controlled studies of Pande *et al.* (2000) and Frye *et al.* (2000) could not prove antimanic efficacy of this drug. A more recent study, however, suggests better efficacy of gabapentin than with carbamazepine or lamotrigine in mixed states (Mokhber *et al.*, 2008).

Controlled data for bipolar depression are missing. As gabapentin appears to also have anxioloytic properties (Mula, Pini, and Cassano, 2007) it may still be helpful in selected bipolar patients with anxiety comorbidity or mixed depression and anxiety (Carta *et al.*, 2003). In line with these findings, an open prospective study demonstrated that the utility of this agent in refractory bipolar disorder can be accounted to its anxiolytic effects in patients with comorbid alcohol problems.

A small double blind, placebo controlled add-on study to ongoing treatment investigated the prophylactic effects of gabapentin in euthymic bipolar I and II patients (Vieta *et al.*, 2006). The investigators found a significant advantage for gabapentin compared to placebo for the primary outcome, a change in the Clinical Global Impression Scale for Bipolar Illness, modified version Clinical Global Impression rating Scale, Bipolar version (CGI-BP); however, this study (n = 25) is too small for definite recommendations, but warrants reproduction in larger samples.

5.1.10   RETIGABINE

Retigabine has shown antimanic activity in an animal model (Dencker and Husum, 2009) and in a small pilot trial (Amann *et al.*, 2006). No information has been published on antidepressant or prophylactic efficacy in bipolar disorder.

5.1.11   TIAGABINE

Only open studies exist so far for tiagabine in bipolar disorder. No antimanic effect was observed in an open study by Grunze *et al.* (1999). No convincing effects neither for mania nor depression were seen in a case series of Suppes *et al.* (2002). In the studies of both Grunze and Suppes significant adverse events (provocation of seizures) were observed. The clinical utility of tiagabine, however, may be different when used in low doses for long-term treatment. Case reports of LC Schaffer and CB Schaffer (Schaffer and Schaffer, 1999) showed some degree of stabilization in outpatients previously not responding satisfactorily to standard medication. With the severe side effects which may be provoked by tiagabine, however, it appears unlikely that further controlled studies will be conducted in bipolar disorder.

5.2   CONCLUSIONS

In this chapter, the author has attempted to provide a comprehensive review about treatment options with anticonvulsants other than valproate and lamotrigine in bipolar

Table 5.1 Efficacy of different anticonvulsants in bipolar disorder.

Substance	Mania	Mixed states	Bipolar depression	Maintenance
Carbamazepine	+++	++	+++	++
Oxcarbazepine	++[a]	0	(+)	(+)
Eslicarbazepine	0[b]	0	0	0
Phenytoin	++	0	0	++
Fosphenytoin	-	0	0	0
Clonazepam	+++	0	+	0
Lorazepam	++[c]	0	0	0
Levetiracetam	(+)	(+)	0	(+)
Zonisamide	+	0	+	0
Topiramate	--	0	++	+
Gabapentin	--	+	0	++
Retigabine	+	0	0	0
Tiagabine	-	0	-	(+)
For comparison (not part of this chapter)				
Valproate	+++	++	+++[d]	0[e]
Lamotrigine	--	+	+++[f]	+++

[a] For adolescents with mania.

[b] Inconclusive data: Missed significance for YMRS reduction, but beats placebo for remission rates in mania.

[c] For injectable lorazepam, otherwise 0.

[d] Based on a meta-analysis of four small, Placebo (PLC)-controlled studies (Bond *et al.*, 2010).

[e] Based on the so far only DB, R, PLC-controlled study which failed. However, secondary analyses of this study (Bowden *et al.*, 2000) and open trials are supportive of some prophylactic efficacy of valproate.

[f] Based on single patient data set reanalysis of five failed studies (Geddes, Calabrese, and Goodwin, 2009).

+++ proof of efficacy based on at least one well powered, double blind, randomized, placebo controlled (DB, R, PLC-controlled) study or a high quality metaanalysis, ++ proof of efficacy based on at least one well powered, double blind, randomized study with a well established comparator substance or an underpowered DB, R, PLC-controlled study or a post-hoc analysis of a DB, R, PLC-controlled study, + proof of efficacy based on single blind or open randomized studies, (+) efficacy suggested by open case series, case reports, retrospective chart analysis, 0 inconclusive data or no data available or failed studies, - no efficacy based on open studies, case reports, comparator trials, -- no efficacy based on a negative study (inferiority to placebo or non-separation from placebo in the presence of a comparator showing significance vs. placebo). In the case of contradicting data, for example, positive open, but negative controlled studies, priority was given to the methodological more valuable and reliable study.

disorder. Some treatment options covered in this chapter have only been evaluated in small case series or open studies. Table 5.1 briefly summarizes the main findings for efficacy of the different anticonvulsants in bipolar disorder.

For the future, we may expect more explorative and possibly also controlled studies with currently emerging anticonvulsants (see Luszczki, 2009) not yet considered in this chapter, such as

- Brivaracetam
- Carabersat
- Carisbamate
- DP-Valproic acid (the phosphatidylcholine estric conjugate of valproic acid)
- Fluorofelbamate
- Ganaxolone
- Lacosamide
- Losigamone
- Remacemide
- Rufinamide
- Safinamide
- Seletracetam
- Soretolide
- Stiripentol
- Talampanel
- Valrocemide.

With this increasing portfolio of treatment options not only in epilepsies, but possibly also in bipolar disorder, every review might be already outdated when published. Thus, in a subsequent edition of this book some years from now, this chapter is quite likely to be substantially revised and expanded.

References

Adler, L.W. (1986) Mixed bipolar disorder responsive to lithium and clonazepam. *J. Clin. Psychiatry*, **47**, 49–50.

Amann, B., Sterr, A., Vieta, E. *et al.* (2006) An exploratory open trial on safety and efficacy of the anticonvulsant retigabine in acute manic patients. *J. Clin. Psychopharmacol.*, **26**, 534–536.

Anand, A., Bukhari, L., Jennings, S.A. *et al.* (2005) A preliminary open-label study of zonisamide treatment for bipolar depression in 10 patients. *J. Clin. Psychiatry*, **66**, 195–198.

Andreasen, A.H., Brosen, K., and Damkier, P. (2007) A comparative pharmacokinetic study in healthy volunteers of the effect of carbamazepine and oxcarbazepine on cyp3a4. *Epilepsia*, **48**, 490–496.

Applebaum, J., Levine, J., and Belmaker, R.H. (2003) Intravenous fosphenytoin in acute mania. *J. Clin. Psychiatry*, **64**, 408–409.

Ballenger, J.C. and Post, R.M. (1980) Carbamazepine in manic-depressive illness: a new treatment. *Am. J. Psychiatry*, **137**, 782–790.

Benedetti, A., Lattanzi, L., Pini, S. *et al.* (2004) Oxcarbazepine as add-on treatment in patients with bipolar manic, mixed or depressive episode. *J. Affect. Disord.*, **79**, 273–277.

Bond, D.J., Lam, R.W., and Yatham, L.N. (2010) Divalproex sodium versus placebo in the treatment of acute bipolar depression: a systematic review and meta-analysis. *J. Affect. Disorders*, **124**, 228–234.

Bottai, T., Hue, B., Hillaire-Buys, D. *et al.* (1995) Clonazepam in acute mania: time-blind evaluation of clinical response and concentrations in plasma. *J. Affect. Disord.*, **36**, 21–27.

Bowden, C.L., Calabrese, J.R., McElroy, S.L. *et al.*, Divalproex Maintenance Study Group (2000) A randomized, placebo-controlled 12-month trial of divalproex and lithium in treatment of outpatients with bipolar I disorder. *Arch. Gen. Psychiatry*, **57**, 481–489.

Bradwejn, J., Shriqui, C., Koszycki, D., and Meterissian, G. (1990) Double-blind comparison of the effects of clonazepam and lorazepam in acute mania. *J. Clin. Psychopharmacol.*, **10**, 403–408.

Brambilla, P., Barale, F., and Soares, J.C. (2001) Perspectives on the use of anticonvulsants in the treatment of bipolar disorder. *Int. J. Neuropsychopharmacol.*, **4**, 421–446.

Bräunig, P. and Krüger, S. (2003) Levetiracetam in the treatment of rapid cycling bipolar disorder. *J. Psychopharmacol.*, **17**, 239–241.

Brown, D., Silverstone, T., and Cookson, J. (1989) Carbamazepine compared to haloperidol in acute mania. *Int. Clin. Psychopharmacol.*, **4**, 229–238.

Calabrese, J.R., Keck, P.E. Jr., McElroy, S.L., and Shelton, M.D. (2001) A pilot study of topiramate as monotherapy in the treatment of acute mania. *J. Clin. Psychopharmacol.*, **21**, 340–342.

Carta, M.G., Hardoy, M.C., Hardoy, M.J. *et al.* (2003) The clinical use of gabapentin in bipolar spectrum disorders. *J. Affect. Disord.*, **75**, 83–91.

Chou, J.C., Czobor, P., Charles, O. *et al.* (1999) Acute mania: haloperidol dose and augmentation with lithium or lorazepam. *J. Clin. Psychopharmacol.*, **19**, 500–505.

Chouinard, G. (1985) Antimanic effects of clonazepam. *Psychosomatics*, **26** (Suppl. 12), 7–12.

Chouinard, G. (1987) Clonazepam in acute and maintenance treatment of bipolar affective disorder. *J. Clin. Psychiatry*, **48**, 29–37.

Chouinard, G., Annable, L., Turnier, L. *et al.* (1993) A double-blind randomized clinical trial of rapid tranquilization with I.M. clonazepam and I.M. haloperidol in agitated psychotic patients with manic symptoms. *Can. J. Psychiatry*, **38** (Suppl. 4), 114–121.

Chouinard, G., Young, S.N., and Annable, L. (1983) Antimanic effect of clonazepam. *Biol. Psychiatry*, **18**, 451–466.

Coxhead, N., Silverstone, T., and Cookson, J. (1992) Carbamazepine versus lithium in the prophylaxis of bipolar affective disorder. *Acta Psychiatr. Scand.*, **85**, 114–118.

Curtin, F. and Schulz, P. (2004) Clonazepam and lorazepam in acute mania: a Bayesian meta-analysis. *J. Affect. Disord.*, **78**, 201–208.

Dardennes, R., Even, C., Bange, F., and Heim, A. (1995) Comparison of carbamazepine and lithium in the prophylaxis of bipolar disorders. A meta-analysis. *Br. J. Psychiatry*, **166**, 378–381.

Dencker, D. and Husum, H. (2009) Antimanic efficacy of retigabine in a proposed mouse model of bipolar disorder. *Behav. Brain Res.*, **207**, 78–83.

Denicoff, K.D., Smith-Jackson, E.E., Disney, E.R. *et al.* (1997) Comparative prophylactic efficacy of lithium, carbamazepine, and the combination in bipolar disorder. *J. Clin. Psychiatry*, **58**, 470–478.

Desarkar, P., Das, B., and Sinha, V.K. (2007) Adjuvant levetiracetam in adolescent mania. *J. Clin. Psychopharmacol.*, **27**, 215–216.

Dietrich, D.E., Kropp, S., and Emrich, H.M. (2001) Oxcarbazepine in affective and schizoaffective disorders. *Pharmacopsychiatry*, **34**, 242–250.

El-Mallakh, R.S., Salem, M.R., Chopra, A.S. *et al.* (2009) Adverse event load in bipolar participants receiving either carbamazepine immediate-release or extended-release capsules: a blinded, randomized study. *Int. Clin. Psychopharmacol.*, **24**, 145–149.

Elphick, M. (1985) An open clinical trial of carbamazepine in treatment-resistant bipolar and schizo-affective psychotics. *Br. J. Psychiatry*, **147**, 198–200.

Emrich, H.M. (1990) Studies with Oxcarbazepine (Trileptal) in acute mania. *Int. Clin. Psychopharmacol.*, **5** (Suppl. 1), 83–88.

Emrich, H.M. (1994) Experiences with oxcarbazepine in acute mania, in *Anticonvulsants in Psychiatry* (eds K. Modigh, O.H. Robak, and P. Vestergaard), Wrightson Biomedical Publishing, Ltd, Petersfield, pp. 23–35.

Emrich, H.M., Dose, M., and von Zerssen, D. (1984) Action of sodium-valproate and of oxcar-bazepine in patients with affective disorders, in *Anticonvulsants in Affective Disorders* (eds H.M. Emrich, T. Okuma, and A.A. Müller), Excerpta Medica, Amsterdam, pp. 45–55.

Emrich, H.M., Dose, M., and von Zerssen, D. (1985) The use of sodium valproate, carbamazepine and oxcarbazepine in patients with affective disorders. *J. Affect. Disord.*, **8**, 243–250.

Fenn, H.H., Sommer, B.R., Ketter, T.A., and Alldredge, B. (2006) Safety and tolerability of mood-stabilising anticonvulsants in the elderly. *Expert. Opin. Drug Saf.*, **5**, 401–416.

Frye, M., Ketter, T., Kimbrell, T.A. *et al.* (2000) A placebo controlled study of lamotrigine and gabapentin monotherapy in refractory mood disorders. *J. Clin. Psychopharmacol.*, **20**, 607–614.

Gajwani, P., Forsthoff, A., Muzina, D. *et al.* (2005) Antiepileptic drugs in mood-disordered patients. *Epilepsia*, **46** (Suppl. 4), 38–44.

Geddes, J.R., Calabrese, J.R., and Goodwin, G.M. (2009) Lamotrigine for treatment of bipolar depression: independent meta-analysis and meta-regression of individual patient data from five randomised trials. *Br. J. Psychiatry*, **194**, 4–9.

Ghaemi, N.S., Ko, J.Y., and Katzow, J.J. (2002) Oxcarbazepine treatment of refractory bipolar disorder: a retrospective chart review. *Bipolar Disord.*, **4**, 70–74.

Ghaemi, S.N., Manwani, S.G., Katzow, J.J. *et al.* (2001) Topiramate treatment of bipolar spectrum disorders: a retrospective chart review. *Ann. Clin. Psychiatry*, **13**, 185–189.

Ghaemi, S.N., Shirzadi, A.A., Klugman, J. *et al.* (2008) Is adjunctive open-label zonisamide effective for bipolar disorder? *J. Affect. Disord.*, **105**, 311–314.

Ghaemi, S.N., Zablotsky, B., Filkowski, M.M. *et al.* (2006) An open prospective study of zon-isamide in acute bipolar depression. *J. Clin. Psychopharmacol.*, **26**, 385–388.

Goldberg, J.F. and Burdick, K.E. (2002) Levetiracetam for acute mania. *Am. J. Psychiatry*, **159**, 148.

Goncalves, N. and Stoll, K.-D. (1985) Carbamazepin bei manischen Syndromen. Eine kontrollierte Doppelblind-Studie. *Nervenarzt*, **56**, 43–47.

Greil, W. and Kleindienst, N. (1999a) Lithium versus carbamazepine in the maintenance treatment of bipolar II disorder and bipolar disorder not otherwise specified. *Int. Clin. Psychopharmacol.*, **14**, 283–285.

Greil, W. and Kleindienst, N. (1999b) The comparative prophylactic efficacy of lithium and car-bamazepine in patients with bipolar I disorder. *Int. Clin. Psychopharmacol.*, **14**, 277–281.

Greil, W., Ludwig-Mayerhofer, W., Erazo, N. *et al.* (1997a) Lithium vs carbamazepine in the maintenance treatment of schizoaffective disorder: a randomised study. *Eur. Arch. Psychiatry Clin. Neurosci.*, **247**, 42–50.

Greil, W., Ludwig-Mayerhofer, W., Erazo, N. *et al.* (1997b) Lithium versus carbamazepine in the maintenance treatment of bipolar disorders–a randomised study. *J. Affect. Disord.*, **43**, 151–161.

Grunze, H., Erfurth, A., Marcuse, A. *et al.* (1999) Tiagabine appears not to be efficacious in the treatment of acute mania. *J. Clin. Psychiatry*, **60**, 759–762.

Grunze, H., Langosch, J., Born, C. *et al.* (2003) Levetiracetam in the treatment of acute mania: an open add-on study with an on-off-on design. *J. Clin. Psychiatry*, **64**, 781–784.

Grunze, H.C., Normann, C., Langosch, J. *et al.* (2001) Antimanic efficacy of topiramate in 11 patients in an open trial with an on-off-on design. *J. Clin. Psychiatry*, **62**, 464–468.

Haefely, W. (1983) The biological basis of benzodizepine actions. *J. Psychoactive Drugs*, **15**, 19–39.

Hartong, E.G., Moleman, P., Hoogduin, C.A. *et al.* (2003) Prophylactic efficacy of lithium versus carbamazepine in treatment-naive bipolar patients. *J. Clin. Psychiatry*, **64**, 144–151.

Hellewell, J.S. (2002) Oxcarbazepine (Trileptal) in the treatment of bipolar disorders: a review of efficacy and tolerability. *J. Affect. Disord.*, **72** (Suppl. 1), 23–34.

Hirschfeld, R.M. and Kasper, S. (2004) A review of the evidence for carbamazepine and oxcarbazepine in the treatment of bipolar disorder. *Int. J. Neuropsychopharmacol.*, **7**, 507–522.

Hovinga, C.A. (2001) Levetiracetam: a novel antiepileptic drug. *Pharmacotherapy*, **21**, 1375–1388.

Hummel, B., Walden, J., Stampfer, R. *et al.* (2002) Acute antimanic efficacy and safety of oxcarbazepine in an open trial with an on-off-on design. *Bipolar Disord.*, **4**, 412–417.

Juruena, M.F., Ottoni, G.L., Machado-Vieira, R. *et al.* (2009) Bipolar I and II disorder residual symptoms: oxcarbazepine and carbamazepine as add-on treatment to lithium in a double-blind, randomized trial. *Prog. Neuropsychopharmacol. Biol. Psychiatry*, **33**, 94–99.

Kakkar, A.K., Rehan, H.S., Unni, K.E. *et al.* (2009) Comparative efficacy and safety of oxcarbazepine versus divalproex sodium in the treatment of acute mania: a pilot study. *Eur. Psychiatry*, **24**, 178–182.

Kanba, S., Yagi, G., Kamijima, K. *et al.* (1994) The first open study of zonisamide, a novel anticonvulsant, shows efficacy in mania. *Prog. Neuropsychopharmacol. Biol. Psychiatry*, **18**, 707–715.

Kaufman, K.R. (2004) Monotherapy treatment of bipolar disorder with levetiracetam. *Epilepsy Behav.*, **5**, 1017–1020.

Kishimoto, A., Kamata, K., Sugihara, T. *et al.* (1988) Treatment of depression with clonazepam. *Acta Psychiatr. Scand.*, **77**, 81–86.

Klein, E., Bental, E., Lerer, B., and Belmaker, R.H. (1984) Carbamazepine and haloperidol v placebo and haloperidol in excited psychoses. A controlled study. *Arch. Gen. Psychiatry*, **41**, 165–170.

Krüger, S., Sarkar, R., Pietsch, R. *et al.* (2008) Levetiracetam as monotherapy or add-on to valproate in the treatment of acute mania-a randomized open-label study. *Psychopharmacology (Berl.)*, **198**, 297–299.

Kushner, S.F., Khan, A., Lane, R., and Olson, W.H. (2006) Topiramate monotherapy in the management of acute mania: results of four double-blind placebo-controlled trials. *Bipolar Disord.*, **8**, 15–27.

Kyomen, H.H. (2006) The use of levetiracetam to decrease mania in elderly bipolar patients. *Am. J. Geriatr. Psychiatry*, **14**, 985.

Lamberty, Y., Margineanu, D.G., and Klitgaard, H. (2001) Effect of the new antiepileptic drug levetiracetam in an animal model of mania. *Epilepsy Behav.*, **2**, 454–459.

Lenox, R.H., Newhouse, P.A., Creelman, W.L., and Whitaker, T.M. (1992) Adjunctive treatment of manic agitation with lorazepam versus haloperidol: a double-blind study. *J. Clin. Psychiatry*, **53**, 47–52.

Lerer, B., Moore, N., Meyendorff, E. *et al.* (1987) Carbamazepine versus lithium in mania: a double-blind study. *J. Clin. Psychiatry*, **48**, 89–93.

Leverich, G., McElroy, S., Altshuler, L. *et al.* (2005) The anticonvulsant zonisamide in bipolar illness: Clinical response and weight loss. *Aspects Affect*, **1**, 53–56.

Lima, L. (1991) Region-selective reduction of brain serotonin turnover rate and serotonin agonist- induced behavior in mice treated with clonazepam. *Pharmacol. Biochem. Behav.*, **39**, 671–676.

Lung, F.W., Liu, C.L., Wang, C.S., and Tzeng, D.S. (2009) Adjunctive topiramate treatment for a refractory familial adolescent mania. *World J. Biol. Psychiatry*, **10**, 74–77.

Luszczki, J.J. (2009) Third-generation antiepileptic drugs: mechanisms of action, pharmacokinetics and interactions. *Pharmacol. Rep.*, **61**, 197–216.

Lusznat, R.M., Murphy, D.P., and Nunn, C.M. (1988) Carbamazepine vs lithium in the treatment and prophylaxis of mania. *Br. J. Psychiatry*, **153**, 198–204.

Marcotte, D. (1998) Use of topiramate, a new anti-epileptic as a mood stabilizer. *J. Affect. Disord.*, **50**, 245–251.

Mazza, M., Di, N.M., Martinotti, G. *et al.* (2007) Oxcarbazepine in bipolar disorder: a critical review of the literature. *Expert. Opin. Pharmacother.*, **8**, 649–656.

McCormack, P.L. and Robinson, D.M. (2009) Eslicarbazepine acetate. *CNS Drugs*, **23**, 71–79.

McElroy, S.L., Suppes, T., Keck, P.E. *et al.* (2000) Open-label adjunctive topiramate in the treatment of bipolar disorders. *Biol. Psychiatry*, **47**, 1025–1033.

McElroy, S.L., Suppes, T., Keck, P.E. Jr. *et al.* (2005) Open-label adjunctive zonisamide in the treatment of bipolar disorders: a prospective trial. *J. Clin. Psychiatry*, **66**, 617–624.

McIntyre, R.S., Mancini, D.A., McCann, S. *et al.* (2002) Topiramate versus bupropion SR when added to mood stabilizer therapy for the depressive phase of bipolar disorder: a preliminary single-blind study. *Bipolar Disord.*, **4**, 207–213.

Meehan, K., Zhang, F., David, S. *et al.* (2001) A double-blind, randomized comparison of the efficacy and safety of intramuscular injections of olanzapine, lorazepam, or placebo in treating acutely agitated patients diagnosed with bipolar mania. *J. Clin. Psychopharmacol.*, **21**, 389–397.

Migliardi, G., D'Arrigo, C., Santoro, V. *et al.* (2007) Effect of topiramate on plasma concentrations of clozapine, olanzapine, risperidone, and quetiapine in patients with psychotic disorders. *Clin. Neuropharmacol.*, **30**, 107–113.

Mishory, A., Winokur, M., and Bersudsky, Y. (2003) Prophylactic effect of phenytoin in bipolar disorder: a controlled study. *Bipolar Disord.*, **5**, 464–467.

Mishory, A., Yaroslavsky, Y., Bersudsky, Y., and Belmaker, R.H. (2000) Phenytoin as an antimanic anticonvulsant: a controlled study. *Am. J. Psychiatry*, **157**, 463–465.

Mokhber, N., Lane, C.J., Azarpazhooh, M.R. *et al.* (2008) Anticonvulsant treatments of dysphoric mania: a trial of gabapentin, lamotrigine and carbamazepine in Iran. *Neuropsychiatr. Dis. Treat.*, **4**, 227–234.

Morishita, S. and Aoki, S. (1999) A trial of clonazepam treatment for manic-depressive psychoses. *Nihon Shinkei Seishin Yakurigaku Zasshi*, **19**, 127–132.

Morrow, J., Russell, A., Guthrie, E. *et al.* (2006) Malformation risks of antiepileptic drugs in pregnancy: a prospective study from the UK Epilepsy and Pregnancy Register. *J. Neurol. Neurosurg. Psychiatr.*, **77**, 193–198.

Mula, M., Pini, S., and Cassano, G.B. (2007) The role of anticonvulsant drugs in anxiety disorders: a critical review of the evidence. *J. Clin. Psychopharmacol.*, **27**, 263–272.

Müller, A.A. and Stoll, K.-D. (1984) Carbamazepine and oxcarbamazepine in the treatment of manic syndromes: studies in Germany, in *Anticonvulsants in Affective Disorders* (eds H.M. Emrich, T. Okuma and A.A. Müller), Excerpta Medica, Amsterdam, pp. 139–147.

Nemets, B., Bersudsky, Y., and Belmaker, R.H. (2005) Controlled double-blind trial of phenytoin vs. fluoxetine in major depressive disorder. *J. Clin. Psychiatry*, **66**, 586–590.

Normann, C., Langosch, J., Schaerer, L.O. *et al.* (1999) Treatment of acute mania with topiramate. *Am. J. Psychiatry*, **156**, 2014.

Okada, M., Hirano, T., Kawata, Y. *et al.* (1999) Biphasic effects of zonisamide on serotonergic system in rat hippocampus. *Epilepsy Res.*, **34**, 187–197.

Okada, M., Kaneko, S., Hirano, T. *et al.* (1995) Effects of zonisamide on dopaminergic system. *Epilepsy Res.*, **22**, 193–205.

Okuma, T., Inanaga, K., Otsuki, S. *et al.* (1979) Comparison of the antimanic efficacy of carbamazepine and chlorpromazine: a double-blind controlled study. *Psychopharmacology*, **66**, 211–217.

Okuma, T., Inanaga, K., Otsuki, S. *et al.* (1981) A preliminary double-blind study on the efficacy of carbamazepine in prophylaxis of manic-depressive illness. *Psychopharmacology (Berl.)*, **73**, 95–96.

Okuma, T., Kishimoto, A., Inoue, K. *et al.* (1973) Anti-manic and prophylactic effects of carbamazepine (Tegretol) on manic depressive psychosis. A preliminary report. *Folia Psychiatr. Neurol. Jpn.*, **27**, 283–297.

Okuma, T., Yamashita, I., Takahashi, R. *et al.* (1990) Comparison of the antimanic efficacy of carbamazepine and lithium carbonate by double-blind controlled study. *Pharmacopsychiatry*, **23**, 143–150.

Oommen, K.J. and Mathews, S. (1999) Zonisamide: a new antiepileptic drug. *Clin. Neuropharmacol.*, **22**, 192–200.

Pande, A.C. (1988) Clonazepam treatment of atypical bipolar disorder. *Psychosomatics*, **29**, 333–335.

Pande, A.C., Crockatt, J.G., Janney, C.A. *et al.*, Gabapentin Bipolar Disorder Study Group (2000) Gabapentin in bipolar disorder: a placebo-controlled trial of adjunctive therapy. *Bipolar Disord.*, **2**, 249–255.

Placidi, G.F., Lenzi, A., Lazzerini, F. *et al.* (1986) The comparative efficacy and safety of carbamazepine versus lithium: a randomized, double-blind 3-year trial in 83 patients. *J. Clin. Psychiatry*, **47**, 490–494.

Popova, E., Leighton, C., Bernabarre, A. *et al.* (2007) Oxcarbazepine in the treatment of bipolar and schizoaffective disorders. *Expert. Rev. Neurother.*, **7**, 617–626.

Post, R.M., Ketter, T.A., Uhde, T., and Ballenger, J.C. (2007) Thirty years of clinical experience with carbamazepine in the treatment of bipolar illness: principles and practice. *CNS Drugs*, **21**, 47–71.

Post, R.M., Uhde, T.W., Roy-Byrne, P.P., and Joffe, R.T. (1987) Correlates of antimanic response to carbamazepine. *Psychiatry Res.*, **21**, 71–83.

Pratoomsri, W., Yatham, L.N., Bond, D.J. *et al.* (2006) Oxcarbazepine in the treatment of bipolar disorder: a review. *Can. J. Psychiatry*, **51**, 540–545.

Pratoomsri, W., Yatham, L.N., Sohn, C.H. *et al.* (2005) Oxcarbazepine add-on in the treatment of refractory bipolar disorder. *Bipolar Disord.*, **7** (Suppl. 5), 37–42.

Reinstein, M.J., Sonnenberg, J.G., Hedberg, T.G. *et al.* (2003) Oxcarbazepine versus divalproex sodium for the continuing treatment of mania. *Clin. Drug Investig.*, **23**, 671–677.

Robertson, B., Grunze, H., Versavel, M. *et al.* (2010) Results of a double-blind, randomized, dose-titration, placebo controlled multicenter trial (SCO/BIA-2093-203 Study) on Safety and Efficacy of eslicarbazepine acetate (BIA 2-093) for acute manic episodes associated with bipolar I disorder. *Bipolar Disord.*, (Suppl. 12), 46.

Roy Chengappa, K.N., Schwarzman, L.K., Hulihan, J.F. *et al.* (2006) Adjunctive topiramate therapy in patients receiving a mood stabilizer for bipolar I disorder: a randomized, placebo-controlled trial. *J. Clin. Psychiatry*, **67**, 1698–1706.

Sachs, G.S. (1990) Use of clonazepam for bipolar affective disorder. *J. Clin. Psychiatry*, **51**, 31–34.

Sachs, G.S., Rosenbaum, J.F., and Jones, L. (1990) Adjunctive clonazepam for maintenance treatment of bipolar affective disorder. *J. Clin. Psychopharmacol.*, **10**, 42–47.

Sachs, G.S., Weilburg, J.B., and Rosenbaum, J.F. (1990) Clonazepam vs. neuroleptics as adjuncts to lithium maintenance. *Psychopharmacol. Bull.*, **26**, 137–143.

Schaffer, L.C. and Schaffer, C.B. (1999) Tiagabine and the treatment of refractory bipolar disorder. *Am. J. Psychiatry*, **156**, 2014–2015.

Schneck, C.D. (2002) Bipolar disorder in neurologic illness. *Curr. Treat. Options Neurol.*, **4**, 477–486.

Small, J.G., Klapper, M.H., Milstein, V. *et al.* (1996) Comparison of therapeutic modalities for mania. *Psychopharmacol. Bull.*, **32**, 623–627.

Spina, E., Pisani, F., and Perucca, E. (1996) Clinically significant pharmacokinetic drug interactions with carbamazepine. An update. *Clin. Pharmacokinet.*, **31**, 198–214.

Stephen, L.J., Maxwell, J.E., and Brodie, M.J. (1999) Transient hemiparesis with topiramate. *Br. Med. J.*, **318**, 845.

Stoll, K.D., Bisson, H.E., Fischer, E. *et al.* (1986) Carbamazepine versus haloperidol in manic syndromes, in *Biological Psychiatry 1985* (eds C. Shagass, R.C. Josiassen, W.H. Bridger *et al.*), Elsevier, New York, pp. 332–334.

Suppes, T., Chisholm, K.A., Dhavale, D. *et al.* (2002) Tiagabine in treatment refractory bipolar disorder: a clinical case series. *Bipolar Disord.*, **4**, 283–289.

Suppes, T., Kelly, D.I., Hynan, L.S. *et al.* (2007) Comparison of two anticonvulsants in a randomized, single-blind treatment of hypomanic symptoms in patients with bipolar disorder. *Aust. N.Z. J Psychiatry*, **41**, 397–402.

Thase, M.E., Jonas, A., Khan, A. *et al.* (2008) Aripiprazole monotherapy in nonpsychotic bipolar I depression: results of 2 randomized, placebo-controlled studies. *J. Clin. Psychopharmacol.*, **28**, 13–20.

Thies-Flechtner, K., Müller-Oerlinghausen, B., Seibert, W. *et al.* (1996) Effect of prophylactic treatment on suicide risk in patients with major affective disorders. Data from a randomized prospective trial. *Pharmacopsychiatry*, **29**, 103–107.

Tohen, M., Bowden, C.L., Smulevich, A.B. *et al.* (2008) Olanzapine plus carbamazepine v. carbamazepine alone in treating manic episodes. *Br. J. Psychiatry*, **192**, 135–143.

Vasudev, K., Goswami, U., and Kohli, K. (2000) Carbamazepine and valproate monotherapy: feasibility, relative safety and efficacy, and therapeutic drug monitoring in manic disorder. *Psychopharmacology (Berl.)*, **150**, 15–23.

Vasudev, A., Macritchie, K., Watson, S. *et al.* (2008) Oxcarbazepine in the maintenance treatment of bipolar disorder. *Cochrane Database Syst. Rev.* (doi: 10.1002/14651858.CD005171.pub2), CD005171.

Vieta, E., Cruz, N., Garcia-Campayo, J. *et al.* (2008) A double-blind, randomized, placebo-controlled prophylaxis trial of oxcarbazepine as adjunctive treatment to lithium in the long-term treatment of bipolar I and II disorder. *Int. J. Neuropsychopharmacol.*, **11**, 445–452.

Vieta, E., Manuel, G.J., Martinez-Aran, A. *et al.* (2006) A double-blind, randomized, placebo-controlled, prophylaxis study of adjunctive gabapentin for bipolar disorder. *J. Clin. Psychiatry*, **67**, 473–477.

Vieta, E., Sanchez-Moreno, J., Goikolea, J.M. *et al.* (2004) Effects on weight and outcome of long-term olanzapine-topiramate combination treatment in bipolar disorder. *J. Clin. Psychopharmacol.*, **24**, 374–378.

Wagner, K.D., Kowatch, R.A., Emslie, G.J. *et al.* (2006) A double-blind, randomized, placebo-controlled trial of oxcarbazepine in the treatment of bipolar disorder in children and adolescents. *Am. J. Psychiatry*, **163**, 1179–1186.

Wang, P.W., Yang, Y.S., Chandler, R.A. *et al.* (2008a) Adjunctive zonisamide for weight loss in euthymic bipolar disorder patients: a pilot study. *J. Psychiatr. Res.*, **42**, 451–457.

Wang, T.Y., Shiah, I.S., Chen, C.K. *et al.* (2008b) Topiramate monotherapy in the maintenance treatment of juvenile bipolar disorder. *Prog. Neuropsychopharmacol. Biol. Psychiatry*, **32**, 306–307.

Watkins, S.E., Callender, K., Thomas, D.R. *et al.* (1987) The effect of carbamazepine and lithium on remission from affective illness. *Br. J. Psychiatry*, **150**, 180–182.

Weisler, R.H., Kalali, A.H., and Ketter, T.A. (2004) A multicenter, randomized, double-blind, placebo-controlled trial of extended-release carbamazepine capsules as monotherapy for bipolar disorder patients with manic or mixed episodes. *J. Clin. Psychiatry*, **65**, 478–484.

Weisler, R.H., Keck, P.E. Jr., Swann, A.C. *et al.* (2005) Extended-release carbamazepine capsules as monotherapy for acute mania in bipolar disorder: a multicenter, randomized, double-blind, placebo-controlled trial. *J. Clin. Psychiatry*, **66**, 323–330.

Wilson, M.S. and Findling, R.L. (2007) Zonisamide for bipolar depression. *Expert. Opin. Pharmacother.*, **8**, 111–113.

Winkler, D., Willeit, M., Wolf, R. *et al.* (2003) Clonazepam in the long-term treatment of patients with unipolar depression, bipolar and schizoaffective disorder. *Eur. Neuropsychopharmacol.*, **13**, 129–134.

Wolfsperger, M., Greil, W., Rossler, W., and Grohmann, R. (2007) Pharmacological treatment of acute mania in psychiatric in-patients between 1994 and 2004. *J. Affect. Disord.*, **99**, 9–17.

Yatham, L.N., Grossman, F., Augustyns, I. *et al.* (2003) Mood stabilisers plus risperidone or placebo in the treatment of acute mania. International, double-blind, randomised controlled trial. *Br. J. Psychiatry*, **182**, 141–147.

Yerevanian, B.I., Koek, R.J., and Mintz, J. (2003) Lithium, anticonvulsants and suicidal behavior in bipolar disorder. *J. Affect. Disord.*, **73**, 223–228.

Zhang, Z.J., Kang, W.H., Li, Q., and Tan, Q.R. (2007a) The beneficial effects of the herbal medicine Free and Easy Wanderer Plus (FEWP) for mood disorders: double-blind, placebo-controlled studies. *J. Psychiatr. Res.*, **41**, 828–836.

Zhang, Z.J., Kang, W.H., Tan, Q.R. *et al.* (2007b) Adjunctive herbal medicine with carbamazepine for bipolar disorders: a double-blind, randomized, placebo-controlled study. *J. Psychiatr. Res.*, **41**, 360–369.

Zimbroff, D.L., Marcus, R.N., Manos, G. *et al.* (2007) Management of acute agitation in patients with bipolar disorder: efficacy and safety of intramuscular aripiprazole. *J. Clin. Psychopharmacol.*, **27**, 171–176.

6

Olanzapine in Treatment for Bipolar Disorder

Mauricio Tohen[1], Giedra Campbell[2] and Juan-Carlos Gómez[3]
[1]Department of Psychiatry, Division of Mood and Anxiety Disorders,
University of Texas Health Science Center at San Antonio, TX, USA
[2]Scientific Communications, Lilly Research Laboratories,
Lilly Corporate Center, IN, USA
[3]Psychosis Global Development Team, Lilly Research Laboratories,
Lilly Corporate Center, IN, USA

6.1 INTRODUCTION

Over the past several decades, significant advances have been made in the pharmacologic treatment of bipolar disorder. Yet a significant proportion of patients with this condition are not responsive or only partially responsive to existing treatments, and among those who do obtain symptomatic relief, the majority subsequently experience relapse. This unmet medical need is being addressed by the introduction of novel medications and strategies for adjunctive therapy.

Typical antipsychotic agents such as haloperidol have been used extensively, either alone or in combination with other agents, to treat bipolar disorder. A meta-analysis of published reports through the year 2000 (Tohen *et al.*, 2001) found that 89% of hospitalized patients with mania and 64% of outpatients with mania were treated with typical antipsychotics. While the efficacy of conventional antipsychotic agents for this condition has been well established, considerable concerns have been raised regarding their associated side effects, especially long-term side effects (Kane and Smith, 1982). The most prominent of these are extrapyramidal symptoms (EPSs), of which tardive dyskinesia is the most serious. More importantly, some studies have reported an increased risk of relapse into depression and higher rates of discontinuation in patients with mania who received mood stabilizer combined with a typical antipsychotic, compared with mood stabilizers alone (Zarate and Tohen, 2004; Morgan, 1972). Thus, the clinical benefits of typical antipsychotic use in bipolar disorder are frequently offset by poor tolerability and the risk of noncompliance.

Bipolar Psychopharmacotherapy: Caring for the patient, Second Edition. Edited by Hagop S. Akiskal and Mauricio Tohen.
© 2011 John Wiley & Sons, Ltd. Published 2011 by John Wiley & Sons, Ltd.

Atypical or second generation antipsychotics are a heterogeneous group of medications that were introduced in the 1990s. Olanzapine was the first atypical antipsychotic medication to be approved in the United States (US) and the European Union (EU) to treat acute bipolar mania. It was also the first atypical antipsychotic to be approved both in the US and the EU for maintenance treatment and relapse prevention in bipolar disorder. It is also approved as an adjunct to lithium or valproate in the treatment of acute mania. In addition, it has been approved in the US to treat bipolar mania in adolescents, and to treat bipolar depression in adults when used in combination with fluoxetine (that is, olanzapine/fluoxetine combination).

Olanzapine has a broad range of action, binding with high affinity to dopaminergic, serotonergic, adrenergic, muscarinic, and histaminergic receptors. The binding characteristics of olanzapine to dopamine D2 receptors are consistent with the hypothesis that functional D2 receptor antagonism is an important factor in antipsychotic efficacy. Olanzapine's higher dissociation constant at the D2 receptor, relative to haloperidol and other typical antipsychotic medications, may account for its lower risk of EPS or tardive dyskinesia (Seeman and Kapur, 2000). The unique pattern of binding of olanzapine to other receptor sites may provide multiple potential mechanisms of therapeutic action and may account for the efficacy of olanzapine in treating the complex symptoms of bipolar disorder (Bymaster *et al.*, 1996).

This chapter reviews the rationale behind the study design and the data from double-blind randomized controlled trials that have evaluated the efficacy of olanzapine alone and of olanzapine in combination with other agents and olanzapine combination therapy in treating bipolar disorder. The safety and tolerability of olanzapine is also briefly reviewed.

6.2 RATIONALE IN THE CLINICAL TRIAL DEVELOPMENT OF OLANZAPINE

Considering the complex nature of bipolar disorder, it is essential to evaluate the potential value of new therapies in all phases of the illness: mania, depression, and maintenance of euthymia. The approach adopted in the evaluation of olanzapine was to establish first the safety and efficacy of the medication as a treatment for acute mania in adults. The value of adjunctive therapy to improve efficacy when treating acute mania was also explored using olanzapine in combination with existing drug therapies, such as lithium or valproate. This was followed by evaluations of efficacy and safety for treating acute bipolar depression with olanzapine and olanzapine/fluoxetine combination. Once efficacy and safety were determined for the acute phases of the disorder, olanzapine was studied as a treatment for relapse prevention or maintenance of response. Finally, the efficacy and safety of olanzapine in adolescents with bipolar disorder was assessed. Thus, a comprehensive evaluation of olanzapine – either alone or in combination with other treatments – has led to regulatory approvals for all phases of bipolar disorder and has increased the number of options available to clinicians to treat patients with this disorder.

6.3 EFFICACY IN THE TREATMENT OF ACUTE MANIA

6.3.1 PLACEBO-CONTROLLED TRIALS

The initial approval of olanzapine in the treatment of bipolar disorder by the US Food and Drug Administration (FDA) was based on two randomized, double-blind, placebo-controlled trials comparing olanzapine with placebo in adult patients having diagnosis of bipolar disorder according to the Diagnostic and Statistical Manual of Mental Disorders, 4th edition (DSM-IV). The first trial (Tohen *et al.*, 1999) investigated 139 patients for three weeks, and the second trial (Tohen *et al.*, 2000) investigated 115 patients for four weeks. In both trials, patients treated with olanzapine showed significantly greater mean improvements in Young Mania Rating Scale (YMRS) total score, the primary efficacy measure, than placebo-treated patients (olanzapine 10.3 versus placebo -4.9, $p < 0.019$ (Tohen *et al.*, 1999) and olanzapine -14.8 versus placebo -8.1, $p < 0.001$ (Tohen *et al.*, 2000)). Based on clinical response criteria, defined as an improvement of $\geq 50\%$ in YMRS total score from baseline to endpoint and an endpoint YMRS total score ≥ 12, significantly more olanzapine-treated patients than placebo-treated patients responded to therapy in both trials (olanzapine 49% versus placebo 24%, $p < 0.004$ (Tohen *et al.*, 1999) and olanzapine 65% versus placebo 43%, $p = 0.02$ (Tohen *et al.*, 2000)). In both trials, the mean modal dose was similar (14.9 mg (Tohen *et al.*, 1999) and 16.4 mg (Tohen *et al.*, 2000)), even though the starting dose was 10 mg in the (Tohen *et al.*, 1999) trial and 15 mg for the (Tohen *et al.*, 2000) trial. There were no significant differences with respect to measures of parkinsonism, akathisia, and dyskinesia between olanzapine- and placebo-treated patients in either study. The results from these two studies confirm that relative to placebo, olanzapine had superior efficacy for the treatment of acute mania symptoms and was generally well tolerated.

As noted previously, the two trials differed in the starting dose of olanzapine, with patients starting on 10 mg/day in the first trial (Tohen *et al.*, 1999) and 15 mg/day in the second trial (Tohen *et al.*, 2000). Significant differences in mania symptoms relative to placebo were observed at week 3 in the first study (Tohen *et al.*, 1999) and at week 1 in the second (Tohen *et al.*, 2000). The benefits of early response to therapy may be partially reflected in a significantly lower rate of premature discontinuation due to lack of efficacy in the first trial (olanzapine 29% versus placebo 48% during three weeks, $p = 0.02$). Notably, there were no clinically meaningful differences in adverse events between the two studies. Based on the observations of an earlier onset of action and the lack of increased adverse event risk, subsequent acute mania studies used a starting dose of 15 mg/day.

In another placebo-controlled trial of olanzapine conducted in Japan, 221 patients experiencing an acute manic or mixed episode of bipolar disorder were randomly assigned to receive olanzapine (5–20 mg/day, n = 104), placebo (n = 97), or haloperidol (2.5–10 mg/day, n = 20) (Katagiri *et al.*, 2010). Patients assigned to the olanzapine and haloperidol groups were treated for six weeks; patients assigned to the placebo group received placebo for three weeks and then were switched to olanzapine after three weeks. The olanzapine-placebo comparison was based on mean change in YMRS after three weeks of therapy. (The haloperidol comparison results, based on remission rates at six weeks, are discussed later in this review.) Mean changes in YMRS total score from baseline to endpoint after three weeks of therapy were −12.6 for the olanzapine group and −6.8 for the placebo group (p < 0.001).

6.3.2   STUDIES WITH ACTIVE CONTROLS

The efficacy of olanzapine for the treatment of acute mania has also been examined in relation to other psychotropic agents. This review will describe studies of olanzapine compared with lithium, risperidone, haloperidol, valproate, and asenapine, followed by studies of olanzapine as adjunctive therapy with valproate, lithium, or carbamazepine. Very few studies have directly compared olanzapine to lithium. In an early small trial (N = 30) comparing olanzapine and lithium (Berk, Ichim, and Brook, 1999), there were no significant outcome differences between the two groups on any of the primary outcome measures. In a more recent trial conducted in China, olanzapine (5–20 mg/day, n = 69) and lithium (600–1800 mg/day, n = 71) were compared in adult patients with a manic or mixed episode of bipolar mania (Niufan et al., 2008). The primary efficacy measure was mean change from baseline on the Clinical Global Impressions (Bipolar Version) Overall Severity of Illness (CGI-BP) score; the YMRS and Brief Psychiatric Rating Scale were also assessed as secondary measures. Significantly greater improvements were observed in patients assigned to olanzapine relative to those assigned to lithium on the CGI-BP overall severity score (olanzapine −2.83 versus lithium −2.22, p = 0.009), YMRS (olanzapine −24.63 versus lithium −20.15, p = 0.013), Brief Psychiatric Rating Scale (olanzapine −11.16 versus lithium −9.04, p = 0.032), and CGI-BP severity of mania score (olanzapine −2.91 versus lithium −2.33, p = 0.012). A significantly greater percentage of patients experienced clinical response, defined as ≥50% decrease in YMRS score, in the olanzapine group (87%) as compared with lithium group (73.2%) (odds ratio = 2.71 [95% confidence interval (CI): 1.07–6.87], p = 0.035). The mean (± SD) daily dose of olanzapine was 17.8 (± 2.55) mg/day, while the mean (± SD) daily dose of lithium was 1110 (± 257.4) mg/day.

In a three-week, randomized, controlled, double-blind, parallel, multicenter study (Perlis et al., 2006), olanzapine 5–20 mg/day (n = 165) was compared with risperidone 1–6 mg/day (n = 164) among hospital inpatients with nonpsychotic manic or mixed episode. Significantly more patients (p = 0.019) completed the study in the olanzapine group (79%) than in the risperidone group (67%). Changes from baseline to week 3, according to mixed-model repeated measures (MMRMs) analysis, were not significantly different between treatment groups for YMRS (olanzapine −15.03, risperidone −16.62) or CGI-BP (olanzapine −1.64, risperidone −1.46). In all, 62.1% of olanzapine-treated patients achieved response (YMRS reduction ≥50%) compared with 59.5% of risperidone-treated patients; and 38.5% of olanzapine-treated patients remitted (YMRS ≤12 and 21-item Hamilton Rating Scale for Depression scale (HAMD-21) ≤8 at endpoint) compared with 28.5% of risperidone-treated patients. These differences were not significant.

Efficacy, safety, and quality-of-life measures were assessed in a direct comparison between olanzapine (5–20 mg/day, n = 234) and haloperidol (3–15 mg/day, n = 219) in a randomized controlled trial consisting of two successive, six-week, double-blind periods in adult patients with bipolar mania (Tohen *et al.*, 2003a). In addition to assessing mania symptoms, this trial also assessed symptoms of depression using the HAMD-21 to evaluate the potential risk of depressogenic effects associated with these treatments. Rates of remission, defined as YMRS scores ≤12 and HAMD-21 scores ≤8 at week 6 of therapy, were similar (p = 0.15) for olanzapine-treated patients (52.1%) and haloperidol-treated patients (46.1%), suggesting a similar efficacy for both agents. However, for a subgroup of patients whose index episode did not include psychotic features, rates of remission were significantly greater for olanzapine-treated patients (56.7%) relative to haloperidol-treated patients (41.6%) (p = 0.04). For the subset of patients who entered the study not depressed but became depressed during the course of the trial, haloperidol therapy was associated with a significantly shorter time to switch into depression (p = 0.04) (Figure 6.1).

Olanzapine was also compared with haloperidol in the Japanese trial described earlier (Katagiri *et al.*, 2010). In that trial, patients with manic or mixed episode bipolar disorder received olanzapine, haloperidol, or placebo. Patients assigned to olanzapine or haloperidol were treated for six weeks; patients assigned to placebo received placebo for

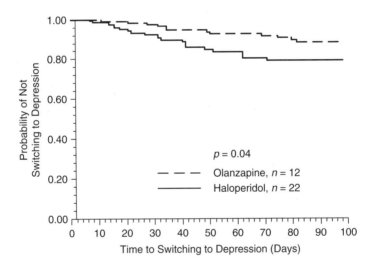

$$p = 0.04$$

– – – Olanzapine, $n = 12$

⎯⎯ Haloperidol, $n = 22$

Figure 6.1 Time to switch to depression for patients who were not clinically depressed at baseline (HAMD-21 ≤ 8). Time to switch to depression (HAMD-21 ≥ 15) was significantly longer (log-rank test $\chi^2_1 = 4.1$; p = 0.04) for the olanzapine group compared with the haloperidol group. During the 12-week period, 22 haloperidol- and 12 olanzapine-treated patients switched to depression. The number of patients who experienced a switch to depression by days 15, 30, and 60 were 3, 9, and 18 for the haloperidol group and 1, 3, and 8 for the olanzapine group. HAMD-21, 21-item Hamilton Depression Rating Scale.

Reprinted by permission from *Archives of General Psychiatry* (Tohen *et al.*, 2002a).

three weeks and then were switched to olanzapine after three weeks. The comparison of olanzapine and haloperidol was based on rates of remission after six weeks of treatment, which were 44.2% for the olanzapine group and 20.0% for the haloperidol group (p = 0.064).

Valproate, an anticonvulsant, has been shown to have efficacy in the treatment of acute bipolar mania (Pope *et al.*, 1991; Bowden *et al.*, 1994). Olanzapine has been compared with valproate in several randomized, double-blind trials. The first, conducted in adult patients hospitalized for acute bipolar manic or mixed episodes (Tohen *et al.*, 2002a), consisted of a three-week acute phase, followed by a 44-week phase to assess maintenance of response. The results of the 44-week extension phase will be discussed at a later point in this review. The primary efficacy measure was baseline to endpoint change in total YMRS score at three weeks. Relative to valproate treatment (500–2500 mg/day, n = 123), olanzapine treatment (5–20 mg/day, n = 125) was more effective in reducing the symptoms of mania. On the primary efficacy measure, YMRS total score, the mean change was −13.4 points for olanzapine-treated patients and −10.4 points for valproate-treated patients (p = 0.03). Response was defined by an improvement of ≥50% in YMRS score from baseline to endpoint. More patients in the olanzapine group (54.4%) responded than did in the valproate group (42.3%), although this difference did not reach statistical significance (p = 0.06). However, a significantly greater number of patients achieved remission, as defined by an endpoint YMRS total score ≤12, in the olanzapine group (47.2%) than in the valproate group (34.1%) (p = 0.04). Patients treated with olanzapine also achieved remission in a significantly shorter period of time than did valproate-treated patients; the estimated 25th percentile for time-to-remission was three days for olanzapine-treated patients and six days for valproate-treated patients (p < 0.04).

In a separate randomized, 12-week, double-blind study powered for safety, olanzapine (5–25 mg/day, n = 57) was compared with valproate (750–3250 mg/day, n = 63) in adult patients with bipolar disorder hospitalized for acute mania (Zajecka *et al.*, 2002). The Mania Rating Scale total scores decreased from baseline to day 21 of therapy in both olanzapine (−17.2) and valproate (−14.8) groups. This difference between groups, however, was not significant (p = 0.210).

Finally, in a third randomized, 12-week, double-blind study, olanzapine (5–20 mg/day, n = 215) was compared with valproate (500–2500 mg/day, n = 201) and placebo (n = 105) in adult patients with mild to moderate nonpsychotic mania (Tohen *et al.*, 2008a). Efficacy was assessed after three weeks of treatment, after which completers could continue in a nine-week double-blind extension study. After three weeks of treatment, olanzapine- and placebo-treated patients significantly differed in YMRS baseline-to-endpoint total score changes (least-squares mean: olanzapine −9.4 versus placebo −7.4, p = 0.034). The differences between olanzapine and valproate or between valproate and placebo were not significant at this time point. After 12 weeks of treatment, however, olanzapine- and valproate-treated patients significantly differed in YMRS baseline-to-endpoint total score changes (least-squares mean: olanzapine −13.3 versus valproate −10.7, p = 0.004). Of observed cases, 35.4% (35/99 at three weeks) to 57.1% (28/49 at 12 weeks) showed that patients had valproate plasma concentrations lower than the recommended valproate therapeutic range; however the YMRS scores of these patients were lower than those of patients with valproate concentrations above or within range. Thus, olanzapine was significantly more efficacious than placebo but not valproate at three weeks and significantly more efficacious than valproate at 12 weeks.

Recently, olanzapine was used as an active control in a pair of three-week, randomized, double-blind, placebo-controlled trials that compared asenapine, olanzapine, and placebo in treatment of acute mania (McIntyre et al., 2009a; McIntyre et al., 2010). In both trials, after a single-blind placebo run-in period, adults experiencing manic or mixed episodes were randomly assigned (2:2:1) to three weeks of flexible-dose sublingual asenapine (10 mg twice daily on day 1, 5, or 10 mg twice daily thereafter), oral olanzapine (15 mg twice daily on day 1, 5–20 mg once daily thereafter), or placebo. In the first study (McIntyre et al., 2009a), 489 adults participated (asenapine n = 194, olanzapine n = 191, and placebo n = 104); the mean daily dosage of asenapine was 18.2 mg and that of olanzapine was 15.8 mg. Significantly greater least-squares mean (SE) changes in YMRS scores were observed at day 21 with both asenapine (−10.8 [0.8]) and olanzapine (−12.6 [0.8]) compared with placebo using last observation carried forward (LOCF) techniques (MMRM results were comparable). Both asenapine- and olanzapine-treated subjects had significantly higher rates of response and remission compared with placebo (p < 0.01 for all comparisons). Direct statistical comparisons between olanzapine and asenapine were not provided in the publication.

In the second study (McIntyre et al., 2010), 488 adults participated (asenapine n = 185, olanzapine n = 205, and placebo n = 98), and mean daily dosages were asenapine 18.4 mg and olanzapine 15.9 mg. Significantly greater least-squares mean (SE) changes in YMRS scores were observed at day 21 with both asenapine (−11.5 [0.8]) and olanzapine (−14.6 [0.8]) compared with placebo using LOCF techniques (MMRM results were comparable). Post hoc analysis indicated that changes in YMRS total score for olanzapine were significantly greater than those for asenapine with LOCF analysis, but not with MMRM analysis. In this study, response and remission rates with asenapine did not differ significantly from placebo; however, olanzapine was superior to placebo in rates of response and remission. Post hoc analysis of YMRS response and remission showed that rates with olanzapine were significantly greater than those with asenapine.

Patients who completed either of these two acute studies were eligible to participate in a nine-week double-blind extension study (McIntyre et al., 2009b). In all, 504 patients participated. Patients who had been randomized to asenapine or olanzapine in the acute study continued the same treatment in the extension period; patients who had been randomized to placebo began receiving asenapine. The mean (± SD) change from baseline to day 84 on the YMRS total score was −24.4 (± 8.7) for asenapine and −23.9 (± 7.9) for olanzapine. A noninferiority analysis indicated no significant difference between therapy groups. The percentages of patients taking asenapine and olanzapine who met response and remission criteria were not significantly different at any assessment during the study period. During an ensuing 40-week extension period (n = 218), more than 90% of patients in both treatment groups showed response or remission at study end (McIntyre et al., 2008).

6.3.3 ADJUNCTIVE TRIALS

Historically, antipsychotic agents have been used in combination with mood stabilizers for the treatment of acute mania, and the accumulated evidence supports the contention that adjunctive therapy with these two classes of compounds yields greater efficacy and more rapid onset of response (Klein *et al.*, 1984; Muller-Oerlinghausen *et al.*, 2000). The use of olanzapine in combination with either lithium or valproate for the treatment of acute mania was examined in 344 adult patients in a six-week double-blind, randomized, placebo-controlled study (Tohen *et al.*, 2002b). Patients diagnosed with bipolar disorder presenting with manic or mixed episodes who were inadequately responsive to at least two weeks of lithium or valproate treatment alone at a therapeutic blood level were randomized to receive olanzapine in combination with lithium or valproate (n = 229) (olanzapine, 5–20 mg/day + lithium or valproate) or lithium or valproate alone (n = 115) (placebo + lithium or valproate). Of note, the requirement to be inadequately responsive to two weeks of treatment does not fulfill any formal definition of treatment resistance; included patients could be better described as early partial nonresponders. The design of this study was intended to address a common treatment dilemma faced by practitioners. Namely, should a physician continue treatment with the original agent under careful observation, even if patients do not demonstrate a response within the first two weeks, or should another drug be added? Patients who received olanzapine in combination with lithium or valproate had significantly greater mean improvements in YMRS total scores than those who received lithium or valproate alone (combination therapy −13.1 versus lithium or valproate monotherapy −9.1; p = 0.003). Rates of clinical response, defined as ≥50% improvement in YMRS total scores from baseline to endpoint, were also significantly higher (p < 0.001) with patients taking combination therapy (68%) than those taking lithium or valproate monotherapy (45%). In addition, time to response was significantly shorter (p = 0.002) for patients taking combination therapy, with a median response time of 18 days with combination therapy versus 28 days with lithium or valproate monotherapy.

The results of this study also demonstrated substantial efficacy of olanzapine plus lithium or valproate in treating depressive symptoms present at randomization. For the study population as a whole, HAMD-21 total scores were significantly more improved (p < 0.001) in patients taking combination therapy (5.0 points) than in those on lithium or valproate monotherapy (0.9 points). Furthermore, in a subset of patients presenting with moderate-to-severe depressive symptoms (DSM-IV mixed episode and HAMD-21 ≥20 at baseline), HAMD-21 scores improved by 10.3 points for combination therapy compared with 1.6 points for lithium or valproate monotherapy (p < 0.001). Also, within this subset of patients, more than four times as many patients in the combination therapy group showed at least a 50% improvement in depressive symptoms (combination therapy 43% versus monotherapy 10%, p = 0.006). Compared with the use of lithium or valproate alone, addition of olanzapine provided superior efficacy in the treatment of manic or mixed bipolar episodes.

In another more recent study of adjunctive therapy, adults with a current mixed episode of bipolar disorder who had been taking valproate for at least 14 days at levels of 75–125 μg/ml with inadequate efficacy were randomly assigned to receive augmentation with olanzapine (5–20 mg/day) or placebo (Houston _et al._, 2009). Mean (SE) score changes from baseline across the six-week treatment period for adjunctive olanzapine (n = 100) versus adjunctive placebo (n = 101) treatment groups, respectively, were −9.37 [0.55] versus −7.69 [0.54] (p = 0.022) for the HAMD-21 and −10.15 [0.44] versus −7.68 [0.44] (p < 0.001) for the YMRS. Time to partial response, defined as decreases of at least 25% on the HAMD-21 and the YMRS, was significantly shorter for the adjunctive olanzapine group (median days: olanzapine 7 versus placebo 14); as was time to response, defined as decreases of at least 50% on the HAMD-21 and YMRS (median days: olanzapine 25 versus placebo 49). Thus olanzapine given with valproate was shown to yield greater and earlier reduction of both manic and depressive symptoms than valproate alone in mixed-episode patients with previously inadequate response.

Olanzapine has also been studied in bipolar disorder in combination with the anticonvulsant carbamazepine. In this study (Tohen _et al._, 2008b), adults with a current manic or mixed episode of bipolar disorder received 400–1200 mg/day carbamazepine and were randomly assigned to receive augmentation with olanzapine (n = 58) or placebo (n = 60). Because carbamazepine substantially induces the cytochrome P450 1A2 metabolism of olanzapine (Lucas, Gilfillan, and Bergstrom, 1998), the dose range for olanzapine was 10–30 mg/day rather than the usual 5–20 mg/day. Efficacy was assessed after six weeks of double-blind treatment, after which patients could participate in a six-month open-label safety evaluation of olanzapine plus carbamazepine. After six weeks of treatment, there were no significant differences in efficacy measures between the two groups. Carbamazepine was shown to reduce olanzapine concentrations.

6.3.4   ASSESSMENT OF INTRAMUSCULAR OLANZAPINE

Patients who suffer from mania with severe agitation are in need of immediate treatment to avoid harm to themselves or others. For pharmacokinetic reasons, the intramuscular administration of a molecule provides a faster onset of action than the oral use of the drug. For this reason, the efficacy and safety of intramuscular injections of olanzapine to treat acutely agitated patients with bipolar mania were examined in a double-blind randomized study (Meehan _et al._, 2001). In this study, 201 agitated adult patients with bipolar mania were randomly assigned to receive one to three injections of olanzapine (n = 99), lorazepam (n = 51), or placebo (n = 51) within a 24-hour period. The doses of olanzapine for the first and second injections were 10 mg and for the third injection, 5 mg. The doses of lorazepam for the first and second injections were 2 mg, and for the third injection, 1 mg. For placebo-treated patients, the first and second injections were placebo, and the third injection was olanzapine 10 mg. Agitation was measured at baseline, every 30 minutes for the first 2 hours, and at 24 hours after the first injection using the Positive and Negative Syndrome Scale-Excited Component subscale (PANSS-EC) as the primary scale, and two additional scales, the Agitated Behavior Scale (ABS), and the Agitation-Calmness Evaluation Scale (ACES). At two hours after the first injection, patients treated with olanzapine showed a significantly greater reduction in scores on the PANSS-EC (Figure 6.2), ABS, and ACES agitation scales compared with patients treated with either lorazepam (p = 0.001) or placebo (p < 0.001). At 24 hours after the

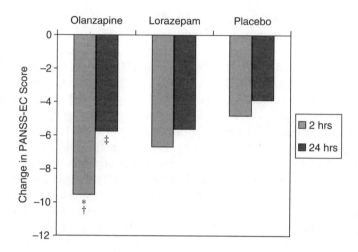

Figure 6.2 Last-observation-carried forward mean change in Positive and Negative Syndrome Scale-Excited Component (PANSS-EC) scores at 2 and 24 hours after an intramuscular injection of olanzapine (n = 99), lorazepam (n = 51), or placebo (n = 51) in acutely agitated patients with bipolar mania (*olanzapine versus placebo, p < 0.001; †olanzapine versus lorazepam, p = 0.001; ‡olanzapine versus placebo, p = 0.025) (Meehan *et al.*, 2001). PANSS-EC, Positive and Negative Syndrome Scale-Excited Component.

first injection, olanzapine remained significantly superior to placebo in reducing agitation in patients with acute mania (PANSS-EC, p = 0.025), whereas such improvements in patients treated with lorazepam were not significantly different from those treated with placebo or olanzapine (PANSS-EC, lorazepam versus placebo, p = 0.080; lorazepam versus olanzapine, p = 0.808). There were no significant differences among the three groups in safety measures, including treatment-emergent EPS, the incidence of acute dystonia, or QTc interval changes.

6.3.5 ADOLESCENTS

Bipolar disorder is particularly disabling for adolescent patients; compared with adult bipolar disorder, adolescent-onset of bipolar disorder is associated with greater severity of illness (for example, psychosis, mixed mania, high rates of self-injury, and drug abuse) and more functional impairment (McClellan, Werry, and Ham, 1993; Strober *et al.*, 1995; Wozniak *et al.*, 1995). The rate of completed suicide among adolescent patients with bipolar disorder ranges from 3 to 25% (Goldstein, 2009). Twenty percent of all patients with bipolar disorder experienced their first manic episode during adolescence, with the most common age of onset in these patients between 15 and 19 years (Goodwin and Jamison, 1990).

Further, adolescent bipolar disorder is much more likely to go undiagnosed for a year or more (Todd *et al.*, 1993). Diagnosis of bipolar disorder in the young is more difficult than in adults, as the clinical presentation of the disease differs (Biederman *et al.*, 2000).

Higher rates of comorbidity with attention-deficit/hyperactivity disorder (ADHD) (57%) (Wozniak *et al.*, 1995; West *et al.*, 1995) and panic disorder (21%) (Chen and Dilsaver, 1995) may further impede correct diagnosis. Many adolescents with bipolar disorder are misdiagnosed as having schizophrenia or ADHD (Geller, Fox, and Clark, 1994; Biederman *et al.*, 1995). Early identification of the disease and initiation of effective drug treatment may improve long-term outcomes (Tohen, 1997).

Until the 2000s, the only approved drug treatment for bipolar disorder for pediatric patients in the US was lithium; in this decade a number of compounds, including olanzapine, have been studied and subsequently approved (in the US) for use in adolescents 13–17 years of age. The approval of olanzapine as a treatment for bipolar disorder in adolescents was based on a three-week, multicenter, parallel, double-blind, randomized, placebo-controlled trial of outpatient, and inpatient adolescents ages 13–17 with an acute manic or mixed episode. Subjects received either olanzapine (2.5–20 mg/day, n = 107) or placebo (n = 54) (Tohen *et al.*, 2007). The mean baseline-to-endpoint change in the YMRS total score was significantly greater (p < 0.001) for patients receiving olanzapine (−17.65) relative to patients receiving placebo (−9.99), and a greater proportion of olanzapine-treated patients met response and remission criteria: 48.6% of olanzapine-treated versus 18.5% of placebo-treated patients met response criteria, and 35.2% of olanzapine-treated versus 11.1% of placebo-treated patients met remission criteria. The mean modal dose (± SD) of olanzapine during the double-blind period was 10.7 mg/day (± 4.5), and the mean daily dose was 8.9 mg. When deciding among the alternative treatments available for adolescents, clinicians should consider the increased potential (in adolescents as compared with adults) for weight gain and hyperlipidemia. Clinicians should consider the potential long-term risks when prescribing to adolescents, and in many cases this may lead them to consider prescribing other drugs first in adolescents (Eli Lilly and Company, 2009).

6.4 EFFICACY IN THE TREATMENT OF BIPOLAR DEPRESSION

In the treatment of bipolar disorder, the major challenge is perhaps not the management of manic episodes, but rather the management of episodes of depression. Bipolar depression, or the depressive phase of bipolar disorder, is a particularly difficult condition to treat.

The potential efficacy of olanzapine monotherapy or combination therapy with the antidepressant fluoxetine to treat bipolar depression was explored in a randomized, double-blind, placebo-controlled study (Tohen *et al.*, 2003b). In this eight-week trial, olanzapine (5–20 mg/day) was compared with placebo and an olanzapine/fluoxetine combination (olanzapine/fluoxetine (mg/day): 6/25, 6/50, or 12/50) in 833 patients with bipolar depression (baseline Montgomery-Asberg Depression Rating Scale (MADRS) scores of ≥20). Starting at week 1, both olanzapine- and olanzapine/fluoxetine combination-treated patients showed significant improvements in depressive symptoms compared with placebo, and the effect was also significantly larger with olanzapine/fluoxetine combination therapy compared with olanzapine monotherapy beginning at week 4 through the end of eight weeks (Figure 6.3). The mean changes in MADRS total

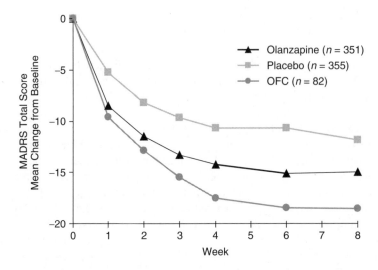

Figure 6.3 Least-squares mean change in Montgomery-Asberg Depression Rating Scale (MADRS) scores for patients with bipolar depression treated with olanzapine, olanzapine/fluoxetine combination, or placebo. Improvements in MADRS scores with olanzapine and olanzapine/fluoxetine combination were significantly greater than that with placebo throughout the study period (p < 0.001). Improvement in MADRS scores with olanzapine/fluoxetine combination was significantly greater than that with olanzapine at weeks 4–8 (p < 0.02) (Tohen *et al.*, 2003b). MADRS, Montgomery-Asberg Depression Rating Scale; OFC, olanzapine/fluoxetine combination.

Reprinted by permission from *Archives of General Psychiatry* (Tohen *et al.*, 2003b).

score between baseline and endpoint were −18.5 for olanzapine/fluoxetine combination, −15.0 for olanzapine, and −11.9 for placebo. The reduction for olanzapine/fluoxetine combination was significantly greater than those for olanzapine (p = 0.01) and placebo (p < 0.001); and the reduction for olanzapine was significantly greater than that for placebo (p = 0.002). The response rate, defined as a ≥50% reduction in MADRS total score, was significantly higher for the olanzapine/fluoxetine combination therapy group (56%) relative to both olanzapine (39%, p = 0.006) and placebo (30%, p < 0.001). Similarly, the rate of remission, as defined by a MADRS total score ≤12 at endpoint and completion of at least four weeks of study, was significantly higher for patients treated with olanzapine/fluoxetine combination (49%) relative to those treated with olanzapine (33%, p = 0.007) and placebo (25%, p < 0.001). Time to remission was significantly shorter for the olanzapine group compared with the placebo group (p = 0.02) and again significantly shorter for the olanzapine/fluoxetine combination group compared with olanzapine (p = 0.01) and placebo (p < 0.001) groups. The results of this study led to the approval by the FDA of olanzapine in combination with fluoxetine to treat bipolar depression, both as a single capsule or as olanzapine and fluoxetine given separately.

In the Tohen *et al.* study (Tohen *et al.*, 2003b), the incidence of treatment-emergent mania was low, and there were no significant differences among the three treatment groups (olanzapine/fluoxetine combination 6.4%, olanzapine 5.7%, and placebo 6.7%).

Thus, neither olanzapine nor the olanzapine/fluoxetine combination induced switches to mania or hypomania, an effect known to occur with some antidepressant drugs when they are given alone (Altshuler et al., 1995; Wehr and Goodwin, 1987). The results of this study suggest that although olanzapine appears to be effective for treating patients with bipolar depression, cotherapy with fluoxetine greatly enhanced its therapeutic effects. Importantly, the enhanced efficacy of olanzapine/fluoxetine combined therapy was not associated with a greater risk of treatment-emergent mania.

An open-label trial evaluated the effectiveness of olanzapine/fluoxetine combination and olanzapine treatment in outpatients with bipolar depression (Tamayo et al., 2009). A total of 161 outpatients experiencing a depressive episode received open-label olanzapine/fluoxetine combination treatment for seven weeks. Responders were then randomized to receive either olanzapine/fluoxetine combination continuation treatment (n = 49) or olanzapine alone starting at 10 mg/day (n = 48) for 12 weeks. During the 12-week period, significantly more patients in the olanzapine/fluoxetine combination group than patients in the olanzapine group maintained response (olanzapine/fluoxetine combination 31.3% versus olanzapine 12.5%) and remission (olanzapine/fluoxetine combination 71.4% versus olanzapine 39.6%). Mania emergence rates were <2% in both groups. Rates of relapse, defined as MADRS score ≥ 20 plus a CGI-BP score ≥ 3 or hospitalization for depression, were 28.1% for the olanzapine arm versus 10.5% for the olanzapine/fluoxetine combination arm (p < 0.05). Although the study findings are limited by the open-label design, they suggest that improvements resulting from 7 weeks of olanzapine/fluoxetine combination treatment of a bipolar depressive episode are maintained for an additional 12 weeks with olanzapine/fluoxetine combination; but that discontinuation of fluoxetine resulting in switching to olanzapine monotherapy may result in worsening of depressive symptoms.

The olanzapine/fluoxetine combination has also been evaluated in comparison to lamotrigine. In a randomized, double-blind study, patients with a current depressed episode of bipolar disorder were randomized to receive either olanzapine/fluoxetine combination (olanzapine/fluoxetine (mg/day): 6/25, 6/50, 12/25, or 12/50; n = 205) or lamotrigine (titrated to 200 mg/day, n = 205) for 25 weeks. Acute, double-blind efficacy was evaluated after 7 and 26 weeks of treatment (Brown et al., 2006, 2009). After seven weeks of treatment (Brown et al., 2006), patients treated with olanzapine/fluoxetine combination had significantly greater mean improvement than lamotrigine-treated patients on baseline-to-endpoint MADRS scores (least-squares means (SE), MMRM: -14.91 [0.49] versus -12.92 [0.50], p = 0.002), Clinical Global Impression of Severity (CGI-S) scores (-1.43 [0.06] versus -1.18 [0.06], p = 0.002), and YMRS scores (-1.68 [0.18] versus -0.94 [0.18], p = 0.001). Rates of response, defined as $\geq 50\%$ reduction in MADRS score, did not significantly differ between treatment groups (olanzapine/fluoxetine combination 68.8% versus lamotrigine 59.7%). Time to response was significantly shorter for patients treated with olanzapine/fluoxetine combination (median [95% CI]: olanzapine/fluoxetine combination 17 days (Pope et al., 1991; Bowden et al., 1994; Tohen et al., 2002a, 2008a; Zajecka et al., 2002; McIntyre et al., 2008, 2009a, 2009b, 2010) versus lamotrigine 23 days (McIntyre et al., 2008, 2009b; Klein et al., 1984; Muller-Oerlinghausen et al., 2000; Tohen et al., 2002b, 2008b; Houston et al., 2009; Lucas, Gilfillan, and Bergstrom, 1998; Meehan et al., 2001;

McClellan, Werry, and Ham, 1993; Strober *et al.*, 1995; Wozniak *et al.*, 1995; Goldstein, 2009; Goodwin and Jamison, 1990)).

After 26 weeks of treatment (Brown *et al.*, 2009), patients treated with the olanzapine/fluoxetine combination had significantly greater mean improvement than lamotrigine-treated patients on baseline-to-endpoint MADRS scores (least-squares mean (SE), MMRM: -16.63 [0.52] versus -14.70 [0.52], $p = 0.005$), CGI-S scores (-1.70 [0.07] versus -1.46 [0.07], $p = 0.008$), and YMRS scores (-1.92 [0.17] versus -1.05 [0.17], $p < 0.001$). Because lamotrigine titration was not complete until week 5, major efficacy outcome data are analyzed from randomization to the end of the 26-week study; patients treated with olanzapine/fluoxetine combination had significantly greater improvement than lamotrigine-treated patients on all three measures during this period as well. Although the study was not powered to study relapse, this outcome was also explored. Of patients in remission after the seven-week acute phase (olanzapine/fluoxetine combination 56.4%, lamotrigine 49.2%), there was no significant difference between groups in the incidence of relapse, defined as MADRS ≥ 15 (olanzapine/fluoxetine combination 13.7% versus lamotrigine 18.2%, $p = 0.528$). Rates of treatment-emergent mania were not significantly different between treatments.

6.5 EFFICACY IN BIPOLAR MAINTENANCE/RELAPSE PREVENTION

Until the late 1990s, the long-term efficacy and relapse prevention of most pharmacotherapies used in bipolar disorder was poorly studied. Yet, there remained then and remains now a great need for prophylactic treatments to minimize the risk of relapse because bipolar disorder is a chronic recurring condition. Repeated relapses into manic, mixed, or depressive phases of bipolar disorder have negative implications for disease progression and patients' responsiveness to subsequent treatments; essentially, patients with a history of multiple relapses are likely to be less responsive to pharmacotherapeutics. Several studies have been performed to explore the role of olanzapine in long-term prophylactic treatment of bipolar disorder.

The efficacy of olanzapine for relapse prevention in bipolar disorder was assessed in a year-long randomized double-blind placebo-controlled study (Tohen *et al.*, 2006). Patients with acute manic or mixed episodes of bipolar disorder received open-label treatment with olanzapine (5–20 mg/day) for 6–12 weeks. Those patients who achieved symptomatic remission, defined as a YMRS total score ≤ 12 and a HAMD-21 total score ≤ 8, were randomized to receive olanzapine (5–20 mg/day, $n = 225$) or placebo ($n = 136$) for 52 weeks. Relative to placebo, olanzapine significantly increased time to relapse to an affective episode (that is, manic, depressive, or mixed episode), defined as a YMRS total score ≥ 15 and/or a HAMD-21 total score ≥ 15 and/or psychiatric hospitalization ($p < 0.001$). Relapse to an affective episode occurred in 46.7% of olanzapine-treated and 80.1% of placebo-treated patients ($p < 0.001$). Compared with the placebo-treated patients, olanzapine-treated patients had a significantly lower rate of relapse into a manic episode (olanzapine 16.4% versus placebo 41.2%, $p < 0.001$). Olanzapine-treated patients also had lower rates of relapse into a depressive episode (olanzapine 30.2% versus placebo 39.0%) or into a mixed episode (olanzapine 4.4% versus placebo 8.8%), but these differences were not significant (p = 0.11 for both comparisons). Significantly more patients in the olanzapine group completed the 52-week trial than those in the placebo group (olanzapine 23.6% versus placebo 9.6%, p = 0.001) with approximately twice as many placebo-treated patients discontinuing due to lack of efficacy (olanzapine 28% versus placebo 57%, p = 0.001). A secondary, post hoc analysis of this study including only patients with a mixed index episode also showed that olanzapine was superior to placebo in the prevention of relapse into either mania or depression (Figure 6.4) (Tohen *et al.*, 2009b).

For over 30 years, lithium has been the "gold standard" for relapse prevention in bipolar disorder. To demonstrate a clear value for new treatments, comparisons to lithium are essential. Olanzapine was compared with lithium in a randomized, double-blind study of relapse prevention in bipolar disorder (Tohen *et al.*, 2005). Patients with a diagnosis of bipolar disorder, manic, or mixed type, with a history of at least two manic or mixed episodes within six years, and a YMRS total score ≥20 received open-label treatment with a combination of olanzapine and lithium for 6–12 weeks. By using a combination of both agents to treat the acute episode (that is, using an "enriched" design) rather than just one of the treatments, the potential bias of including patients who were not tolerant of either treatment or who might improve with only one of the drugs during the acute phase, was avoided. Furthermore, a past history of nontolerance or nonresponse to either treatment was an important exclusion criterion. Patients who achieved symptomatic remission, defined as a YMRS total score ≤12 and a HAMD-21 total score ≤8, were randomly assigned to receive monotherapy with either olanzapine (5–20 mg/day,

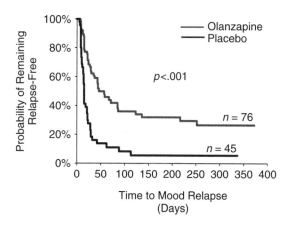

Figure 6.4 Kaplan-Meier analysis of time to symptomatic relapse for subjects with mixed index episodes. Patients had presented with a mixed index episode, responded to open-label olanzapine, and were then randomly assigned to olanzapine (n = 76) or placebo (n = 45). Olanzapine-treated subjects had a longer time to relapse compared with placebo-treated subjects (p < 0.001). The median time to relapse for olanzapine-treated subjects was 46 days compared with 15 days for placebo-treated subjects.

Reprinted by permission from *Journal of Affective Disorders* (Tohen *et al.*, 2009b).

n = 217) or lithium (300–1800 mg/day, n = 214) for 52 weeks. Relapse to an affective episode, defined as a YMRS total score ≥ 15 and/or a HAMD-21 total score ≥ 15, occurred in 30% of olanzapine-treated and 39% of lithium-treated patients (p = 0.055). The incidence of relapse into a manic episode was significantly lower (p = 0.02) in olanzapine-treated patients (14%) than in lithium-treated patients (23%), whereas the incidence of relapse into a depressive episode was higher for olanzapine than lithium (olanzapine 16% versus lithium 11%, p = 0.15). Of note, the definitions of remission and relapse used in this study and the previously described placebo-controlled study for the most part follow those recommended by an international task force that was recently published (Tohen *et al.*, 2009a). The incidence of hospitalization for an affective episode was significantly lower (p < 0.03) for olanzapine-treated patients (14%) compared with lithium-treated patients (23%). Significantly more (p = 0.004) olanzapine-treated patients (47%) completed the 52-week trial than those on lithium (33%). Time to discontinuation for any reason was longer for olanzapine-treated patients than for lithium-treated patients (log-rank analysis p = 0.017), with median times to discontinuation of 303 days for olanzapine and 207 days for lithium (Figure 6.5). The rates of discontinuation due to adverse events were 19% for the olanzapine group and 26% for the lithium group (p = 0.105).

Olanzapine's efficacy in relapse prevention has also been assessed when given in combination with mood stabilizers. The relative efficacy of olanzapine cotherapy (olanzapine in combination with lithium or valproate) versus monotherapy (either lithium or valproate alone) in preventing relapse was evaluated in an 18-month, double-blind study (Tohen

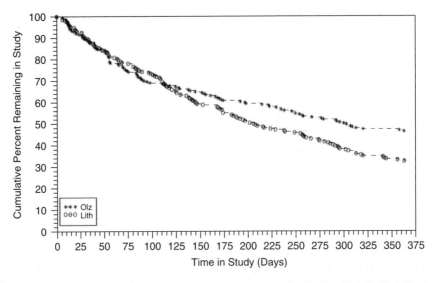

Figure 6.5 Time to discontinuation for any reason during double-blind treatment in relapse prevention study of olanzapine (n = 217) versus lithium (n = 214) (Tohen *et al.*, 2005).

_et al._, 2004). Patients who had previously achieved syndromic remission (DSM-IV) after six weeks' treatment with olanzapine cotherapy (Tohen _et al._, 2004) were re-randomized to either olanzapine cotherapy or to monotherapy (lithium or valproate) and followed double-blind for up to 18 months. No significant differences occurred between the treatment groups for time to relapse into an affective episode (based on DSM-IV criteria) or for rates of relapse into either mania or depression when relapse was defined using a symptom-rating scale. However, in a subset of patients who met both symptomatic and syndromic remission criteria, the latter defined as YMRS ≤ 12 and HAMD-21 ≤ 8, at the outset of the study, the median time to symptomatic relapse into either mania (YMRS ≥ 15) or depression (HAMD-21 ≥ 15) was significantly longer ($p = 0.023$) for the olanzapine cotherapy group (163 days) relative to that in the monotherapy group (42 days).

Finally, in a randomized double-blind study, described previously (Tohen _et al._, 2002a), the long-term efficacy of flexibly dosed olanzapine (5–20 mg/day) was compared with valproate (500–2500 mg/day) in 251 patients with bipolar disorder during 47 weeks (Tohen _et al._, 2003c). Relative to valproate-treated patients, olanzapine-treated patients had a significantly greater mean improvement at endpoint in YMRS total score, the primary efficacy measure ($p = 0.03$). The median time to symptomatic remission of mania (YMRS total score ≤ 12) was significantly shorter ($p = 0.05$) for olanzapine-treated patients (14 days) than for those treated with valproate (62 days). However, no significant differences between treatments were observed for the rates of remission during the 47 weeks (olanzapine 56.8% and valproate 45.5%) or subsequent rates of relapse into mania or depression (olanzapine 42.4% and valproate 56.5%). Note that the study was not powered to assess relapse prevention.

6.6   SAFETY AND TOLERABILITY

With respect to safety, it is important to highlight that in patients treated with olanzapine, weight gain is common, as are increases in blood glucose and lipid levels (2009). To characterize the incidence of weight gain and changes in metabolic parameters in patients treated with olanzapine, Lilly conducted pooled analyses of 86 clinical trials of the oral and depot formulations of olanzapine including more than 12 000 adult patients (Eli Lilly and Company, 2009). Although the studies included patients with numerous diagnoses, the majority of patients in the database had schizophrenia, with bipolar mania the next most common diagnosis. Despite the inclusion of diagnoses other than bipolar disorder, these data provide valuable information for clinicians about metabolic safety changes that may be seen with long-term olanzapine treatment. Unless otherwise indicated, results of the analyses described later in this review are compiled from the olanzapine product insert (2009), from a comprehensive brochure on olanzapine in bipolar disorder, that is, available from Lilly upon request (Eli Lilly and Company, 2009), and from unpublished sources (unpublished data, Eli Lilly Research Laboratories, December 2007).

6.6.1 WEIGHT

Among patients in the 86-study database with at least 48 weeks of exposure to olanzapine, mean weight gain was 5.6 kg (12.3 lb; median exposure of 573 days, n = 2021). The rate of discontinuation due to weight gain in this patient group was 0.4% (8/2034). The percentages of patients who gained at least 7, 15, or 25% of their baseline body weight with long-term exposure represented 64, 32, and 12% of the patients treated, respectively. To provide information on the pattern of weight changes over time with long-term treatment, all weight data from the 86-study database were analyzed using a MMRM analysis (Millen, Campbell and Beasley, 2010). This analysis method appropriately addresses the issue of missing data that may result from early patient discontinuation or lack of weight measurements from continuing patients in clinical trials. Clinically important weight gain was observed over 48 weeks across all body mass index (BMI) categories (that is, underweight, normal, overweight, and obese). The rate of weight gain tended to be greatest early in treatment and slowed within 2–4 months after the start of treatment (Figure 6.6).

Predictors of substantial weight gain, defined as 5 kg or 7% of initial weight in 30 ± 2 weeks, during treatment of bipolar disorder with olanzapine were studied in a database that pooled four long-term studies of adult patients with bipolar mania or mixed mania (n = 948 at initiation of olanzapine) (Lipkovich *et al.*, 2006). Baseline characteristics significantly associated with substantial weight gain included younger age, nonwhite ethnicity, lower BMI, nonrapid cycling status, and psychotic features. Weight gain of 2 kg or more in the first three weeks of therapy predicted substantial weight gain by 30 weeks (sensitivity 57%, specificity 71%). A classification system with thresholds for early weight gain, baseline BMI, and ethnicity further improved predictability for substantial weight gain (sensitivity 79%, specificity 70%). The authors concluded that early weight

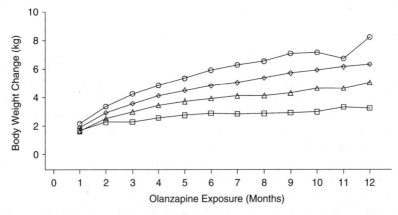

Figure 6.6 Mixed-model repeated-measure (MMRM) analyses of least-squares mean changes in weight (kg) in adult patients treated with the oral or depot formulations of olanzapine over 12 months (48 weeks) by baseline body mass index (BMI). ⌒, Underweight (month 1 n = 302, month 12 n = 21); ◇, Normal (month 1, n = 3652, month 12, n = 312); ∧, Overweight (month 1, n = 2985, month 12, n = 289); ⊏, Obese (month 1, n = 2440, month 12, n = 195).

Reprinted by permission from *Journal of Psychopharmacology* (Millen, Campbell and Beasley, 2010).

gain (that is, 2–3 kg in first three weeks of olanzapine treatment) is a strong predictor of substantial weight gain. Patients with less pronounced early weight gain were still at risk for later substantial weight gain if they had close to normal BMI (≤ 27 kg/m^2) at baseline.

6.6.2 GLUCOSE AND LIPIDS

For patients from the 86-study database described above with at least 48 weeks of exposure, mean change in fasting glucose was 4.2 mg/dl (n = 487). Patients had mean increases from baseline in fasting total cholesterol (5.6 mg/dl), fasting low-density lipoprotein (LDL) cholesterol (2.5 mg/dl), and fasting triglycerides (18.7 mg/dl), and a mean decrease in fasting high-density lipoprotein (HDL) cholesterol (0.16 mg/dl). Table 6.1 summarizes proportions of patients with shifts from normal or borderline to high (or low, as appropriate) in lipid and glucose parameters.

Similar weight, glucose, and lipids analyses of adolescents aged 13–17 in a pooled database of 489 patients across six studies (all in either schizophrenia or bipolar I disorder) demonstrated that adolescent patients treated with olanzapine also experience undesirable changes in weight, glucose, and lipids. In a subset of adolescents who had had at least 24 weeks of exposure (approximately six months), mean changes included weight gain of 11.2 kg (24.6 lb; n = 179, with median exposure of 201 days); increases in fasting total cholesterol of 5.5 mg/dl, LDL cholesterol of 5.4 mg/dl, triglycerides of 20.5 mg/dl, and glucose of 3.1 mg/dl (n = 121 or 122 in all cases); and a decrease in fasting HDL cholesterol of 4.5 mg/dl (n = 122). The percentages of adolescent patients who gained at least 7, 15, or 25% of their baseline body weight with at least 24 weeks of exposure represented 89, 55, and 29% of the patients treated, respectively. Proportions of adolescent patients with shifts from normal or borderline to high (or low, as appropriate) in lipid and glucose parameters are included in Table 6.1.

6.6.3 SAFETY IN BIPOLAR STUDIES

In the short- and long-term studies for the treatment of bipolar I disorder described in the efficacy sections above, treatment with olanzapine or olanzapine/fluoxetine combination was generally well tolerated, with low proportions of patients discontinuing due to adverse events (0–14% in short-term studies and 8–25% in longer-term studies). The adverse events observed significantly more often in patients treated with olanzapine- or olanzapine/fluoxetine combination than in patients treated with comparators in almost all studies include somnolence/sedation, increased weight, increased appetite, dry mouth, and dizziness. Mean weight gain was generally higher for patients treated with olanzapine or olanzapine/fluoxetine combination than for comparator-treated patients; likewise, higher proportions of patients treated with olanzapine or with olanzapine/fluoxetine combination had clinically significant, treatment-emergent weight gain of at least 7% over baseline. In many studies, patients treated with olanzapine and olanzapine/fluoxetine combination had mean increases in glucose and lipid levels, and clinically significant treatment-emergent elevations for these analytes. Elevations in prolactin, uric acid, LDL cholesterol, alanine transaminase, and aspartate transaminase were also observed in some studies. Table 6.2 summarizes these findings from the bipolar I studies in more detail.

Table 6.1 Proportions of adult patients with at least 48 weeks' olanzapine exposure and adolescent patients with at least 24 weeks' olanzapine exposure with treatment-emergent shifts in fasting glucose and lipids.

Analyte		Shift (definition)	Proportion (95% CI)	N
Glucose	Adults	Normal → high (<100 to ≥126 mg/dl)	12.8% (9.4, 16.7)	345
		Borderline → high (≥100 and <126 to ≥126 mg/dl)	26.0% (18.6, 34.5)	127
	Adolescents	Normal → high (<100 to ≥126 mg/dl)	0.9% (0.0, 5.1)	108
		Borderline → high (≥100 and <126 to ≥126 mg/dl)	23.1% (5, 53.8)	13
Total cholesterol	Adults	Normal → high (<200 to ≥240 mg/dl)	14.8% (10.9, 19.5)	283
		Borderline → high (≥200 and <240 to ≥240 mg/dl)	55.2% (46.0, 64.1)	125
	Adolescents	Normal → high (<170 to ≥200 mg/dl)	7.7% (2.9, 16.0)	78
		Borderline → high (≥170 and <200 to ≥200 mg/dl)	57.6% (39.2, 74.5)	33
LDL cholesterol	Adults	Normal → high (<100 to ≥160 mg/dl)	7.3% (3.4, 13.4)	123
		Borderline → high (≥100 and <160 to ≥160 mg/dl)	31.0% (25.7, 36.7)	284
	Adolescents	Normal → high (<110 to ≥130 mg/dl)	10.9% (5.3, 19.1)	92
		Borderline → high (≥110 and <130 to ≥130 mg/dl)	47.6% (25.7, 70.2)	21
Triglycerides	Adults	Normal → high (<150 to ≥200 mg/dl)	32.4% (27.1, 38.1)	293
		Borderline → high (≥150 and <200 to ≥200 mg/dl)	70.7% (59.0, 80.6)	75
	Adolescents	Normal → high (<90 to ≥130 mg/dl)	36.4% (24.9, 49.1)	66
		Borderline → high (≥90 and <130 to ≥130 mg/dl)	64.5% (45.4, 80.8)	31
HDL cholesterol	Adults	Normal → low (≥40 to <40 mg/dl)	44.0% (38.1, 50.1)	277
	Adolescents	Normal → low (>65 to <35 mg/dl)	0% (0.0, 28.5)	11
		Borderline → low (≥35 and ≤65 to <35 mg/dl)	21.0% (13.5, 30.0)	100

CI, confidence interval; HDL, high-density lipoprotein; LDL, low-density lipoprotein; N, number of patients in analysis.Zyprexa United States (US) Package Insert (2009) and Eli Lilly Research Laboratories data on file, December 2007 (for confidence intervals).

Table 6.2 Summary of safety findings in studies of olanzapine in bipolar disorder.

Study	Treatment (N)	Adverse event discontinuations (%)	Weight Mean change (kg)	Weight Change ≥7% (%)	Adverse events, laboratory measures, or vital signs with significant treatment group differences in favor of comparator[a]
Acute mania studies					
Placebo-controlled					
Tohen et al. (1999)	olz (70)	0	+1.65[b]	NR	Incidence of somnolence, dry mouth, dizziness, elevated ALT
	pla (69)	2.9	−0.44	NR	
Tohen et al. (2000)	olz (55)	3.6	+2.11[b]	NR	Mean change in supine systolic blood pressure; Incidence of somnolence, elevated ALT, elevated AST
	pla (60)	1.7	−0.45	NR	
Katagiri et al. (2010)	olz (105)	8.6	+0.70	6.7	Incidence of somnolence, dizziness, thirst, high AST, high ALT, high prolactin; mean change in RBC, hemoglobin, hematocrit, stab cell, eosinophils, AST, ALT, GGT, alkaline phosphatase, total bilirubin, HbA1c, prolactin, urine specific gravity.
	pla (96)	7.3	−0.86	1.0	
Tohen et al. (2007) (Note: Adolescents)	olz (107)	2.8	+3.66[b]	41.9[b]	Mean change in supine systolic blood pressure, supine pulse, standing pulse, fasting glucose, fasting cholesterol, AST, ALT, uric acid; incidence of increased appetite, somnolence, sedation, elevated cholesterol, elevated LDL cholesterol, elevated triglycerides, elevated prolactin
	pla (54)	1.9	+0.30	1.9	
Active-controlled					
McIntyre et al. (2009)	olz (126)	9.6	+2.49[b]	NR	Incidence of high ALT, dry mouth, increased appetite, somnolence
	val (125)	7.1	+0.92	NR	

(Continued Overleaf)

Table 6.2 (Continued)

Study	Treatment (N)	Adverse event discontinuations (%)	Weight Mean change (kg)	Weight Change ≥7% (%)	Adverse events, laboratory measures, or vital signs with significant treatment group differences in favor of comparator[a]
Zajecka et al. (2002)	olz (57)	8.8	$+4.0^b$	NR	Mean changes in total cholesterol, LDL cholesterol, albumin, alkaline phosphatase, total protein, platelet count, and neutrophils (all increases for olanzapine and decreases for valproate); eosinophils (decrease for olz and increase for valproate); and monocytes (greater increase for valproate); and incidence of somnolence, rhinitis, edema, slurred speech
	val (63)	11.1	$+2.5$	NR	
Tohen et al. (2003a)	olz (234)	8.1	$+2.82^b$	39.7^b	Incidence of somnolence, infection, dizziness, and fever
	hal (219)	11.4	$+0.02$	16.1	
Perlis et al. (2006)	olz (165)	5.4	$+2.46^b$	NR	Mean changes in alkaline phosphatase, ALT, AST, and GGT
	risp (164)	8.5	$+1.60$	NR	
Tohen et al. (2008a) 3 wk	olz (215)	7.4	$+1.3^{b,c}$	6.4	Mean changes that were significantly different between olanzapine and both dival AND placebo include those for fasting uric acid, fasting glucose, fasting triglycerides, fasting cholesterol, and prolactin; other changes that were worse for olz versus placebo included changes in bilirubin, alkaline phosphatase, creatinine, calcium, albumin, and potassium. Also, olz had greater incidence than valproate of shift from normal to high fasting triglycerides, and somnolence.
	val (201)	3.0	$+0.3$	2.7	
	pla (105)	1.0	$+0.4$	1.0	

Study	Group (n)				Notes
12 wk	olz (196)	7.5	+2.3[b]	18.8[b]	Mean changes in fasting uric acid, glucose, triglycerides, and prolactin; and incidence of somnolence and shifts to elevated glucose, elevated cholesterol, and elevated triglycerides
	val (187)	8.7	+0.5	8.5	
Niufan et al. (2008)	olz (69)	NR	+1.85[b]	16.2[b]	No statistical comparisons made for individual events; common adverse events for olanzapine (incidence ≥5%) included constipation, nausea, somnolence, nasopharyngitis, vomiting, diarrhea, dizziness, and restlessness.
	lith (71)	NR	+0.73	2.9	
Katagiri et al. (2010)	olz (105)	9.5	+1.22	13.3	Incidence of high ALT; and mean changes in RBC, eosinophils, AST, ALT, LDH, GGT, total protein, total bilirubin, uric acid
	hal (20)	25.0	−0.68	5.3	
Olanzapine as adjunctive therapy					
Tohen et al. (2002b)	olz + lith or val (229)	10.9[b]	+3.08[b]	NR	Incidence of somnolence, dry mouth, increased appetite, tremor, slurred speech
	lith or val (115)	1.7	+0.23	NR	
Tohen et al. (2008b)	olz + carb (58)	8.6	+2.96[b]	24.6[b]	Incidence of shift from normal to high triglycerides and the adverse events ALT increased and constipation. Of note, patients on olanzapine/carbamzepine combination had significantly higher increase in triglycerides levels than those on carbamazepine alone.
	carb (60)	8.3	+0.36	3.4	
Houston et al. (2009)	olz + val (101)	5.9	+3.34[b]	22[b]	Mean change in fasting glucose; incidence of sedation, somnolence, dry mouth, tremor.
	val (101)	4.0	+0.7	3	
Acute bipolar depression					
Tohen et al. (2003b)	olz (370)	9.2[b,c]	+2.59[b]	18.7[b]	Olanzapine and OFC versus placebo: mean increases in cholesterol and nonfasting glucose, and incidence of somnolence, increased appetite, dry mouth, and asthenia. OFC versus placebo: incidence of diarrhea, nausea, high supine systolic blood pressure, and potentially clinically significant orthostatic hypotension.
	olz + flx (86)	2.3	+2.79[b]	19.5[b]	
	pla (377)	5.0	−0.47	0.3	

(Continued Overleaf)

Table 6.2 (Continued)

Study	Treatment (N)	Adverse event discontinuations (%)	Weight Mean change (kg)	Weight Change ≥7% (%)	Adverse events, laboratory measures, or vital signs with significant treatment group differences in favor of comparator[a]
Brown et al. (2009)	olz + flx (205)	8.3	+3.1[b]	23.4[b]	Mean change in HbA1c, prolactin, total cholesterol, HDL, LDL, triglycerides; incidence of somnolence, increased appetite, dry mouth, sedation, tremor, elevated total cholesterol, LDL, and prolactin.
	lam (205)	7.3	−0.3	0	
Tamayo et al. (2009)	olz (57)	1.8	+4.85	11.1	The only between-group differences were for mean change in alkaline phosphatase (greater for OFC), and incidence of elevated AST and depressed mood (both greater for olanzapine).
	olz + flx (57)	5.3	+2.86	5.7	
Longer-term studies					
Tohen et al. (2003c) (47 wk)	olz (125)	24.8	+2.79[b]	23.6	Mean increase in total cholesterol and QTc interval; Incidence of somnolence, dry mouth, increased appetite, akathisia, and elevated ALT
	val (126)	19.8	+1.22	17.9	
Tohen et al. (2004) (78 wk)	olz + lith or val (51)	9.8	+2.0	27[b]	Incidence of weight gain was only significant difference
	lith or val (48)	16.7	−1.8	6	
Tohen et al. (2005) (52 wk)	olz (217)	18.9	+1.79[b]	29.8[b]	Note: pts gained 2.74 kg during open-label olanzapine acute treatment; mean weight changes shown to left are after randomization. Mean increase in cholesterol; incidence of depression, hypersomnia
	lith (214)	25.7	−1.38	9.8	

Tohen et al. (2006) (48 wk)	olz (225)	7.6[b]	+1.0	>35[b]	Note: pts gained 3.0 kg during open-label olanzapine acute treatment; mean weight changes shown to left are after randomization. Incidence of dry mouth, appetite increased, somnolence, sedation, fatigue, elevated prolactin.
	pla (136)	0.0	−2.0	2.3	
Brown et al. (2006) (25 wk)	olz + flx (205)	18.0	+4.4[b]	33.8[b]	Mean change in HbA1c, prolactin, total cholesterol, LDL cholesterol; incidence of somnolence, increased appetite, dry mouth, sedation, tremor, lethargy, disturbance in attention, peripheral edema, and elevated total cholesterol, triglycerides, prolactin, ALT, and AST
	lam (205)	13.2	−0.9%	2.1	
Tohen et al. (2008c) 26 wk (Note: adolescents)	olz (146)	16.4	+7.5	69.0	No statistical comparisons, but events with incidence of >10% included increased appetite, somnolence, sedation; elevations of ALT, AST, CPK, creatinine, calcium, albumin, uric acid; and shifts from normal to borderline and borderline to high cholesterol, normal to borderline and borderline to high LDL cholesterol, normal to low HDL, and normal to borderline and normal to high triglycerides

[a] Note that significant differences in weight or weight-related adverse events are not included in this column because more specific weight-related information is provided to left.

[b] Statistically significant difference at $p > 0.05$ from comparator (or from placebo, if there are multiple comparators).

[c] Statistically significant difference at $p > 0.05$ from non-placebo comparator.

ALT, alanine aminotransferase; AST, aspartate aminotransferase; carb, carbamazepine; CPK, creatine phosphokinase; flx, fluoxetine; GGT, gamma glutamyl transferase; hal, haloperidol; HbA1c, hemoglobin A1c; HDL, high-density lipoprotein; lam, lamotrigine; LDH, lactate dehydrogenase; LDL, low-density lipoprotein; lith, lithium; N/n, number; NR, not reported; OFC, olanzapine/fluoxetine combination; olz, olanzapine; pla, placebo; risp, risperidone; val, valproate.

It is important to note that compared with adult patients, adolescents treated with olanzapine were likely to gain more weight, experience increased sedation, and have greater increases in total cholesterol, triglycerides, LDL cholesterol, prolactin, and hepatic aminotransferase levels. Clinicians should consider the long-term risks of these findings, particularly weight gain and hyperlipidemia, and in many cases may consider prescribing other drugs first in adolescents.

6.7 SUMMARY

In summary, data based on multiple randomized double-blind controlled trials suggest that olanzapine monotherapy has efficacy in the treatment of acute mania and the prevention of relapse into both mania and depression. Olanzapine alone and in combination with fluoxetine has efficacy in the treatment of acute bipolar depressive episodes, although for this use it appears more effective in combination with fluoxetine than alone. Olanzapine in monotherapy has not been approved for the treatment of bipolar depression by regulatory authorities. All of the available evidence positions olanzapine, whether alone or in combination with mood stabilizers or fluoxetine, as a valuable therapeutic tool for the treatment of different phases of bipolar disorder. These efficacy results should be balanced with the safety profile of olanzapine. In trials in patients with bipolar disorder, the adverse events that were seen most commonly in patients treated with olanzapine or olanzapine/fluoxetine combination at significantly greater rates than in comparator-treated patients were events related to sedation and weight gain. The incidence of weight gain and changes in metabolic parameters in short- and long-term studies should also be taken into consideration. Patients treated with olanzapine should be monitored appropriately with respect to weight and metabolic parameters to achieve good treatment outcomes in the long term.

References

Altshuler, L.L., Post, R.M., Leverich, G.S. *et al.* (1995) Antidepressant-induced mania and cycle acceleration: a controversy revisited. *Am. J. Psychiatry*, **152** (8), 1130–1138.

Berk, M., Ichim, L., and Brook, S. (1999) Olanzapine compared to lithium in mania: a double-blind randomized controlled trial. *Int. Clin. Psychopharmacol.*, **14** (6), 339–343.

Biederman, J., Mick, E., Faraone, S.V. *et al.* (2000) Pediatric mania: a developmental subtype of bipolar disorder? *Biol. Psychiatry*, **48** (6), 458–466.

Biederman, J., Wozniak, J., Kiely, K. *et al.* (1995) CBCL clinical scales discriminate prepubertal children with structured interview-derived diagnosis of mania from those with ADHD. *J. Am. Acad. Child Adolesc. Psychiatry*, **34** (4), 464–471.

Bowden, C.L., Brugger, A.M., Swann, A.C. *et al.* (1994) Efficacy of divalproex vs lithium and placebo in the treatment of mania. The Depakote mania study group. *J. Am. Med. Assoc.*, **271** (12), 918–924.

Brown, E., Dunner, D.L., McElroy, S.L. *et al.* (2009) Olanzapine/fluoxetine combination vs. lamotrigine in the 6-month treatment of bipolar I depression. *Int. J. Neuropsychopharmacol.*, **12** (6), 773–782.

Brown, E.B., McElroy, S.L., Keck, P.E. Jr. *et al.* (2006) A 7-week, randomized, double-blind trial of olanzapine/fluoxetine combination versus lamotrigine in the treatment of bipolar I depression. *J. Clin. Psychiatry*, **67** (7), 1025–1033.

Bymaster, F.P., Calligaro, D.O., Falcone, J.F. *et al.* (1996) Radioreceptor binding profile of the atypical antipsychotic olanzapine. *Neuropsychopharmacology*, **14** (2), 87–96.

Chen, Y.W. and Dilsaver, S.C. (1995) Comorbidity of panic disorder in bipolar illness: evidence from the Epidemiologic Catchment Area Survey. *Am. J. Psychiatry*, **152** (2), 280–282.

Eli Lilly and Company (2009) *Zyprexa Integrated Benefit/Risk Considerations for Patients with Bipolar I Disorder*, Eli Lilly and Company, Indianapolis.

Geller, B., Fox, L.W., and Clark, K.A. (1994) Rate and predictors of prepubertal bipolarity during follow-up of 6- to 12-year-old depressed children. *J. Am. Acad. Child Adolesc. Psychiatry*, **33** (4), 461–468.

Goldstein, T.R. (2009) Suicidality in pediatric bipolar disorder. *Child Adolesc. Psychiatr. Clin. N. Am.*, **18** (2), 339–352, viii.

Goodwin, F.K. and Jamison, K.R. (1990) *Manic-depressive illness*, Oxford Press, New York.

Houston, J.P., Tohen, M., Degenhardt, E.K. *et al.* (2009) Olanzapine-divalproex combination versus divalproex monotherapy in the treatment of bipolar mixed episodes: a double-blind, placebo-controlled study. *J. Clin. Psychiatry*, **70** (11), 1540–1547.

Kane, J.M. and Smith, J.M. (1982) Tardive dyskinesia: prevalence and risk factors, 1959 to 1979. *Arch. Gen. Psychiatry*, **39** (4), 473–481.

Katagiri, H., Takita, Y., Tohen, M. *et al.* (2010) Efficacy and safety of olanzapine in the treatment of Japanese patients with a bipolar manic or mixed episode – a multicenter, randomized double-blind, parallel, placebo- and haloperidol-controlled study. Poster presented at the International College of Neuropsychopharmacology 2010 World Congress, 6–10 June, 2010, Hong Kong. [abstract].

Klein, E., Bental, E., Lerer, B. *et al.* (1984) Carbamazepine and haloperidol v placebo and haloperidol in excited psychoses. A controlled study. *Arch. Gen. Psychiatry*, **41** (2), 165–170.

Lipkovich, I., Citrome, L., Perlis, R. *et al.* (2006) Early predictors of substantial weight gain in bipolar patients treated with olanzapine. *J. Clin. Psychopharmacol.*, **26** (3), 316–320.

Lucas, R.A., Gilfillan, D.J., and Bergstrom, R.F. (1998) A pharmacokinetic interaction between carbamazepine and olanzapine: observations on possible mechanism. *Eur. J. Clin. Pharmacol.*, **54** (8), 639–643.

McClellan, J.M., Werry, J.S., and Ham, M. (1993) A follow-up study of early onset psychosis: comparison between outcome diagnoses of schizophrenia, mood disorders, and personality disorders. *J. Autism Dev. Disord.*, **23** (2), 243–262.

McIntyre, R.S., Alphs, L., Cohen, M. *et al.* (2008) Long-term double blind extension studies of asenapine versus olanzapine in patients with bipolar mania. *J. Affect. Disord.*, **107**, S91–S92. [abstract].

McIntyre, R.S., Cohen, M., Zhao, J. *et al.* (2009a) A 3-week, randomized, placebo-controlled trial of asenapine in the treatment of acute mania in bipolar mania and mixed states. *Bipolar Disord.*, **11** (7), 673–686.

McIntyre, R.S., Cohen, M., Zhao, J. *et al.* (2009b) Asenapine versus olanzapine in acute mania: a double-blind extension study. *Bipolar Disord.*, **11** (8), 815–826.

McIntyre, R.S., Cohen, M., Zhao, J. *et al.* (2010) Asenapine in the treatment of acute mania in bipolar I disorder: a randomized, double-blind, placebo-controlled trial. *J. Affect. Disord.*, **122** (1–2), 27–38.

Meehan, K., Zhang, F., David, S. *et al.* (2001) A double-blind, randomized comparison of the efficacy and safety of intramuscular injections of olanzapine, lorazepam, or placebo in treating acutely agitated patients diagnosed with bipolar mania. *J. Clin. Psychopharmacol.*, **21** (4), 389–397.

Millen, B.A., Campbell, G.M., and Beasley, C.M. (2010) Weight changes over time in adults treated with the oral or depot formulations of olanzapine: a pooled analysis of 86 clinical trials. *J. Psychopharmacol.*, [ePub before print], doi: 10.1177/0269881110370505.

Morgan, H.F. (1972) The incidence of depressive symptoms during recovery from hypomania. *Br. J. Psychiatry*, **120**, 537–539.

Muller-Oerlinghausen, B., Retzow, A., Henn, F.A. *et al.*, European Valproate Mania Study Group (2000) Valproate as an adjunct to neuroleptic medication for the treatment of acute episodes of mania: a prospective, randomized, double-blind, placebo-controlled, multicenter study. *J. Clin. Psychopharmacol.*, **20** (2), 195–203.

Niufan, G., Tohen, M., Qiuqing, A. *et al.* (2008) Olanzapine versus lithium in the acute treatment of bipolar mania: a double-blind, randomized, controlled trial. *J. Affect. Disord.*, **105** (1–3), 101–108.

Perlis, R.H., Baker, R.W., Zarate, C.A. Jr. *et al.* (2006) Olanzapine versus risperidone in the treatment of manic or mixed states in bipolar I disorder: a randomized, double-blind trial. *J. Clin. Psychiatry*, **67** (11), 1747–1753.

Pope, H.G. Jr., McElroy, S.L., Keck, P.E. Jr., *et al.* (1991) Valproate in the treatment of acute mania. A placebo-controlled study. *Arch. Gen. Psychiatry* **48** (1), 62–68.

Seeman, P. and Kapur, S. (2000) What makes olanzapine an atypical antipsychotic? in *Olanzapine (Zyprexa): A Novel Antipsychotic?* (eds P. Tran, F.P. Bymaster, N.C. Tye *et al.*), Lippincott Williams and Wilkens, Philadelphia, pp. 3–24.

Strober, M., Schmidt-Lackner, S., Freeman, R. *et al.* (1995) Recovery and relapse in adolescents with bipolar affective illness: a five-year naturalistic, prospective follow-up. *J. Am. Acad. Child Adolesc. Psychiatry*, **34** (6), 724–731.

Tamayo, J.M., Sutton, V.K., Mattei, M.A. *et al.* (2009) Effectiveness and safety of the combination of fluoxetine and olanzapine in outpatients with bipolar depression: an open-label, randomized, flexible-dose study in Puerto Rico. *J. Clin. Psychopharmacol.*, **29** (4), 358–361.

Todd, R.D., Neuman, R., Geller, B. *et al.* (1993) Genetic studies of affective disorders: should we be starting with childhood onset probands? *J. Am. Acad. Child Adolesc. Psychiatry*, **32** (6), 1164–1171.

Tohen, M. (1997) Mania, in *Acute Care Psychiatry Diagnosis and Treatment* (eds L.I. Sederer and A.J. Rotchschild), Williams & Wilkens, Baltimore, pp. 141–165.

Tohen, M., Baker, R.W., Altshuler, L.L. *et al.* (2002a) Olanzapine versus divalproex in the treatment of acute mania. *Am. J. Psychiatry*, **159** (6), 1011–1017.

Tohen, M., Chengappa, K.N., Suppes, T. *et al.* (2002b) Efficacy of olanzapine in combination with valproate or lithium in the treatment of mania in patients partially nonresponsive to valproate or lithium monotherapy. *Arch. Gen. Psychiatry*, **59** (1), 62–69.

Tohen, M., Vieta, E., Goodwin, G.M. *et al.* (2008a) Olanzapine versus divalproex versus placebo in the treatment of mild to moderate mania: a randomized, 12-week, double-blind study. *J. Clin. Psychiatry*, **69** (11), 1776–1789.

Tohen, M., Bowden, C.L., Smulevich, A.B. *et al.* (2008b) Olanzapine plus carbamazepine v. carbamazepine alone in treating manic episodes. *Br. J. Psychiatry*, **192** (2), 135–143.

Tohen, M., Kryzhanovskaya, L., Carlson, G. *et al.* (2008c) Open-label treatment with olanzapine in adolescents with bipolar mania. Poster presented at the Winter Workshop on Schizophrenia and Bipolar Disorders – 14th Biennial, February 3, 2008, Montreux, Switzerland.

Tohen, M., Calabrese, J.R., Sachs, G.S. *et al.* (2006) Randomized, placebo-controlled trial of olanzapine as maintenance therapy in patients with bipolar I disorder responding to acute treatment with olanzapine. *Am. J. Psychiatry*, **163** (2), 247–256.

Tohen, M., Chengappa, K.N., Suppes, T. *et al.* (2004) Relapse prevention in bipolar I disorder: 18-month comparison of olanzapine plus mood stabiliser v. mood stabiliser alone. *Br. J. Psychiatry*, **184**, 337–345.

Tohen, M., Frank, E., Bowden, C.L. *et al.* (2009a) The International Society for Bipolar Disorders (ISBD) Task Force report on the nomenclature of course and outcome in bipolar disorders. *Bipolar Disord.*, **11** (5), 453–473.

Tohen, M., Sutton, V.K., Calabrese, J.R. *et al.* (2009b) Maintenance of response following stabilization of mixed index episodes with olanzapine monotherapy in a randomized, double-blind, placebo-controlled study of bipolar 1 disorder. *J. Affect. Disord.*, **116** (1–2), 43–50.

Tohen, M., Goldberg, J.F., Gonzalez-Pinto Arrillaga, A.M. *et al.* (2003a) A 12-week, double-blind comparison of olanzapine vs haloperidol in the treatment of acute mania. *Arch. Gen. Psychiatry*, **60** (12), 1218–1226.

Tohen, M., Vieta, E., Calabrese, J. *et al.* (2003b) Efficacy of olanzapine and olanzapine-fluoxetine combination in the treatment of bipolar I depression. *Arch. Gen. Psychiatry*, **60** (11), 1079–1088.

Tohen, M., Ketter, T.A., Zarate, C.A. *et al.* (2003c) Olanzapine versus divalproex sodium for the treatment of acute mania and maintenance of remission: a 47-week study. *Am. J. Psychiatry*, **160** (7), 1263–1271.

Tohen, M., Greil, W., Calabrese, J.R. *et al.* (2005) Olanzapine versus lithium in the maintenance treatment of bipolar disorder: a 12-month, randomized, double-blind, controlled clinical trial. *Am. J. Psychiatry*, **162** (7), 1281–1290.

Tohen, M., Jacobs, T.G., Grundy, S.L. *et al.*, The Olanzapine HGGW Study Group (2000) Efficacy of olanzapine in acute bipolar mania: a double-blind, placebo-controlled study. *Arch. Gen. Psychiatry*, **57** (9), 841–849.

Tohen, M., Kryzhanovskaya, L., Carlson, G. *et al.* (2007) Olanzapine versus placebo in the treatment of adolescents with bipolar mania. *Am. J. Psychiatry*, **164** (10), 1547–1556.

Tohen, M., Sanger, T.M., McElroy, S.L. *et al.*, Olanzapine HGEH study Group (1999) Olanzapine versus placebo in the treatment of acute mania. *Am. J. Psychiatry*, **156** (5), 702–709.

Tohen, M., Zhang, F., Taylor, C.C. *et al.* (2001) A meta-analysis of the use of typical antipsychotic agents in bipolar disorder. *J. Affect. Disord.*, **65** (1), 85–93.

Wehr, T.A. and Goodwin, F.K. (1987) Can antidepressants cause mania and worsen the course of affective illness? *Am. J. Psychiatry*, **144** (11), 1403–1411.

West, S.A., McElroy, S.L., Strakowski, S.M. *et al.* (1995) Attention deficit hyperactivity disorder in adolescent mania. *Am. J. Psychiatry*, **152** (2), 271–273.

Wozniak, J., Biederman, J., Kiely, K. *et al.* (1995) Mania-like symptoms suggestive of childhood-onset bipolar disorder in clinically referred children. *J. Am. Acad. Child Adolesc. Psychiatry*, **34** (7), 867–876.

Zajecka, J.M., Weisler, R., Sachs, G. *et al.* (2002) A comparison of the efficacy, safety, and tolerability of divalproex sodium and olanzapine in the treatment of bipolar disorder. *J. Clin. Psychiatry*, **63** (12), 1148–1155.

Zarate, C.A. Jr. and Tohen, M. (2004) Double-blind comparison of the continued use of antipsychotic treatment versus its discontinuation in remitted manic patients. *Am. J. Psychiatry*, **161** (1), 169–171.

Haloperidol and Other First Generation Antipsychotics in Mania

John Cookson

The Royal London Hospital, Mile End Hospital,
London, UK

7.1 INTRODUCTION

Mania is a clearly defined condition that can present in different levels of severity varying from the mild (hypomanic) to the florid, raging, and psychotic. Only the mildest forms can be left untreated without risking harm to either the patient's welfare, relationships and job, or to the well-being of those who are close to them (relatives, carers, or staff). Severe forms constitute a psychiatric emergency, demanding immediate control including rapid tranquillization with medication. The milder forms may be accompanied by high levels of energy, productivity, and creativity. But even these carry a risk of subsequently switching into a phase of depression and incapacity that might have been avoided by treatment of the preceding hypomania. Mania is one of the most insightless forms of mental disorder and for treatment to be very useful it must be not only effective but also acceptable to the patient, easy to use, and not produce unpleasant side effects.

Surveys of clinical practice have shown that antipsychotics are the most commonly used drugs in patients hospitalized with mania, whether in Britain, Scandinavia, other parts of Europe, or North America. Classical antipsychotics produce unpleasant extrapyramidal side effects (EPS) such as akathisia, dystonia, and Parkinsonism which (although partially preventable by anticholinergic medication) are resented by patients and which limit their adherence to treatment.

The occurrence of neurological (Parkinsonian) side effects with the phenothiazines such as chlorpromazine (discovered in 1952) had indicated that these drugs affected neurones, and the name "neuroleptic" ("seizes neurones") was used to describe the phenothiazines and later haloperidol; the term "antipsychotic" is now preferred. Chlorpromazine, other phenothiazines, haloperidol, and the thioxanthine zuclopenthixol are the first generation antipsychotics that are most used in mania. They are also called "typical" or "classical" antipsychotics. Later, newer drugs were developed to avoid "extra-pyramidal" side effects, and were called "atypical," "second generation," or "new generation" antipsychotics. Owens (2008) and others have argued that the use of the term "atypical" to describe the newer antipsychotics is unhelpful. He questioned also whether

Bipolar Psychopharmacotherapy: Caring for the patient, Second Edition. Edited by Hagop S. Akiskal and Mauricio Tohen.
© 2011 John Wiley & Sons, Ltd. Published 2011 by John Wiley & Sons, Ltd.

they have advantages in efficacy, other than by producing fewer EPSs. Cookson (2008b) argued that views about antipsychotics should be "triangulated" to appreciate efficacy trials, effectiveness studies, and naturalistic data together.

In 1958 the creative genius of Paul Janssen, the Belgian clinician and chemist, and founder of the Janssen pharmaceutical company, led to the introduction of haloperidol, a butyrophenone with antipsychotic properties. This had been synthesized as a variant of the pethidine molecule and it was observed to antagonize the effects of amphetamines in animals. The fact that amphetamines were associated with psychotic reactions in cyclists, who were taking them to enhance their performance, led Janssen to study the effects of haloperidol in schizophrenia and mania.

Clopenthixol is a more sedative drug than haloperidol and has been used in mania, especially in its cis(zu)-clopenthixol isomer (Bjørndal, 1990).

7.1.1 ASSESSING THE EVIDENCE

To prove that a drug is efficacious for a psychiatric condition, it is essential to show that it is superior to placebo, by conducting randomized double-blind placebo-controlled trials. The challenges of conducting such trials in mania have been met only in recent years, in the course of developing novel anticonvulsant and new generation antipsychotic treatments in trials since 1994. These trials are therefore providing answers to questions that have long remained unresolved about the treatment of mania. Analysis of the results of these trials requires attention not only to the statistical significance of differences in special rating scales, but also to the size of the effect, and to the generalizability of results derived from highly selected patients in clinical trials centers, to patients with mania in routine practice. It is also important to consider how drop-outs from the studies may have biased the interpretation of results.

7.1.2 MECHANISMS OF ANTIMANIC ACTIONS OF ANTIPSYCHOTICS

It is thought that antipsychotics owe their antimanic effects mainly to blockade of receptors for dopamine (DA), but additionally to some extent to blockade of noradrenaline at alpha-1 receptors (as in the case of haloperidol), and blockade of histamine at H-1 receptors (causing sedation as in the case of chlorpromazine) (Peroutka and Snyder, 1980; Cookson, 2001). Alpha-1 receptor blockade is also thought to contribute to transient sedative effects of antipsychotics (Peroutka and Snyder, 1980). It may account for the early transient sedative effects seen in mania with haloperidol (Cookson, 1985; Cookson *et al.*, 1983).

7.2 ACUTE TRANQUILLIZATION IN MANIA

The acutely manic patient presents an immediate challenge to medical and nursing staff, and usually requires medication to reduce aggressive or violent behavior, agitation, and the behavioral consequences of psychotic thinking. The violent patient presents the most extreme challenge to the psychiatrist of how to combine psychology and pharmacology, compassion, and safety in effective proportion. Drugs are used both to treat the underlying manic state and to reduce aggression and arousal (Royal College of Psychiatrists, 1998; Cookson, Taylor, and Katona, 2002a). The aim of acute tranquillization is to calm or sedate the patient sufficiently to minimize the risk posed to the patient and to others. Often it is used for sedation, but sometimes it addresses also the underlying illness, particularly mania. When an antipsychotic is used, haloperidol is often the drug of first choice, especially if intramuscular administration is necessary. Five milligrams to 10 mg may be given intramuscularly for the first injection and repeated. In some countries, a lower dose is started.

A combination of haloperidol with a benzodiazepine such as lorazepam (LZP), which may also be given intramuscularly (1–2 mg), has been the commonest approach for rapid tranquillization of acutely disturbed patients, many of whom have mania. There is little evidence concerning the optimal dose of haloperidol for this use. Mania may improve rapidly following parenteral haloperidol. Ratings of mania improved by 30% within 20 minutes after intravenous injection of 2.5–5 mg, and such improvement was seen before patients slept (Cookson et al., 1983).

7.2.1 LONG-ACTING INJECTIONS OF ANTIPSYCHOTICS

For patients who continue to refuse oral medication, and if excitement or aggression persist, the use of a longer acting intramuscular (IM) injection of zu-clopenthixol as acetate (Acuphase) helps to reduce the need for frequent injections. This has an effect lasting for about three days. Fifty milligrams to 150 mg is given by deep IM injection. The onset of action takes 2–8 hours during which time another drug may be required. The injection should not be repeated for 24 hours, and the maximum amount for a course is 400 mg in total. Subsequently the longer acting zu-clopenthixol decanoate may be used (Nolen, 1983). This has a duration of one to two weeks.

7.3 SEDATION IS NOT REQUIRED FOR ANTIPSYCHOTICS TO IMPROVE MANIA

Chlorpromazine was the most widely investigated antipsychotic in early comparative trials in mania, but drugs with more specific DA-receptor blocking actions have antimanic properties. These drugs – such as pimozide and haloperidol – are less sedative, being without blocking actions at histamine receptors. The efficacy of these less sedative drugs in mania highlights the importance of DA receptor blockade in the antimanic effects of antipsychotic drugs (Cookson et al., 1981; Post et al., 1980), and indicates that antimanic activity can occur independently of sedation (Cookson, 2008a).

7.4 CHLORPROMAZINE IN MANIA

The first antipsychotic drug, chlorpromazine, was effective in mania in a placebo-controlled trial (Klein, 1967). It was also the first such agent to be widely compared with

112 _____ **Bipolar Psychopharmacotherapy**

lithium in randomized, double-blind controlled trials. A summary by Davis, Wang, and Janicak (1993), of trials in which categorical outcomes were given, showed a response rate in four trials (145 patients) of 23% with chlorpromazine, compared with 63% for lithium, an "effect size" or absolute difference in risk of 39%, which would correspond to an Number Needed to Treat (NNT) of 2.6, in favor of lithium. This difference appears impressive, but the original studies had many shortcomings. They did not use rating scales specific for mania, and lacked a clear definition of response ("remission or marked improvement"). There was also potential for unblinding because of the faster effects of chlorpromazine and its sedative properties. The number of patients included was usually small by current standards.

7.5 HALOPERIDOL IN MANIA

In the 1990s, the preferences of American (New York) psychiatrists for high potency antipsychotics such as haloperidol in mania was illustrated in a study by Chou *et al.* (1996) of 528 manic patients in New York state hospitals in 1990. Ninety-two percent received antipsychotic medication, 61% lithium, 54% both, and 22% benzodiazepines – mainly lorazepam – during the first three weeks of hospitalization for mania. Haloperidol (38% of prescriptions) was the most widely used antipsychotic drug, followed by fluphenazine (20%) and chlorpromazine (18%).

Since haloperidol was the most commonly prescribed antipsychotic in mania, the study by Shopsin *et al.* (1975) is important. This compared haloperidol (up to 36 mg per day) with chlorpromazine (up to 1800 mg per day) and lithium in a three-week study with only 10 patients in each treatment group. Lithium appeared to produce a broader improvement in manic symptoms than the antipsychotics; seven patients were well enough to be discharged after treatment with lithium compared to only one patient on chlorpromazine and two patients on haloperidol. However the clinical ratings (Clinical Global Impression (CGI)) showed almost identical levels of improvement at three weeks for lithium and haloperidol, both of which were superior to chlorpromazine. The authors described haloperidol as more effective than lithium in reducing hyperactivity, while lithium produced greater effects on mood and ideation; however, the Brief Psychiatric Rating Scale did not show significant differences in individual items for the three treatments. Haloperidol had a more pronounced antimanic effect than chlorpromazine and this was not accompanied by sedation. The authors argued that the control of symptoms by haloperidol was "a suppressive lid," as opposed to the "more total normalization of affect, ideation, and behavior" on lithium. An alternative view was expressed as early as 1973 by Prien *et al.*, who found " . . . no evidence the treatments worked differently on the underlying manic process" and were " . . . unable to confirm . . . the claims that lithium treats the underlying manic process while chlorpromazine controls . . . behavior through sedation without affecting underlying mood and ideation."

The high rate of remission within three weeks on lithium in this study by Shopsin *et al.* (1975) is in contrast to the lower rates seen in more recent studies such as that by Bowden *et al.* (1994). Conversely, the very low rate of remission on haloperidol contrasts with the dose-finding study of 47 severely ill manic patients by Rifkin *et al.* (1994), in which 45% of patients, treated with haloperidol, remitted within six weeks. The latter study was important in failing to show a significantly greater improvement with doses of haloperidol above 10 mg per day and up to 80 mg per day. However, the numbers involved were small and the confidence limits overlapped in all three dose ranges. There was a distinct trend for patients on 30 mg per day or more to do better than those on only 10 mg per day. Further studies are needed to identify the optimal doses for haloperidol in mania.

In patients who remain disturbed on standard doses of haloperidol, additional sedation may be achieved by benzodiazepines, especially lorazepam, a practice that carries less risk of cardiotoxicity than using higher doses of antipsychotics (Lenox *et al.*, 1992; Busch, Miller, and Weiden, 1989). However, a combination of two antimanic drugs from different classes should also be considered, for example, an antipsychotic with lithium.

7.5.1 COMBINATION TREATMENT WITH LITHIUM AND HALOPERIDOL

If, as Shopsin *et al.* (1975) found, lithium is superior to haloperidol, and acts through different mechanisms to exert its antimanic effect, one would expect that patients treated with a combination of lithium and haloperidol would respond significantly better than patients treated with either drug alone. One small study (with seven patients in each group and therefore not sufficiently powered to explore the question conclusively) addressed this comparison in mania (Garfinkel, Stancer, and Persaud, 1980). Haloperidol appeared superior to lithium alone, and the combination gave no additional advantage during three weeks of treatment.

One of the recent combination studies of new generation antipsychotics plus "mood stabilizers" included haloperidol as an active comparator (see below, Table 7.2).

7.5.2 DEPRESSION IN MANIA

Depressive symptoms are very common during mania, and if amounting to a major depressive syndrome the condition is classified as mixed mania in Diagnostic Statistical Manual Version IV (DSM–IV) (American Psychiatric Association, 1994). However, at least 12 forms of bipolar mixed states have been described and are likely to respond differently to treatments (Cookson and Ghalib, 2004). Some patients develop depressive syndromes after mania has improved ("post-manic depression"), and this is described as a "switch" into depression.

It has been suggested, but never proved, that classical antipsychotics may worsen or induce depression apart from their obvious EPSs. For example, the use of perphenazine in mania without an anticholinergic drug has been associated with a high rate of development of depressive symptomatology, with accompanying signs of Parkinsonism, particularly akinesia (Zarate and Tohen, 2004). Used in this way for schizophrenia, the older antipsychotics such as haloperidol are known to induce "akinetic depression," which is best viewed as an EPS (van Putten and May, 1978).

7.6 HORMONE CHANGES AND MECHANISMS OF ANTIMANIC EFFECTS OF ANTIPSYCHOTICS

7.6.1 CORTISOL

Elevated serum cortisol levels are found in mania. During treatment with haloperidol, there is dissociation between an early normalization of cortisol levels within three days, and a more gradual clinical improvement during two weeks of treatment (Cookson et al., 1985). This may occur because haloperidol blocks noradrenaline alpha-1 receptors in man (Szabadi, Gaszner, and Bradshaw, 1981).

7.6.2 PROLACTIN

DA-2 receptors in the prolactin-secreting cells of the anterior pituitary gland are blocked by classical antipsychotic agents, and by risperidone. The resulting elevation of serum prolactin levels provides a biological marker of this DA receptor blockade; it may also have clinical consequences including side effects such as galactorrhoea, amenorrhoea, reduced libido, and reduced bone density. During treatment with haloperidol, prolactin levels increase in the plasma over the course of 14 days, with a pattern of rise similar to the timecourse of clinical improvement. However, more detailed analysis using intravenous "test doses" of haloperidol, shows an initial rise in serum prolactin levels, which is partly transient after the first intravenous dose and cannot be exceeded by giving larger doses of haloperidol (Cookson et al., 1983). This is followed by a gradual rise during the following two to four weeks. Within two weeks, prolactin secretion by the pituitary becomes sensitive over a wider range of doses of haloperidol than in the drug-naive patient. These compensatory changes, in the control of prolactin secretion, are thought to include changes in the level of DA in the portal pituitary blood supply during prolonged treatment with haloperidol. If similar compensatory changes occur in the DA pathways of the limbic system, doses of haloperidol that are effective in the drug-naive manic patient may not be sufficient to control patients in later stages of mania, who have received prolonged treatment with antipsychotic drugs.

Comparison of haloperidol with new generation antipsychotics in mania have shown that risperidone produces a larger rise in prolactin levels than haloperidol (Smulevich et al., 2005), but that quetiapine (McIntyre et al., 2005) and aripiprazole (Young et al., 2009) produce much less increase in prolactin than haloperidol.

7.7 ANTIPSYCHOTICS AS MOOD STABILIZERS

Antipsychotic drugs are used extensively in the maintenance treatment of bipolar patients (Sernyak et al., 1994; Sernyak and Woods, 1998; Cookson and Sachs, 1999; Cookson, 2001). For patients who are unresponsive to lithium (and anticonvulsants), and particularly for those whose compliance with oral medication is poor, depot formulations of antipsychotic drugs including haloperidol decanoate have the advantage of providing a sustained and reliable delivery of a drug for periods of weeks. For rapid cycling bipolar patients, the depot antipsychotics haloperidol decanoate stabilized mood swings (Lowe and Batchelor, 1990). In a minority of bipolar outpatients, depot antipsychotic medication is used and can reduce the time spent in both manic and depressed phases (Littlejohn, Leslie, and Cookson, 1994). Seemingly poorly responding patients, who were switched from lithium to flupentixol decanoate, then had less time ill with mania but more time ill with depression (Ahlfors, Baastrup, and Dencker, 1981).

7.8   PLACEBO-CONTROLLED STUDIES IN MANIA

7.8.1   PLACEBO-CONTROLLED MONOTHERAPY TRIALS OF HALOPERIDOL IN MANIA

Three of the recent parallel-group randomized placebo-controlled monotherapy studies of new generation antipsychotics in mania have included haloperidol as an active comparator, the risperidone study reported by Smulevich _et al._ (2005), the quetiapine study of McIntyre _et al._ (2005), and the aripiprazole trial reported by Young _et al._ (2009). Table 7.1 summarizes these international studies using a "NNT" analysis and showing the dropouts rates for reasons of adverse events, lack of efficacy, and other reasons. A study with ziprasidone was also conducted (Dunn _et al._, 2005), but the results for the haloperidol arm (mean dose 16 mg/day) have not as yet been fully published (Scherk _et al._, 2007).

NNT is calculated by dividing the difference in response rate between active drug and placebo into 100 and correcting to the next highest integer. It represents the number of patients who must be treated in order for one patient to achieve the defined response – usually a 50% reduction in score on a scale such as the 11-item Young Mania Rating Scale (YMRS) – as a result of the pharmacological effect of the drug. NNT thus provides a measure of the size of effect that can be expected of the drug in a clinical situation. For a drug to be useful monotherapy as a first-line treatment in a common and severe disorder such as mania, the NNT for 50% improvement in severity should be in the order of two to four (Cookson, Taylor, and Katona, 2002b).

The studies, of three weeks duration, had placebo response rates of 33, 35, and 39%, reflecting the effects of a variety of possible non-specific factors such as hospitalization, extra medication with benzodiazepines or chloral allowed during the first 10–14 days, and bias in the raters.

Haloperidol compared favorably with the new drugs, regarding dropouts. Total dropout rates on the new drug in the three studies were 11% on risperidone, 46% on quetiapine, and 25% on aripiprazole. Total dropout rates on placebo were 15, 59, and 29%, and on haloperidol were 10, 46, and 27%. Dropout rates for inefficacy on new generation antipsychotic (risperidone, quetiapine, and aripiprazole) were 3, 18, and 5%. On haloperidol they were 1, 10, and 6%. On placebo dropout rates for inefficacy were 6, 29, and 9%. Dropouts through adverse events (including suspected side effects) were 4, 5, and 8% on risperidone, quetiapine, and aripiprazole, compared with 3, 10, and 5% on haloperidol. They were 5, 6, and 11% on placebo.

In the study with risperidone (Smulevich _et al._, 2005), the dose of haloperidol started at 4 mg/day and was adjusted to 2–12 mg/day by day 5. The timecourse of improvement

Table 7.1 Placebo-controlled parallel-group randomized trials of monotherapy with risperidone, quetiapine or aripiprazole, or haloperidol in mania.

Treatment mean dose numbers for ITT	Duration Authors Extra drugs	Inclusion criteria Criterion for response	Dropouts for inefficacy (%)	Dropouts for adverse events (%)	Other dropouts (%)	Response (%)	Difference from placebo	Number-needed-to-treat
Risperidone N = 154 Mean modal 4.2 mg/d	3 wk (extended to 12 wk without placebo) Smulevich et al. (2005) LZP, chloral, or diazepam for 10 d	DSM-IV Manic YMRS ≥ 20 MADRS < or = 20 50% reduction YMRS	3	4	4	48	15	95% CI 7 (4–26)
Placebo N = 140			6	5	4	33		
Haloperidol N = 144 Mean modal 8 mg/d			1	3	6	47	14	8 (4–36)
Quetiapine N = 102 Responders day 21: Mean 559 mg/d	3 wk (extended to 12 wk) McIntyre et al. (2005) LZP for 10 d Hypnotics for insomnia	DSM-IV Manic YMRS ≥ 20 50% reduction YMRS	17.6	4.9	23.5	3/52: 42 12/52: 60	3/52: 7 12/52: 21	3/52: NSD 15 (5–∞ to −16) 12/52: 5 (3–14)

Study arm	Design / reference	Criteria						
Placebo N = 100			28.7	5.9	23.9	3/52: 35 12/52: 39		
Haloperidol N = 98 Mean day 21: 5.2 mg/d			10.1	10.1	25.3	3/52: 55 12/52: 70	8.8	3/52: 5 (3–16) 12/52: 4 (3–6)
Aripiprazole N = 166 15 to 30 mg/d	3 wk (extended to 12 wk without placebo) Young et al. (2009) LZP up to 14 d	DSM-IV manic or mixed YMRS ≥20 MADRS <or =17 50% reduction YMRS	5	8	12	47		NSD 12 (5– ∞ to –50)
Placebo N = 152			9	11	9	38.2		
Haloperidol N = 161 5 to 15 mg/d Mean 8.5 mg/d by week 3			6	5	16	49.7	11.5	9 (5–174)

ITT, intention to treat.

on haloperidol was similar to that with risperidone, and by day 21 the NNT for 50% improvement on haloperidol was 8 (95% confidence interval (CI) 4–36). This is far larger than one would usually associate with the most commonly used antimanic drug of the previous decade; this might be because the mean modal dose of haloperidol was only 8 mg/day, or because the patients in the trial were in some way not typical of routine clinic patients and were more resistant to treatment.

Montgomery–Åsberg Depression Rating Scale (MADRS) depression scores, low at the start, fell more on risperidone than on placebo from week 1, and on haloperidol only at week 2 (Smulevich *et al.*, 2005). Side effects on risperidone included extrapyramidal symptoms (17% compared with 40% on haloperidol). In this study, the improvement in mania occurred in patients with or without psychotic symptoms. The improvement on active treatments compared with placebo was continuing to develop during the third week of treatment; the extension to 12 weeks demonstrated further improvement in YMRS scores with active treatment, suggesting that the dose initially administered may not have been sufficient to achieve maximum improvement.

A comparator group on haloperidol (up to 8 mg/day) was also included in the study reported by McIntyre *et al.* (2005) of quetiapine (up to 800 mg/day) and placebo, analyzed at 3 and 12 weeks. At three weeks the response rate (50% reduction in YMRS score) on haloperidol, on a mean dose of only 5.2 mg/day, was 55% compared with 35% on placebo, giving a NNT of 5 (95% confidence interval 3–16). The response rate on quetiapine was 42%, not significantly greater than on placebo. There were more dropouts on placebo than on haloperidol or quetiapine, so that the analysis using last observations carried forward was biased in favor of the active drugs, and especially so in favor of quetiapine after three weeks when more patients on placebo or haloperidol than on quetiapine dropped out. By 12 weeks the response rate on haloperidol was 70% and on placebo 39%, giving a NNT of 4 (3–6). The response rate on quetiapine was 60%; the NNT was 5 (3–14). Depression scores (MADRS) improved by day 21 on both quetiapine and haloperidol more than on placebo. On the other hand, the switch rates into depression over 12 weeks were similar for haloperidol (8.1%) and placebo (8.9%), and tended to be lower for quetiapine (2.9%). Side effects in the form of extrapyramidal symptoms were much more common on haloperidol (59.6%) than on placebo (15.8%), as was akathisia (33.3% on haloperidol and 5.9% on placebo). Anticholinergic medication was permitted and used in 52.5% on haloperidol, 9.8% on quetiapine, and 11.9% on placebo. Somnolence occurred more often with haloperidol (9.1%) than placebo (5%)

Young *et al.* (2009) reported the findings of a study comparing haloperidol with aripiprazole or placebo in mania or mixed mania (20% of cases). Anticholinergic medication was permitted and used in 44.2% on haloperidol, 15.1% on aripiprazole, and 6.5% on placebo. Haloperidol produced statistically significant improvements at all post-baseline assessments from day two to three weeks. By contrast, aripiprazole produced slower or less improvement, which was statistically significant at weeks 2 and 3. At three weeks the NNT was significant for haloperidol at 9 (5–174), but not significant for aripiprazole at 12 (5 − ∞ to −50).

There was no significant difference in the rate of emergent depression (MADRS total score >or = 18 plus >or = 4-point increase from baseline for any two consecutive assessments) between either aripiprazole (6.0%) or haloperidol (1.9%) vs. placebo (4.6%) at week 3. At week 12, rates of emergent depression were 4.3% for haloperidol and 9.6% for aripiprazole, not significantly different (ratio of incidence rates 2.2, 95% CI 0.9–5.3).

Serious adverse events were reported in 19 (11.4%) aripiprazole-treated patients and 5 (3%) haloperidol-treated patients. Fourteen (8.4%) of the aripiprazole-treated patients experienced at least one serious adverse event categorized as "psychiatric disorder," including worsening of mania, depression, and insomnia.

7.8.2 HALOPERIDOL EFFICACY IN MONOTHERAPY: CONCLUSIONS

Based upon these three placebo-controlled monotherapy studies, haloperidol was consistently efficacious with respect to 50% improvement in mania scores within three weeks, whereas two of the new drugs (aripiprazole and quetiapine) were not. Although there was a need for additional anticholinergic medication in many patients on haloperidol, it compared favorably with the new drugs regarding overall discontinuation for adverse events. The rather disappointing NNT for haloperidol (8, 5, and 9 at three weeks) should be seen in the context of placebo response rates of 33, 35, and 38%, high numbers but typical of most randomized controlled trials (RCTs) in mania, where the placebo group could receive benzodiazepines in the first 10–14 days. The dropouts for reasons other than lack of efficacy would also limit the benefits that could be obtained with drug treatment. In the case of haloperidol, anticholinergic medication can be given from the start in normal clinical practice, but was not given until EPSs developed in these trials, a factor that would detract from the efficacy of haloperidol, if it led to drop out from the trial.

7.8.3 HALOPERIDOL WITH LITHIUM OR VALPROATE: TRIALS OF COMBINATION THERAPY VS MONOTHERAPY

Since lithium and valproate are thought to have mechanisms of action other than receptor blockade, and probably reduce DA release, it may be expected that combination of an antipsychotic with lithium or valproate will produce a greater antimanic effect than the lithium or valproate alone. Two earlier trials found carbamazepine together with a typical antipsychotic (haloperidol) more effective than an antipsychotic alone (Klein *et al.*, 1984; Moller *et al.*, 1989).

The benefit off adding antipsychotic to lithium or valproate has been confirmed in trials in which an antipsychotic or placebo was given in addition to lithium or valproate. The effect is clearest when patients had previously shown only partial response to the lithium or valproate. The antipsychotics for which this added benefit has been shown are haloperidol, olanzapine, risperidone, quetiapine, and aripiprazole, but not ziprasidone (Scherk *et al.*, 2007).

Table 7.2 summarizes RCTs of combining haloperidol or other first generation antipsychotics with lithium or valproate.

A large study of risperidone (1–6 mg daily) added for three weeks to treatment with lithium or valproate included a group on haloperidol (2–12 mg/day) (Sachs *et al.*, 2002). In this study, response rates based on a CGI-I of much or very much improvement were

Table 7.2 NNTs for combination of haloperidol (or risperidone) with "mood stabilizer" (lithium or valproate).

Authors Treatment Duration Sites Extra drugs	Treatments Mean Modal dose Numbers	Inclusion criteria Criterion of response	Dropouts for inefficacy (%)	Dropouts for adverse events (%)	Other dropouts (%)	Response (%)	Difference from placebo (%)	Number-needed-to-treat (95% C.I.)
Sachs et al. (2002) Combination with Li or valproate. Three weeks, USA Benzodiazepines for sleep, LZP 4 mg/d for seven days	Haloperidol 6.2 mg/d N = 53	Manic or mixed YMRS ≥ 20 CGI much or very much improved	6	2	45	50	20	5 (3–64)
	Placebo N = 51		10	4	35	30		
	Risperidone 3.8 mg/day N = 52		6	4	25	53	23	5 (3–23)
Combination with antipsychotics Three weeks Muller-Oerlinghausen et al. (2000)	Valproate n = 69	50% less Y-MRS	1	9	—	70	24	5 (3–13)
	Placebo n = 67		3	13	—	46		

30% on mood stabilizer plus placebo and 53% on combination of mood stabilizer with risperidone (in a mean modal dose of only 3.8 mg/day); this difference corresponds to a NNT of 5 (95% confidence interval 3–23) for response to risperidone. Combination with haloperidol (mean modal dose 6.2 mg/day) and lithium or valproate also showed a NNT of 5 (95% confidence interval 3–64). The higher total dropout rate on haloperidol (53%) than on placebo combination (49%), or risperidone combination (35%) would bias the analysis of efficacy against haloperidol. Sixty-three percent of patients had already received lithium or valproate before randomization to risperidone or placebo, and might therefore be considered non-responders to the mood stabilizer; the rest commenced on lithium or valproate at the same time as being randomized to start on risperidone or placebo. The benefit of additional antipsychotic medication was much less apparent in the latter group. Significant improvement in response to haloperidol was limited to patients with pure mania and was not evident in those with mixed manic states, who comprised 21% of patients. No patients achieved a CGI rating of very much improved on lithium or valproate plus placebo, but 16% of those receiving additional haloperidol did so. The antipsychotics (risperidone or haloperidol) were effective in patients with or without psychotic features. A rating scale for depression was not used. Although dropouts due directly to side effects were few in all groups (2–4%), among patients receiving haloperidol plus lithium or valproate, 28% reported EPSs, and 38% received antiparkinsonian medication, compared with 13 and 17% on risperidone in combination, and 4 and 8% on placebo in combination with lithium or valproate. Weight gain was greater on risperidone than on haloperidol or placebo, plus mood stabilizer. Somnolence was slightly more common on haloperidol (30%) than on risperidone (25%) or on placebo (12%), plus mood stabilizer.

Conversely, in a three-week study with 136 patients, the addition of valproate to classical antipsychotics (mainly haloperidol) has been shown to produce greater improvement than addition of placebo (Muller-Oerlinghausen et al., 2000). Seventy percent responded (at least 50% reduction in Y-MRS score) compared with 46% on antipsychotic plus placebo (NNT = 5; 95% C.I. 3–13).

7.8.4 HALOPERIDOL EFFICACY IN COMBINATION THERAPY: CONCLUSIONS

Thus, on the basis of the little data available from RCTs, it seems that either adding haloperidol to patients already receiving lithium or valproate, or adding valproate to patients with mania already receiving a first generation antipsychotic, results in further improvement, with NNT of 5 for "response." Ketter (2009) concludes that physicians should exercise caution when treating patients with a combination of medications and strive to use monotherapy when feasible.

7.9 RECENT COMPARATIVE TRIALS WITHOUT PLACEBO

Questions arise about the relative efficacy of the new generation antipsychotics compared either with haloperidol or with valproate, and whether they should be used initially as monotherapy or combined with valproate or lithium. Also, since treatment often needs to commence with rapid tranquillization, and there is limited experience with the three new generation antipsychotics that can be given intramuscularly (olanzapine, aripiprazole, and in some countries ziprasidone), haloperidol remains widely used despite its propensity to cause unpleasant EPSs.

7.9.1 TRIALS OF CLASSICAL ANTIPSYCHOTICS VS. VALPROATE IN MANIA

Haloperidol has been compared directly with valproate in psychotic mania by McElroy *et al.* (1996). If a sufficiently large dose of valproate (as semisodium valproate 20 mg/kg/day) is used from the start, a similar improvement occurs with valproate or haloperidol (0.2 mg/kg/day). However, the generalizability of this finding may be limited, since haloperidol did not show its usual rapid onset of effect. Furthermore, a second study of valproate loading by Hirschfeld *et al.* (1999) showed a delay of about 48 hours in onset of the antimanic effect with valproate. Consistent with this delay, intravenous valproate (20 mg/kg) was not associated with an improvement in mania within 2 hours (Phrolov *et al.*, 2004), suggesting a different mechanism of action from that of antipsychotics.

7.9.2 COMPARATIVE RCTs OF HALOPERIDOL VS. NEW GENERATION ANTIPSYCHOTICS IN MANIA

The three studies described in Table 7.1, comparing a new drug with placebo or haloperidol for three weeks, had continuation phases in which the new drug (risperidone, quetiapine, or aripiprazole), was compared with haloperidol, but without a placebo group (except the trial with quetiapine) for a total of 12 weeks. The comparisons of quetiapine (McIntyre *et al.*, 2005), risperidone (Smulevich *et al.*, 2005), and aripiprazole (Young *et al.*, 2009) with haloperidol over 12 weeks has been described above and in Table 7.1.

Three additional studies compared a new drug (risperidone, olanzapine, or aripiprazole) with haloperidol without a placebo phase. In a comparative trial in mania, haloperidol showed similar efficacy to risperidone or lithium; however adjunctive lorazepam was permitted, making the effectiveness of the two antipsychotics difficult to judge (Segal, Berk, and Brook, 1998). Aripiprazole was compared with haloperidol (mean 11 mg per day) over 12 weeks (Vieta *et al.*, 2005). In this study, patients were discontinued from the trial if they required anticholinergic medication. The trial was therefore biased in favor of aripiprazole, which did indeed result in fewer total discontinuations; however haloperidol gave a slight faster improvement in mania ratings and led to fewer dropouts through lack of efficacy.

In the largest randomized comparative study of haloperidol (219 patients on haloperidol), it was compared with olanzapine over 12 weeks (Tohen *et al.*, 2003). Among patients on haloperidol (up to 15 mg/day; at week 6 mean dose 7 mg/day), the proportion responding (50% reduction in YMRS score) by six weeks was 74%. The proportion showing syndromal remission (according to DSM–IV) was 44%, a figure similar to that found on haloperidol in consecutive admissions for mania by Rifkin *et al.* (1994). In patients with low levels of depressive symptoms at commencement on haloperidol, a total of 16.8% switched into depression within 12 weeks. However, as there was no placebo group, it is not clear whether this represents the natural history of the patients' mood cycles, perhaps accelerated by effective treatment of mania, or some additional depressant effect of haloperidol. The switch rate among patients on olanzapine was non-significantly lower at 12 weeks (9.4%), but the switch to depression occurred significantly sooner with haloperidol (Tohen *et al.*, 2003).

Thus, both olanzapine and quetiapine tended to produce a (nonsignificantly) lower rate of switching into depression than did haloperidol. Both drugs (in the doses used) seemed also to lead to slower improvement in mania than did haloperidol. There is also the problem that haloperidol is prescribed in double-blind trials without a prophylactic anticholinergic drug, and is therefore liable to induce "akinetic depression," as described by van Putten and May (1978) in schizophrenia. When this occurs, some studies allow that an anticholinergic be added; others discontinued the patient from the trial (Vieta *et al.*, 2005).

These studies confirm the efficacy of haloperidol in reducing the symptoms of mania. None of the newer drugs has been shown to be more effective in this regard. Most (risperidone is the exception) appear to be less effective than haloperidol (Scherk *et al.*, 2007). However, the doses used in the trials for both the new generation antipsychotics and for haloperidol may be less than sufficient to produce optimal improvement. The clear superiority of the newer antipsychotics is that they produce far fewer EPSs than haloperidol. For example, the potentially very unpleasant side effect of akathisia was reported by 30% of patients on haloperidol and 6% on olanzapine (Tohen *et al.*, 2003), by 33% on haloperidol and 5.9% on quetiapine (McIntyre *et al.*, 2005), by 11.4% on aripiprazole and 24.8% on haloperidol (Young *et al.*, 2009), and hyperkinesia by 19% on haloperidol and by (10%) on risperidone (Smulevich *et al.*, 2005).

Patients with bipolar disorder are prone to develop EPSs with antipsychotic drugs. Cavazzoni *et al.* (2006) analyzed data on EPSs in patients with schizophrenia or bipolar disorder in clinical trials with olanzapine or haloperidol. Haloperidol-treated patients with bipolar disorder appeared to be more vulnerable to the development of EPS than those with schizophrenia.

7.9.3   DEPRESSION IN MANIA IN CLINICAL TRIALS

In the trials of new generation antipsychotics in mania, changes in symptoms of depression have usually been monitored. For example, in one study (Smulevich *et al.*, 2005), depression scores (on the MADRS) fell more on risperidone than on placebo from week 1, and on haloperidol only from week 2. Likewise, on both quetiapine and haloperidol, depression scores improved by day 21 more than on placebo (McIntyre *et al.*, 2005). In a pooled analysis, depressive symptoms improved more with Second Generation Antipsychotics than with haloperidol (Scherk *et al.*, 2007). However, the more recent study of haloperidol and aripiprazole found no such difference (Young *et al.*, 2009).

7.9.4 SWITCHING TO DEPRESSION IN NATURALISTIC STUDIES

The European Mania in Bipolar Longitudinal Evaluation of Medication (EMBLEM) study, in 14 European countries, followed the progress of 2390 patients with a manic episode for up to 24 months. At baseline each patient had medication initiated or changed according to the clinician's practice, with a requirement that half of the patients enrolled should be prescribed olanzapine. About 25% of patients were prescribed a first generation antipsychotic from baseline, often in combination with other drugs. One hundred and twenty (5.0% of the total) switched to depression within the first 12 weeks. Factors associated with greater switching to depression included more previous depressive episodes, substance abuse, greater overall severity, and benzodiazepine use at baseline. One factor associated with lower switching rates was atypical antipsychotic use at the start (Vieta *et al.*, 2009). Of course, naturalistic studies involve a bias due to selection of certain types of patient for particular treatments by the clinician.

7.10 PHARMACOECONOMICS

McGarry *et al.* (2003, 2004) used a Markov model to evaluate the cost-effectiveness in the UK and the USA of new generation antipsychotics and competing treatment strategies in the treatment of mania, employing published costs and probabilities of outcomes, and the standard-gamble method to estimate total quality-adjusted life-years (QALYs). The monotherapy model was based on the United Kingdom National Health Service (NHS) and included costs of initial hospitalization, drugs, and laboratory tests for monitoring but did not include costs of adverse events. Risperidone monotherapy was dominant relative to both olanzapine and haloperidol monotherapy by being both less costly and more effective in the treatment of acute mania from the perspective of the NHS in the United Kingdom. These results must be considered with caution because of the noninclusion of adverse effects in the model (Fleurence, Dixon, and Revicki, 2006; Fleurence, Chatterton, and Dixon, 2007).

The combination-therapy model used a United States payer perspective (see Fleurence, Dixon, and Revicki, 2006; Fleurence, Chatterton, and Dixon, 2007). Costs in this model included 2003 costs for drugs, hospitalization, outpatient care, and adverse events (tardive dyskinesia and weight gain). Results showed that the 24-week costs of treating acute mania were lowest with risperidone monotherapy ($6643) compared to haloperidol ($6896) and olanzapine ($7221). Though haloperidol plus mood stabilizer was the least costly treatment option, risperidone plus mood stabilizer was the most effective. Risperidone plus mood stabilizer cost an additional $3300, and olanzapine plus mood stabilizer an additional $8700 per QALY, compared to haloperidol + mood stabilizer (MS). This compares with the customary threshold of less than £30 000 per QALY to justify new treatments in the UK.

7.11 CONCLUSIONS

The clinical trials of new generation antipsychotics and anticonvulsants in mania, sponsored by the pharmaceutical manufacturers, have answered many important questions about bipolar disorder that had been unresolved for 50 years. In particular, they have shown that antipsychotics generally have broad and specific antimanic properties that are independent of sedation or psychosis. The speed of action and size of effect of antipsychotics makes them especially useful for control of emergent (hypomanic) symptoms and for acute tranquillization in mania. None of the new generation antipsychotics is more effective than haloperidol in reducing manic symptoms, but all produce fewer EPSs than haloperidol and may therefore be more acceptable to patients. Although the trials do not show that patients on haloperidol are more likely to drop out through recognized adverse events than patients on new generation drugs, troublesome EPSs occur in the majority of patients on haloperidol and require treatment with additional anticholinergic medication.

In these studies, even the "gold standard" antimanic drug haloperidol had a rather small effect size with NNTs of 5–9 for response by three weeks, perhaps reflecting that the patients taking part in the trials were resistant to treatment, or that inadequate doses of haloperidol were used in the trials.

Haloperidol would still be considered appropriate as the first-line treatment for severe mania (often combined with a benzodiazepine), especially if rapid tranquillization is required. For less severe mania, an atypical antipsychotic might be preferred to avoid EPSs (National Collaborating Centre for Mental Health, 2006; Goodwin, 2009). However, for patients with mania, that is, not adequately controlled by olanzapine, quetiapine, aripiprazole, or ziprasidone, additional treatment with a more effective antipsychotic such as haloperidol or risperidone should be considered.

Many patients with mania will require combination treatment with an antipsychotic and lithium or valproate. The trial of such combination therapy with haloperidol indicates that for patients who have not responded to two weeks treatment with lithium or valproate, additional treatment with haloperidol conveys further efficacy. The NNT for this improvement is rather large (about 5), but the trials include patients who started on the antipsychotic and mood stabilizer at the same time. The trials do not provide evidence to support commencing patients with mania on a combination of antipsychotic with lithium or valproate, if their responsiveness to individual drug treatments is not already known.

For manic patients with depressive symptoms, a new generation antipsychotic may be more effective than haloperidol in reducing depressive symptoms. However haloperidol should always be used in conjunction with an anticholinergic drug to reduce the risk of EPSs including "akinetic depression." Likewise, there is tentative evidence from comparative efficacy trials that new generation antipsychotics may be associated with a lower rate of switching from mania into depression in the first 12 weeks of treatment, and this impression is also gained from naturalistic data.

Thus the efficacy trials indicate that some newer antipsychotics (other than risperidone) may be less efficacious than haloperidol in improving manic symptoms, but may have advantages in producing fewer EPSs and better control of depressive symptoms. It should however be noted that the optimal dose of antipsychotics for treating mania has never been firmly established, in contrast to their use in schizophrenia.

The use of antipsychotics for long-term treatment in bipolar disorder is an area of growing evidence and changing clinical practice. Whether new generation antipsychotics are superior in prophylaxis to older drugs, such as haloperidol, in either efficacy or tolerability and effectiveness, is an important theme for further studies, where longer-term side effects such as tardive dyskinesia, weight gain, and metabolic problems would also need consideration. In particular, further information is needed from naturalistic studies, and from randomized "effectiveness trials" or "pragmatic trials," which follow the progress of broader categories of large numbers of patients treated over long periods, and using wider outcome measures, to determine the relative advantages of newer versus older antipsychotics. These three perspectives can contribute to a "triangulated" view on the use of antipsychotics in bipolar disorder (Cookson, 2008b).

DECLARATION OF INTEREST

J. C. has provided advice and lectures at meetings sponsored by the manufacturers of several atypical antipsychotics, including those mentioned in this article.

References

Ahlfors, U.G., Baastrup, P.C., and Dencker, S. (1981) Flupenthixol decanoate in recurrent manic depressive illness: a comparison with lithium. *Acta Psychiatr. Scand.*, **64**, 226–237.
Bjørndal, F. (1990) Review of treating mania with zuclopenthixol: looking for a therapeutic window. *Nord. J. Psychiatry*, **44**, 383–386.
Bowden, C.L., Brugger, A.M., Swann, A.C. *et al.*, The Depakote Mania Study Group (1994) Efficacy of Divalproex vs lithium and placebo in the treatment of mania. *J. Am. Med. Assoc.*, **271**, 918–924.
Busch, F.N., Miller, F.T., and Weiden, P.J. (1989) A comparison of two adjunctive treatment strategies in acute mania. *J. Clin. Psychiatry*, **50**, 453–455.
Cavazzoni, P.A., Berg, P.H., Kryzhanovskaya, L.A. *et al.* (2006) Comparison of treatment-emergent extrapyramidal symptoms in patients with bipolar mania or schizophrenia during olanzapine clinical trials. *J. Clin. Psychiatry*, **67**, 107–113.
Chou, J.C., Zito, J.M., Vitrai, J. *et al.* (1996) Neuroleptics in acute mania: a pharmacoepidemiologic study. *Ann. Pharmacother.*, **30**, 1396–1398.
Cookson, J.C. (1985) The neuroendocrinology of mania. *J. Affect. Disord.*, **8**, 233–241.
Cookson, J.C. (2001) Use of antipsychotic drugs and lithium in mania. *Br. J. Psychiatry*, **178** (Suppl. 41), s148–s156.
Cookson, J.C. (2008a) Atypical antipsychotics in bipolar disorder: the treatment of mania. *Adv. Psychiatr. Treat.*, **14**, 330–338.
Cookson, J.C. (2008b) Triangulating views on antipsychotics. *Adv. Psychiatr. Treat.*, **14**, 17.
Cookson, J.C. and Ghalib, S. (2004) The treatment of bipolar mixed states. In *Mixed States* (eds A. Mameros and F.K. Goodwin), pp. 324–352. Cambridge University Press.
Cookson, J.C., Moult, P.J.A., Wiles, D. *et al.* (1983) The relationship between prolactin levels and clinical ratings in manic patients treated with oral and intravenous test doses of haloperidol. *Psychol. Med.*, **13**, 279–285.
Cookson, J.C. and Sachs, G.S. (1999) Lithium: clinical use in mania and prophylaxis of affective disorders, in *Schizophrenia and Mood Disorders: The New Drug Therapies in Clinical Practice* (eds P.F. Buckley and J.L. Waddington), pp. 155–178, Butterworth Heinemann, Oxford.
Cookson, J.C., Silverstone, T., and Wells, B. (1981) A double-blind comparative clinical trial of pimozide and chlorpromazine in mania: a test of the dopamine hypothesis. *Acta Psychiatr. Scand.*, **64**, 381–397.

Cookson, J.C., Silverstone, T., Williams, S. *et al.* (1985) Plasma cortisol levels in mania: associated clinical ratings and change during treatment with haloperidol. *Br. J. Psychiatry*, **146**, 498–502.

Cookson, J.C., Taylor, D., and Katona, C. (2002a) Violence: assessing risk and acute tranquillisation, *Use of Drugs in Psychiatry: The Evidence From Psychopharmacology*, Chapter 14, Gaskell Press, London, pp. 117–131.

Cookson, J.C., Taylor, D., and Katona, C. (2002b) Placebo effects, evaluating evidence, and combining psychotherapy, *Use of Drugs in Psychiatry: The Evidence From Psychopharmacology*, Chapter 5, Gaskell Press, London, pp. 117–131.

Davis, J.M., Wang, Z., and Janicak, P.G. (1993) A quantitative analysis of clinical trials for the treatment of affective disorders. *Psychopharmacol. Bull.*, **29**, 175–181.

Dunn, J., Ramey, T.S., Giller, E.L. *et al.* (2005). Efficacy and tolerability of ziprasidone in acute bipolar mania: twelve week, double-blind study. Poster presented at the Association of European Psychiatrists Congress, Munich.

Fleurence, R.L., Chatterton, M.L., Dixon, J.M. *et al.* (2007) Economic outcomes associated with atypical antipsychotics in bipolar disorder: a systematic review. *Prim. Care Companion J. Clin. Psychiatry*, **9**, 419–428.

Fleurence, R.L., Dixon, J.M., and Revicki, D.A. (2006) Economics of atypical antipsychotics in bipolar disorder: a review of the literature. *CNS Drugs*, **20**, 591–599.

Garfinkel, P.E., Stancer, H.C., and Persaud, E. (1980) A comparison of haloperidol, lithium carbonate and their combination in the treatment of mania. *J. Affect. Disord.*, **2**, 279–288.

Goodwin, G.M., The Consensus Group of the British Association for Psychopharmacology (2009) Evidence-based guidelines for treating bipolar disorder: revised second edition – recommendations from the British association for psychopharmacology. *J. Psychopharmacol.*, 1–43. Available at http://www.bap.org.uk/consensus/FinalBipolarGuidelines.pdf.

Hirschfeld, R.M.A., Allen, M.H., McEvoy, J.P., *et al.* (1999) Safety and tolerability of oral loading divalproex sodium in acutely manic bipolar patients. *Journal of Clinical Psychiatry*, **60**, 815–818.

Ketter, T.A. (2009) Treating bipolar disorder: monotherapy versus combination therapy. *J. Clin. Psychiatry*, **70**, e42 (Review).

Klein, D.F. (1967) Importance of diagnosis in prediction of clinical drug effects. *Arch. Gen. Psychiatry*, **16**, 118–126.

Klein, E., Bental, E., Lerer, B. *et al.* (1984) Carbamazepine and haloperidol v placebo and haloperidol in excited psychoses. A controlled study. *Arch. Gen. Psychiatry*, **41**, 165–170.

Lenox, R.H., Newhouse, P.A., Creelman, W.L. *et al.* (1992) Adjunctive treatment of manic agitation with lorazepam versus haloperidol: a double-blind study. *J. Clin. Psychiatry*, **53**, 47–52.

Littlejohn, R., Leslie, F., and Cookson, J. (1994) Depot antipsychotics in the prophylaxis of bipolar affective disorder. *Br. J. Psychiatry*, **165**, 827–829.

Lowe, M.R. and Batchelor, D.H. (1990) Lithium and neuroleptics in the management of manic-depressive psychosis. *Hum. Psychopharmacol.*, **5**, 267–274.

McElroy, S.L., Keck, P.E. Jr, Stanton, S.P., *et al.* (1996) A randomized comparison of divalproex oral loading versus haloperidol in the initial treatment of acute psychotic mania. *J. Clin. Psychiatry*, **57**, 142–146.

McGarry, L.J., Bird, A., Thompson, D. *et al.* (2003) Cost-effectiveness of atypical antipsychotics in acute bipolar mania. Poster Presented at the 8th Annual International Meeting of the International Society for Pharmacoeconomics and Outcomes Research, May 18–21, Arlington, VA.

McGarry, L.J., Thompson, D., Knudsen, A.P. *et al.* (2004) Cost-effectiveness of competing antipsychotic monotherapies in acute bipolar mania in the UK. Poster Presented at the 7th Annual European Congress of the International Society for Pharmacoeconomics and Outcomes Research, October 24–26, Hamburg, Germany.

McIntyre, R.S., Brecher, M.,Paulsson, B. *et al.* (2005) Quetiapine or haloperidol as monotherapy for bipolar mania – a 12-week, double-blind, randomised, parallel group, placebo-controlled trial. *Eur. Neuropsychopharmacol.*, **15**, 573–585.

Moller, H.J., Kissling, W., Riehl, T. *et al.* (1989) Double-blind evaluation of the antimanic properties of carbamazepine as a comedication to haloperidol. *Prog. Neuropsychopharmacol. Biol. Psychiatry*, **13**, 127–136.

Muller-Oerlinghausen, B., Retzow, A., Henn, F.A., *et al.* (2000) Valproate as an adjunct to neuroleptic medication for the treatment of acute episodes of mania: a prospective, randomized, double-blind, placebo-controlled, multicentre study. *J. Clin. Psychopharmacol.*, **20**, 195–203.

National Collaborating Centre for Mental Health (2006) *Guideline 38: Management of Bipolar Disorder in Adults, Children and Adolescents, in Primary and Secondary Care*, National Institute for Health and Clinical Excellence.

Nolen, W.A. (1983) Dopamine and mania. The effects of trans- and cis-clopenthixol in a double-blind pilot study. *J. Affect. Disord.*, **5**, 91–96.

Owens, D.C. (2008) How CATIE brought us back to Kansas: a critical re-evaluation of the concept of atypical antipsychotics and their place in the treatment of schizophrenia. *Adv. Psychiatr. Treat.*, **14**, 17–28.

Peroutka, S.J. and Snyder, S.H. (1980) Relationship of neuroleptic drug effects at brain dopamine, serotonin, alpha-adrenergic, and histamine receptors to clinical potency. *Am. J. Psychiatry*, **137**, 1518–1522.

Post, R.M., Jimerson, D.C., Bunney, W.F. *et al.* (1980) Dopamine and mania: behavioural and biochemical effects of the dopamine receptor blocker pimozide. *Psychopharmacology*, **67**, 297–305.

Phrolov, K., Applebaum, J., Levine, J., *et al.* (2004) Single dose intravenous valproate in acute mania. *J. Clin. Psychiatry*, **65**, 6, 70.

van Putten, T. and May, R.P. (1978) "Akinetic depression" in schizophrenia. *Arch. Gen. Psychiatry*, **35**, 1101–1107.

Rifkin, A., Doddi, S., Karajgi, B. *et al.* (1994) Dosage of haloperidol for mania. *Br. J. Psychiatry*, **165**, 113–116.

Royal College of Psychiatrists (1998) *Management of Imminent Violence. Clinical Practice Guidelines To Support Mental Health Services (Occasion paper OP41)*, The Royal College of Psychiatrists, London.

Sachs, G.S., Grossman, F., Ghaemi, S.N. *et al.* (2002) Combination of a mood stabilizer with Risperidone or Haloperidol for treatment of acute mania: a double-blind, placebo-controlled comparison of efficacy and safety. *Am. J. Psychiatry*, **159**, 1146–1154.

Scherk, H., Pajonk, F.G., and Leucht, S. (2007) Second-generation antipsychotic agents in the treatment of acute mania: a systematic review and meta-analysis of randomized controlled trials. *Arch. Gen. Psychiatry*, **64**, 442–455.

Segal, J., Berk, M., and Brook, S. (1998) Risperidone compared with both lithium and haloperidol in mania: a double blind randomized controlled trial. *Clin. Neuropharmacol.*, **21**, 176–180.

Sernyak, M.J., Griffin, R.A., Johnson, R.M. *et al.* (1994) Neuroleptic exposure following inpatient treatment of acute mania with lithium and neuroleptic. *Am. J. Psychiatry*, **151**, 133–135.

Sernyak, M.J. and Woods, S.W. (1998) Chronic neuroleptic use in manic-depressive illness. *Psychopharmacol. Bull.*, **29**, 375–381.

Shopsin, B., Gershon, S., Thompson, H. *et al.* (1975) Psychoactive drugs in mania: a controlled comparison of lithium carbonate, chlorpromazine, and haloperidol. *Arch. Gen. Psychiatry*, **32**, 34–42.

Smulevich, A.B., Khanna, S., Eerdekens, M. *et al.* (2005) Acute and continuation risperidone monotherapy in bipolar mania: a 3-week placebocontrolled trial followed by a 9-week double-blind trial of risperidone and haloperidol. *Eur. Neuropsychopharmacol.*, **15**, 75–84.

Szabadi, E., Gaszner, P., and Bradshaw, C.M. (1981) An investigation of the alpha-adrenoceptor blocking properties of neuroleptics in the human iris in vivo. *Br. J. Clin. Pharmacol.*, **11**, 416–417.

Tohen, M., Goldberg, J.F., Gonzalez-Pinto, A.M. *et al.* (2003) A 12-week double-blind comparison of olanzapine versus haloperidol in the treatment of acute mania. *Arch. Gen. Psychiatry*, **60**, 1218–1226.

Vieta, E., Angst, J., Reed, C. *et al.*, The EMBLEM Advisory Board (2009) Predictors of switching from mania to depression in a large observational study across Europe (EMBLEM). *J. Affect. Disord.*, **118**, 118–123.

Vieta, E., Bourin, M., Sanchez, R. *et al.* (2005) Effectiveness of aripiprazole v. haloperidol in acute bipolar mania: double-blind, randomised, comparative 12-week trial. *Br. J. Psychiatry*, **187**, 235–242.

Young, A.H., Oren, D.A., Lowy, A. *et al.* (2009) Aripiprazole monotherapy in acute mania: 12-week randomised placebo- and haloperidol-controlled study. *Br. J. Psychiatry*, **194**, 40–48.

Zarate, C.A. and Tohen, M. (2004) Double-blind comparison of the continued use of antipsychotic treatment versus its discontinuation in remitted manic patients. *Am. J. Psychiatry*, **161**, 169–171.

8

Clinical Utility of Clozapine in Bipolar Disorder

V.E. Cosgrove[1,2], J.S. Seo[1,2], H. Yang[1,2] and Trisha Suppes[1,2]

[1]VA Palo Alto Health Care System, Palo Alto, CA, USA
[2]Stanford School of Medicine, Stanford University Medical Center, Stanford, CA, USA

8.1 INTRODUCTION

Clozapine, a second-generation atypical antipsychotic with an unusually complex pharmacologic profile, has demonstrated efficacy in improving symptoms in treatment-resistant schizophrenia. Although research examining clozapine's role in the treatment of bipolar disorders is limited, several retrospective reviews and prospective, open-label studies indicate that clozapine has pronounced antimanic and mood-stabilizing effects for episodes of dysphoric or psychotic mania and may exceed chlorpromazine in effectiveness. Clozapine may also be a desirable clinical option for treatment-refractory patients who have failed trials of lithium or valproate. This chapter will first briefly present the complicated history of clozapine. Next the clinical pharmacology of clozapine and risks associated with administration will be explored. Clozapine has been associated with agranulocytosis in 1–2% of patients in addition to increased risk of seizure, myocarditis, and metabolic syndrome. Despite this risk profile, our critical review will argue clozapine's utility as an adjunctive or sole agent in the management of treatment-resistant bipolar disorder. Suggestions for future explorations of clozapine's effects on affective symptomatology will be presented.

8.2 HISTORY

Clozapine has served as the prototype for a new group of medications referred to as second generation, or atypical, antipsychotics since its synthesis by the Swiss pharmaceutical company Wander AG in 1958. Examining its history as well as its inception in US markets sheds light on its role in contemporary psychopharmacology for bipolar disorders.

By the time Sandoz Ltd had acquired Wander AG in 1967, clozapine's clinical effectiveness in reducing both positive and negative symptoms associated with schizophrenia had already been observed in non-Western countries. Furthermore, its administration appeared to cause no debilitating neurological side effects like tardive dyskinesia,

Bipolar Psychopharmacotherapy: Caring for the patient, Second Edition. Edited by Hagop S. Akiskal and Mauricio Tohen.
© 2011 John Wiley & Sons, Ltd. Published 2011 by John Wiley & Sons, Ltd.

commonly seen with first generation or typical neuroleptics. Crilly (2007) describes how clozapine's benign side effect profile ironically discredited its face validity as an effective second generation antipsychotic medication. During the 1950s and 1960s, effective antipsychotic agents were thought to uniformly and necessarily have extreme extrapyramidal side effects. Because side effects were believed to be related to efficacy, clozapine was not given serious consideration as a marketable agent for schizophrenia until the 1970s (Hippius, 1989).

Research and Development for clozapine was initiated in the United States in 1973. Only shortly after, in September 1975, the National Board of Health in Finland reported that 16 patients had developed agranulocytosis, a severe blood disorder, and eight of these had died as a result (Idanpaan-Heikkila *et al.*, 1977). All worldwide, clinical R&D efforts were abruptly curtailed by Sandoz Ltd in 1976.

However, Sandoz continued to provide clozapine to clinical populations in the US and abroad for compassionate use. Widespread reports of its clinical effectiveness in severely ill populations continued, and after successful schizophrenia clinical trials in the US (Kane *et al.*, 1988), the U.S. Food and Drug Administration (FDA) formally approved Sandoz's second New Drug Application for "Clozaril," its brand name for clozapine, in September 1989. Clozaril entered the US market in February 1990 with five years of protected marketing exclusivity (Crilly, 2007).

With FDA approval, Sandoz began marketing Clozaril for what was considered at the time as prohibitively high prices. Public outcry, Senate antitrust hearings, and class action lawsuits because of its high cost plagued Sandoz's dissemination of Clozaril. By the time Sandoz was finally free of all lawsuits in 1992, less than three years of its marketing exclusivity remained. Rival pharmaceutical giants like Eli Lilly and Pfizer were developing second generation antipsychotics meant to directly compete with clozapine. Sandoz decided that initiating strong marketing efforts at such a late stage would not provide a good return. Clozaril marketing was largely abandoned, and generic versions of clozapine became available in 1997 (Crilly, 2007). As a result, Clozaril never benefited from the kind of robust marketing campaigns that its second generation antipsychotic counterparts risperidone, olanzapine, or quetiapine eventually did.

During the next decade, clozapine became a "gold standard" antipsychotic for patients with treatment-resistant schizophrenia (Hippius, 1999). Treatment-resistance in psychopathology is generally defined by persistence of symptomatology despite trials of multiple adequate treatments (Elkis, 2007). Research reports, systematic reviews, and meta-analyses have repeatedly demonstrated clozapine's superior effectiveness for treatment-refractory positive and negative symptoms of schizophrenia. Meta-analysis comparing clozapine with first generation antipsychotics in schizophrenia has demonstrated that clozapine-treated patients experience clinical improvement and fewer relapses than those treated with first generation antipsychotics (Wahlbeck, Cheine, and Essali 1999; Essali *et al.*, 2009). When compared with newer second generation antipsychotics, research has demonstrated that clozapine superiorly treats positive symptoms (Tuunainen, Wahlbeck, and Gilbody, 2002) and is often the best option for individuals who have already failed a trial with another antipsychotic (McEvoy *et al.*, 2006).

Prior to clozapine, lithium had generally been combined with first-generation antipsychotics to treat acute manic states. Tohen *et al.* (2001) reported via meta-analysis that 91% of inpatients and 65% of outpatients with bipolar mania were treated with first-generation antipsychotics before the advent of second-generation antipsychotics. However, extrapyramidal symptoms caused by first-generation medications were commonplace occurrences often leading to premature discontinuation of adjunctive first generation agents that were otherwise ameliorating manic symptomatolgoy. With its FDA approval in 1990, clozapine became a new possibility for psychopharmacological management of acute mania and other affective states associated with bipolar disorder. Clinical trials examining the effectiveness of clozapine in bipolar disorder were soon to follow. We critically review this literature later in this chapter.

8.3 CLINICAL PHARMACOLOGY OF CLOZAPINE

8.3.1 MECHANISM OF ACTION

As noted in previous chapters, therapeutic actions of first-generation antipsychotics are believed to result from blockade of D2 receptors in the mesolimbic dopamine pathway. This D2 blockade counters hyperactivity in the pathway thought to be associated with hallucinations and delusions (for example, positive symptoms) of psychosis. Unfortunately, first generation antipsychotics are nonspecific in their blockade, and D2 receptors are blocked through the entire brain. As a result, cognitive and negative symptoms of schizophrenia often worsen due in part to D2 blockage in the mesocortical dopamine pathway. Movement disorders or tardive dyskinesia may result in part from blockage in the nigrostriatal dopamine pathway. Hyperprolactinemia due to dopamine blockage in the tuberoinfundibular pathway may interfere with fertility in female patients.

See Figure 8.1 for clozapine's chemical structure. Clozapine's pharmacologic profile is notable, earning its classification as a second-generation antipsychotic because of its role

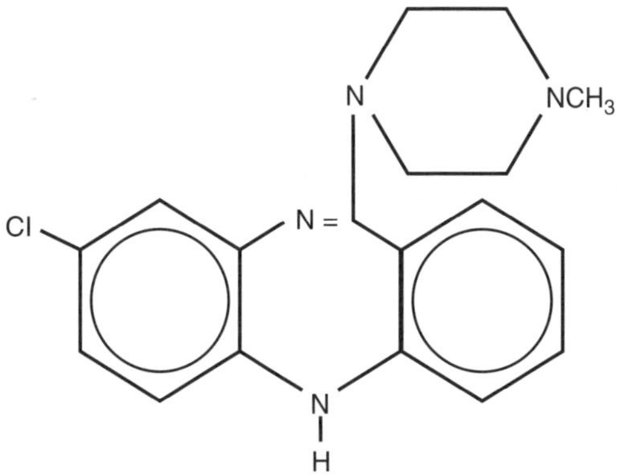

$C_{18}H_{19}ClN_4$ Molecular weight = 326.83

Figure 8.1 Chemical structure of clozapine.

as a serotonin 2A-dopamine 2 antagonist. Clozapine's binding profile includes much more than just antagonism at serotonin2A and dopamine 2 sites. Clozapine is thought to interact with multiple other receptor subtypes for both dopamine and serotonin including 5HT1A, 5HT2C, 5HT3, 5HT6, 5HT7, D1, D3, and D4. Antimuscarinic and antihistaminic as well as alpha 1 adrenergic plus alpha 2 adrenergic blockade are also likely to be involved (Iqbal *et al.*, 2003). This complex binding profile may result in its differentially supreme effectiveness as an antipsychotic agent.

8.3.2   PHARMACOKINETICS

Generic clozapine is available in 25, 50, 100, and 200 mg oral tablets. The range of steady state peak plasma concentrations is 102–771 ng/ml occurring at one to 6 hours, respectively. Clozapine plasma level in schizophrenia is correlated with dose, and threshold for efficacy is considered near 350–420 ng/ml (Khan and Preskorn, 2005). The relationship of dose and plasma levels has not been studied in bipolar disorder. Degree of sedation, degree of hypotension, and risk of developing seizures may be related to dose and plasma levels of clozapine (Khan and Preskorn, 2005). The bioavailability of clozapine is not affected by food, and 95% of the drug is bound to serum proteins (Iqbal *et al.*, 2003). Clozapine is almost fully metabolized before excretion. Fifty percent of the dose is excreted in the urine and 30% in the feces. Mean elimination half-life for 100 mg bid is 12 hours (Thomson Corporation, 2006).

8.3.3   ADVERSE EFFECTS AND MANAGEMENT

It is important to discuss clozapine's profile of adverse effects since estimates of clozapine discontinuation resulting from adverse side effects are close to 20% (Young, Bowers, and Mazure 1998; Meltzer, 1992). We will discuss serious adverse effects – agranulocytosis, seizure disorder, myocarditis, and metabolic syndrome – that often lead to termination of a trial with clozapine. The Federal Drug Administration in the United States requires that all three are listed as "black box" warnings on package labels for clozapine. Generally, clozapine interacts with other similar psychotropic agents (that is, first- and second-generation antipsychotics) additively or synergistically. Therefore, pharmacological or side effects of clozapine are usually enhanced during such interactions (Edge, Markowitz, and Devane, 1999).

8.3.3.1   Agranulocytosis

Agranulocytosis is an acute leucopenia whereby the concentration of granulocytes (white blood cells containing neutrophils, basophils, and eosinophils) drops dangerously low. Specifically, a diagnosis of agranulocytosis is defined as a neutropenia with absolute neurophil count (ANC) below 500 cells/mm^3. The immune system's functioning is subsequently severely compromised, inviting acute infection. In the United States, 1.3%

of clozapine patients will develop agranulocytosis (Thomson Corporation, 2006). Agranulocytosis is considered a medical emergency as its mortality rate is 3–4% if untreated (Iqbal *et al.*, 2003). Ninety-five percent of agranulocytosis cases develop within six months of clozapine initiation (Lieberman and Safferman, 1992). Agranulocytosis in most cases is reversed by discontinuation of clozapine and is often treated with bone marrow stimulating medications.

Sandoz's final FDA approval for clozapine in 1990 was contingent upon their creating a Clozaril National Registry (CNR) system in the U.S. (Bastani, Alphs, and Meltzer 1989). Its primary purpose was to prevent cases of agranulocytosis by requiring regular monitoring of blood counts of any patient taking clozapine (Honigfeld *et al.*, 1998). When agranulocytosis data from the 1990–1994 CNR database was compared with data from the pre-CNR period, a dramatically reduced death rate was observed (Honigfeld *et al.*, 1998). Based on pre-CNR death rates, 149 deaths from agranulocytosis were expected from 99 502 patients. Instead, only 12 deaths occurred.

Today, participation in the CNR (www.clozaril.com) or the Clozapine Patient Registry (CPR; www.clozapineregistry.com) is required for safe administration of clozapine. FDA-required frequency of monitoring is identical for the CNR and the CPR. At clozapine initiation, patient white blood count (WBC) must exceed 3500/mm^3 and ANC must exceed 2000/mm^3. Clozapine should not be initiated for patients with histories of clozapine-induced agranulocytosis. Both WBC and ANC must be monitored weekly for six months followed by every two weeks for an additional six months. After 12 months with no incident, WBC and ANC must be monitored every four weeks until treatment is discontinued.

8.3.3.2 Seizure Disorder

Seizures occur in 3–5% of patients treated with clozapine (Devinsky, Honigfeld, and Patin, 1992). Seizures occur more frequently in clozapine-treated patients than in patients treated with first-generation antipsychotics (Toth and Frankenburg 1994). Risk factors for seizures are higher clozapine doses, rapid titration, and history of seizure disorder, however neither presence of risk factors or occurrence of seizures is necessarily contraindication for clozapine prescription (Iqbal *et al.*, 2003).

8.3.3.3 Myocarditis

Myocarditis is defined by inflammation and infection in the heart resulting in damage to the heart muscle without blockage of coronary arteries that characterizes traditional heart attacks. Based on data from the World Health Organization, the rate of myocarditis in clozapine patients is between 17 and 322 times higher than the general population (Thomson Corporation, 2006). Multiple case reports (Bandelow *et al.*, 1995) and at least one study from Australia (Kilian *et al.*, 1999) have definitively linked clozapine to myocarditis. While myocarditis is rare, clinicians prescribing clozapine should be aware of its potentially fatal effects.

8.3.3.4 Metabolic Syndrome and Weight Gain

Significant weight gain can be associated with clozapine treatment. One-fifth of clozapine-treated patients gain over 10% of their baseline body weight in the initial months of treatment (Bustillo *et al.*, 1996). Hypertension, heart disease, and diabetes are all associated with weight gain in clinical and nonclinical populations. Furthermore, treatment with clozapine as well as other second generation antipsychotics has been specifically linked to development of Type II diabetes (Wirshing *et al.*, 1998). Weight gain with clozapine and olanzapine has been shown to be higher than that associated with risperidone (Guille, Sachs, and Ghaemi, 2000). Longevity as well as quality of life are deeply affected by the presence of these metabolic effects of treatment with clozapine. However since quality of life is also severely affected by a severe bipolar disorder, risks associated with side effects must be measured against benefits of treatment with clozapine. Routine monitoring for glucose irregularities and weight gain accompanies administration of clozapine (Suppes *et al.*, 2005). The American Diabetes Association recommends that patients taking second generation antipsychotic medications receive regular monitoring for cardiovascular and diabetes risk factors by checking weight, body mass index, waist circumference, blood pressure, hemoglobin A1C, fasting glucose, and lipid profiles every three months (American Diabetes Association, 2004).

8.4 CLOZAPINE IN BIPOLAR DISORDERS

Clozapine's demonstrated effectiveness in treatment-resistant schizophrenia led to speculation from the psychiatric community regarding the possible utility of clozapine in severely ill bipolar patients. Initially, researchers attempted to categorize and define patients with affective symptomatology who were treated with clozapine under compassionate use protocols preceding FDA approval in 1990. Naturalistic and open-label trials have sought to prospectively validate long-held clinical hypotheses supporting clozapine's effectiveness in treating psychotic and dysphoric or mixed mania. Probably in part because of clozapine's profile of adverse effects and frequency of costly blood counts required by the CNR and CPR, no randomized, single- or double-blind trials with clozapine in bipolar disorder have been completed. Two randomized trials have compared clozapine with chlorpromazine or treatment-as-usual, respectively, in bipolar mania.

Previous reviews have concluded that clozapine was effective and well-tolerated in severe affective disorders (Zarate, Tohen, and Baldessarini, 1995; Frye *et al.*, 1998). While the following review is not comprehensive, we attempt to underscore primary contributions to the clozapine-bipolar disorder literature. Investigations are best subdivided by study design and methodology into three categories of descending strength: (i) randomized, controlled trials; (ii) retrospective chart reviews and case studies; and (iii) naturalistic, prospective, open-label trials. See Table 8.1 for all included studies.

8.4.1 RANDOMIZED, CONTROLLED TRIALS

To date, no double- or single-blind, randomized, controlled trials exist with clozapine in bipolar disorder (see Section 8.5.4). However, two randomized trials have examined

Table 8.1 Summary of reviewed studies with clozapine and bipolar disorder.

	Sample type	N	Outcome measure	Methodology	Methodological limitations	Conclusions
Retrospective chart reviews and case studies						
McElroy et al. (1991)	Bipolar disorder w/psychotic features	14	BPRS	Retrospective chart review	Missing data	Significant reduction in BPRS
	Schizoaffective disorder, bipolar or depressed type	25				
Suppes et al. (1992)	Mixed bipolar disorder (dysphoric mania)	7	Chart review and patient review	Case series	Small N, descriptive	Bidirectional mood stabilization
Banov et al. (1994)	Refractory affective disorders	BP = 52 SchizAff = 81 Unipolar = 14	CGI-I rehospitalization	Naturalistic, follow-up interview; Retrospective chart review	Heterogeneous sample	Decreased rehospitalization and CGI-I with bipolar manic and SchizAff, bp subtype

(Continued Overleaf)

Table 8.1 (Continued)

	Sample type	N	Outcome measure	Methodology	Methodological limitations	Conclusions
Zarate et al. (1995)	Manic or mixed bipolar disorder	17	CGI-I rehospitalization rates	Case series	No control group	88% response to clozapine
Chang et al. (2006)	Bipolar I or II disorder	51	Hospitalization patterns	Retrospective chart review	No comparison group	Decreased hospital days/year
Guille, Sachs, and Ghaemi (2000)	Bipolar I disorder	42	CGI weight change	Naturalistic comparison of second generation antipsychotics	Small clozapine subgroup	Risperidone = olanzapine = clozapine
Suppes, Phillips and Judd (1994)	Rapid cycling bipolar I disorder	3	Psychosocial functioning	case series	Small N, descriptive	Substantial mood-stabilizing effects
Prospective, open-label trials						
Calabrese et al. (1996)	tx-refractory bipolar I disorder	10	YMRS BPRS	Prospective, open-label	Heterogeneous sample; no control group	Decreased YMRS and BPRS in bipolar patients
	Schizoaffective bipolar disorder type	15				

Study	N	Population	Measures	Design	Limitations	Results
Green et al. (2000)	22	tx-refractory bipolar I disorder with psychotic mania	BPRS YMRS CGI	Prospective, open-label	High dropout rate (8/22)	Significant improvements in YMRS, BPRS, CGI
Ciapparelli et al. (2000, 2003, 2004)	34	Schizophrenia	BPRS GAF	Prospective, open-label, naturalistic	No parallel comparison group	Reduction in BPRS scores and increase in GAF scores in bipolar disorder compared with other subgroups
	30	Chizoaffective, bipolar type				
	37	Bipolar with psychosis				
Randomized, controlled trials						
Barbini et al. (1997)	30	Bipolar I disorder, current mania	YMRS	Open-label, randomized, adjunctive clozapine v. chlorpromazine	Unblinded; non-standard titration scheulde; three-week trial	Decreased YMRS scores in both treatment groups
Suppes et al. (1999)	26	Bipolar I disorder	BPRS	Naturalistic, open-label, randomized	Open treatment Unblinded	Greater decrease in clozapine-treated BPRS scores; positive mood-stabilizing properties for clozapine
	12	Schizoaffective disorder, bipolar type	CGI			

effectiveness in bipolar disorder samples with open-label designs. Results from these randomized trials provide some information about clozapine's comparative utility in bipolar disorder.

Barbini and colleagues (1997) prospectively compared adjunctive chlorpromazine treatment to adjunctive clozapine treatment in 30 acutely manic bipolar patients. Study physicians were aware of patient treatment assignment. Patients were randomly assigned to a chlorpromazine (n = 15) or clozapine (n = 15) group. While the study duration was only three weeks in duration, significant decreases in Young Mania Rating Scale (YMRS) scores were observed in both conditions with clozapine patients exhibiting symptom reduction more rapidly than the chlorpromazine group. Adjunctive clozapine appears to be as effective as and quicker than an adjunctive first generation antipsychotic in the treatment of acute mania.

Secondly, Suppes *et al.* (1999) compared adjunctive clozapine with treatment as usual (that is, no clozapine) in a sample of patients diagnosed with bipolar I disorder (n = 26) or schizoaffective disorder, bipolar type (n = 12) with a history of mania in a prospective, naturalistic, randomized, one-year study. Clinical response was defined as 30% reduction in 18-item Brief Psychiatric Rating Scale (BPRS) scores. After three months, 65% of clozapine-treated subjects had responded compared with 48% of treatment-as-usual subjects. By six months, those numbers increased to 82 and 57%, respectively. The authors suggest that the substantially greater reduction in BPRS scores in the clozapine-treated group versus the treatment-as-usual group demonstrates mood-stabilizing in addition to anti-manic properties for clozapine. Furthermore, when response to clozapine was subsequently analyzed in psychotic versus nonpsychotic bipolar patients, similar reductions in BPRS scores were observed. Clozapine may be an effective treatment in nonpsychotic bipolar disorders.

8.4.2   PROSPECTIVE, OPEN-LABEL TRIALS

Prospective, open-label trials with clozapine in bipolar disorder are substantially fewer than are retrospective chart reviews and case series. Even after the FDA approved clozapine with an indication for treatment-resistant schizophrenia in 1990, clozapine's reputation as a cumbersome, expensive agent with multiple serious side effects prevailed in medical communities. This likely deterred potential researchers from designing adequate clinical trials to test its effectiveness in subpopulations of seriously mentally ill individuals. To our knowledge, there have been only three methodologically-sound, prospective, open-label studies with clozapine in bipolar disorder.

Calabrese *et al.* (1996) recruited 25 patients with treatment-refractory bipolar disorder or schizoaffective disorder with at least one episode of mania during the past two years for an open-label trial of clozapine monotherapy. Treatment with clozapine was preceded by a seven-day washout period from any concomitant medications. Of the 25 patients, 88% (22) completed a 13-week clozapine trial and 72% (18) manifested significant improvement (>50% decrease in score) on the Young Mania Rating Scale. Additionally, patients with bipolar disorder improved more on the BPRS than did schizoaffective patients. The authors cautioned that bipolar patients seemed to respond negatively to rapid titration of clozapine.

A second, open-label, prospective trial (Green *et al.*, 2000) recruited 22 inpatients diagnosed with treatment-refractory bipolar disorder to receive a 12-week trial with clozapine monotherapy. Included patients had experienced at least three episodes of mania in the past two years or recent mania with psychotic symptoms lasting at least six months. Outcome measures BPRS, YMRS, and Clinical Global Impressions (CGI) saw reductions of 56.7, 56.6, and 39.1%, respectively, for the entire group of 22 patients. Most of this clinical improvement was observed in the first eight weeks of clozapine treatment. A significant consideration when interpreting results from this study was its high dropout rate. Eight of 22 subjects (36.4%) dropped out before week 10 in the study. The authors suggested that the observed dropouts may have resulted from a rigid study design. Nonetheless, they conclude that clozapine is effective for treatment-refractory psychotic mania.

Three published reports detail results from a 48-month, prospective, open, naturalistic trial with clozapine in 101 treatment-refractory patients diagnosed with schizophrenia (N = 34), schizoaffective disorder (N = 30); or bipolar disorder with psychotic features (N = 37; (Ciapparelli *et al.*, 2000, 2003, 2004)). Enrolled subjects were required to be depot neuroleptic-free for at least eight weeks before beginning adjunctive treatment or monotherapy with clozapine. Patients with bipolar disorder demonstrated the most accelerated improvement in both BPRS and Global Assessment of Functioning (GAF) scores. More than 50% of bipolar patients responded to clozapine (>50% reduction in BPRS) within six months of treatment inception. By 48 months, 83.6% of patients with bipolar disorder had responded to clozapine. While female gender, university education, and early age at onset were related to psychosocial functioning (GAF scores) at 48 months, only a diagnosis of bipolar disorder was a significantly predicted clinical response (Ciapparelli *et al.*, 2004). The authors contend that clozapine is a useful treatment for treatment-refractory bipolar disorder in addition to schizophrenia and schizoaffective disorder however cautioned that theirs is only preliminary evidence since adequate parallel control groups were not available for analyses.

8.4.3 RETROSPECTIVE CHART REVIEWS AND CASE STUDIES

As mentioned earlier, Sandoz continued supplying clozapine for clinical compassionate use protocols both in the U.S. and abroad after R&D was temporarily abandoned in 1975 following the Finnish agranulocytosis epidemic. During this time, mental health care professionals observed the clinical usefulness of clozapine in treating patients with schizophrenia as well as individuals with severe or refractory affective illnesses. Early reports attempted to systematically evaluate patient outcomes during compassionate use protocols. Many examined clozapine in bipolar disorder samples alongside schizoaffective disorder and schizophrenia.

McElroy *et al.* (1991) identified 85, severely ill patients who received clozapine for six weeks or longer within a compassionate use protocol at McLean Hospital from March 1975 to November 1989. Fourteen were diagnosed as having treatment-resistant bipolar disorder with psychotic features and 25 with treatment-resistant schizoaffective disorder, bipolar, or depressed type. Forty-one percent of the patients receive clozapine monotherapy while clozapine was adjunctive to other psychotropic agents for the remaining 59%. Baseline BPRS scores were 52.2 ± 12.9 and 56.0 ± 21.4 for bipolar disorder and schizoaffective groups, respectively. After 20.4 ± 4.3 (bipolar disorder) and 34.7 ± 44.8 (schizoaffective disorder) months of treatment with clozapine, substantial reductions in BPRS scores were observed (-21.8 ± 14.7 for bipolar disorder and -27.9 ± 22.4 for schizoaffective disorder). The authors concluded that both adjunctive clozapine and clozapine monotherapy may be effective in acute and maintenance treatment of treatment-resistant affective psychosis.

Subsequently, a case series (Suppes *et al.*, 1992) from the parent McElroy *et al.* (1991) study described seven patients with treatment-resistant bipolar disorder characterized by dysphoric mania (that is, mixed states) and psychosis. The authors noted that all seven patients demonstrated reductions in affective and psychotic symptoms. Furthermore, clozapine seemed to have "bidirectional" effects on mood whereby both dysphoria and mania symptoms were ameliorated.

Banov *et al.* (1994) conducted follow-up interviews with 183 severely ill patients treated with clozapine during previous inpatient hospitalizations at McLean Hospital circa 1992. Comparisons on Clinical Global Impressions-Improvement (CGI-I) and rehospitalization rates were made among patients with bipolar disorder, schizoaffective illness, unipolar depression, and schizophrenia. Thirty-seven percent of the entire sample had discontinued clozapine by follow-up. Favorable clinical outcome and low hospitalization rates were observed in the bipolar mania subgroup.

Zarate, Tohen, and Baldessarini (1995) evaluated clozapine's effectiveness as a mood stabilizer by studying 17 patients from Banov *et al.*'s cohort who were initially discharged on clozapine monotherapy and whose diagnosis was manic or mixed bipolar disorder. At follow-up, 88% of patients were considered responders to clozapine based on statistically significant improvement in their CGI-I scores from hospital discharge. Hospitalizations were less likely to occur during the period after discharge on clozapine than before hospital admission. In fact, 65% of this severely ill sample had no further hospitalizations or relapses of affective episodes from discharge to follow-up. Clozapine seemed to be a sound maintenance treatment for manic or mixed bipolar disorder. Bipolar patients developed neither manic nor depressive episodes during follow-up. This suggests that clozapine may be effective at stabilizing mood in affectively disordered individuals.

Chang *et al.* (2006) retrospectively reviewed medical records from 51 patients with bipolar disorder who received adjunctive clozapine at the Refractory Bipolar Disorders Clinic of Seoul National University from 1995 to 2004. Forty-six (90.2%) of the patients had fewer days per year in the hospital after adjunctive clozapine was added to their treatment regimen. Adjunctive clozapine led to significant reduction in both manic and depressive episodes leading to hospitalizations, supporting a bidirectional, mood-stabilizing role for clozapine (McElroy *et al.*, 1991; Zarate, Tohen, and Baldessarini, 1995).

One report (Guille, Sachs, and Ghaemi, 2000) attempted a naturalistic comparison of clozapine, risperidone, and olanzapine in 42 patients with bipolar disorder, type I treated at the Massachusetts General Hospital Bipolar Clinic. Treatment trials were defined as one or more dose of an antipsychotic. Of the 50 trials (eight patients had >1 trial), 5, 25, and 20 were with clozapine, risperidone, and olanzapine, respectively. No differences in CGI-I were observed between treatment groups, suggesting similar clinical efficacy across second generation antipsychotics in bipolar disorder. Weight gain was higher in both olanzapine-treated and clozapine-treated groups, however the clozapine-treated group's small sample size hampered purposeful interpretation of some statistical analyses. Here bipolar patients faired equally well on risperidone, olanzapine, or clozapine.

Finally, we will briefly mention a case series and two case studies. These three were chosen to further emphasize the manifold ways that clozapine is utilized in clinical practice. While chart reviews and case series reviewed above generally investigated clozapine's role as an antimanic or mood-stabilizing agent in bipolar mania, these cases suggest alternative mood-stabilizing and anti-suicidal uses for clozapine add-on and monotherapy.

One case series (Suppes, Phillips, and Judd, 1994) chronicled response to adjunctive clozapine in three individuals with treatment-resistant, nonpsychotic, rapid cycling bipolar I disorder. In all three cases, severely ill patients with frequent affective shifts experienced substantial abatement of cycling and increased periods of euthymia after clozapine treatment. Additionally, all three performed activities of daily living (that is, work, school) with increased efficacy and reported better quality of life. This series suggests that clozapine may have considerable mood stabilizing properties for rapid cyclers.

A decade-old case study addressed the utility of clozapine in combination therapy of bipolar disorder (Calabrese and Gajwani, 2000). The authors described the care of a severely treatment-resistant patient who had relapsed into mania. Addition of clozapine to a regimen of divalproex and lamotrigine allowed the patient to achieve mania-free euthymia for a full seven-month period. This case again suggests that clozapine exhibits both antimanic and mood-stabilizing properties even in combination with other psychotropic medications.

A recent case study suggested that clozapine may reduce the risk of suicidal thoughts in an individual with a severe, treatment resistant bipolar disorder and history of multiple suicide attempts and multiple hospitalizations (Gupta, 2009). After initiation of clozapine monotherapy, the patient had experienced no further affective episodes of mania or depression, no additional hospitalizations, and no self-reported suicidal ideation. While research has documented anti-suicidal properties of clozapine in treatment-resistant schizophrenia (Meltzer *et al.*, 2003), this case study suggests that clozapine may relieve suicidal ideation and suicide attempts in treatment-resistant bipolar disorder.

8.4.4   CONSIDERATIONS WITH UNIQUE POPULATIONS

8.4.4.1   Pregnant and Lactating Females

Clozapine crosses the placenta with relative ease. However, studies with clozapine in rats with twice the human dose suggest no harm to the fetus or increased risk of infertility as a result of clozapine administration (Thomson Corporation, 2006). Individual clinical case reports suggest that clozapine utilization during pregnancy does not have adverse effects on the fetus. However, these same case reports detail accounts of sedation, decreased suckling, irritability, and cardiovascular instability in a nursing infant that may be a result of clozapine in the mother (Barnas *et al.*, 1994; Waldman and Safferman, 1993). While other antipsychotic medications have been linked to hyperprolactinemia (that is, elevated prolactic production), clozapine does not appear to elevate plasma prolactin levels (Byerly *et al.*, 2007). Prolactin-sensitive issues include milk production and sexual side effects. Given that no studies to date have specifically examined clozapine and fertility, women diagnosed with bipolar disorder and currently treated with clozapine who are considering becoming pregnant should consult their physician (Iqbal *et al.*, 2003). The ultimate decision should weight relative risk of clozapine administration to the fetus or breast-feeding infant with severity of bipolar symptoms in the mother.

8.4.4.2 Older Adults

Shulman, Singh, and Shulman (1997) used clozapine to prospectively treat three elderly, institutionalized, male patients (mean age 72 ± 2.5 years) diagnosed with acute, psychotic mania. All three patients responded to clozapine with mood stabilization and reduction in psychotic symptoms within seven weeks. While lithium remains a first-line treatment of bipolar disorder in elderly patients (Baldessarini, Tondo, and Suppes, 1996), clozapine may be considered as a safe alternative in patients refractory to lithium or other traditional mood-stabilizers for bipolar disorder. Although clozapine was tolerated well in these three patients, other reports have detailed an increased risk of agranulocytosis with increasing age (Salzman *et al.*, 1995). All package inserts for clozapine contain a black box warning that elderly patients with dementia-related psychosis are at increased risk of death when treated with clozapine or other second generation antipsychotics due to cardiovascular or infectious complications (Gareri *et al.*, 2008). When considering clozapine therapy in elderly populations, risks, and benefits should be evaluated on an individualized basis before beginning treatment.

8.4.4.3 Children and Adolescents

Bipolar disorder in children and adolescents has received considerable attention in the past decade and is associated with irritable manias as well as significant depressive symptoms (Chang, 2009). Clinicians often treat children and adolescents with similar pharmacological strategies used with adults (Danielyan and Kowatch, 2005). Clozapine has been reported to be effective in children and adolescents with acute manic or mixed symptomatology who had not responded to other psychotropic agents (that is, mood stabilizers, other first- and second-generation antipsychotics, and so on) at relatively low doses (75–300 mg/day; Masi, Mucci, and Millepiedl, 2002; Kowatch, Suppes, and Gilfillan, 1995).

8.4.4.4 Asian Populations

Earlier in this chapter, we reviewed the literature examining the effectiveness of clozapine in bipolar disorder. All reviewed reports were from North American or European reports with the exception of one. Chang *et al.* (2006) presented results from a trial of long-term adjunctive clozapine in bipolar disorder, however the authors did not address cross-cultural considerations. Tang *et al.* (2008) present data on clozapine's widespread and popular use in China via critical examination of Chinese-written empirical reports. Traditionally, China and Western nations have not shared their scientific and medical literatures. Tang and colleagues maintain that clozapine is the most commonly used antipsychotic agent in China for schizophrenia. Given that generic clozapine is relatively inexpensive, Tang *et al.* suggest that clozapine's use in China may in part reflect the nation's economic trials and tribulations. Nevertheless, Chinese psychiatrists overall believe in the effectiveness of clozapine in difficult-to-treat disorders such as schizophrenia, mania, and depression (Tang *et al.*, 2008). Risk of agranulocytosis with clozapine in China appears similar to that in the United States (Honigfeld *et al.*, 1998).

8.5 EFFECTIVE PHARMACOTHERAPY FOR BIPOLAR DISORDER?

8.5.1 ANTIMANIC, ANTIPSYCHOTIC, AND MOOD-STABILIZING PROPERTIES

Although clozapine received FDA approval nearly two decades ago, investigations of clozapine's utility in bipolar disorders has received limited focus. A preponderance of reports, retrospective in nature, has attempted to describe clinical and psychosocial outcomes in bipolar patients after short- and long-term trials with clozapine. A handful of prospective reports and two randomized studies further clarified its clinical profile under controlled conditions.

Results of published reports in our review appear to be relatively consistent and unambiguous. Clozapine is an effective pharmacotherapy for bipolar disorders. However, less certainty is available when clarifying clozapine's putative role (that is, antimanic, antipsychotic, and/or mood-stabilizing) for different subgroups of patients (that is, manic, depressed, psychotic).

Clozapine appears an effective treatment option for patients with treatment-refractory bipolar disorder. Given robust evidence of clozapine's effectiveness in treatment-resistant schizophrenia (Meltzer, 1992, 1994), most bipolar disorder research has focused on treatment-refractory samples (McElroy *et al.*, 1991; Suppes *et al.*, 1992, 1999; Chang *et al.*, 2006; Suppes, Phillips, and Judd, 1994; Calabrese *et al.*, 1996; Green *et al.*, 2000; Ciapparelli *et al.*, 2000, 2003, 2004). Patients in these studies responded to clozapine with reductions in mood symptoms or rehospitalization rates.

Clozapine may have distinctive antipsychotic effects for patients with psychotic mania. Several reports (Suppes *et al.*, 1992, 1999; Ciapparelli *et al.*, 2000, 2003, 2004; Green *et al.*, 2000) describe reductions in overall psychiatric symptomatology including psychotic symptoms after treatment with adjunctive clozapine or clozpaine monotherapy.

Clozapine may be most effective at treating acute mania. A majority of reports (Suppes *et al.*, 1992, 1999; Banov *et al.*, 1994; Zarate, Tohen, and Baldessarini, 1995; Calabrese *et al.*, 1996; Green *et al.*, 2000; Barbini *et al.*, 1997) studied clinical outcome in patients whose bipolar disorders were characterized by frequent manic episodes. Antimanic effects for clozapine were observed across all samples. It appears to be effective regardless of whether the patient has psychiatric symptoms.

Finally, clozapine may have mood-stabilizing effects. While there is minimal evidence for clozapine's effectiveness in treating depression alone (Banov *et al.*, 1994), mood-stabilizing effects have been observed in multiple reports (Suppes *et al.*, 1992, 1999; Zarate, Tohen, and Baldessarini, 1995; Chang *et al.*, 2006). When clozapine was used to treat acute mania, subsequent episodes of either mania or depression were often significantly minimized during a follow-up period. This effect has been observed equally in psychotic and nonpsychotic bipolar disorder.

8.5.2 METHODOLOGICAL LIMITATIONS IN EXISTING RESEARCH

Randomized, double-blind, controlled designs are viewed as the gold standard for clinical treatment trial research. No trials of this nature examine clozapine's effectiveness in bipolar disorder. In fact, no single-blind trials have been conducted to date. Because of this important methodological constraint, conclusions about clozapine's utility in patients with bipolar disorder must be drawn with caution.

The most methodologically sound studies to date examining clozapine's utility in bipolar disorder are two controlled, prospective, randomized treatment trials comparing clozapine with an alternative treatment (Barbini *et al.*, 1997; Suppes *et al.*, 1999). Results suggest strong antimanic and possible mood-stabilizing properties for clozapine in patients currently manic or by history resistant to treatment. However, though randomized, non-tandard titration (that is, rapid) (Barbini *et al.*, 1997) and open, add-on treatment (Suppes *et al.*, 1999) designs must be considered when interpreting their conclusions.

While results from retrospective chart reviews and open label trials with clozapine provide compelling evidence about clozapine's utility in bipolar disorder, they too must be considered with caution. Small sample sizes, missing data, and heterogeneous samples were common in all retrospective reports (McElroy *et al.*, 1991; Suppes *et al*, 1992; Banov *et al.*, 1994; Zarate, Tohen, and Baldessarini, 1995; Chang *et al.*, 2006; Guille, Sachs, and Ghaemi, 2000; Suppes, Phillips, and Judd, 1994). Absence of a control group (Calabrese *et al.*, 1996; Ciapparelli *et al.*, 2000, 2003, 2004) generally characterized open-label trials.

8.5.3 ADMINISTRATION

Clozapine appears to be effective as monotherapy (McElroy *et al.*, 1991; Zarate, Tohen, and Baldessarini, 1995; Gupta, 2009; Calabrese *et al.*, 1996; Green *et al.*, 2000) or as an adjunctive agent (McElroy *et al.*, 1991; Banov *et al.*, 1994; Chang *et al.*, 2006; Calabrese and Gajwani, 2000; Suppes, Phillips, and Judd, 1994; Barbini *et al.*, 1997; Suppes *et al.*, 1999). Additionally, clozapine seems to be effective in patients with bipolar patients at lower doses than in patients with schizophrenia (Fehr, Ozcan, and Suppes, 2005). Effective doses of clozapine in bipolar disorder are often between 200 and 300 mg

Table 8.2 Mean clozapine doses across bipolar disorder studies.

Study	Mean dose (mg/d)
Retrospective chart reviews	
McElroy *et al.* (1991)	350–900
Suppes *et al.* (1992)	75–900
Banov *et al.* (1994)	341 ± 160
	Range = 125–800
Zarate *et al.* (1995)	304.4 ± 163 at followup
	182 ± 94 at discharge
Chang *et al.* (2006)	201.6 ± 75.9
Guille, Sachs, and Ghaemi (2000)	210 ± 119.4
Suppes, Phillips, and Judd (1994)	150–400
Open-label, prospective trials	
Calabrese *et al.* (1996)	494 ± 145
Green *et al.* (2000)	289 ± 162
Ciapparelli *et al.* (2000, 2003, 2004)	137–184
Randomized trials	
Barbini *et al.* (1997)	175 at day 8
Suppes *et al.* (1999)	355 ± 248

(see Table 8.2) and considerably lower than first generation clozapine dosing in schizophrenia (Meltzer, 1992, 1994). Individuals taking clozapine should be monitored every three months for weight gain, fasting glucose, and lipid profile (American Diabetes Association, 2004). Decisions concerning administration of clozapine in patients with bipolar disorder are best made on an individualized, patient-specific basis.

8.5.4 CONCLUSION

While randomized, controlled, double-blind trials examining clozapine's differential effectiveness in treating the various affective episodes characteristic of bipolar disorder are indeed needed, they are unlikely to be completed in the near future. With the advent of generic versions of clozapine in 1997, Sandoz (now Novartis) lost any incentive to fund such expensive investigations. The National Institute of Mental Health has recently announced a Strategic Plan (http://www.nimh.nih.gov/about/strategic-planning-reports, National Institute of Mental Health Strategic Plan, 2008) focused on the multiplex developmental etiologies (that is, genetic, neurobiological, behavioral, environmental) of mental illnesses. As a result, National Institute of Mental Health (NIMH) is unlikely to continue funding agent-to-agent treatment trials of psychotherapeutic drugs with modest effectiveness at best for complex, mental illnesses.

In this chapter, we have demonstrated that clozapine is an effective medication for bipolar disorder. Adverse effects associated with its administration can be avoided with careful monitoring. Treating physicians should consider clozapine a reliable option for patients struggling with bipolar disorder's affective storms.

8.6 CASE STUDIES

8.6.1 MS. J

Ms. J is a 36-year-old Caucasian female. She presented to the Bipolar Disorders Clinic after becoming frustrated with care after lengthy unsuccessful treatment with another psychiatrist. Onset of bipolar disorder was in her early teens. Her first manic episode occurred at age 18 and was severe with psychotic symptoms. Since then, she has experienced at least two manic episodes every year. Manias last approximately 12–14 days and are characterized by auditory hallucinations, 2–3 hours of sleep/night, excessive energy, excessive spending, racing thoughts, and pressured speech. Ms. J experiences episodes of depression lasting 15–25 days at least four times a year. She has attempted suicide 13 times and has been hospitalized as a result of these attempts at least five times. Her longest period of euthymia since onset has been one month at age 26 when she was married. Her psychosis generally consists of delusions of grandeur (that is, she is a close descendant of God and Jesus) and low-level voices encouraging her to travel long distances by foot.

Over the course of her illness, she has had several trials with mood-stabilizing agents (for example, carbamazepine, lithium, valproate) with adjunctive antipsychotic medication (for example, chlorpromazine, risperidone, olanzapine). She continued to experience episodes of depression and mania as well as experiencing significant psychosis. Ms. J has not maintained employment of any kind since age 18. Her marriage ended in divorce when she was 27 years old.

Given the severe psychosis and treatment resistant nature of Ms. J's bipolar disorder as well as the significant impairment resulting from her illness, her psychiatrist recommended clozapine as the next psychopharmacological treatment option. After risks and benefits were carefully discussed, Ms. J agreed to close monitoring, and provided consent. After checking her white blood cell count with differential, metabolic panel including fasting glucose, hemoglobin A1C, lipid profile, blood pressure, weight, body mass index, and waist circumference (all fell within reference ranges), her psychiatrist registered her case with the CPR and started her on 12.5 mg daily. Despite some sedation, Ms. J was able to tolerate a subsequent dose increase of 12.5–25 mg every two to three days. By the end of week 2, she was on 75 and 100 mg daily by week 3.

Since initiation of treatment with clozapine six months ago, her mood has become more stable. Clozapine was eventually titrated to a target dose of 150–300 mg daily in concordance with her response and tolerability. Ms. J has charted her mood daily and has incorporated more physical activities and healthy diet into her daily routines. In these six months, Ms. J estimates that she has been euthymic for nearly four. She has not attempted suicide while taking clozapine. While she has experienced brief hypomanic symptoms and anhedonia, these symptoms have lasted only one to two days and have included no psychosis.

8.6.2 MR. K

Mr. K is a 45-year old Caucasian man with a 30-year history of bipolar disorder and significant exposure to sexual and physical abuse as a child and adolescent. He was referred to the Bipolar Disorders Clinic after being discharged from the hospital following a suicide attempt. He remembers feeling symptoms of depression when he was in middle school but does not report a full-blown episode of depression until he was a senior in high school. He has attempted suicide four times by self-report and been hospitalized for two of these attempts. Mr. K remembers no periods of euthymia lasting longer than one week in duration. His manic episodes typically occur five times per year and are characterized by hypersexuality and excessive, irrational impulsive behavior. Hypersexual behavior during previous manic episodes led to his acquiring HIV and fathering three children. Mr. K reports never experiencing psychosis.

Mr. K remained ummedicated until age 20 because his family believed that medication would hurt him. From age 20 to 30, he received trials with lithium and valproate monotherapy as well as adjunctive risperidone, olanzapine, and haloperidol. He continued to experience manic and depressive episodes at similar rates to his pre-medication period. He attempted suicide less frequently, however attempts were more severe and most required hospitalization.

Since Mr. K had proven resistant to many pharmacotherapy regimens, clozapine was initiated. White blood cell count with differential and metabolic panels were collected, and Mr. K was registered with the CPR after normal ranges were confirmed. Clozapine was begun and gradually increased to 350 mg/day. However, Mr. K reported severe sedation so his dose was gradually decreased to 250 mg/day. During the past seven months of clozapine treatment, Mr. K averaged only 11 days of depression per month, though not at a severity consistent with full episode criteria. He reported experiencing periods of euthymia lasting two to three weeks for the first time since his mood symptoms began. His family noticed that his productivity and psychosocial functioning were substantially improved. He has started a romantic relationship and held a part-time job since being stabilized on clozapine.

References

American Diabetes Association (2004) Consensus development conference on antipsychotic drugs and obesity and diabetes. *J. Clin. Psychiatry*, **65** (2), 267–272.

Baldessarini, R., Tondo, L., and Suppes, T. (1996) Pharmacological treatment of bipolar disorder throughout the life-cycle, in *Mood Disorders Across the Life Span* (eds K. Shulman, M. Tohen, and S.E. Kutcher), John Wiley & Sons, Inc., New York, pp. 299–338.

Bandelow, B., Degner, D., Kreusch, U. *et al.* (1995) Myocarditis under therapy with clozapine. *Schizophr. Res.*, **17**, 293–294.

Banov, M., Zarate, C., Tohen, M. *et al.* (1994) Clozapine therapy in refractory affective disorders: polarity predicts response in long-term follow-up. *J. Clin. Psychiatry*, **55** (7), 295–300.

Barbini, B., Scherillo, P., Benedetti, F. *et al.* (1997) Response to clozapine in acute mania is more rapid than that of chlorpromazine. *Int. Clin. Psychopharmacol.*, **12**, 109–112.

Barnas, C., Bergant, A., Hummer, M. *et al.* (1994) Clozapine concentrations in maternal and fetal plasma, amniotic fluid, and breast milk. *Am. J. Psychiatry*, **151** (6), 945.

Bastani, B., Alphs, L., and Meltzer, H. (1989) Development of the Clozaril patient management system. *Psychopharmacology*, **99**, S122–S125.

Bustillo, J., Buchanan, R., Irish, D. *et al.* (1996) Differential effect of clozapine on weight: a controlled study. *Am. J. Psychiatry*, **153** (6), 817–819.

Byerly, M., Suppes, T., Tran, Q. *et al.* (2007) Clinical implications of antipsychotic-induced hyperprolactinemia in patients with schizophrenia spectrum or bipolar spectrum disorders: recent developments and current perspectives. *J. Clin. Psychopharmacol.*, **27** (6), 639–661.

Calabrese, J. and Gajwani, P. (2000) Lamotrigine and clozapine for bipolar disorder. *Am. J. Psychiatry*, **157** (9), 1523.

Calabrese, J., Kimmel, S., Woyshville, M. *et al.* (1996) Clozapine for treatment-refractory mania. *Am. J. Psychiatry*, **153** (6), 759–764.

Chang, K. (2009) Challenges in the diagnosis and treatment of pediatric bipolar disorder. *Diaglogues Clin. Neurosci.*, **11** (1), 73–80.

Chang, J., Ha, K., Lee, K. *et al.* (2006) The effects of long-term clozapine add-on therapy on the rehospitalization rate and the mood polarity patterns in bipolar disorders. *J. Clin. Psychiatry*, **67** (3), 461–467.

Ciapparelli, A., Dell'Osso, L., Bandettini di Poggio, A. *et al.* (2003) Clozapine in treatment-resistant patients with schizophrenia, schizoaffective disorder, or psychotic bipolar disorder: a naturalistic, 48-month follow-up study. *J. Clin. Psychiatry*, **64**, 451–458.

Ciapparelli, A., Dell'Osso, L., Pini, S. *et al.* (2000) Clozapine for treatment-refractory schizophrenia, schizoaffective disorder, and psychotic bipolar disorder: a 24-month naturalistic study. *J. Clin. Psychiatry*, **61** (5), 329–334.

Ciapparelli, A., Ducci, F., Carmassi, C. *et al.* (2004) Predictors of response in a sample of treatment-resistant psychotic patients on clozapine. *Eur. Arch. Psychiatry Clin. Neurosci.*, **254**, 343–346.

Crilly, J. (2007) The history of clozapine and its emergence in the US market: a review and analysis. *Hist. Psychiatry*, **18** (1), 39–60.

Danielyan, A. and Kowatch, R. (2005) Management options for bipolar disorder in children and adolescents. *Pediatr. Drugs*, **7** (5), 277–294.

Devinsky, O., Honigfeld, G., and Patin, J. (1992) Clozapine-related seizures. *Neurology*, **41**, 369–371.

Edge, S., Markowitz, J., and Devane, C. (1999) Clozapine drug-drug interactions: a review of the literature. *Hum. Psychopharmacol. Clin. Exp.*, **12** (1), 5–20.

Elkis, H. (2007) Treatment-resistant schizophrenia. *Psychiatr. Clin. N. Am.*, **30**, 511–533.

Essali, A., Al-Haj Haasan, N., Li, C. *et al.* (2009). Clozapine versus typical neuroleptic medication for schizophrenia. *Cochrane Database Syst. Rev.* (1) CD000059.

Fehr, B., Ozcan, M., and Suppes, T. (2005) Low doses of clozapine may stabilize treatment-resistant bipolar disorder. *Eur. Arch. Psychiatry. Clin. Neurosci.*, **255**, 10–14.

Frye, M., Ketter, T., Altshuler, L. *et al.* (1998) Clozapine in bipolar disorder: treatment implications for other atypical antipsychotics. *J. Affect. Disord.*, **48** (2–3), 91–104.

Gareri, P., De Faxio, P., Russo, E. *et al.* (2008) The safety of clozapine in the elderly. *Exp. Opin. Drug Saf.*, **7** (5), 525–538.

Green, A., Tohen, M., Patel, J. *et al.* (2000) Clozapine in the treatment of refractory psychotic mania. *Am. J. Psychiatry*, **157** (6), 982–986.

Guille, C., Sachs, G., and Ghaemi, S. (2000) A naturalistic comparison of clozapine, risperidone, and olanzapine in the treatment of bipolar disorder. *J. Clin. Psychiatry*, **61** (9), 638–642.

Gupta, M. (2009) Clozapine monotherapy for 66 months in treatment resistant bipolar disorder: a case report. *J. Clin. Psychopharmacol.*, **29** (5), 501–503.

Hippius, H. (1989) The history of clozapine. *Psychopharmacology*, **99**, S3–S5.

Hippius, H. (1999) A historical perspective of clozapine. *J. Clin. Psychiatry*, **60** (Suppl. 12), 22–23.

Honigfeld, G., Arellano, F., Sethi, J. *et al.* (1998) Reducing clozapine-related morbidity and mortality: 5 years of experience with the Clozaril National registry. *J. Clin. Psychiatry*, **59** (Suppl. 3), 3–7.

Idanpaan-Heikkila, J., Alhava, E., Olkinuora, M. *et al.* (1977) Agranulocytosis during treatment with clozapine. *Eur. J. Clin. Psychopharmacol.*, **11**, 193–198.

Iqbal, M., Rahman, A., Husain, Z. *et al.* (2003) Clozapine: a clinical review of adverse effects and management. *Ann. Clin. Psychiatry*, **15** (1), 33–48.

Kane, J., Honigfeld, G., Singer, J. *et al.* (1988) Clozapine for the treatment-resistant schizophrenic: a double-blind comparison with chlorpromazine. *Arch. Gen. Psychiatry*, **45**, 789–797.

Khan, A. and Preskorn, S. (2005) Examining concentration-dependent toxicity of clozapine: role of therapeutic drug monitoring. *J. Psychiatr. Pract.*, **11** (5), 289–301.

Kilian, J., Kerr, K., Lawrence, C. *et al.* (1999) Myocarditis and cardiomyopathy associated with clozapine. *Lancet*, **354**, 1841–1845.

Kowatch, R., Suppes, T., and Gilfillan, S. K. (1995) Clozapine treatment of children and adolescents with bipolar disorder and schizophrenia: a clinical case series. *J. Child Adolesc. Psychopharmacol.*, **5**, 241–253.

Lieberman, J. and Safferman, A. (1992) Clinical profile of clozapine: adverse reactions and agranulocytosis. *Psychiatr. Q.*, **63**, 51–70.

Masi, G., Mucci, M., and Millepiedl, S. (2002) Clozapine in adolescent inpatients with acute mania. *J. Child Adolesc. Psyhopharmacol.*, **12** (2), 9309.

McElroy, S., Dessain, E., Pope, H. *et al.* (1991) Clozapine in the treatment of psychotic mood disorders, schizoaffective disorder, and schizophrenia. *J. Clin. Psychiatry*, **52**, 41–414.

McEvoy, J., Lieberman, J., Stroup, T. *et al.* (2006) Effectiveness of clozapine versus olanzapine, quetiapine, and risperidone in patients with chronic schizophrenia who did not respond to prior atypical antipsychotic treatment. *Am. J. Psychiatry*, **163** (4), 600–610.

Meltzer, H.Y. (1992) The mechanism of action of Clozapine in relation to its clinical advantages, in *Novel Antipsychotic Drugs* (eds H.Y. Meltzer), Raven Press, New York, pp. 1–13.

Meltzer, H. (1994) An overview of the mechanism of action of clozapine. *J. Clin. Psychiatry*, **55** (Suppl. B), 47–52.

Meltzer, H., Alphs, L., Green, A. *et al.* (2003) Clozapine treatment for suicidality in schizophrenia: international suicide prevention trial (InterSePT). *Arch. Gen. Psychiatry*, **60**, 82–91.

National Institute of Mental Health Strategic Plan (2008) http://www.nimh.nih.gov/about/strategic-planning-reports. Accessed in 2008.

Salzman, C., Vaccaro, B., Lieff, J. *et al.* (1995) Clozapine in older patients with psychosis and behavioral disruption. *Am. J. Geriatr. Psychaitry*, **3**, 26–33.

Shulman, R., Singh, A., and Shulman, K. (1997) Treatment of elderly inststitutionalized bipolar patients with clozapine. *Psychopharmacol. Bull.*, **33** (1), 113–118.

Suppes, T., Dennehy, E., Hirschfeld, R. *et al.* (2005) The Texas implementation of treatment algorithms: update to the algorithms for treatment of bipolar I disorder. *J. Clin. Psychiatry*, **66** (7), 870–886.

Suppes, T., McElroy, S.G., Dessain, E. *et al.* (1992) Clozapine in the treatment of dysphoric mania. *Biol. Psychiatry*, **32**, 270–280.

Suppes, T., Phillips, K., and Judd, C. (1994) Clozapine treatment of nonpsychotic rapid cycling bipolar disorder: a report of three cases. *Biol. Psychiatry*, **36**, 338–340.

Suppes, T., Webb, A., Paul, B. *et al.* (1999) Clinical outcome in a randomized 1-year trial of clozapine versus treatment as usual for patients with treatment-resistant illness and a history of mani. *Am. J. Psychiatry*, **156** (8), 1164–1169.

Tang, Y.-I., Mao, P.-X., Jiang, F. *et al.* (2008) Clozapine in China. *Pharmacopsychiatry*, **41**, 1–9.

Thomson Corporation (2006) Miscellaneous antipsychotic agents, *Physicians Desk Reference Psychotropic Prescribing Guide*, Thomson Corporation, Toronto, pp. 286–295.

Tohen, M. and Vieta, E. (2009) Antipsychotic agents in the treatment of bipolar mania. *Bipolar Disord.*, **11** (Suppl. 2), 45–54.

Tohen, M., Zhang, F. Taylor, C. *et al.* (2001) A meta-analysis of the use of typical antipsychotic agents in bipolar disorder. *J. Affect. Disord.*, **65**, 85–93.

Toth, P. and Frankenburg, F. (1994) Clozapine and seizures: a review. *Can. J. Psychiatry*, **39**, 236–238.

Tuunainen, A., Wahlbeck, K., and Gilbody, S. (2002) Newer atypical antipsychotic medication in comparison to clozapine: a systematic review of randomized trials. *Schizophr. Res.*, **56** (1–2), 1–10.

Wahlbeck, K., Cheine, M., Essali, A. *et al.* (1999) Evidence of clozapine's effectiveness in schizophrenia: a systematic review and meta-analysis of randomized trials. *Am. J. Psychiatry*, **156** (7), 990–999.

Waldman, M.S. and Safferman, A.Z. (1993) Pregnancy and clozapine. *Am. J. Psychiatry*, **150** (1), 168–169.

Wirshing, D., Spellberg, B., Erhart, S. *et al.* (1998) Novel antipsychotics and new onset diabetes. *Biol. Psychiatry*, **44**, 778–783.

Young, C., Bowers, M., and Mazure, C. (1998) Management of the adverse effects of clozapine. *Schizophr. Bull.*, **24** (3), 381–390.

Zarate, C., Tohen, M., and Baldessarini, R.J. (1995) Clozapine in severe mood disorders. *J. Clin. Psychiatry*, **56** (9), 411–417.

Zarate, C., Tohen, M., Banov, M.W. *et al.* (1995) Is clozapine a mood stabilizer?. *J. Clin. Psychiatry*, **56** (3), 108–112.

Risperidone and Paliperidone in the Treatment of Bipolar Disorder

L. Ivo Caers and Joris Berwaerts

Johnson & Johnson Pharmaceutical Research & Development, LIC, Beerse, Belgium; NJ, USA

9.1 INTRODUCTION

Risperidone is a selective mono-aminergic antagonist belonging to the class of benzisoxazole derivatives with a high affinity for serotoninergic 5-HT2A and dopaminergic D2 receptors. Risperidone binds also to alpha1-adrenergic receptors, and, with lower affinity, to H1-histaminergic and alpha2-adrenergic receptors (Kalkman and Loetscher, 2003; Leysen *et al.*, 1994). It was the first atypical or second generation antipsychotic to become available for first line use, initially in schizophrenia, later on in a variety of psychiatric diseases including bipolar disorder.

Paliperidone or 9-hydroxyrisperidone belongs to the same class of compounds. Similar to other atypical antipsychotics, it is a centrally active dopamine D2 and 5HT2A antagonist. Paliperidone Extended Release (ER) tablets utilize patented osmotic drug-release (OROS®) technology, whereby osmotic pressure delivers paliperidone from the dosage form at a controlled rate. Paliperidone ER exhibits a slowly ascending plasma concentration-time profile (Cleton *et al.*, 2007), allowing initiation of treatment with a potentially effective dose without the need for dose titration. This ER technology also allows a substantial reduction of the peak to through plasma levels after administration of a fixed dose on consecutive days compared to conventional immediate release tablets (Cleton *et al.*, 2007).

Both oral risperidone and paliperidone ER have been studied in placebo-controlled studies in acute manic and mixed episodes associated with bipolar I disorder, both as monotherapy and as adjunctive treatment to mood stabilizers such as lithium and valproate. Maintenance of the antimanic effect has been documented with reference to established compounds in randomized, double-blind studies of 12 weeks duration. Risperidone has also been studied in children and adolescents with manic or mixed episodes associated with bipolar I disorder.

Bipolar Psychopharmacotherapy: Caring for the patient, Second Edition. Edited by Hagop S. Akiskal and Mauricio Tohen.
© 2011 John Wiley & Sons, Ltd. Published 2011 by John Wiley & Sons, Ltd.

With the availability of atypical antipsychotics, interest in the therapeutic use of these compounds for the maintenance treatment of bipolar disorder, that is, for the prevention of recurrence of mood episodes, has increased substantially. Several atypical antipsychotics have been documented to be effective in the maintenance treatment of bipolar disorder (Smith *et al.*, 2007). One of the well-documented factors contributing to frequent relapses of mood episodes in bipolar disorder patients is poor treatment adherence (Lingam and Scott, 2002; Sajatovic *et al.*, 2006). Long-acting injectable (LAI) formulations of atypical antipsychotics combine the benefits of oral atypical antipsychotics with the assurance of steady medication delivery and the potential of improved adherence (Chue and Emsley, 2007; McEvoy, 2006). Risperidone LAI has been studied in the maintenance treatment of bipolar disorder, both as monotherapy and as adjunctive therapy to treatment as usual.

This chapter reviews the principal clinical studies available for oral risperidone and paliperidone ER as well as for risperidone LAI in the management of patients with bipolar disorder.

9.2 ORAL RISPERIDONE IN BIPOLAR MANIA

Shortly after risperidone became available for the treatment of schizophrenia, investigators started exploring the usefulness of this new compound in bipolar disorder.

Open-label studies of risperidone as adjunctive treatment to mood stabilizers in bipolar mania patients suggested a beneficial effect with good tolerance and no cases of worsened mood symptoms (Tohen *et al.*, 1996; Paik *et al.*, 1995; Ghaemi *et al.*, 1997). Equivocal results were reported with monotherapy, particularly in treatment resistant subjects, suggesting some antidepressant effect but also a potential of overstimulation (Sajatovic *et al.*, 1996; Dwight *et al.*, 1994; Schaffer and Schaffer, 1996).

Risperidone as monotherapy has been studied in three double-blind placebo-controlled studies in acute mania. Two three weeks studies, both followed by a nine-week, open-label safety follow-up period (Hirschfeld *et al.*, 2004; Khanna *et al.*, 2005). One 12-week study with haloperidol as active comparator in which the placebo patients were switched to risperidone after the third week (Smulevich *et al.*, 2005). The 12-week statistical comparisons included only those patients randomly assigned to risperidone or haloperidol at the start of the study to document maintenance of antimanic effect of risperidone versus an established reference compound. Two additional studies were performed to assess the efficacy and safety of risperidone in combination with mood stabilizers (Yatham *et al.*, 2003). One of these studies also included a haloperidol plus mood stabilizer arm (Sachs *et al.*, 2002). Both these studies lasted for 3 weeks and were followed by a 10-week open-label risperidone safety follow-up period. All studies were done in patients who had bipolar I disorder and were in a manic episode. Three studies also included patients with mixed episodes. In all studies, risperidone was administered in a flexible dose range of 1–6 mg/day starting from 2 or 3 mg/day with 1-mg increments if required over the first four days. The primary efficacy parameter in all controlled studies was the change from baseline of the Young Mania Rating Scale (YMRS) total score. See Table 9.1 for an overview of the risperidone studies in acute mania.

Table 9.1 Clinical studies with oral risperidone in bipolar mania.

Study	Design	Sample	Dose	Primary outcome	Results	Secondary outcome measures
Smulevich *et al.*, (2005)	Double-blind 3 wk vs. placebo, 12 wk vs. haloperidol	n = 140 Plac n = 154 Ris n = 144 Hal	Flexible 1–6 mg Ris 2–12 mg Hal	YMRS	Ris significantly better than placebo (3 wk) No difference Ris and Hal at 12 wk	YMRS responder rate BPRS CGI-S GAS MADRS
Hirschfeld *et al.*, (2004)	Double-blind *vs.* placebo 3 wk	n = 125 Plac n = 134 Ris	Flexible 1–6 mg Ris	YMRS	Ris significantly better than placebo	YMRS responder rate CGI-S GAS MADRS PANSS
Khanna *et al.*, (2005)	Double-blind *vs.* placebo 3 wks	n = 144 Plac n = 146 Plac	Flexible 1–6 mg Ris	YMRS	Ris significantly better than placebo	YMRS responder rate CGI-S GAS MADRS PANSS

(Continued Overleaf)

Table 9.1 (Continued)

Study	Design	Sample	Dose	Primary outcome	Results	Secondary outcome measures
Sachs et al., (2002)	Double-blind vs. placebo, haloperidol 3 wk in combination with lithium or valproate + 10 wk open-label risperidone	n = 51 Plac n = 52 Ris n = 53 Hal	Flexible 1–6 mg Ris 2–12 mg Hal	YMRS	Ris significantly better than placebo No difference Ris and Hal at 3 wk	YMRS responder rate BPRS CGI-C HAM-D
Yatham et al., (2003)	Double-blind vs. placebo, 3 wk in combination with lithium, valproate, or carbamazepine + 10 wk open-label risperidone	n = 75 Plac n = 75 Ris	Flexible 1–6 mg Ris	YMRS	Ris not significantly different from placebo	YMRS responder rate BPRS CGI-C HAM-D
Hirschfeld et al., (2006)	Open-label for 9 wk (follow-up of Hirschfeld et al., (2004) and Khanna et al., (2005)	n = 283 that is, 123 Plac/Ris 160 Ris/Ris	Flexible 1–6 mg Ris	YMRS	Significant improvement at endpoint vs. open-label baseline	GCI-S GAS MADRS PANSS

YMRS, Young Mania Rating Scale; BPRS, Brief Psychiatric Rating Scale; GAS, Global Assessment Scale; MADRS, Montgomery Asberg Depression Rating Scale; PANSS, Positive and Negative Syndrome Scale; CGI-S, Clinical Global Impression Scale of Severity; CGI-C, Clinical Global Impression Scale of Change; HAM-D, Hammilton Rating Scale for Depression.

9.2.1 RISPERIDONE MONOTHERAPY IN BIPOLAR MANIA

In all three studies, risperidone was shown to be significantly superior to placebo on the prespecified primary endpoint, the change from baseline in the YMRS total score at week 3 (Table 9.2).

Risperidone was also shown to be significantly more effective than placebo after one and two weeks of treatment. In one of the two studies that also performed a YMRS assessment at day 3, a significant difference from placebo was seen at that timepoint (Hirschfeld *et al.*, 2004). In all three studies, the antimanic effects of risperidone were supported by the YMRS responder rates, that is, the proportion of patients with a ≥50% improvement from baseline in total YMRS total score at the three-week endpoint. Outcomes on other secondary efficacy measures, including Clinical Global Impression (CGI) change, Global Assessment Scale (GAS) change, and Brief Psychiatric Rating Scale (BPRS) or Positive and Negative Syndrome Scale (PANSS) change, further confirmed the superiority of risperidone over placebo in treating bipolar mania and associated symptoms. The improvements on the secondary efficacy measures also indicate that risperidone has a clinically relevant effect.

Gopal *et al.* (2005) assessed rates of symptomatic remission in the patient population studied by Khanna *et al.* (2005). Sixty-one (42%) risperidone-treated patients achieved remission, as defined by a YMRS total score of ≤8 within three weeks from baseline

Table 9.2 Risperidone oral monotherapy in bipolar mania: change from baseline in YMRS total score by study (Week 3 LOCF/endpoint).

Study Treatment	N[a]	LS mean change (SD)	Comparison with Placebo	
			Diff in LS mean change (95% CI)	p value
Smulevich *et al.*, (2005)				
Placebo	138	−8.4 (9.65)	—	
Risperidone	153	−13.9 (9.65)	−5.6 (−7.8, −3.3)	—
Haloperidol	144	−13.3 (9.65)	−5.0 (−7.2, −2.7)	<0.001
				<0.001
Hirschfeld *et al.*, (2004)	119		—	
Placebo	127	−4.8 (9.52)	−5.9 (−8.3, −3.4)	
Risperidone		−10.6 (9.52)		—
				<0.001
Khanna *et al.*, (2005)	142		—	
Placebo	144	−10.8 (13.45)	−12.4 (−15.6, −9.3)	
Risperidone		−23.2 (13.45)		—
				<0.001

[a]N, number of patients with both baseline and postbaseline timepoint measurements.
CI, confidence interval; LOCF, last observation carried forward; LS, least squares; SD, standard deviation; YMRS, Young Mania Rating Scale.

and for the remainder of the trial duration, versus 18 (13%) of patients given placebo. Treatment with risperidone was associated with a significantly shorter time to remission (hazard ratio = 3.7; $p < 0.0001$). Additional evaluations determined that both treatment with risperidone and absence of psychosis at baseline were significant independent predictors of remission ($p < 0.0001$ and $p < 0.01$, respectively).

Risperidone did not appear to induce or worsen coexisting subsyndromal depressive symptoms. In two studies (Smulevich *et al.*, 2005; Khanna *et al.*, 2005), risperidone-treated patients showed significantly greater mean changes from baseline in the Montgomery Åsberg Depression Rating Scale (MADRS) score than patients receiving placebo. In the study by Hirschfeld *et al.* (2004), significance was shown at weeks 1 and 2, with a numerical advantage for risperidone at the three-week endpoint.

Both risperidone and haloperidol were effective relative to placebo for the change from baseline in YMRS total score at the three-week endpoint (Smulevich *et al.*, 2005). Between weeks 3 and 12, there was further mean improvement on the YMRS that was similar on both risperidone and haloperidol. At the 12-week endpoint, difference in change from baseline in YMRS total score between risperidone and haloperidol was -1.5 (95% confidence interval: -3.94, 1.03), showing a slight numerical advantage for risperidone. The results at 12 weeks also showed that risperidone continued to increase the proportion of responders, with good control of comorbid depressive symptoms in line with that observed on haloperidol. Among the 54 risperidone and 37 haloperidol responders at the end of 3 weeks who continued into the 9-week double-blind maintenance period, all but 1 risperidone patient were also responders at the 12-week endpoint.

The mean modal risperidone dose was 4.2 mg/day (Smulevich *et al.*, 2005), 5.6 mg/day (Khanna *et al.*, 2005), and 4.1 mg/day (Hirschfeld *et al.*, 2004). The mean modal dose of haloperidol was 8.0 mg/day in the (Smulevich *et al.*, 2005) study. The mean baseline body weight in the (Khanna *et al.*, 2005) study was 1.2 times (Smulevich *et al.*, 2005), and 1.6 times (Hirschfeld *et al.*, 2004) lower than in the two other studies, respectively. Patients in the (Khanna *et al.*, 2005) study had more severe manic symptoms at baseline (mean YMRS total score = 37.5 and 37.1 (placebo and risperidone, respectively), compared to 31.3–32.1 (Smulevich *et al.*, 2005), or 29.2 and 29.1 (placebo and risperidone, respectively) (Hirschfeld *et al.*, 2004). In these more severely affected manic patients, changes from baseline in both the risperidone and placebo group as well as the differentiation between risperidone and placebo were more pronounced compared to the two other monotherapy studies (Table 9.2).

9.2.2 RISPERIDONE IN COMBINATION WITH MOOD STABILIZERS IN BIPOLAR MANIA

In the (Sachs *et al.*, 2002) study, risperidone in addition to lithium or valproate was superior to lithium or valproate alone for the change in YMRS total score at Week 3 (Table 9.3). In the (Yatham *et al.*, 2003) study, risperidone combined with lithium, valproate, or carbamazepine was not significantly superior to lithium, valproate, or carbamazepine alone in the reduction of YMRS total score. However, risperidone versus placebo results in the carbamazepine subgroup qualitatively differed from results seen in

Table 9.3 Risperidone oral adjunctive therapy in bipolar disorder; change from baseline in YMRS total score by study (LOCF/Endpoint).

Study	N^a	Mean change (SD)	p value vs. plac
Sachs *et al.*, (2002)			
Placebo	50	−8.2 (10.4)	—
Risperidone	51	−14.3 (9.3)	0.0009
Haloperidol	52	−13.4 (10.0)	<0.03
Yatham *et al.*, (2003)			
All patients	73	−10.3 (11.8)	—
Placebo	69	−14.5 (12.6)	0.089
Risperidone			
Excluding carbamazepine	62	−9.8 (12.1)	—
subgroup	55	−15.2 (12.4)	0.047
Placebo			
Risperidone			

^{a}N, Number of patients with both baseline and post baseline timepoint measurements.
SD, standard deviation; YMRS, Yound Mania Rating Scale; LOCF, last observed carried forward.

the lithium and valproate subgroups. In addition, patients assigned to risperidone in the carbamazepine subgroup showed markedly lower plasma concentrations of risperidone and its metabolite 9-hydroxyrisperidone combined. Because of the evidence of a pharmacokinetic interaction between carbamazepine and risperidone, an additional analysis was performed on the primary efficacy parameter for the population of patients who had either lithium or valproate as mood stabilizer treatment. When the carbamazepine group was excluded from the analysis, there was a significant difference at the double-blind endpoint between the two treatment groups in the mean change from baseline in YMRS total score.

The mean modal dose of risperidone in these studies was 3.8 and 3.7 mg/day respectively (Sachs *et al.*, 2002; Yatham *et al.*, 2003).

In both of these studies, the 10-week open-label risperidone treatment resulted in an improvement of the remaining mania symptoms, especially in the group of patients who were treated with placebo in the double-blind treatment phase.

9.2.3 DRUG–DRUG INTERACTIONS RELEVANT FOR THE TREATMENT OF BIPOLAR DISORDERS WITH RISPERIDONE

Risperidone is extensively metabolized in the liver through hydroxylation to 9-hydroxyrisperidone by the CYP2D6 enzyme. Since 9-hydroxyrisperidone has similar pharmacological activity as risperidone, the clinical effect of the drug results from the combined concentrations of risperidone plus 9-hydroxyrisperidone (Vermeulen, Piotrovsky, and Ludwig, 2006).

Inhibitors of CYP2D6 interfere with the conversion of risperidone to 9-hydroxy-risperidone. Fluoxetine and paroxetine have been shown to increase the plasma concentration of risperidone 2-5–2-9- and 3-9-fold respectively, whereas the concentrations of 9-hydroyrisperidone were either not affected or lowered by about 13% (Bondolfi *et al.*, 2002; Spina *et al.*, 2001). The overall effect on the combined risperidone and 9-hydroxyrisperidone concentrations was in the order of magnitude of +45%. The dosing of risperidone should be re-evaluated when fluoxetine or paroxetine or other antidepressants with CYP2D6 inhibiting properties are initiated or discontinued.

Carbamazepine co-administration decreased the steady-state plasma concentrations of risperidone and 9-hydroxyrisperidone by about 50% which could lead to decreased efficacy of risperidone treatment (Vermeulen, Piotrovsky, and Ludwig, 2006). The dose of risperidone may need to be titrated up or down during initiation or discontinuation of concomitant carbamazepine therapy. Oxcarbazepine does not affect the elimination of risperidone (Muscatello *et al.*, 2005). Lamotrigine or valproate do not affect the plasma levels of risperidone and 9-hydroxyrisperidone (Spina *et al.*, 2000, 2006). Plasma concentrations of carbamazepine or lithium were not affected by repeated doses of risperidone (Demling *et al.*, 2006; Gupta *et al.*, 2006).

Similarly, risperidone did not affect the overall exposure of valproate at steady state although there was a 20% increase in valproate peak plasma concentration after concomitant administration of risperidone (Ravindran *et al.*, 2004). Risperidone does not affect the clearance of drugs that are metabolized by CYP2D6 or other liver enzymes.

9.2.4 SAFETY AND TOLERABILITY

The adverse events reported with risperidone in acute mania are largely consistent with those reported in patients with schizophrenia.

Adverse drug reactions reported by $\geq 2\%$ of risperidone treated patients with bipolar mania in double-blind placebo-controlled monotherapy and adjuvant studies are summarized in Tables 9.4 and 9.5 respectively. The overall incidence of extrapyramidal symptom (EPS)-related adverse events was somewhat higher than that reported in schizophrenia. This is consistent with clinical experience that manic patients in general may display EPS more frequently than patients treated with antipsychotics for other psychiatric disorders (Gao *et al.*, 2008a). The rate of extrapyramidal disorder in the (Khanna *et al.*, 2005) study in the risperidone group was more than double that in the other two studies (Hirschfeld *et al.*, 2004; Smulevich *et al.*, 2005), most likely because of the higher doses used while body weights were lower in this study population.

In both studies with haloperidol as the active comparator, the incidence of extrapyramidal disorder was substantially lower in the risperidone groups (17 and 13%) than in the haloperidol groups (40 and 28%) in the Hirschfeld *et al.* (2004) and Sachs *et al.* (2002) studies respectively.

Weight changes from baseline were minimal in the three-week studies and ranged on average from +0.9 to +1.4 kg across risperidone treatment groups in the 9- or 12-week treatment periods vs. +0.8 kg on haloperidol (Hirschberg *et al.*, 2006; Smulevich *et al.*, 2005). Patients treated with risperidone or haloperidol had modest elevations of serum

Table 9.4 Adverse drug reactions in ≥2% of oral risperidone-treated patients with bipolar mania in double-blind, placebo-controlled monotherapy studies[a].

Adverse reaction	Risperidone (n = 448) %	Placebo (n = 424) %
Parkinsonism[b]	25.4	8.7
Akathisia[b]	8.9	3.1
Tremor[b]	6.0	3.3
Dizziness	5.8	5.0
Sedation	5.8	1.7
Somnolence	5.4	1.9
Dystonia[b]	4.7	0.7
Nausea	4.5	1.9
Diarrhea	2.5	2.4
Salivary hypersecretion	2.5	0.5
Dyspepsia	2.0	1.7

[a]Includes RIS-USA-240, a study discontinued for business reasons after approximately 10% of the planned number of patients had enrolled.
[b]Parkinsonism includes extrapyramidal disorder, Parkinsonism, musculoskeletal stiffness, hypokinesia, muscle rigidity, muscle tightness, bradykinesia, cogwheel rigidity. Akathisia includes akathisia and restlessness. Tremor includes tremor and Parkinsonian rest tremor. Dystonia includes dystonia, muscle spasms, oculogyration, toritcollis. Dyskinesia includes muscle twitching and dyskinesia.

prolactin levels. Treatment-emergent potentially prolactin-related adverse events were rare (Smulevich *et al.*, 2005) or absent (Khanna *et al.*, 2005), however.

9.2.5 ADDITIONAL STUDIES ORAL RISPERIDONE IN BIPOLAR DISORDER

Segal, Berk, and Brook (1998) compared risperidone 6 mg/day with 10 mg/day haloperidol and 800–1200 mg/day lithium in a double-blind randomized trial in 45 subjects with bipolar mania for 28 days. Similar improvements were seen in all three groups on overall psychiatric symptoms, manic symptoms, and global assessment of functioning and clinical impression.

Perlis *et al.* (2006) compared risperidone (n = 164; 1–6 mg/day) to olanzapine (n = 165; 5–20 mg/day) in manic or mixed states of bipolar I disorder in a three-week randomized double-blind study. Mean modal doses were 3.9 mg/day risperidone and 14.7 mg/day olanzapine. There were no differences in mean change from baseline in YMRS, MADRS, or functional outcome measures, and no differences in response or remission rates. Significantly more olanzapine patients completed the study (78.9% vs. 67.0%). Olanzapine-treated patients had greater Hamilton Rating Scale for Depression (HAM-D) and CGI-BP score improvements and experienced more weight gain. More risperidone subjects had prolactin elevation and experienced sexual dysfunction, as determined by a clinician-rated assessment scale of sexual functioning. Analysis of

Table 9.5 Adverse drug reactions in ≥2% of oral risperidone-treated patients with bipolar mania in double-blind, placebo-controlled adjuvant therapy studies.

Adverse reaction	Risperidone (n = 127) %	Placebo (n = 126) %
Nasopharyngitis	2.4	3.2
Urinary tract infection	2.4	0.8
Insomnia	3.9	7.9
Anxiety	3.1	2.4
Parkinsonism[a]	14.2	4.0
Headache	14.2	15.1
Akathisia[a]	7.9	0
Dizziness	7.1	2.4
Sedation	6.3	3.2
Tremor	5.5	2.4
Somnolence	3.1	0.8
Lethargy	2.4	0.8
Palpitations	2.4	0
Pharyngolaryngeal pain	4.7	1.6
Cough	2.4	0
Dyspepsia	9.4	7.9
Nausea	6.3	4.0
Diarrhea	5.5	4.0
Dry mouth	3.9	4.0
Vomiting	3.9	5.6
Constipation	3.1	3.2
Salivary hypersecretion	2.4	0
Chest pain	2.4	0.8
Fatigue	2.4	1.6
Weight increased	2.4	1.6

[a]Parkinsonism includes extrapyramidal disorder, Parkinsonism, musculoskeletal stiffness, hypokinesia, muscle rigidity, muscle tightness, bradykinesia, cogwheel rigidity. Akathisia includes akathisia and restlessness. Tremor includes tremor and Parkinsonian rest tremor. Dystonia includes dystonia, muscle spasms, oculogyration, toritcollis. Dyskinesia includes muscle twitching and dyskinesia.

EPSs via the Simpson-Angus Scale (SAS) or Barnes Akathisia Rating Scale (BARS) did not find significant differences between the two treatments.

Long-term efficacy and safety in bipolar mania were studied in six-months open label studies, either as monotherapy (Vieta *et al.*, 2004) or adjunctive therapy (Vieta *et al.*, 2002). At a mean dose of 4.2 mg/day monotherapy in 96 acutely manic patients, risperidone produced significant reductions from baseline on all efficacy measures from week 1 (YMRS) and 4 (PANSS and CGI) onwards, for a six-month period. Risperidone did not induce depressive symptoms, as mean depression scores actually improved significantly from baseline, and exacerbation of mania was rare (4.2%). There was a significant increase from baseline in the number of subjects reporting extrapyramidal adverse events by week 4 and a significant decrease from baseline at endpoint. The average weight increase was 3.2 ± 2.1 kg. Nine patients (9.4%) had an increase of more than 7% in body weight. Eighty-three (83.3%) patients completed the study (Vieta *et al.*, 2004).

In a similar open-label study in 174 manic, hypomanic, or mixed episode subjects, risperidone, at a mean dose of 4.9 mg/day as adjunctive therapy to treatment as usual reduced YMRS, PANSS and HAM-D scores, and CGI ratings at endpoint. Risperidone was generally well tolerated with no significant increments in the severity of EPSs (Vieta *et al.*, 2002).

9.3 PALIPERIDONE EXTENDED RELEASE (ER) IN BIPOLAR MANIA

The clinical development program of paliperidone ER in acute mania evaluated its efficacy and safety in the treatment of subjects with acute manic or mixed episodes associated with Bipolar I Disorder. The clinical program in acute mania consisted of three Phase 3 clinical studies (Table 9.6).

The subjects enrolled in the studies were acutely symptomatic based on clinical diagnosis and YMRS total scores, and had a significant psychiatric history. Mean baseline YMRS total scores ranged from 26.7 to 28.4 across studies. Approximately two-thirds of the subjects in each of the studies had a DSM-IV diagnosis of Bipolar I Disorder, most recent episode manic; for the remaining one-third, the most recent episode was mixed.

9.3.1 FIXED-DOSE MONOTHERAPY STUDY

In this study, the assigned doses of paliperidone ER (3, 6, or 12 mg) remained fixed throughout the three week, double-blind treatment period. From baseline to endpoint (last observed carried forward, LOCF), median and mean YMRS total score decreased in all treatment groups (Table 9.7), indicating improvement in the severity of manic symptoms. This improvement was dose-related in the paliperidone ER groups. Based on LOCF analysis with the Dunnett-Bonferroni-based parallel gatekeeping procedure to control for multiplicity, the improvement in the paliperidone ER 12-mg group (mean (SD): -13.9 (9.19)) reached statistical significance (p $= 0.005$) compared with the placebo group (-9.9 (10.22)). The 3 and 6 mg groups were not statistically significantly different from placebo. The unusually large treatment effect in subjects assigned to placebo may have contributed to the lack of statistically significant separation between the 6-mg dose group and placebo group (Berwaerts *et al.*, in press).

Onset of effect was determined based on the earliest occurrence of a statistically significant difference in the change from baseline in YMRS total score relative to placebo that was maintained at all subsequent time points. Onset of effect was observed as early as day 2 for paliperidone ER 12 mg. Response was defined a priori as a reduction from baseline of at least 50% in YMRS total score. Remission represents a reduction in mania symptoms to near-normal levels, and is therefore a clinically important outcome. Remission was defined as YMRS total score of 12 or less at endpoint. Dose-related increases in the percentage of both responders and remitters were observed (38.4–53.5% for rates of response and 36.6–44.7% for rates of remission across paliperidone ER dose

Table 9.6 Clinical studies with paliperidone ER in acute mania.

Study	Design	Sample[a]	Dose	Primary outcome	Results	Secondary outcome measures
Monotherapy studies						
Berwaerts et al., (in press)	Double-blind, 3 wk vs. placebo, three fixed doses of paliperidone	n = 121 Plac n = 112 Pal 3 mg n = 119 Pal 6 mg n = 115 Pal 12 mg	Fixed: 3, 6, or 12 mg Pal	YMRS	Pal 12 mg significantly better than placebo Pal 3 and 6 mg not significantly different from placebo Change in YMRS total score increases with Pal dose	YMRS responder rate GAF CGI-BP-S PANSS MADRS
Vieta et al., (2010)	Double-blind 3 wk vs. placebo, 12 wk vs. quetiapine	n = 105 Plac n = 194 Pal n = 192 Que	Flexible 3–12 mg Pal 400–800 mg Que	YMRS	Pal significantly better than placebo at 3 wk Pal non-inferior to Que at 12 wk	YMRS responder rate GAF CGI-BP-S PANSS MADRS
Adjunctive therapy study						
Berwaerts et al., (in press)	Double-blind vs. placebo, 6 wk in combination with lithium or valproate	n = 150 Plac n = 149 Pal	Flexible 3–12 mg Pal	YMRS	Pal not significantly different from placebo	YMRS responder rate GAF CGI-BP-S PANSS MADRS

[a]Includes all subjects who were evaluable for safety.
YMRS, Young Mania Rating Scale; GAF, Global assessment Scale; CGI-BP-S, Clinical Global Impression for Bipolar Disorder-Severity; PANSS, Positive and Negative Syndrome Scale; MADRS, Montgomery Asberg Depression Rating Scale.

Table 9.7 Paliperidone ER in acute mania; change from baseline in YMRS total score (week 3 LOCF/endpoint).

| Study | N^a | Mean change (SD) | Comparison with placebo | |
			Diff in LS mean change (95% CI)	p value
Berwaerts *et al.*, (in press)				
Placebo	121	−9.9 (10.22)	—	—
Paliperidone ER 3 mg	112	−9.6 (11.30)	0.3 (−2.24, 2.82)	0.992
Paliperidone ER 6 mg	118	−11.7 (10.04)	−1.9 (−4.43, 0.58)	0.302
Paliperidone ER 12 mg	114	−13.9 (9.19)	−4.0 (−6.56, −1.52)	0.005
Vieta *et al.*, (2010)				
Placebo	104	−7.4 (10.74)	—	—
Paliperidone ER	190	−13.2 (8.68)	−5.5 (−7.57, −3.35)	<0.001
Quetiapine	192	−11.7 (9.28)	−4.2 (−6.45, −1.95)	<0.001
Berwaerts *et al.*, (in press)				
Placebo	150	−13.2 (10.91)	—	—
Paliperidone ER	149	−14.3 (10.01)	−1.36 (−3.27, 0.54)	0.160

[a] Includes subjects who were evaluable for efficacy (intent-to-treat analysis set).
CI, confidence interval; LOCF, last observation carried forward; LS, least squares; SD, standard deviation; YMRS. Young Mania Rating Scale.

groups). None of the differences between paliperidone ER and placebo (rate of response, 42.1%; rate of remission, 37.2%) reached statistical significance.

9.3.2 FLEXIBLE-DOSE MONOTHERAPY STUDY

During the initial, three-week acute treatment phase, the median mode doses of paliperidone ER and quetiapine were 9 and 600 mg, respectively. Over the 12-week period, the median mode dose of paliperidone ER was 6 mg in the placebo/paliperidone ER group, and 9 mg in the paliperidone ER/paliperidone ER group. The median mode dose of quetiapine was 600 mg during the combined acute and maintenance phases of the study (Vieta *et al.*, 2010).

From baseline to three-week endpoint (LOCF), median and mean YMRS total score decreased in all treatment groups (Table 9.7), indicating improvement in the severity of manic symptoms. Based on LOCF analysis of the primary efficacy variable, paliperidone ER was statistically superior to the placebo group (−13.2 (8.68) vs. −7.4 (10.74); p<0.001).

Onset of effect was observed as early as day 2 for paliperidone ER. In the acute phase of this flexible-dose study, the percentage of responders was 55.8% for paliperidone ER, 34.6% for placebo, and 49% for quetiapine. The corresponding percentage of remitters was 52.1, 28.8, and 47.4%, respectively. Paliperidone ER was statistically superior to placebo with respect to the percentage of both responders and remitters (p < 0.001). The mean change (SD) in YMRS total score from baseline to the 12-week endpoint (LOCF) was −15.2 (10.26) in the paliperidone ER group and −13.5 (11.02) in the quetiapine group. Non-inferiority of paliperidone ER to quetiapine was demonstrated based on the difference in least squares (LS) means between treatments for the change from baseline in YMRS total score. The point estimate was 1.7 (95% of −0.47, 3.96) for the per-protocol analysis set. The lower limit of the 95% confidence interval (CI) was greater than the prespecified non-inferiority margin of −4.

9.3.3 ADJUNCTIVE THERAPY STUDY

During the six-week double-blind period, the median mode dose of paliperidone ER was 6 mg, that is, lower than the median dose for the 3- and 12-week treatment periods in the paliperidone ER/paliperidone ER group in the flexible-dose monotherapy study (Berwaerts et al., in press).

The change from baseline to endpoint in YMRS total score was −13.2 (10.91) for the placebo group and −14.3 (10.01) for the paliperidone ER group (Table 9.7). Based on the intent-to-treat LOCF analysis, the difference was not statistically significant (p = 0.160). The type of mood stabilizer used (lithium or valproate) did not differentially affect the change from baseline to endpoint in YMRS total score across treatment groups. There were no statistically significant differences between paliperidone ER and placebo with regard to the rate of response or remission.

In each of the three Phase 3 studies that evaluated the efficacy and safety of paliperidone ER for the treatment of acute mania, the consistency of the treatment effect of paliperidone ER versus placebo with regard to the primary efficacy variable was analyzed in subgroups defined by demographic characteristics and baseline disease characteristics. In a subgroup analysis by region, paliperidone ER appeared more effective than placebo in subjects enrolled at sites in Asia, Eastern Europe, and other regions. Paliperidone ER did not appear to be more effective than placebo in subjects enrolled at sites in North America (71 and 54% of subjects enrolled in the fixed-dose and flexible-dose monotherapy studies, respectively). Exploratory analyses did not reveal any additional factors that may have contributed to the observed interaction.

9.3.4 DRUG–DRUG INTERACTIONS RELEVANT FOR BIPOLAR DISORDER

Paliperidone is not expected to cause clinically important pharmacokinetic interactions with drugs that are metabolized by cytochrome P450 isozymes. *In vitro* studies in human liver microsomes showed that paliperidone does not substantially inhibit the metabolism of drugs metabolized by cytochrome P450 isozymes, including CYP1A2, CYP2A6, CYP2C8/9/10, CYP2D6, CYP2E1, CYP3A4, and CYP3A5 (INVEGA® United States Prescribing Information, 2010). Therefore, paliperidone is not expected to inhibit clearance of drugs that are metabolized by these metabolic pathways in a clinically relevant manner. Paliperidone is also not expected to have enzyme inducing properties.

Paliperidone is not a substrate of CYP1A2, CYP2A6, CYP2C9, and CYP2C19 (INVEGA® United States Prescribing Information, 2010), so that an interaction with inhibitors or inducers of these isozymes is unlikely. While *in vitro* studies indicate that CYP2D6 and CYP3A4 may be minimally involved in paliperidone metabolism, *in vivo* studies show that these isozymes only contribute to a small fraction of total body clearance (INVEGA® United States Prescribing Information, 2010).

A randomized, crossover study evaluated the effects of the potent CYP2D6 inhibitor, paroxetine, on the pharmacokinetics of a single dose of paliperidone ER in healthy subjects (Berwaerts *et al.*, 2009). The mean maximum plasma concentration (Cmax) and area under the curve (AUC) of paliperidone were slightly higher and paliperidone clearance was slightly lower following coadministration of a single dose of paliperidone ER (3 mg) with paroxetine (20 mg/day for consecutive 13 days). The ratio of geometric treatment means for AUC_∞ was 116.48 [90% CI: 104.49–129.84]. These results suggest that there is no clinically relevant pharmacokinetic interaction when paroxetine and paliperidone ER are coadministered and, therefore, initiation or discontinuation of concomitant treatment with CYP2D6-inhibiting drugs does not appear to warrant an adjustment in paliperidone ER dosage. Hence, paliperidone ER may offer a valuable alternative to other atypical antipsychotics in patients with bipolar disorder who are at particular risk of metabolic drug-drug interactions while they receive treatment with SSRIs, which are often potent CYP2D6 inhibitors.

No effect of lithium on paliperidone pharmacokinetics is expected when lithium and paliperidone ER are coadministered. Observations by Demling *et al.* (2006) indicated that plasma concentrations of risperidone, 9-hydroxyrisperidone (paliperidone), and the active moiety (risperidone plus 9-hydroxyrisperidone) in the presence of lithium were comparable to those reported when risperidone was administered alone. These data are supportive for the absence of an effect on the pharmacokinetics of paliperidone. Likewise, no effect of paliperidone on lithium pharmacokinetics is expected, as repeated oral doses of risperidone (3 mg twice daily) did not affect the AUC or Cmax of lithium (Demling *et al.*, 2006).

Coadministration of paliperidone ER 6 mg once daily with carbamazepine 200 mg twice daily caused a decrease of approximately 37% in the mean steady-state Cmax and AUC of paliperidone (INVEGA® United States Prescribing Information, 2010). This decrease is caused, to a substantial degree, by a 35% increase in renal clearance of paliperidone. A minor decrease in the amount of drug excreted unchanged in the urine suggests that there was little effect on the CYP metabolism or bioavailability of paliperidone during carbamazepine coadministration. On initiation of carbamazepine, the dose of paliperidone ER should be reevaluated and increased if necessary. Conversely, on discontinuation of carbamazepine, the dose of paliperidone ER should be reevaluated and decreased if necessary. No effect of paliperidone on carbamazepine pharmacokinetics is expected (INVEGA® United States Prescribing Information, 2010).

In an open-label, two-treatment, single-sequence drug-drug interaction study in healthy subjects, coadministration of a single dose of paliperidone ER 12 mg with divalproex sodium extended-release tablets (two 500 mg tablets once daily) resulted in an increase of approximately 50% in the Cmax and AUC of paliperidone (INVEGA® United States Prescribing Information, 2010). Dosage reduction for paliperidone ER should be considered after clinical assessment when paliperidone ER is coadministered with valproate.

In the adjunctive therapy study (Berwaerts *et al.*, in press), scheduled pharmacokinetic blood samples for paliperidone were taken for all subjects in the combination treatment and mood stabilizer only groups. The median dose-normalized paliperidone plasma concentrations on day 6 were similar between subjects who received valproate and those who received lithium in combination with paliperidone ER, suggesting that valproate and lithium have a similar effect on paliperidone plasma concentrations in subjects with bipolar I disorder. Subjects on a stable dose of valproate showed comparable valproate average plasma concentrations when paliperidone ER (3–15 mg/day) was added to their existing valproate treatment (INVEGA® United States Prescribing Information, 2010).

9.3.5 SAFETY AND TOLERABILITY

Paliperidone ER, administered in daily doses ranging from 3 to 12 mg, either as monotherapy or as adjunctive therapy to the mood stabilizers lithium or valproate, was generally well tolerated for a period of 3–12 weeks. The types and incidences of adverse events observed in adult subjects with acute mania were consistent with those reported in the six-week, placebo-controlled Phase 3 studies of paliperidone ER in the treatment of schizophrenia (Meltzer *et al.*, 2008). There was no evidence of a new safety signal compared to the adverse event profile of paliperidone ER in subjects with schizophrenia.

In all studies, adverse events occurred in a higher percentage of subjects administered paliperidone ER than placebo. The difference was more pronounced in the adjunctive therapy study (69.8% vs. 54.0%) (Berwaerts *et al.*, in press), than in the fixed-dose (74.3% across paliperidone ER dose groups vs. 70.2%) (Berwaerts *et al.*, in press) and flexible-dose monotherapy studies (65.5% vs. 62.9) (Vieta *et al.*, 2010).

In the fixed-dose monotherapy study (Berwaerts *et al.*, in press), most of the frequently reported adverse events showed no apparent dose relationship among paliperidone ER treatment groups. The treatment-emergent adverse events that occurred with a higher incidence (that is, a difference of at least 3%) in at least one of the paliperidone ER dose groups than in the placebo group were headache, somnolence, dizziness, sedation, akathisia, hypertonia, dystonia, nausea, and dyspepsia. Akathisia and extrapyramidal disorder occurred at higher rates in the paliperidone ER 12 mg group compared to lower dose paliperidone ER groups.

In the flexible-dose monotherapy study, the overall incidence of adverse events was higher in the quetiapine-treated subjects than in paliperidone ER-treated subjects both during the acute phase (76.6% vs. 65.5%) and during combined 12-week treatment (81.8% vs. 70.1%). During the three-week acute treatment phase, common treatment-emergent adverse events (that is, events that occurred in at least 5% of subjects in any treatment group) that occurred with a higher incidence (that is, a difference of at least 3%) in the paliperidone ER group compared to placebo included somnolence, akathisia, constipation, and dyspepsia. Of the common treatment-emergent adverse events, akathisia, drooling, and depression occurred at higher rates in the paliperidone ER group compared to the quetiapine group during the full 12 weeks of treatment. Common treatment-emergent adverse events that occurred more frequently in subjects who received quetiapine than those who received paliperidone ER over the 12-week period included somnolence, sedation, dizziness, lethargy, dry mouth, and weight increased.

In the adjunctive therapy study, adverse events occurred in a higher percentage of subjects administered paliperidone ER vs. placebo (69.8% vs. 54.0%). Subjects who used lithium or valproate as the background mood stabilizer differentially reported adverse events consistent with the respective safety profiles of these drugs (for example, weight gain and increased appetite for valproate, extrapyramidal disorder for lithium). The proportion of subjects who reported at least one adverse event was higher in the subgroup of subjects treated with valproate, as opposed to lithium.

Across all studies, EPS-related adverse events were reported at a higher rate in subjects treated with paliperidone ER compared to placebo or quetiapine. Individual adverse events reported at a higher rate (that is, difference of $\geq 3\%$) in paliperidone ER-treated subjects compared to placebo included extrapyramidal disorder, hypertonia, drooling, akathisia, dystonia, and muscle spasms in the monotherapy studies and extrapyramidal disorder and akathisia in the adjunctive therapy study. The incidences of extrapyramidal disorder, akathisia, dystonia, and dyskinesia were higher in the paliperidone ER 12-mg group than in the lower dose groups (3- or 6-mg) in the fixed-dose monotherapy study.

Across all studies, a total of 15 paliperidone ER-treated subjects experienced potentially prolactin-related adverse events. Most of these subjects had confirmed prolactin elevations above the upper limit of the normal range. These events did not show a dose-related pattern in the fixed-dose monotherapy study. None of the potentially prolactin-related adverse events was severe, serious, or resulted in discontinuation of study treatment.

Based on baseline body mass index (BMI) values, over one-half of the subjects in the Phase 3 studies were overweight ($25 - <30$ kg/m^2) or obese (≥ 30 kg/m^2) at study entry. Across studies, body weight showed mean increases from baseline in all treatment groups. No dose-related trend was apparent in the fixed-dose monotherapy study (mean percent increase in body weight, 1.3–1.5% across paliperidone ER groups vs. 0.2% for placebo). Over the course of 12-week flexible-dose monotherapy trial, quetiapine had a more pronounced adverse effect on body weight than paliperidone ER with regard to the mean percent weight increase (quetiapine, 2.5% vs. paliperidone ER, 1.9%), the proportion of subjects with body weight increases of $\geq 7\%$ (quetiapine, 17% vs. paliperidone ER, 8%) and the incidences of adverse events of weight increase and increased appetite. Higher mean percent increases in body weight compared to monotherapy studies were observed in the adjunctive study, both for the paliperidone ER group (2.4%) and for the placebo group (1.0%), suggesting an additive effect of the background therapy with mood stabilizers over the six-week, double-blind treatment period.

9.4 RISPERIDONE LONG-ACTING INJECTABLE (LAI) IN THE MAINTENANCE TREATMENT OF BIPOLAR DISORDER

Bipolar disorder is characterized in the vast majority of cases by recurrent episodes of manic and/or depressive episodes. Hence, in addition to safe and effective treatment of the acute episodes, there is a clear need for long-term treatments to prevent or delay the onset of these recurrent mood episodes. Several mood stabilizer and antipsychotic compounds have shown efficacy in such maintenance treatment of bipolar disorder.

One of the well-documented factors contributing to frequent relapse of mood episodes in these patients is poor treatment adherence. The median non-adherence rate to long-term maintenance treatment in bipolar disorder is 41%, with a range of 20–60% across studies (Lingam and Scott, 2002). Nearly half of the bipolar patients were found to be partially or completely nonadherent to their prescribed oral antipsychotic treatment (Sajatovic *et al.*, 2006). A review of six randomized controlled trials reported that subjects who discontinued lithium had a 28-fold increased risk of relapses compared with subjects who were maintained on medication (Suppes *et al.*, 1991). Keck *et al.* (1996) reported that 64% of subjects hospitalized for treatment of a manic episode were nonadherent with prescribed pharmacotherapy in the month prior to admission. Among patients who were previously hospitalized for treatment of bipolar disorder, those who were adherent to their antipsychotic medication at least 75% of the time had lower risks of all-cause and mental-health-related hospitalization (Hassan and Lage, 2009).

One treatment modality that aims to address the problem of adherence is the LAI or "depot" medication. The most commonly cited advantages for LAI treatment are adherence and more rapid detection of nonadherence (Vasile *et al.*, 2006; El-Mallakh, 2007). Another potential advantage of LAI treatment is a steadier release of medication into the systemic circulation, resulting in more constant plasma concentrations of the drug. Fluctuations in plasma levels of risperidone and 9-hydroxyrisperidone combined were 32–42% lower with the intramuscular than oral immediate-release formulation of risperidone (Eerdekens *et al.*, 2004). Few studies are available on first-generation antipsychotic LAI formulations in bipolar disorder (Bond, Pratoomsri, and Yatham, 2007). Risperidone LAI is an aqueous suspension containing risperidone in a copolymer matrix. Gradual copolymer hydrolysis at the injection site ensures slow and steady risperidone release over a period of several weeks enabling continuous treatment with stable plasma risperidone concentrations. After a single intramuscular (IM) injection, the release profile consists of a small initial release of drug (<1% of the dose), followed by a lag time of approximately three weeks. The mean release of drug starts from week 3 onwards, is maintained from four to six weeks, and subsides by week 7. Risperidone LAI can be administered in either the gluteal or deltoid muscle. Studies in patients with schizophrenia have demonstrated that risperidone LAI is associated with clinically significant efficacy and is generally safe and well tolerated during long-term use (Kane *et al.*, 2003; Fleischhacker *et al.*, 2003).

9.4.1 RISPERIDONE LAI STUDIES

Three long-term, placebo-controlled studies have been performed with risperidone LAI in bipolar disorder patients to evaluate its efficacy and safety for the prevention of mood episodes, administered as monotherapy (Quiroz *et al.*, 2010; Montgomery *et al.*, 2010) or as adjunctive therapy to treatment as usual in patients with bipolar disorder who relapse frequently (Bipolar I cohort, that is, 124 patients of 139 randomized patients; Macfadden *et al.*, 2009). The design of these studies is summarized in Table 9.8. Randomization and recurrence criteria as used in these studies are described in Table 9.9.

Patients who entered the study published by Quiroz *et al.* (2010) were either currently experiencing a manic or mixed episode or were between mood episodes and stabilized on either oral risperidone or another antipsychotic agent. Subjects must have had at least two bipolar mood episodes, exclusive of the current episode if applicable, during the last two years. Similar patients were recruited in the study of Montgomery *et al.* (2010) except that two bipolar mood episodes were required over the last year. The latter study had olanzapine as active comparator during the double-blind maintenance period. Both studies were designed to evaluate the safety and efficacy of risperidone LAI as monotherapy for its capacity to delay the occurrence of any mood episodes (that is, elevated as well as depressive) in patients who had previously shown a maintained response to risperidone long-term treatment on the basis of various pre-specified criteria (Table 9.9) during a 26- or 12-week, open-label treatment period, respectively. For subjects who had an acute episode at study entry and who were randomized to double-blind treatment, most had a history of their most recent episode being manic (80 and 92%) with a much smaller number of subjects having their most recent episode mixed (20 and 8%) in the Quiroz *et al.* (2010) and Montgomery *et al.* (2010) study, respectively.

The Macfadden *et al.* (2009) study evaluated risperidone LAI as adjunctive therapy to treatment as usual. Patients were diagnosed as having either bipolar I or II disorder (Bipolar II patient cohort not covered in publication) and had to have at least four mood episodes during the 12 months prior to enrollment requiring psychiatric intervention, two of which occurred in the 6 months prior to enrollment. Subjects could be enrolled during any phase of the illness, including depressive episodes, irrespective of their ongoing therapy.

The primary efficacy variable in all three studies was the time to recurrence of a mood episode in the double-blind period, from the first injection of double-blind treatment in the maintenance period to the date of termination for subjects whose reason for discontinuation was recurrence (see Table 9.9 for recurrence criteria). All other randomized subjects were considered censored for time to relapse on the date of termination of the double-blind period.

In the study of Montgomery *et al.* (2010), the primary pre-specified analysis carried out by log-rank test stratified by patient type at screening and region showed a qualitative interaction between stratification factors, suggesting that the pre-specified statistical method was not the most appropriate approach. Visual inspection of Kaplan-Meier curves revealed qualitative differences for time to recurrence for acute and nonacute patients across different regions. Hence, a post-hoc adjusted log-rank test stratified by region only was carried out. Additional analyses of time to recurrence of a mood episode were conducted for either type of episode (that is, elevated or depressive). Change in YMRS, MADRS, and Clinical Global Impression for Bipolar Disorder-Severity (CGI-BP-S) scores from the relevant baselines during open-label and double-blind treatment was evaluated.

Across the three studies, risperidone LAI was effective as monotherapy and adjunctive therapy in delaying the recurrence of any mood episode in subjects with bipolar disorder,

Table 9.8 Controlled studies with risperidone long-acting injectable (LAI) in the prevention of mood episodes in bipolar I disorder.

Study	Design	Sample	Dose	Primary outcome measures	Results	Secondary outcome measures
Quiroz et al., (2010)	26 wk open-label Ris LAI, 24 mo double-blind, placebo-controlled for patients showing maintained response during OL phase (monotherapy)	n = 501 OL n = 154 DB Ris LAI n = 149 DB plac	Flexible 25–50 mg Ris LAI every 2 wk (OL). DB; fixed dose Ris LAI as at OL endpoint	Time to any mood episode during DB period	Time to any episode Ris LAI significantly longer than placebo	Time to depression/ manic epidose. YMRS MADRS CGI-S
Montgomery et al., (2010)	12 wk open label Ris LAI, 18 mo double-blind, placebo/active controlled.for patients showing response during OL phase (monotherapy)	n = 585 OL n = 137 DB Ris LAI n = 140 DB plac. n = 138 DB Olanz	Flexible 25–50 mg Ris LAI every 2 wk (OL). DB; fixed dose Ris LAI as at OL endpoint 10 mg/d oral olanz	Time to any mood episode during DB period	No significant delay of time to firstrecurrence of any mood episode Ris LAI vs. plac. Time to recurrence of any mood episode significantly longer Ris LAI vs. placebo (adjusted analysis)	Time to depression/ manic episode Time to SF-36 decline YMRS MADRS CGI-S PSP

| Macfadden et al., (2009)[a] | 16 wk open label Ris LAI, 52 wk double-blind, placebo-controlled for patients showing remission during OL phase. Adjunctive to therapy as usual in bipolar I patients who relapse frequently | n = 240 OL n = 59 Ris LAI n = 65 plac | Flexible 25–50 mg Ris LAI every 2 wk | Time to relapse | Time to relapse Ris LAI significantly longer than placebo | YMRS MADRS CGI-BP-S CGI-BP-C GAF SDS |

[a]Not including 35 (OL), 13 (Ris LAI), and 2 (plac) bipolar II patients.

OL, Open-label; DB, Double-blind; YMRS, Young Mania Rating Scale; BPRS, Brief Psychiatric Rating Scale; GAF, Global Assessment of Function Scale; MADRS, Montgomery Asberg Depression Rating Scale; PANSS, Positive and Negative Syndrome Scale; CGI-S,Clinical Global Impression Scale of Severity; CGI-C, Clinical Global Impression Scale of Change; HAM-D, Hammilton Rating Scale for Depression; CGI-BP-S/C, Clinical Global Impression for Bipolar Disorder-Severity/-Change; PSP, Personal and Social Performance Scale; SDS, Sheeham Disability Scale; SF-36, Short Form 36 Health Survey.

Table 9.9 Risperidone LAI in the prevention of mood episodes in bipolar I disorder: randomization and recurrence criteria.

Study	End open-label phase – randomization criteria	Double-blind phase – recurrence criteria
Quiroz et al., (2010)	Maintained response for the 26 wk of open-label treatment with risperidone LAI, that is, The subject does not meet DSM-IV-TR criteria for a manic, hypomanic, mixed, or depressive episode. No need for treatment intervention with any mood stabilizer, antipsychotic medication (other than study drug), benzodiazepine (beyond the dosage allowed), or antidepressant medication. The subject did not require hospitalization for any bipolar mood episode. The subject has a YMRS total score ≤ 15, a MADRS score ≤ 15, and a CGI-S score ≤ 5	Any of the following Fulfilled DSM-IV-TR criteria for a manic, hypomanic, mixed, or depressive episode; Required treatment intervention with any mood stabilizer, antipsychotic medication (other than study drug), benzodiazepine (beyond the dosage allowed), or antidepressant medication; Hospitalization for any bipolar mood episode; Had YMRS total score > 12, MADRS score > 12, or CGI-S scale score > 4 at any visit; or Needed an increase in risperidone LAI dosage or supplementation with oral risperidone
Montgomery et al., (2010)	Subjects who maintain efficacy during the 12-wk open-label risperidone LAI stabilization period, that is, The subject does not meet DSM-IV-TR criteria for a hypomanic, manic, mixed, or depressive episode. No need for treatment intervention with any mood stabilizer, antipsychotic medication (other than study drug), benzodiazepine (beyond the dosage allowed), or antidepressant medication. The subject did not require hospitalization for any bipolar mood episode. The subject has a YMRS total score ≤ 12 or MADRS score ≤ 12 and/or CGI-S score < 4	Any one of the following: The subject met DSM-IV-TR criteria for a hypomanic, manic, mixed, or depressive episode. The subject needed treatment intervention with any mood stabilizer, antipsychotic medication (other than study medication), benzodiazepine (beyond the dose allowed) or antidepressant medication. The subject required hospitalization for any bipolar mood episode. The subject either had YMRS >12 in combination with CGI-S ≥ 4 or MADRS > 12 in combination with CGI-S ≥4. Dosage increase or supplementation with oral risperidone or other antipsychotic or mood stabilizer, is needed in the opinion of the investigator.

| Macfadden et al., (2009) | Met all of the following criteria for at least the last 4 wk before randomization:

Absence of full DSM-IV-TR criteria for active mood disorder;

  No crisis intervention (e.g., hospitalization)
  YMRS ≤ 10, and CGI-BP-S ≤ 3
  Stable risperidone LAI dose
  Stable TAU medications and doses | For the primary analysis, relapse was determined by an independent relapse monitoring board. The investigator considered a patient to have relapsed if the patient met DSM-IV-TR criteria for an acute mood episode in the setting of adequate compliance with oral treatment-as-usual. Additionally, at least one of the following three conditions was satisfied:

  Clinical worsening, with the addition of a new mood stabilizer, antidepressant, or antipsychotic or a >20% dose increase of existing oral TAU medication, and meeting the following criteria:

  YMRS total score > 15 or MADRS score > 15 and
  CGI-BP-S score ≥ 4 or CGI-BP-C score ≥ 6 or GAF score decreased by >10 points from baseline;
  Hospitalization for worsening of manic or depressive symptoms and meeting the following criteria:
  YMRS total score > 15 or MADRS score > 15 and
  CGI-BP-S score ≥ 4 or CGI-BP-C score ≥ 6 or GAF score decreased by >10 points from baseline;
  Hospitalization for worsening of manic or depressive symptoms and having significant suicidal ideation; for example, InterSePT Scale for Suicidal Thinking revised score > 7. |

YMRS, Young Mania Rating Sale; MADRS, Montgomery Åsberg Depression Raging Scale; CGI-S, Clinical Global Impression Scale of Severity; CGI-BP-S/C, Clinical Global Impression for Bipolar Disorder-Severity/-Change; TAU, Treatment-as-usual.

and maintaining the clinical improvement achieved during an initial open-label stabilization period.

In both monotherapy studies (Quiroz *et al.*, 2010; Montgomery *et al.*, 2010), time to recurrence of any mood episode during double-blind treatment was significantly delayed with risperidone LAI compared with placebo (Table 9.10). Subjects in the placebo group were twice as likely to experience a recurrence than subjects in the risperidone LAI group. The estimated hazard ratios (95% CI) were 0.40 (0.27, 0.59) and 0.67 (0.47, 0.96) for comparison of risperidone LAI to placebo. Most subjects who experienced a recurrence had more severe symptomatology than the minimum required by the symptom severity criteria for recurrence.

Risperidone LAI as adjunctive therapy to treatment as usual showed a significant delay in time to recurrence of any mood episode compared with treatment as usual alone (Table 9.10). Subjects in the placebo group were twice as likely to experience a recurrence than subjects in the risperidone LAI group with an estimated hazard ratio for risperidone to placebo of 0.439 (0.233, 0.826). Results in the bipolar I and II population combined were very similar to the bipolar I patient cohort published by Macfadden *et al.* (2009). The changes in YMRS and MADRS scores for subjects considered to have a clinically meaningful recurrence by the blinded, independent Recurrence Monitoring Board generally had more severe symptomatology than the minimum required by the symptom severity criterion (>15 for both scales).

In both monotherapy studies, any recurrence that occurred during double-blind treatment was classified as an elevated mood episode (manic, hypomanic, or mixed) or a depressive mood episode based on the subject's presentation at the time of the event (Table 9.10). The percentage of subjects with an elevated mood episode in the risperidone LAI group was approximately half of that in the placebo group (Quiroz *et al.*, 2010), and approximately a third of that in the placebo group (Montgomery *et al.*, 2010), during the double-blind period. Most of the elevated mood episodes were manic in the risperidone LAI and placebo groups in both studies. These data demonstrate unequivocally that risperidone LAI is effective in delaying time to recurrence of elevated mood episodes. In the Montgomery *et al.* (2010) study, the percentage of subjects with a depressive episode in the risperidone LAI group was similar to that in the placebo group (19 and 17%, respectively). In the Quiroz *et al.* (2010) study, there was a slightly higher percentage of subjects who experienced a depressive episode in the risperidone LAI group (14%) than in the placebo group (10%). In the adjunctive therapy study, more subjects in the placebo group (21%) experienced a depressive recurrence than in the risperidone LAI group (12%). In many of the subjects with depressive recurrences, their prior bipolar history was notable for a higher number of past depressive episodes than manic episodes. Based on bipolar disorder history, the monotherapy study included subjects with, on average, more prior manic episodes than prior depressive episodes, while the adjunctive therapy study also included subjects with depressive episodes at screening.

The Montgomery *et al.* (2010) study included olanzapine as an active control. In the olanzapine group 32 (23%) subjects experienced a recurrence of a mood episode. The percentage of subjects with elevated mood episodes was similar in both active groups whereas the percentage of subjects with a depressive episode in the risperidone long-acting LAI group was 18.5% versus 9% in the olanzapine group.

Table 9.10 Summary of recurrence percentages for all mood episodes and individual type of episode during double-blind treatment in risperidone LAI maintenance of efficacy studies.

Study	Quiroz et al., (2010)		Montgomery et al., (2010)			Macfadden et al., (2009)[a]	
Treatment group	Ris LAI	Plac	Ris LAI	Plac	Ola	Ris LAI	Plac
No. of patients	140	135	135	138	137	72	67
25% quantile, days (95% CI)	173 (113; 435)	82 (71; 112)	98 (50; 192)	97 (66; 126)	459 (275;–)	ND (129;–)	134 (77; 207)
Median days (95% CI)	ND (–;–)	219 (170; 271)	ND (323;–)	206 (171; 354)	ND (–;–)	ND (–;–)	305 (207;–)
p-value vs.placebo	<0.001	—	0.032	—	<0.001	0.004	—
Mood episodes (%)	42 (30)	76 (56)	52 (39)	77 (56)	32 (23)	16 (22)	32 (48)
Elevated mood	22 (16)	62 (46)	27 (20)	54 (39)	20 (15)	7 (10)	18 (27)
(Hypo) manic	20 (14)	53 (39)	19 (13)	47 (34)		5 (7)	14 (21)
Mixed	2 (1)	9 (7)	8 (6)	7 (5)		2 (3)	4 (6)
Depressive mood	20 (14)	14 (10)	25 (18.5)	23 (17)	12 (9)	9 (12.5)	14 (21)

[a]Figures include patients with bipolar II disorder (n = 15).
ND, not defined as the percentile had not been reached.

The results of the secondary efficacy endpoints during double-blind treatment in all three studies support the effectiveness of risperidone LAI in maintaining the clinical improvement achieved during an initial open-label stabilization period in subjects with bipolar disorder.

Except for patients already stable on risperidone LAI who continued to receive the same dose when entering the open-label phase, patients began treatment with 25 mg risperidone LAI on day 1 and every two weeks thereafter with appropriate open-label oral risperidone supplementation for the first three weeks until release of risperidone from the microspheres occurred. Dose titration in 12.5 mg increments was allowed at four-week intervals up to a maximum of 50 mg every two weeks. Oral supplementation after the first three weeks was allowed only in conjunction with a dose increase. No dose adjustment was allowed during the last eight weeks (four weeks in Macfadden et al., 2009) of the open label stabilization phases. Treatment with risperidone LAI at this dose was continued or switched to placebo in the subsequent double-blind phase without allowance for dose changes. The majority of subjects in all three studies received a mode dose of 25 mg risperidone LAI every two weeks both during the open-label stabilization period (66–86% of patients) and the double-blind recurrence prevention phase (66–77%). In 10–31% (open-label) and 18–31% (double-blind) of patients, the mode dose was 37.5 mg whereas few patients (2–7%) were treated with the maximum dose of 50 mg every two weeks.

9.4.2 SAFETY AND TOLERABILITY

In the two monotherapy studies combined, the most commonly reported adverse events during open-label treatment were insomnia (14%) and headache (6%). Agitation, anxiety, depression, akathisia, and weight increase were all reported in 5% of subjects during the open-label risperidone LAI period. Few patients (2%) discontinued this open-label phase due to adverse events or death. Only insomnia, weight increase, and fatigue were reasons for discontinuation in more than one subject and occurred in two subjects each. In the double-blind periods, the overall incidence of adverse events was higher in the risperidone LAI treated subjects than in the subjects treated with placebo, predominantly due to the higher incidence of weight increase. The incidence of mania, bipolar I disorder, and agitation was higher in the placebo group while depression was slightly higher in the risperidone treated group. The overall incidence of adverse events was higher in subjects treated with olanzapine than those treated with risperidone LAI or placebo, predominantly due to the higher incidence of weight increase, somnolence, and hypersomnia.

In the adjunctive therapy study (Macfadden et al., 2009), the most frequently reported treatment-emergent adverse events during double-blind treatment in the risperidone LAI and placebo groups respectively, were tremor (24.6 and 10.2%), insomnia (20.0 and 18.6%), muscle rigidity (12.3 and 5.1%), and mania (4.6 and 13.6%). Treatment-emergent adverse events that occurred more frequently in the risperidone LAI group than the placebo group (≥3% difference) in the double-blind period were tremor, muscle rigidity, weight increase, sedation, increased appetite, decreased appetite, disturbance in attention, abnormal gait, and hypokinesia. Events that occurred more frequently (≥3% difference) in the placebo group than the risperidone LAI group were insomnia, headache, fatigue, nausea, pyrexia, depression, mania, suicidal ideation, hypertension, and injury. The adverse event profile of this study reflects the wide range of medications that subjects were taking as treatment as usual in addition to risperidone LAI or placebo.

Treatment-emergent EPS-related adverse events occurred in 9 and 3% of patients who received risperidone LAI in the open-label and double-blind phase of the (Quiroz *et al.*, 2010) study respectively (2% on placebo), and 20 and 17% during these same study periods in the (Montgomery *et al.*, 2010) study (14 and 9% on olanzapine and placebo, respectively, during the double-blind phase). In the adjunctive therapy study, the proportion of patients with at least one EPS-related adverse event was 31 and 17% in the risperidone and placebo treatment groups during the double-blind period (Macfadden *et al.*, 2009). Tardive dyskinesia was reported as a treatment-emergent adverse event in three subjects who were currently receiving treatment with risperidone LAI (two open-label, and one double-blind) in the three studies combined.

In the monotherapy studies, there were no meaningful changes from baseline to study endpoint for mean Extrapyramidal Symptom Rating Scale (ESRS) total score during any study phase. The ESRS scores decreased (improved) in both the open-label (from 1.4 to 1.1) and double-blind (from 0.9 to 0.7) period on risperidone LAI with no changes in the placebo group in the (Quiroz *et al.*, 2010) study. In the adjunctive therapy study, there were no meaningful changes from baseline to endpoint in dyskinetic symptoms (Abnormal Involuntary Movement Scale or AIMS), akathisia symptoms (Barnes Akathisia Scale or BAS) or Parkinsonian symptoms (SAS) during any study phase.

Body weight increased with 1.6–2.6 kg during the open-label phase (Quiroz *et al.*, 2010; Macfadden *et al.*, 2009) with changes from double-blind baseline (randomization) to end point of −1.5 to −2.0 kg on placebo versus +0.7 and +1.1 kg on risperidone during the double-blind periods. In the double-blind period of the (Montgomery *et al.*, 2010) study, 18, 26, and 5% of subjects showed a weight increase of ≥7% in the risperidone, olanzapine, and placebo treatment arms, respectively. Incidences of ≥7% increase in body weight were 12% in the risperidone versus 3% in the placebo treatment arm in the double-blind phase of the study published by Quiroz *et al.* (2010), and 18% versus 31% in the risperidone and placebo treatment arms, respectively, in the adjunctive study (Macfadden *et al.*, 2009).

Potentially prolactin-related adverse events (for example, erectile dysfunction, amenorrhea) occurred in 1–5% of subjects on placebo, 4–14% of subjects on risperidone and in 6% of the olanzapine treated subjects.

Overall, the adverse event profile of risperidone LAI reported during these studies is consistent with the underlying psychiatric disorder and with the known safety profile of the study drug.

9.4.3 ADDITIONAL STUDIES WITH RISPERIDONE LAI IN BIPOLAR DISORDER

Several studies have been published on the use of risperidone LAI in the maintenance treatment of bipolar disorder in settings resembling more the naturalistic setting of clinical practice.

Chengappa *et al.* (2010) randomized bipolar patients in a hypomanic, manic, or mixed episode to either oral risperidone followed by risperidone LAI (n = 23) or another oral atypical antipsychotic (n = 25) for three months. Any mood stabilizers were continued during open-label treatment. Of the 48 patients who participated in the study, 39 patients improved and participated in a one year extension. In total, 47 clinical events were declared by an independent clinician board. The risperidone LAI group experienced significantly fewer clinical events (mean 0.86 ± 0.73) compared with the oral atypical antipsychotic group (1.61 ± 1.29).

Yatham, Fallu, and Binder (2007) randomized 49 bipolar patients taking a mood stabilizer and an atypical antipsychotic in a double-blind fashion to continuation of this antipsychotic (n = 26) or switching to risperidone LAI (n = 23) for six months, while the mood stabilizer was kept unchanged. The risperidone LAI group had significant reduction in symptoms as measured by changes in CGI-S scores and YMRS at endpoint relative to baseline. The oral atypical antipsychotic group had reductions in Hamilton Anxiety Rating Scale Scores relative to baseline. No significant differences were noted between the two treatment groups on any of the efficacy measures. There were no significant differences between the groups in any safety assessments.

Twenty-nine acutely manic bipolar patients with a history of poor or partial adherence to medication received naturalistic treatment for a manic episode plus risperidone LAI for a mean period of two years (Vieta *et al.*, 2008). During the follow-up, in comparison to a similar period before study entry, there was a significant decrease in the total number of hospitalizations per patient, the number of manic or mixed episodes leading to hospitalization but not in the hospitalizations due to a depressive episode, a significant increase in time to any subsequent episode and significant improvement in treatment adherence and hetero-aggressive episodes, but not suicide attempts.

9.5 ELEMENTS OF SPECIAL INTEREST

9.5.1 PEDIATRIC STUDIES

In a randomized double-blind study that included children and adolescents (ages 10–17 years) with a DSM-IV diagnosis of bipolar I disorder, most recent episode manic or mixed, two dose ranges of oral risperidone monotherapy (0.5–2.5 mg/day, n = 50 and 3–6 mg/day, n = 61) were compared to placebo (n = 58) (Haas *et al.*, 2009). Double-blind treatment lasted three weeks. The primary efficacy measure was change in YMRS total score from baseline to end point. Secondary assessments included Clinical Global Impression-Bipolar (CGI-BP) and the Brief Psychiatric Rating Scale for children (BPRS-C).

Once the fixed maximally tolerated target dose was reached, 57% of subjects had a mode dose of 2.5 mg in the 0.5–2.5 mg group. In the 3–6 mg group, 41% of subjects had a mode dose of 6 mg, 15, 19, and 26% had a mode sode of 5, 4, and 3 mg respectively.

Improvement in mean YMRS was significantly greater in the risperidone-treated subjects than in placebo-treated subjects (Table 9.11). Significant improvements over placebo were noted in the two age groups (subjects ≤12 (n = 67) or >12 years of age (n = 102)).

Significantly greater improvements were detected for both risperidone dose groups compared with the placebo group at the first post randomization study time point (day 7) and each time point thereafter. Clinical response rate ($\geq$50% reduction from baseline in total YMRS total score at end point) was significantly higher for both risperidone dose groups versus the placebo group. Changes from baseline to endpoint in CGI-BP demonstrated a statistically significant improvement in both risperidone treatment groups ($p < 0.001$) compared with the placebo group. Mean BPRS-C depression factor scores decreased at end point in both risperidone dose groups, but the differences in changes from baseline were not significantly different from placebo.

The most common treatment-emergent adverse events in risperidone treated subjects were somnolence, headache, and fatigue (Table 9.11). There was a dose dependent increase in the percentage of risperidone-treated subjects who experienced somnolence or fatigue. The rate of adverse events in the gastrointestinal system was similar in the risperidone groups but was approximately twice that of placebo treated subjects. The type and rate of adverse events across the two risperidone groups were generally similar between subjects $\leq$12 and >12 years of age. The percentage of subjects with at least 1 EPS-related adverse event was similar in the placebo and risperidone 0.5–2.5 mg groups, but higher in the risperidone 3–6 mg group (Table 9.11). There were no reports

Table 9.11 Oral risperidone in bipolar mania in children (>10 yr) and adolescents (Haas *et al.*, 2009).

	Placebo	0.5–2.5 mg risperidone	3–6 mg risperidone
No. of patients	58	50	61
$\leq$12 yr/>12 yr	41%/59%	36%/64%	41%/59%
Male/female	48%/52%	56%/44%	43%/57%
Manic/mixed episode	33%/67%	40%/60%	34%/66%
Baseline YMRS, mean total score (SD)	31.0 (7.5)	31.1 (6.0)	30.5 (5.96)
Mean change from baseline (SD)	−9.1 (11.0)	−18.5 (9.7)[a]	−16.5 (10.3)[a]
Response rate (%)	26%	59%[a]	63%[a]
BPRS-C total	−11.6	−17.9[a]	−16.6[a]
Mean changes at endpoint			
Total with AEs (%)	76%	90%	95%
Common AEs (>20%)	19%	42%	56%
Somnolence	33%	40%	38%
Headache	3%	18%	30%
Fatigue	5%	8%	25%
$\geq$1 EPS-related AE (%)	2%	4%	5%
Potentially PRL related AE (%)	2%	2%	3%
Weight increased AE (%)			

[a] Significantly different from placebo.
YMRS, Young Mania Rating Scale; BPRS-C, Brief Psychiatry Rating Scale – Child version; AE, adverse event; EPS, extrapyramidal symptoms; PRL, prolactin; SD, standard deviation.

of tardive dyskinesia. The incidence of potentially prolactin related adverse events is given in Table 9.11. Mean (SD) weight increases from baseline at the three-week end point were 0.7 (1.9), 1.9 (1.7), and 1.4 (2.4) kg in the placebo, 0.5–2.5 and 3–6 mg resperidone – treatment groups, respectively. The percentages of subjects with ≥7% weight increase from baseline were 5.3, 14.3, and 10%, respectively.

Biederman *et al.* (2005) studied 30 children and adolescents, 6–17 years of age, with bipolar disorder currently experiencing a manic, hypomanic, or mixed episode in an open-label study for eight weeks with risperidone (1.25 ± 1.5 mg/day) monotherapy. Twenty-two (73%) subjects completed the study. The responder rate for manic symptoms defined as CGI-I ≤2 at end point was 70%. Weight increased from baseline with on average +2.1 ± 2.0 kg. Responders were subsequently enrolled in a 10-month open-label extension study (Mick and Biederman, 2005). Among these subjects, the rate of relapse defined as a 30% increase in YMRS total score and CGI-I > 2 was 21%. The mean ± SD treatment duration was 25.9 ± 12.5 weeks.

The safety and effectiveness of risperidone (0.25–3 mg/day) used as adjunctve therapy to lithium or valproate was evaluated in a six-month, open label study in 37 children and adolescents (aged 5–18 years) with Diagnostic and Statistical Manual of Mental Disorders, 4th Edition (DSM-IV) diagnosis of bipolar I disorder, most recent episode manic or mixed (Pavuluri *et al.*, 2004). The response rate defined as change from baseline in YMRS total score ≥50% at end point was 81% and similar in both lithium and valproate subgroups. After adjusting to the growth curve of normal weight over six months, all subjects gained some weight (total mean increase of 6 and 6.8 kg in the lithium and valproate subgroup, respectively). There was no clinically relevant difference in safety or tolerability between subjects on lithium or valproate background therapy.

There are no studies available on paliperidone ER in pediatric populations with bipolar disorder. One prospective, open-label study documented the use of risperidone LAI in children and adolescents (aged 10–16 years) with bipolar disorder (Boarati *et al.*, 2009).

9.5.2   BIPOLAR PATIENT SUBPOPULATIONS

9.5.2.1   Rapid Cycling Bipolar Disorder

Ten patients with rapid cycling bipolar I or II disorder refractory to lithium, carbamazepine, and valproate and who had taken typical antipsychotics with no apparent improvement were treated with oral risperidone 2–6 mg for at least six months (Vieta *et al.*, 1998). Mood stabilizers prescribed before study initiation were maintained. Eight of the 10 patients improved. The number of episodes within six months after baseline was significantly reduced from 5.5 (3.7) per six months before study entry to 2.0 (1.7); mean YMRS and HAM-D scores were significantly decreased from baseline; YMRS; from 14.0 (7.3) to 6.1 (5.2) and HAM-D from 17.5 (4.7) to 11.5 (6.5).

9.5.2.2   Bipolar II Disorder

Forty-four DSM-IV bipolar II patients with a YMRS total score > 7 were treated with oral risperidone, mean dose of 2.8 mg/day (n = 14 on monotherapy) (Vieta *et al.*, 2001).

Thirty-four patients completed the open-label trial. Last observation-carried-forward analysis showed a significant reduction of YMRS total score from baseline. At six months follow-up, 60% of patients were asymptomatic according to the CGI. Risperidone appeared to be more protective against hypomanic than depressive recurrences. Nine patients (12%) had a depressive relapse, one (2%) had a hypomanic relapse and another (2%) had both. Only three patients discontinued risperidone because of adverse events.

9.5.2.3 Bipolar Disorder with Comorbid Substance Use Disorder

Nejtek *et al.* (2008) studied oral risperidone (n = 38; 3.1 ± 1.2 mg/day) and quetiapine (n = 42; 303.6 ± 151.9 mg/day) in a 20-week, double-blind, randomized study in patients with bipolar I or II disorder with comorbid cocaine or methamphetamine dependence. In both treatment groups, manic and depressive symptoms significantly improved versus baseline (p < 0.0005), as well as drug cravings as compared to baseline (p < 0.0005). Decreased drug cravings were related to less frequent drug use (p = 0.03). The two medications did not significantly differ in any efficacy parameter.

9.5.2.4 Bipolar Disorder with Comorbid Anxiety Disorder

Risperidone monotherapy (0.5–4 mg/day) was not more effective than placebo on the CGI-21 Anxiety score or other anxiety outcome measures in an eight-week, double-blind, placebo-controlled randomized study in 111 patients with bipolar disorder and co-occurring panic disorder or generalized anxiety disorder (Sheehan *et al.*, 2009).

9.5.3 BIPOLAR DEPRESSION

There are currently no published placebo-controlled trials that evaluated the efficacy and safety of risperidone or paliperidone in the treatment of patients with bipolar disorder who are currently experiencing an acute depressive episode ("bipolar depression") (Cruz *et al.*, 2010). Risperidone was evaluated for the treatment of bipolar depression in two randomized, controlled trials without placebo control. In patients with treatment-resistant bipolar depression in the Systematic Treatment Enhancement Program for Bipolar Disorder (STEP-BD) program, lamotrigine was found to produce a greater recovery rate than risperidone when added in an open-label fashion to a combination of adequate doses of established mood stabilizers and at least one antidepressant over a period of 16 weeks (23.8% vs. 4.6%) (Nierenberg, Ostacher, and Calabrese, 2006). Risperidone was also evaluated relative to paroxetine and the combination of risperidone and paroxetine in a 12-week, double-blind study (Shelton and Stahl, 2004). All patients with bipolar depression in that study continued to receive stable doses of mood stabilizers. The three groups showed decreases from baseline in HAM-D score without any significant between-group differences. However, the improvement was only moderate as remission was achieved in 20% of patients (that is, three patients in the combination group, two patients in the paroxetine group, and one patient in the risperidone group).

The number of patients with a mixed episode in the placebo-controlled studies of oral risperidone in acute mania was too small to draw a meaningful conclusion on a potential antidepressant effect in this population. Changes from baseline in MADRS score are more likely to reflect an effect on subsyndromal depressive symptoms. Risperidone was significantly more effective than placebo for the change from baseline in MADRS score at the three-week endpoint in two of three monotherapy studies (Smulevich et al., 2005; Khanna et al., 2005). In the third study (Hirschfeld et al., 2004), significance was observed at weeks 1 and 2 with a numerical advantage for risperidone at the three-week endpoint. In the 12-week study, which included haloperidol as a control, risperidone was significantly better than placebo at three weeks while haloperidol was not. In the main-tenance period from Week 3 to 12, risperidone was numerically better than haloperidol at all time points (Smulevich et al., 2005).

About one third of all subjects enrolled across placebo-controlled studies of paliperidone ER in acute mania had a mixed episode. This substantial number of subjects who met criteria for a major depressive episode in addition to acute mania allows a more accurate assessment of the proper effect of paliperidone on depressive symptoms in patients with bipolar disorder.

Across studies conducted with paliperidone ER, MADRS scores decreased from base-line in all treatment groups, indicating improvement in the symptoms of depression. There was no dose-related pattern with regard to change from baseline in MADRS score (Berwaerts et al., in press). In both flexible dose studies, paliperidone ER was numerically superior to placebo with regard to the change from baseline in MADRS score; this difference reached statistical significance in the acute phase of the flexible-dose monotherapy study (Vieta et al., 2010). In that study, quetiapine was statistically superior to paliperidone ER based on the 95% CI of the LS mean difference for the change from baseline in MADRS score over 12 weeks of treatment. This finding is in line with the known antidepressant properties of the active metabolite of quetiapine (N-desalkylquetiapine), as reflected in clinical trials of quetiapine in subjects with bipolar depression (Cruz et al., 2010). Across the studies of paliperidone ER, the mean decrease from baseline in MADRS score was greater across all treatment groups in subjects with a baseline diagnosis of bipolar I disorder, most recent episode mixed than in subjects with a diagnosis of most recent episode manic.

In the treatment of patients with bipolar disorder, switching from mania to depression represents a key treatment challenge. During its development for the treatment of acute mania, paliperidone ER was carefully evaluated for its potential to induce depressive symptoms. "Switch to depression" was defined as a MADRS score of at least 18 with an increase from baseline of at least four at any two consecutive assessments or at the last observation. There was no dose-related pattern with regard to switch to depression in the fixed-dose monotherapy study (Berwaerts et al., in press). In the flexible-dose monotherapy, the proportion of subjects who switched to depression was lower for quetiapine (7.5%) than for paliperidone ER (13.9%) (Vieta et al., 2010).

The beneficial effect of risperidone LAI seen in the monotherapy studies in the prevention of recurrence of a mood episode was mainly due to the prevention of manic episodes (Quiroz et al., 2010; Montgomery et al., 2010). In the adjunctive therapy study, the overall observed risk ratio of relapse between treatment groups (2.3) did not differ among relapse episode types (Macfadden et al., 2009).

9.5.4   COMPARISON OF SAFETY PROFILES BETWEEN BIPOLAR DISORDER AND SCHIZOPHRENIA

The overall safety profiles of both formulations of risperidone (that is, oral and LAI) and paliperidone ER as documented in the respective clinical development programs in acute mania and bipolar disorder were generally consistent with the profiles observed in schizophrenia. No new or unexpected safety findings were reported, and there was no evidence of a substantially increased safety risk.

Patients with bipolar disorder have been shown in some studies to possess a greater sensitivity to select side effects of antipsychotics compared to patients with schizophrenia (Chue and Kovacs, 2003). For instance, a review of safety data from placebo-controlled monotherapy studies of typical and atypical antipsychotics across the two indications suggested that there was a greater difference in the risk of experiencing somnolence with risperidone relative to placebo among patients with acute mania than those with schizophrenia, resulting in a higher incidence of somnolence among patients with acute mania (Gao et al., 2008a). The separation in risk difference between the two indications was not statistically significant.

Direct comparison of safety data across studies that evaluated risperidone and paliperidone ER for the treatment of patients with an acute exacerbation of schizophrenia and acute manic episodes associated with bipolar I disorder, respectively, may be confounded by differences in study design such as treatment duration, dose range, use of concomitant medications (for example, benzodiazepines), as well as the inherent differences in patient population and disease characteristics.

Across the studies of oral risperidone, the incidence of adverse events related to EPS was higher in patients with acute mania than in patients with schizophrenia. This raises the question whether patients with bipolar disorder may be more sensitive to EPS than patients with schizophrenia (Gao et al., 2008b). A greater sensitivity to experience EPS by patients with acute mania has been observed with other antipsychotics, especially conventional antipsychotics, but has not been confirmed across all atypical antipsychotics (Cavazzoni et al., 2006). In a review of safety data from placebo-controlled studies of antipsychotics across the two indications, the separation in risk difference for experiencing EPS with risperidone relative to placebo between patients with acute mania and those with schizophrenia was statistically significant while it was not statistically significant for any of the other antipsychotics evaluated (Gao et al., 2008b). This finding may be driven in part by the absolute risk difference of 30% for risperidone relative to placebo in a monotherapy study conducted in India (Khanna et al., 2005), which was larger than the risk difference of EPS observed across the pooled placebo-controlled monotherapy studies of risperidone in acute mania (24%). The high rate of EPS reported by subjects in the study may be related to the high baseline YMRS total scores and the rapid increase in risperidone dosage. The low body weight of subjects (mean 54 kg), together with a mean modal dose of 5.6 mg per day of risperidone, may also have contributed to the EPS-related adverse events.

For paliperidone ER, the rates of EPS reported by subjects with acute mania and schizophrenia can be compared at distinct dose levels as both clinical development programs included fixed-dose studies (Berwaerts et al., in press; Meltzer et al., 2008). Across the studies of paliperidone ER, EPS-related adverse events were reported at a higher overall rate in subjects with acute mania compared to those with schizophrenia. Consistent with the recent observations from clinical trials of aripiprazole (EMEA, 2010), higher rates of akathisia were noted in paliperidone ER-treated subjects with acute mania compared to the rates previously observed in subjects with schizophrenia. However, the rates of other distinct EPS-related adverse events, the rate of anticholinergic medication use, and the dose relationship for EPS-related adverse events were similar for the two study populations.

The safety profile of risperidone LAI in bipolar disorder was generally consistent with the profile observed in schizophrenia. No striking differences in EPS were observed except for a higher incidence of tremor in subjects assigned to risperidone LAI in the adjunctive therapy study (24%), although the incidence in the placebo group was also higher (16%) than that previously observed in schizophrenia studies (Macfadden et al., 2009). This was likely due to the concomitant use of certain medications (for example, lithium). Weight increase was more common in one of the monotherapy studies (Montgomery et al., 2010), most likely as a result of the longer treatment duration than that of the 12-week, placebo controlled study in schizophrenia (Kane et al., 2003).

9.6 SUMMARY AND CONCLUSIONS

The efficacy of oral risperidone in the treatment of bipolar mania and associated symptoms has been demonstrated unequivocally in monotherapy as well as in adjunctive therapy to mood stabilizers. The treatment effect of risperidone emerges early, within the first three to seven days of treatment. The antimanic efficacy of risperidone is maintained over a period of 12 weeks, as documented in comparison with the established reference compound haloperidol. In double-blind, placebo-controlled studies, risperidone showed antimanic efficacy similar to olanzapine and lithium. Risperidone did not appear to induce or worsen coexisting subsyndromal depressive symptoms. Although the number of patients with a mixed episode was limited, depressive symptoms improved in both monotherapy and adjunctive therapy studies. Long-term antimanic efficacy beyond 12 weeks is only documented in open-label studies. In both mono- and adjunctive therapy studies, reductions of manic and depressive symptoms lasted over the six months treatment period.

The recommended starting dose is 2–3 mg per day once daily. Dose adjustments, if indicated should occur at intervals of no less than 24 hours and in dosage increments of 1 mg per day. Efficacy was demonstrated in flexible doses over a range of 1–6 mg per day. The usual mean dosages used in the various studies were around 4 mg per day with exception of a mean modal dose of 5.6 mg in one study in patients with severe manic symptoms and a mean dose of 2.8 mg per day in a population of bipolar II disorder patients.

Dose reductions should be considered with concomitant use of CYP2D6 inhibiting antidepressants such as paroxetine or fluoxetine whereas upwards dose titration may be indicated with concomitant use of carbamazepine. There are no clinically relevant drug-drug interactions with other mood stabilizers such as lithium or valproate.

The adverse events reported with risperidone in bipolar mania are largely consistent with those reported in patients with schizophrenia. Changes on EPS rating scales are generally mild and were comparable to olanzapine in one study and less pronounced than haloperidol in the two randomized controlled studies. EPS may be more pronounced with fast titration to high doses. Patients who are currently experiencing an acute manic episode are more likely to report akathisia than patients with schizophrenia. One should also consider the higher background incidence of distinct EPS such as tremor in patients with bipolar disorder who are receiving background therapy with mood stabilizers such as lithium. Weight changes were minimal in the 3–12-week, controlled studies. The average weight gain over six months was 3.2 ± 2.1 kg (Vieta *et al.*, 2004). Treatment-emergent potentially prolactin-related adverse effects were rare, both in short-term and long-term studies.

Risperidone is effective in acute mania in children (≥ 10 years) and adolescents with bipolar mania. The recommended starting dose is 0.5 mg daily with increments of 0.5 or 1 mg at intervals of not less than 24 hours to a recommended target dose of 2.5 mg. Doses higher than 2.5 mg/day did not reveal any trend towards greater efficacy whereas adverse events such as somnolence, fatigue, and EPS were more common at higher doses. Data on risperidone and body weight in pediatric bipolar patients are limited. Mean weight increases of approximately 6 kg over six months treatment, were reported in one study, exceeding the normal weight gain over such a period of time. In other psychiatric conditions, a mean increase of 7.5 kg after 12 months treatment was observed which was higher than the expected normal weight gain of 3–3.5 kg per year in that age group. The majority of the weight increase was observed within the first six months of exposure to risperidone. When treating pediatric subjects with risperidone, weight gain should be assessed against that expected with normal growth. Prolactin increases are common although treatment-emergent potentially prolactin-related adverse events were $\leq 5\%$.

Data from the completed monotherapy studies support the efficacy and safety of paliperidone ER when used in a flexible dose range of 3–12 mg for the treatment of acute mania. It should be noted that there is currently limited data from placebo-controlled studies to confirm the efficacy of paliperidone ER for the treatment of acute manic episodes in patients recruited at sites in North America. While the efficacy of paliperidone ER as adjunctive therapy in patients experiencing an acute manic episode could not be established, treatment with paliperidone ER was proven safe and well tolerated when used in combination with mood stabilizers. The recommended dose is 9 mg once daily. Initial dose titration is not required. Some patients may benefit from lower or higher doses within the recommended range of 3–12 mg. The overall safety findings were similar to those observed in previous studies with paliperidone ER in schizophrenia. Paliperidone ER may be a valuable addition to the treatment armamentarium for acute mania. It may present an alternative to other atypical antipsychotics in patients who are at risk of metabolic drug-drug interactions, especially those patients who receive concomitant treatment with potent CYP2D6 inhibitors such as many Selective Serotonin Reuptake Inhibitors (SSRIs).

The efficacy and safety of risperidone and paliperidone ER in the treatment of patients with bipolar depression have so far not been formally evaluated in placebo-controlled studies. Data, that is, currently available from placebo-controlled studies in the treatment of acute mania and prevention of recurrences suggests that the effect of either compound used as monotherapy on depressive symptoms is modest. While patients with a mixed episode will benefit from treatment with risperidone or paliperidone ER for improvement of their manic symptoms, it would seem prudent to use either compound in combination with a mood stabilizer, or possibly an antidepressant, in patients who are currently experiencing an acute depressive episode pending the availability of placebo-controlled studies that establish the efficacy in bipolar depression. The currently available data suggest that there is no concern about patients who are experiencing an acute manic episode switching to depression when they are being treated with risperidone or paliperidone ER alone.

There remains a significant unmet need for well-tolerated and effective medications that can be used either alone or as adjunctive therapy in the management of bipolar disorder, specifically for the long-term maintenance phase of treatment, where the key objective is to prevent or delay the recurrence of mood episodes. The data from three placebo-controlled studies provide compelling clinical evidence that risperidone LAI is effective and generally safe and well tolerated both as monotherapy and as adjunctive therapy for maintenance treatment to prevent the recurrence of mood episodes in patients with bipolar I disorder. Although the monotherapy data demonstrated efficacy especially in prevention of elevated mood episodes, the adjunctive data show that the addition of risperidone LAI to other standard bipolar medications was clearly superior to use of those treatments alone in the prevention of both manic and depressive episodes.

The recommended dose for risperidone LAI for the maintenance treatment of bipolar I disorder is 25 mg IM, every two weeks. Some patients may benefit from a higher dose of 37.5 or 50 mg. Upwards dose adjustments should not be made more frequently than every four weeks. Oral risperidone or another antipsychotic medication should be given with the first injection of risperidone LAI and continued for three weeks to ensure that adequate therapeutic plasma concentrations are maintained prior to the main release phase of risperidone from the injection site. Dose adjustments for drug-drug interactions with certain antidepressants or carbamazepine are similar to those with oral risperidone.

Since most patients with bipolar I disorder require polypharmacy in "real world" treatment, it can be assumed that adjunctive treatment will be, in fact, the most common clinical scenario facing the treating psychiatrist. Many of these patients who are receiving mood stabilizers and antidepressants have a suboptimal treatment response and are poorly adherent to treatment.

The LAI formulation of risperidone offers clear advantages over currently available oral medication treatments for bipolar I disorder. The expected benefits of LAI treatment are at least partially related to improved adherence and more rapid detection of nonadherence. Patients who fail to return for their scheduled injection are readily identified and can be contacted early, thereby allowing earlier intervention to prevent worsening of symptoms and escalation to a full-blown bipolar episode. Risperidone LAI offers a new opportunity to maintain clinical stability in patients with bipolar I disorder and is therefore likely to offer advantage particularly in the treatment of this serious psychiatric disorder where treatment nonadherence is recognized as one of the most important predictors of recurrence and poor prognosis.

References

Berwaerts, J., Cleton, A., Herben, V. *et al.* (2009) The effects of paroxetine on the pharmacokinetics of paliperidone extended-release tablets. *Pharmacopsychiatry*, **42**, 158–163.

Berwaerts, J., Lane, R., Nuamah, I. *et al.* Paliperidone extended-release as adjunctive therapy to lithium or valproate in the treatment of acute mania: a randomized, placebo-controlled study. *J. Affect. Disord.*, in press.

Berwaerts, J., Xu, H., Nuamah, I. *et al.* Evaluation of the efficacy and safety of paliperidone extended-release in the treatment of acute mania: a randomized, double-blind, dose-response study. *J. Affect. Disord.*, in press.

Biederman, J., Mick, E., Wozniak, J. *et al.* (2005) An open-label trial of risperidone in children and adolescents with bipolar disorder. *J. Child Adolesc. Psychopharmacol.*, **15**, 311–317.

Boarati, M., Wang, Y.-P., Pereira, A. *et al.* (2009) An open-label study of treatment of the early-onset bipolar disorders with risperidone long-acting injection. Abstract of the 9th World Congress of Biological Psychiatry (WCBP), June28–July 2, 2009, Paris, France.

Bond, D.J., Pratoomsri, W., and Yatham, L.N. (2007) Depot antipsychotic medications in bipolar disorder: a review of the literature. *Acta Psychiatr. Scand.*, **116** (Suppl. 434), 3–16.

Bondolfi, G., Eap, C.B., Bertschy, G. *et al.* (2002) The effect of fluoxetine on the pharmacokinetics and safety of risperidone in psychotic patients. *Pharmacopsychiatry*, **35**, 50–56.

Cavazzoni, P.A., Berg, P.H., Kryzhanovskaya, L.A. *et al.* (2006) Comparison of treatment-emergent extrapyramidal symptoms in patients with bipolar mania or schizophrenia during olanzapine clinical trials. *J. Clin. Psychiatry*, **67**, 107–113.

Chengappa, K.N.R., Turkin, S.R., Schlicht, P.J. *et al.* (2010) A pilot, 15-month, randomized effectiveness trial of risperidone long-acting injection (RLAI) versus oral atypical antipsychotic agents (AAP) in persons with bipolar disorder. *Acta Neuropsychiatr.*, **22**, 68–80.

Chue, P. and Emsley, R. (2007) Long-acting formulations of atypical antipsychotics: Time to reconsider when to introduce depot antipsychotics. *CNS Drugs* **21** (6), 441–448.

Chue, P. and Kovacs, C.S. (2003) Safety and tolerability of atypical antipsychotics in patients with bipolar disorder: prevalence, monitoring and management. *Bipolar Disord.*, **5** (Suppl. 2), 62–79.

Cleton, A., Rossenu, Z., Talluri, K. *et al.* (2007) Evaluation of the pharmacokinetics of an extended-release formulation of paliperidone with an immediate-release formulation of risperidone. Annual Meeting of the American Society For Clinical Pharmacology and Therapeutics, March 21–24, 2007, California; *Nature*, **81**, S62.

Cruz, N., Sanchez-Moreno, J., Torres, F. *et al.* (2010) Efficacy of modern antipsychotics in placebo-controlled trials in bipolar depression: a meta-analysis. *Int. J. Neuropsychopharmacol.*, **13**, 5–14.

Demling, J.H., Huang, M.L., Remmerie, B. *et al.* (2006) Pharmacokinetics and safety of combination therapy with lithium and risperidone. *Pharmacopsychiatry*, **39**, 230–231.

Dwight, M.M., Keck, P.E., Stanton, S.P. *et al.* (1994) Antidepressant activity and mania associated with risperidone treatment of schizoaffective disorder. *Lancet*, **344**, 554–555.

Eerdekens, M., Van Hove, I., Remmerie, B., and Mannaert, E. (2004) Pharmacokinetics and tolerability of long-acting risperidone in schizophrenia. *Schizophr. Res.*, **70**, 91–100.

El-Mallakh, R.S. (2007) Medication adherence and the use of long-acting antipyshotics in bipolar disorder. *J. Psychiatr. Pract.*, **13**, 79–85.

EMEA–The European Agency for the Evaluation of Medicinal Products (2010) Variation Assessment Report for Abilify (aripiprazole). Available from URL: http://www.ema.europa.eu/docs/en_GB/document_library/EPAR_-_Assessment_Report_-_Variation/human/000471/WC50-0020167.pdf (accessed August 14, 2010).

Fleischhacker, W.W., Eerdekens, M., Karcher, K. *et al.* (2003) Treatment of schizophrenia with long-acting injectable risperidone: a 12-month open-label trial of the first long-acting second-generation antipyshcotic. *J. Clin. Psychopharmacol.*, **64**, 1250–1257.

Gao, K., Ganocy, S.J., Gajwani, P. *et al.* (2008a) A review of sensitivity and tolerability of antipsychotics in patients with bipolar disorder or schizophrenia: focus on somnolence. *J. Clin. Psychiat.*, **69**, 302–309.

Gao, K., Kemp, D.E., Ganocy, S.J. *et al.* (2008b) Antipsychotic-induced extrapyramidal side effects in bipolar disorder and schizophrenia: a systematic review. *J. Clin. Psychopharmacol.*, **28**, 203–209.

Ghaemi, S.N., Sachs, G.S., Baldassano, C.F., and Truman, C.J. (1997) Acute treatment of bipolar disorder with adjunctive risperidone in outpatients. *Can. J. Psychiatry*, **42**, 196–199.

Gopal, S., Steffens, D.C., Kramer, M.L., and Olsen, M.K. (2005) Symptomatic remission in patients with bipolar mania: results from a double-blind, placebo-controlled trial of risperidone monotherapy. *J. Clin. Psychiatry*, **66**, 1016–1020.

Gupta, B., Shopra, S.C., Gupta, C. *et al.* (2006) Effects of fluoxetine, risperidone and alprazolam on pharmacokinetics of lithium in patients with psychiatric illness. *Indian J. Pharmacol.*, **38**, 133–134.

Haas, M., DelBello, M.P., Pandina, G. *et al.* (2009) Risperidone for the treatment of acute mania in children and adolescents with bipolar disorder: a randomized, double-blind, placebo-controlled study. *Bipolar Disord.*, **11**, 687–700.

Hassan, M. and Lage, M.J. (2009) Risk of rehospitalization among bipolar disorder patients who are nonadherent to antipsychotic therapy after hospital discharge. *Am. J. Health Syst. Pharm.*, **66**, 358–365.

Hirschfeld, R.M.A., Eerdekens, M., Kalali, A.H. *et al.* (2006) An open-label extension trial of risperidone monotherapy in the treatment of bipolar I disorder. *Int. Clin. Psychopharmacol.*, **21**, 11–20.

Hirschfeld, R.M.A., Keck, P.E., Kramer, M. *et al.* (2004) Rapid antimanic effect of risperidone monotherapy: a 3-week multicenter, double-blind, placebo-controlled trial. *Am. J. Psychiatry*, **161**, 1057–1065.

INVEGA® United States Prescribing Information (2010) Available from URL: http://www.janssen.com/janssen/shared/pi/invega.pdf (accessed August 14, 2010).

Kalkman, H.O. and Loetscher, E. (2003) Alpha2C-adrenoreceptor blockade by clozapine and other antipsychotic drugs. *Eur. J. Pharmacol.*, **462**, 33–40.

Kane, J.M., Eerdekens, M., Lindenmayer, J.-P. *et al.* (2003) Long-acting injectable risperidone: efficacy and safety of the first long-acting atypical antipsychotic. *Am. J. Psychiatry*, **160**, 1125–1132.

Keck, P.E. Jr., McElroy, S.L., Strakowski, S.M. *et al.* (1996) Factors associated with pharmacologic noncompliance in patients with mania. *J. Clin. Psychiatry*, **57**, 292–297.

Khanna, S., Vieta, E., Lyons, B. *et al.* (2005) Risperidone in the treatment of acute mania: double-blind, placebo-controlled study. *Br. J. Psychiatry*, **187**, 229–234.

Leysen, J.E., Janssen, P.M., Megens, A.H., and Schotte, A. (1994) Risperidone: a novel antipsychotic with balanced serotonin-dopamine antagonism receptor occupancy profile, and pharmacologic activity. *J. Clin. Psychiatry*, **55**, 5–12.

Lingam, R. and Scott, J. (2002) Treatment non-adherence in affective disorders. *Acta Psychiatr. Scand.*, **105**, 164–172.

Macfadden, W., Alphs, L., Haskins, J.T. *et al.* (2009) A randomized, double-blind, placebo-controlled study of maintenance treatment with adjunctive risperidone long-acting therapy in patients with bipolar I disorder who relapse frequently. *Bipolar Disord.*, **11**, 827–839.

McEvoy, J.P. (2006) Risks versus benefits of different types of long-acting injectable antipsychotics. *J. Clin. Psychiatry*, **67** (Suppl. 5), 15–18.

Meltzer, H.Y., Bobo, W.V., Nuamah, I. *et al.* (2008) Efficacy and tolerability of oral paliperidone extended-release tablets in the treatment of acute schizophrenia: pooled data from three 6-week, placebo-controlled studies. *J. Clin. Psychiatry*, **69**, 817–829.

Mick, E. and Biederman, J. (2005) One-year open-label trial of risperidone monotherapy in children with bipolar disorder. 6th International Conference on Bipolar Disorder. *Bipolar Disord.*, **7** (Suppl. 2), 78.

Montgomery, S., Vieta, E., Sulaiman, A.H. *et al.* (2010) Randomized, double-blind, placebo-controlled study of risperidone long-acting injectable in relapse prevention in patients with bipolar I disorder. *Eur. Psychiatry*, **25** (Suppl. 1), 974.

Muscatello, M.R., Pacetti, M., Cacciola, M. *et al.* (2005) Plasma concentrations of risperidone and olanzapine during coadministration with oxcarbazepine. *Epilepsia*, **46**, 771–774.

Nejtek, V.A., Avila, M., Chen, L.-A. *et al.* (2008) Do atypical antipsychotics effectively treat co-occurring bipolar disorder and stimulant dependence? A randomized, double-blind trial. *J. Clin. Psychiatry*, **69**, 1257–1266.

Nierenberg, A.A., Ostacher, M.J., and Calabrese, J.R. (2006) Treatment-resistant bipolar depression. A STEP-BD equipoise randomized effectiveness trial of antidepressant augmentation with lamotrigine, inositol, or risperidone. *Am. J. Psychiatry*, **163**, 210–216.

Paik, I.H., Lee, C.U., Lee, C. *et al.* (1995) Effects of risperidone in acute manic patients: an open clinical trial. *J. Korean Soc. Biol. Psychiatry*, **2**, 281–286.

Pavuluri, M.N., Henry, D.B., Carbray, J.A. *et al.* (2004) Open-label prospective trial of risperidone in combination with lithium or divalproex sodium in pediatric mania. *J. Affect. Disord.*, **82S**, S103–S111.

Perlis, R.H., Baker, R.W., Zarate, C.A. *et al.* (2006) Olanzapine versus risperidone in the treatment of manic or mixed states in bipolar I disorder: a randomized, double-blind trial. *J. Clin. Psychiatry*, **67**, 1747–1753.

Quiroz, J.A., Yatham, L.N., Palumbo, J.M. *et al.* (2010) Risperidone long-acting injectable monotherapy in the maintenance treatment of bipolar I disorder. *Biol. Psychiatry*, **68**, 156–162.

Ravindran, A., Silverstone, P., Lacroix, D. *et al.* (2004) Risperidone does not affect steady-state pharmacokinetics of divalproex sodium in patients with bipolar disorder. *Clin. Pharmacokinet.*, **43**, 733–740.

Sachs, G.S., Grossman, F., Ghaemi, S.N. *et al.* (2002) Combination of a mood stabilizer with risperidone or haloperidol for treatment of acute mania: a double-blind, placebo-controlled comparison of efficacy and safety. *Am. J. Psychiatry*, **159**, 1146–1154.

Sajatovic, M., DiGiovanni, S.K., Bastani, B. *et al.* (1996) Risperidone therapy in treatment refractory acute bipolar and schizoaffective mania. *Psychopharmacol. Bull.*, **32**, 55–61.

Sajatovic, M., Valenstein, M., Blow, F.C. *et al.* (2006) Treatment adherence with antipsychotic medications in bipolar disorder. *Bipolar Disord.*, **8**, 232–241.

Schaffer, C.B. and Schaffer, L.C. (1996) The use of risperidone in the treatment of bipolar disorder. *J. Clin. Psychiatry*, **57**, 136.

Segal, J., Berk, M., and Brook, S. (1998) Risperidone compared with both lithium and haloperidol in mania: a double-blind randomized controlled trial. *Clin. Neuropharmacol.*, **21**, 176–180.

Sheehan, D.V., McElroy, S.L., Harnett-Sheehan, K. *et al.* (2009) Randomized, placebo-controlled trial of risperidone for acute treatment of bipolar anxiety. *J. Affect. Disord.*, **115**, 376–385.

Shelton, R.C. and Stahl, S.M. (2004) Risperidone and paroxetine given singly and in combination for bipolar depression. *J. Clin. Psychiatry*, **65**, 1715–1719.

Smith, L.A., Cornelius, V., Warnock, A. *et al.* (2007) Effectiveness of mood stabilizers and antipsychotics in the maintenance phase of bipolar disorder: a systemic review of randomized controlled trials. *Bipolar Disord.*, **9**, 394–412.

Smulevich, A.B., Khanna, S., Eerdekens, M. *et al.* (2005) Acute and continuation risperidone monotherapy in bipolar mania: a 3-week placebo-controlled trial followed by a 9-week double-blind trial of risperidone and haloperidol. *Eur. Neuropsychophamacol.*, **15**, 75–84.

Spina, E., Avenoso, A., Facciolà, G. *et al.* (2000) Plasma concentrations of risperidone and 9-hydroxyrisperidone: effect of comedication with carbamazepine or valproate. *Ther. Drug Monit.*, **22**, 481–485.

Spina, E., Avenoso, A., Facciola, G. *et al.* (2001) Plasma concentrations of risperidone and 9-hydroxyrisperidone during combined treatment with paroxetine. *Ther. Drug Monit.*, **23**, 223–227.

Spina, E., D'Arrigo, C., Migliardi, G. *et al.* (2006) Effect of adjunctive lamotrigine treatment on the plasma concentrations of clozapine, risperidone and olanzapine in patients with schizophrenia or bipolar disorder. *Ther. Drug Monit.*, **28**, 599–602.

Suppes, T., Baldessarini, R.J., Faedda, G.L., and Tohen, M. (1991) Risk of recurrence following discontinuation of lithium treatment in bipolar disorder. *Arch. Gen. Psychiatry*, **48**, 1082–1088.

Tohen, M., Zarate, C.A., Centorrino, F. *et al.* (1996) Risperidone in the treatment of mania. *J. Clin. Psychiatry*, **57**, 249–253.

Vasile, D., Vasiliu, O., Ojog, D., and Gheorghe, M.D. (2006) Risperidone long acting im formulation in high risk of noncompliance bipolar patients. *Eur. Neuropsychopharmacol.*, **16** (Suppl. 4), S413–S414.

Vermeulen, A., Piotrovsky, V., and Ludwig, E.A. (2006) Population pharmacokinetics of risperidone and 9-hydroxyrisperidine in patients with acute episodes associated with bipolar I disorder. *J.Pharmacokin. Pharmacodyn.*, **34**, 183.

Vieta, E., Brugué, E., Goikolea, J.M. *et al.* (2004) Acute and continuation risperidone monotherapy in mania. *Hum. Psychopharmacol. Clin. Exp.*, **19**, 41–45.

Vieta, E., Gasto, C., Colom, F. *et al.* (1998) Treatment of refractory rapid cycling bipolar disorder with rhisperidone. *J. Clin. Psychopharmacol.*, **18**, 172–174.

Vieta, E., Gasto, C., Colom, F. *et al.* (2001) Role of risperidone in bipolar II: an open 6-month study. *J. Affect. Disord.*, **67**, 213–219.

Vieta, E., Herraiz, M., Parramon, G. *et al.* (2002) Risperidone in the treatment of mania: efficacy and safety results from a large multicentre, open study in Spain. *J. Affect. Disord.*, **72**, 15–19.

Vieta, E., Nieto, E., Autet, A. *et al.* (2008) A long-term prospective study on the outcome of bipolar patients treated with long-acting injectable risperidone. *World J. Biol. Psychiatry*, **9**, 219–224.

Vieta, E., Nuamah, I., Lim, P. *et al.* (2010) A randomized, placebo- and active-controlled study of paliperidone extended release for the treatment of acute manic and mixed episodes of bipolar I disorder. *Bipolar Disord.*, **12**, 230–243.

Yatham, L.N., Fallu, A., and Binder, C.E. (2007) A 6-month randomized open-label comparison of continuation of oral atypical antipsychotic therapy or switch to long acting injectable risperidone in patients with bipolar disorder. *Acta Psychiatr. Scand.*, **116** (Suppl. 434), 50–56.

Yatham, L.N., Grossman, F., Augustyns, I. *et al.* (2003) Mood stabilizers plus risperidone or placebo in the treatment of acute mania: international, double-blind, randomized controlled trial. *Br. J. Psychiatry*, **182**, 141–147.

10

Quetiapine in Bipolar Disorder

Mauricio Kunz[1], Svante Nyberg[2] and Lakshmi N. Yatham[3]

[1]University of British Columbia, Vancouver, Canada
[2]Neuroscience TA, AstraZeneca R&D, Södertälje, Sweden
[3]UBC Department of Psychiatry, UBC Hospital, The University
of British Columbia, Vancouver, Canada

10.1 INTRODUCTION

Quetiapine fumarate, marketed by AstraZeneca as **Seroquel** or **Seroquel XR**, is an atypical antipsychotic. It received its initial indication from the US Food and Drug Administration (FDA) for the treatment of schizophrenia in 1997. In 2004, it was approved for the treatment of bipolar mania and, based on more recent studies, quetiapine has also been approved by the FDA for the treatment of acute bipolar depression and for maintenance treatment and is now commonly used in the management of bipolar disorder. The CANMAT guidelines recommend quetiapine as one of the first-line agents in the pharmacological treatment of acute mania, acute bipolar depression, and maintenance pharmacotherapy in bipolar disorder (Yatham *et al.*, 2009).

10.2 PHARMACOLOGY

The pharmacological effects observed following treatment with quetiapine fumarate are thought to be mediated by quetiapine and its main, active human metabolite, norquetiapine (*N*-desalkylquetiapine) (Jensen *et al.*, 2008; Winter, Earley, and Hamer-Maansson, 2008). Pharmacokinetic data in adults show that quetiapine is rapidly absorbed after oral administration, with maximal plasma concentrations at 1–2 hours, and is eliminated with a mean terminal half-life of approximately 7 hours (DeVane and Nemeroff, 2001; Li *et al.*, 2004). Steady state is achieved within 48 hours. Pharmacokinetics are linear within the clinical dose range. Recently, an extended-release formulation with similar bioavailability but later Cmax and slower elimination has been developed, quetiapine XR (Datto *et al.*, 2009; Figueroa *et al.*, 2009). During steady-state conditions, patients treated with quetiapine fumarate have norquetiapine plasma concentrations within the same range as that of quetiapine (Winter, Earley, and Hamer-Maansson, 2008).

    Quetiapine has affinity at multiple neurotransmitter receptors in the brain, including serotonin $5HT_{1A}$, $5HT_{2A}$, and $5HT_{2C}$, dopamine D_1 and D_2, histamine H_1, and adrenergic

Bipolar Psychopharmacotherapy: Caring for the patient, Second Edition. Edited by Hagop S. Akiskal and Mauricio Tohen.
© 2011 John Wiley & Sons, Ltd. Published 2011 by John Wiley & Sons, Ltd.

alpha$_1$ and alpha$_2$ receptors. Interestingly, norquetiapine differs from quetiapine by displaying high affinity for the norepinephrine transporter (NET) and, relative to quetiapine, has higher affinity for several serotonin receptors including the 5HT$_{2C}$ and 5HT$_{1A}$ receptors (Jensen *et al.*, 2008). Both quetiapine and norquetiapine display partial agonism at the 5HT$_{1A}$ receptor, with similar activity.

Studies with positron emission tomography (PET) in patients treated with quetiapine have demonstrated high 5HT$_{2A}$ receptor occupancy throughout the clinical dose range (Kapur *et al.*, 2000). At the time of Cmax, there is moderate dopamine D$_2$ receptor occupancy, while at the end of the dosing interval occupancy is low (Mamo *et al.*, 2008). The antimanic activity of atypical antipsychotics has been repeatedly demonstrated, and is most likely related to their blockade or antagonism of D$_2$ receptors (Yatham *et al.*, 2005). As compared to typical and certain other atypical antipsychotics, the moderate, transient occupancy of D$_2$ receptors by quetiapine is consistent with the low frequency of extrapyramidal side-effects observed in quetiapine-treated patients. Moreover, quetiapine is one of the few medications of this class that has been shown to be effective in bipolar depression (Yatham, 2005). Although several mechanisms are likely to contribute to this broad range of clinical effects, NET inhibition is a distinguishing property not found in other atypical antipsychotics at clinically relevant doses. This view is further supported by the recent PET demonstration of moderate NET occupancy in subjects treated with quetiapine XR 300 mg/day (Nyberg *et al.*, 2008). This chapter reviews double-blind clinical trial data on the efficacy of quetiapine in acute mania, acute bipolar depression, and in continuation and maintenance treatment of bipolar disorder.

10.3   QUETIAPINE IN THE TREATMENT OF ACUTE MANIA

10.3.1   PLACEBO-CONTROLLED MONOTHERAPY STUDIES

The efficacy of quetiapine monotherapy was assessed in three clinical trials in patients with acute mania (Bowden *et al.*, 2005; McIntyre *et al.*, 2005; Cutler *et al.*, 2008; see Table 10.1). The entry criteria included a mania severity score of 20 or higher on the Young Mania Rating Scale (YMRS), and all studies excluded patients with substance abuse. Manic patients with psychotic features were included. All studies used changes in the YMRS score from baseline to the endpoint as the primary measure of efficacy. The studies were all of three weeks' duration; however, two of them also included a 9-week double-blind extension phase with the data analyzed at 12 weeks (Bowden *et al.*, 2005; McIntyre *et al.*, 2005). The third study was a three-week, randomized controlled trial of quetiapine XR, and the results of this study are currently available only in abstract form (Cutler *et al.*, 2008).

All studies showed that quetiapine was significantly superior to placebo in treating acute manic symptoms. The mean difference in the reduction of the primary efficacy measure of YMRS score between quetiapine and placebo in these studies ranged from −3.8 to −7.9 at three weeks, and from −8.0 to −11.3 at 12 weeks.

The earliest day at which a medication separates from placebo might indicate how quickly the medication works in treating manic symptoms. In these studies, a significant improvement over placebo was observed as early as day 4 with quetiapine (Vieta, Mullen, and Brecher, 2005; Cutler *et al.*, 2008) (Figure 10.1).

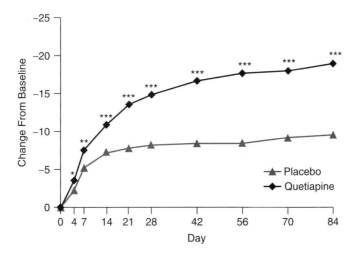

Figure 10.1 Quetiapine in the treatment of acute mania. Combined analysis of two placebo-controlled monotherapy studies (Bowden *et al.*, 2005; McIntyre *et al.*, 2005), showing change from baseline in mean YMRS score over time (LOCF, ITT population). *p < 0.05; **p < 0.01; *** p < 0.001 versus placebo.

From Vieta, Mullen, and Brecher (2005), with permission. Vieta, E., Mullen, J., Brecher. M., Paulsson, B., and Jones, M. Quetiapine monotherapy for mania associated with bipolar disorder: combined analysis of two international, double-blind, randomized, placebo-controlled studies. *Curr. Med. Res. Opin*. 2005, **21**, 923–934.

Response is typically defined as a 50% or greater reduction on the primary efficacy measure score or "much or very much improved" on the Clinical Global Impression-Improvement (CGI-I) Scale. The differences in response rates between the active agent and the placebo from each study should provide an estimate of true response to the medication. The placebo-corrected response rates for quetiapine on the YMRS ranged from 22 to 26% (Bowden *et al.*, 2005; McIntyre *et al.*, 2005; Cutler *et al.*, 2008).

Patients who meet criteria for response may still have significant manic symptoms, because response requires only a 50% reduction in rating scale scores. Remission should be the goal of therapy, but there is no consensus as to what constitutes remission and therefore remission rates may vary depending on the definition used. The quetiapine monotherapy studies used a score of 12 or lower on the YMRS to define remission. Using this definition, remission rates varied from 4 to 25% higher than placebo at week 3 and 23.4 and 35.5% higher at week 12 (Bowden *et al.*, 2005; McIntyre *et al.*, 2005). Remission rates with quetiapine XR monotherapy were 14% higher than placebo at three weeks of follow-up (Cutler *et al.*, 2008).

Patients with current mixed episodes were included in the quetiapine XR trial, but were excluded from the other trials. Nonetheless, all three studies found greater mean reductions in depressive scores in the quetiapine group than in the placebo group and the incidence of treatment-emergent depression was similar in the quetiapine and the placebo groups.

All studies included patients with and without psychotic features. In general, the results suggested that the magnitude of improvement in YMRS scores was similar in patients

Table 10.1 Randomized placebo-controlled trials of quetiapine in the treatment of acute mania.

Study	Study arms	Duration	YMRS change during treatment	Response/remission	Separation from placebo	MADRS change during treatment	Common side effects
McIntyre et al. (2005)	Quetiapine: N = 101 Range: 400–800 mg/d Mean modal dose: N/A Placebo: N = 100	3 wk 12 wk data also presented	Q: −12.3 P: −8.3 Q: −17.5 P: −9.5	Response: Q: 43% P: 35% Remission: Q: 28% P: 24% Response: Q: 61% P: 39% Remission: Q: 61% P: 38%	4 d	3 wk Q: −2.8 P: −0.9 12 wk Q = −3.3 P: −0.7 Treatment emergent depression: Q: 2.9% P: 8.9%	Discontinuation due to AE: Q: 5% P: 6% Weight change (12 wk): Q: 2.1 kg P: −0.1 kg Weight gain ≥ 7%: Q: 13% P: 4% EPS: Q: 13% P: 16% Other common: Somnolence
Bowden et al. (2005)	Quetiapine: N = 107 Range: 400–800 mg/d Mean last-week dose in responders: 3 wk:	3 wk	Q: −14.6 P: −6.7	Response: Q: 53% P: 27% Remission: Q: 47% P: 22%	7 d	3 wk: Q: −1.6 P: −0.1	Discontinuation due to AE: Q: 7% P: 4% Weight change (12 wk): Q: 2.6 kg P: −0.1 kg

Study	Drug/dose	Duration				Adverse effects
	586 mg/d 12 wk: 618 mg/d Placebo: N = 97	12 wk data also presented	Q: −20.3 P: −9.0	Response: Q: 72% P: 41% Remission: Q: 69% P: 34%	12 wk: Q: −1.5 P: 1.2 Treatment emergent depression: Q: 5.6% P: 8.4%	EPS: No different than P Other common: somnolence, dry mouth, dizziness
Cutler et al. (2008)	Quetiapine XR: N = 149 Range: 400–800 mg/d Mean dose: 604 mg/d Placebo: N = 159	3 wk	Q: −14.3 P: −10.5	Response Q: 55% P: 33% Remission: Q: 42% P: 28%	4 d Q: −4.4 P: −1.9	Discontinuation due to AE: Q: 3% P: 8% Weight change: Q: 1.3 kg P: 0.1 kg EPS: Q: 7% P: 4% Other common: somnolence, dry mouth, headache, constipation, dizziness

with and without psychotic features and was significantly greater than the improvement seen with placebo.

10.3.2   DOUBLE-BLIND ACTIVE COMPARATOR STUDIES

One of the previously mentioned studies included a three-week comparison of quetiapine with haloperidol, showing no significant differences in changes on the YMRS score or in response rates between the two medications (McIntyre *et al.*, 2005; see Table 10.2). The incidence of extrapyramidal symptoms (EPS) was higher in the haloperidol group. Quetiapine was also compared with lithium monotherapy, showing that quetiapine monotherapy appeared as effective as lithium in treating acute mania (Bowden *et al.*, 2005).

10.3.3   COMBINATION THERAPY STUDIES

The combination of an atypical antipsychotic and a mood stabilizer is commonly used in clinical practice, and studies suggest that up to 80% of patients receive combination therapy (Miller, Yatham, and Lam, 2001). Three different studies have compared the efficacy of quetiapine plus a mood stabilizer with a mood stabilizer plus placebo for treating acute mania (Sachs *et al.*, 2004; DelBello *et al.*, 2002; Yatham, Vieta, and Young, 2007; see Table 10.3).

One of the studies included a sample of adolescents (12–18 years) who were treated with either divalproex plus placebo or divalproex plus quetiapine for a period of three weeks (DelBello *et al.*, 2002). The other two studies used either lithium or divalproex as a mood stabilizer and had follow up periods of three weeks (Sachs *et al.*, 2004) and six weeks (Yatham, Vieta, and Young, 2007).

Two of the three studies showed that quetiapine plus mood stabilizer therapy was superior to placebo plus mood stabilizer (Sachs *et al.*, 2004; DelBello *et al.*, 2002) while the third study showed only numerical superiority (Yatham, Vieta, and Young, 2007). Further, not surprisingly, the combined analysis of two trials (Sachs *et al.*, 2004; Yatham, Vieta, and Young, 2007) showed that changes in YMRS scores were significantly greater in the combination-therapy group than in the mood stabilizer plus placebo group (Yatham *et al.*, 2004) (Figure 10.2). Mood stabilizer-corrected response rates to quetiapine plus mood stabilizer were on average about 20% (ranging from 7 to 34%) higher than with mood stabilizer plus placebo, indicating that the combination treatment provides a clinically meaningful increase in response rates. Overall, there is evidence that adding quetiapine to a mood stabilizer does provide additional benefit in treating acute manic symptoms.

Combination therapy was generally well tolerated; however, in all studies, side effects such as weight gain, somnolence, and headaches were more common with combination therapy than with mood stabilizer monotherapy.

10.3.4   REVIEWS AND POOLED ANALYSES

A pooled analysis of two monotherapy randomized controlled trials (n = 403) reported significantly higher remission rates with quetiapine at 3 and 12 weeks compared to

Table 10.2 Active-comparator trials of quetiapine in the treatment of acute mania.

Study	Study arms	Duration	YMRS change during treatment	Response/ remission rates	Separation from comparator	MADRS change during treatment	Common side effects
McIntyre et al. (2005)	Quetiapine: N = 101 Range: 400–800 mg/d Haloperidol: N = 98 Range: 2–8 mg/d Placebo: N = 100	3 wk	Q: −12.3 H: −15.7 P: −8.3	Response: Q: 43% H: 56% P: 35% Remission: Q: 28% H: 37% P: 24%	Q vs P: 4 d H vs P: 4 d H vs Q: 21 d	Q: −2.8 H: −2.3 P: −0.9	Discontinuation due to AE: Q: 5% H: 10% P: 6% Weight change (12 wk): Q: 2.1 kg H: 0.2 kg P: −0.1 kg Weight gain ≥7%: Q: 13% H: 5% P: 4% EPS: Q: 13% H: 60% P: 16% Other common: Q: somnolence H: tremor
		12 wk data also presented	Q: −17.5 H: −18.9 P: −9.5	Response: Q: 61% H: 70% P: 39% Remission: Q: 61% H: 63% P: 38%		Q: −3.3 H: −1.9 P: −0.7 Treatment emergent depression: Q: 2.9% H: 8.1% P: 8.9%	

(Continued Overleaf)

Table 10.2 (Continued)

Study	Treatment	Duration	Change	Response/Remission	Onset		Discontinuation
Bowden et al. (2005)	Quetiapine: N = 107	3 wk	Q: −14.6	Response:	Q vs P: Day 7	Q: −1.6	Discontinuation due to AE:
	Mean last week dose in responders:		L: −15.2	Q: 53%	L vs P: Day 7	L: N/R	Q: 7%
	3 wk: 586 mg/d		P: −6.7	L: 53%		P: −0.1	L: 6%
	12 wk: 618 mg/d			P: 27%			P: 4%
	Lithium: N = 98			Remission:			Weight change (12 weeks):
	Mean serum level:			Q: 47%			Q: 2.6 kg
	3 wk: 0.8 mEq/l			L: 49%			L: 0.7 kg
	12 wk: 0.8 mEq/l			P: 22%			P: −0.1 kg
	Placebo: N = 97	12 wk data also presented	Q: −20.3	Response:		Q: −1.5	EPS:
			L: −20.8	Q: 72%		L: −1.8	Q = L = P
			P: −9.0	L: 76%		P: 1.2	Other common:
				P: 41%		Treatment emergent depression:	Q: somnolence, dry mouth, dizziness
				Remission:		Q: 5.6%	L: tremor, insomnia, headache
				Q: 69%		L: 3.1%	
				L: 72%		P: 8.4%	
				P: 34%			

| DelBello et al. (2006) | 4 wk | Quetiapine: N = 25 Dose range: 400–600 mg/d Mean dose at endpoint: 412 mg/d Divalproex: N = 25 Mean serum level at endpoint: 101 µg/ml 96% had therapeutic serum level at endpoint | Change during treatment: Q: −23 D: −19 | Response (CGI-BP score ≤ 2) Q: 72% D: 40% Remission (YMRS score ≤ 12): Q: 60% D: 28% | No significant changes between treatments by endpoint | Change in Childhood Depression Rating Scale – Revised: Q: −21 D: −22 | Discontinuation due to AE: Q: 0% D: 0% Weight change: Q: 4.4 kg D: 3.6 kg Other common: Q: sedation, dizziness, GI upset, dry mouth D: sedation, dizziness, GI upset, insomnia |

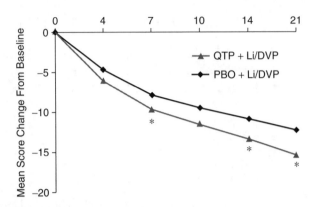

Figure 10.2 Adjunctive quetiapine in the treatment of acute mania. Combined analysis of two placebo-controlled add-on studies with lithium or divalproex (Sachs *et al.*, 2004; Yatham, Vieta, and Young, 2007), showing change from baseline in mean YMRS score over time (LOCF, ITT population). *p < 0.001 versus placebo; QTP, quetiapine; Li, lithium; DVP, divalproex.

From Yatham *et al.* (2004), with permission. Yatham, L.N., Paulsson, B., Mullen, J., and Vagero, A.M. Quetiapine versus placebo in combination with lithium or divalproex for the treatment of bipolar mania. *J. Clin. Psychopharmacol*. 2004, **24**, 599–606.

placebo (Ketter, Jones, and Paulsson, 2007). Similarly, a pooled analysis of two adjunctive therapy randomized controlled trials (n = 370) found significantly higher remission rates with adjunctive quetiapine at three weeks compared to lithium/divalproex alone (Sussman *et al.*, 2007). In addition, reviews of these data have confirmed that the efficacy of quetiapine was superior to placebo and at least comparable to lithium and haloperidol (Brahm, Gutierres, and Carnahan, 2007). Quetiapine was well tolerated, with most adverse events being mild to moderate and discontinuations for adverse events not significantly different from placebo (Adler *et al.*, 2007). Another *post hoc* pooled analysis compared the safety and efficacy of quetiapine in manic patients aged 55 years and older with younger patients, finding significant and similar improvements in symptomatology in both groups when compared to placebo. The most common adverse effects associated with active treatment in the older adults were dry mouth, somnolence, postural hypotension, insomnia, weight gain, and dizziness, while younger adults presented most commonly with dry mouth, somnolence, and insomnia (Sajatovic, Calabrese, and Mullen, 2008). Finally, the efficacy of quetiapine appeared to be independent of baseline disease severity, the presence of psychosis, and treatment-emergent sedation/somnolence (McIntyre *et al.*, 2007).

Two meta-analyses evaluating different treatments for acute mania confirm the efficacy of antipsychotics, lithium, and divalproex (Smith *et al.*, 2007a; Scherk, Pajonk, and Leucht, 2007). A meta-analysis of 13 randomized controlled trials (n = 3089) found that monotherapy with carbamazepine, haloperidol, lithium, olanzapine, quetiapine, risperidone, divalproex, and aripiprazole showed significant benefit compared with placebo for reduction in mania scores. Meta-analysis also found significant reductions in mania scores with adjunctive haloperidol, olanzapine, risperidone, and quetiapine compared

Table 10.3 Combination therapy studies of quetiapine in the treatment of acute mania.

Study	Study arms	Duration	YMRS change during treatment	Response/remission rates	Separation from comparator	Depression rating scale scores	Common side effects
Sachs et al. (2004)	Mood stabilizer+quetiapine (N=91) Dose range: 200–800 mg/d Mean endpoint dose: 504 mg/d Mean endpoint dose in responders: 584 mg/d Mood stabilizer+placebo (N=100)	3 wk	Q: -13.8 P: -10.0	Response: Q: 54% P: 33% Remission (YMRS ≤ 12): Q: 46% P: 26%	N/R	MADRS change during treatment: Q: -3.4 P: -2.8 Treatment emergent depression (MADRS score ≥ 18): Q: 17.3% P: 13.5%	Discontinuation due to AE: Q: 6% P: 6% Weight change: Q: 1.6 kg P: 0.4 kg Weight gain $\geq 7\%$: Q: 4% P: 1% EPS: Q = P Other common: somnolence, headache, dry mouth, asthenia, postural hypotension

(Continued Overleaf)

Table 10.3 (Continued)

Study	Study arms	Duration	YMRS change during treatment	Response/remission rates	Separation from comparator	Depression rating scale scores	Common side effects
Yatham, Vieta, and Young (2007)	Mood stabilizer + quetiapine Dose range: 200–800 mg/d Mean endpoint dose in responders: Day 21: 423 mg/d Day 42: 461 mg/d (N = 106) Mood stabilizer + placebo (N = 105)	3 wk 6 wk data also reported	Q: −15.2 P: −13.2 Q: −17.1 P: −14.3	Q: 57% response: P: 50% response: Remission (YMRS ≤ 12): Q: 51% P: 40% Response: Q: 72% P: 57% Remission: Q: 68% P: 57%	No significant differences between treatments at week 3 or week 6.	Treatment-emergent depression: Q: 6.6% P: 7.8% (Day 42)	Discontinuation due to AE: Q: 2.8% P: 5.8% Weight change: Day 21: Q: 1.6 kg P: 0.1 kg Day 42: Q: 2.2 kg P: 0.2 kg Weight gain ≥ 7%: Q: 21% P: 7% EPS: Q: 17.9% P: 28.2% Other common: somnolence, dry mouth, constipation

Study	Treatment	Duration	Baseline/Change	Response	Efficacy	Adverse events
DelBello et al. (2002)	Divalproex + quetiapine (N = 15) Dose: titrated to 450 mg/d (in all but one patient) Mean dose: 432 mg/d Divalproex + placebo (N = 15)	6 wk	Baseline: Q: N/R Change during treatment: Q: −24.5 P: −14.0 Difference: 10.5	Response: Q: 87% P: 53% Remission: N/R	Week 6 (separated from P at weeks 2 and 3 but not significantly different at weeks 4 and 5)	No difference between groups in change in Children's Depression Rating Scale scores at endpoint	Discontinuation due to AE: Q: 0% P: 0% Weight change: Q: 4.2 kg P: 2.5 kg EPS: Q = P Other common: sedation dry mouth

with lithium/divalproex alone (Smith *et al.*, 2007b). There were no differences in effect sizes between the various antimanic treatments. Another meta-analysis of 24 studies (n = 6187) found that atypical antipsychotics were significantly more efficacious than placebo (12 studies), and as effective as lithium/divalproex (five studies). For adjunctive atypical antipsychotics combined, the pooled difference in mean scores was 4.41. Response rates were significantly higher with combination therapy (relative risk 1.53) compared with lithium/divalproex alone. A meta-analysis of 24 studies (n = 6187) found that adding atypical antipsychotic agents to lithium/divalproex was significantly more effective than treatment with lithium/divalproex alone (six studies) for the treatment of acute mania (Scherk, Pajonk, and Leucht, 2007).

10.4 QUETIAPINE IN THE TREATMENT OF ACUTE BIPOLAR DEPRESSION

Bipolar patients experience depressive symptoms three times more commonly than mania (Judd *et al.*, 2002); however, only recently have studies focused attention on the use of atypical antipsychotics in the treatment of bipolar depression.

A total of five large randomized controlled trials have assessed the efficacy of quetiapine monotherapy in bipolar depression. Of these, four used quetiapine, that is, BOLDER I (Calabrese *et al.*, 2005), BOLDER II (Thase *et al.*, 2006), EMBOLDEN I (Young *et al.*, 2010) and EMBOLDEN II (McElroy *et al.*, 2010), and one used quetiapine XR (Suppes *et al.*, 2010) (see Table 10.4).

BOLDER I included both bipolar I (66.4%) and bipolar II (33.6%) depressed patients, who were randomly assigned to treatment with quetiapine 300 mg/day (n = 172), quetiapine 600 mg/day (n = 170), or placebo (n = 169) for eight weeks. Patients in the quetiapine groups were started on 50 mg/day and titrated upwards so that the target dose was reached by day 4 in the 300 mg group and by day 8 in the 600 mg group. Both quetiapine groups significantly separated from the placebo group on the primary efficacy measure of change in Montgomery-Asberg Depression Rating Scale (MADRS) score from week 1 to endpoint. Response rates were significantly greater for the quetiapine groups (58%) compared with the placebo group (36%). The incidence of treatment-emergent mania was similar in the three groups (2.2, 3.9, and 3.9%, respectively). Treatment-emergent adverse events, such as dry mouth, sedation, somnolence, and dizziness, were more common in both quetiapine groups than in the placebo groups, but no differences in EPS or sexual adverse events were observed among the groups (Calabrese *et al.*, 2005).

BOLDER II confirmed these results with a similar design and a sample of 509 patients (bipolar I and II), of whom 59% completed the study. Improvements from baseline in mean MADRS total score were significantly greater with quetiapine 300 mg/day and 600 mg/day than with placebo from week 1 through week 8. Improvements in mean Hamilton Rating Scale for Depression (HAM-D) scores were also significantly greater with both quetiapine doses than with placebo as early as week 1 and throughout the study. The MADRS response and remission rates were also significantly greater in both quetiapine dose groups. Improvements in

Table 10.4 Randomized controlled trials of quetiapine in the treatment of acute bipolar depression.

Study	Study arms	Duration	MADRS scores	Separation from comparator	Response/ remission rates	Treatment-emergent mania	Side effects
Calabrese et al. (2005)	Quetiapine 300 mg/d: N = 172 Quetiapine 600 mg/d: N = 170 Placebo: 169 (BDI and BDII)	8 wk	Baseline: Q300 mg: 30.4 Q600 mg: 30.3 P: 30.6 Change during treatment: Q300 mg: −16.4 Q600 mg: −16.7 P: −10.3 Difference vs P: Q300 mg: 6.1 Q600 mg: 6.5	Q300 mg: week 1 Q600 mg: week 1	Response: Q300 mg: 57.6% Q600 mg: 58.2% P: 36.1% Remission: Q300 mg: 52.9% Q600 mg: 52.9% P: 28.4%	Q300 mg: 3.9% Q600 mg: 2.2% P: 3.9%	Weight gain: Q300 mg: 1.0 kg Q600 mg: 1.6 kg P: 0.2 kg Weight gain ≥ 7% Q300 mg: 8.5% Q600 mg: 9.0% P: 1.7% Sedation, somnolence, dry mouth, dizziness, constipation significantly more common in both QTP groups.

(Continued Overleaf)

Table 10.4 (Continued)

Study	Study arms	Duration	MADRS scores	Separation from comparator	Response/ remission rates	Treatment- emergent mania	Side effects
Thase et al. (2006)	Quetiapine 300 mg/d: N = 155 Quetiapine 600 mg/d: N = 151 Placebo: N = 161 (BDI and BDII)	8 wk	Baseline: Q300 mg: 31.1 Q600 mg: 29.9 P: 29.6 Change during treatment: Q300 mg: −16.9 Q600 mg: −16.9 P: −11.9 Difference vs P: Q300 mg: 5.0 Q600 mg: 4.0	Q300 mg: week 1 Q600 mg: week 1	Response: Q300 mg: 60.0% Q600 mg: 58.3% P: 44.7% Remission: Q300 mg: 51.6% Q600 mg: 52.3% P: 37.3%	Q300 mg: 1.8% Q600 mg: 3.6% P: 6.6%	Weight gain: Q300 mg: 1.4 kg Q600 mg: 1.3 kg P: 0.3 kg Sedation, somnolence, dry mouth, dizziness, constipation more common in both QTP groups.
Young et al. (2010)	Quetiapine 300 mg/d: N = 265 Quetiapine 600 mg/d: N = 268 Lithium: N = 136 Mean median	8 wk	Baseline: Q300 mg: 28.1 Q600 mg: 28.3 L: 28.5 P: 28.2 Change during treatment: Q300 mg: −15.4	Q300 mg: week 1 Q600 mg: week 1 L: did not separate	Response: Q300 mg: 69% Q600 mg: 70% L: 63% P: 56% Remission: Q300 mg:	Q300 mg: 4% Q600 mg: 2% L: 1% P: 2%	Weight gain: Q300 mg: 0.6 kg Q600 mg: 0.8 kg L: 0.2 kg P: −0.7 kg Weight gain ≥ 7%: Q300 mg: 5% Q600 mg: 8% L: 2%

Study	Duration					Adverse effects
dose: 981 mg/d Mean serum level: 0.61 mEq/l Placebo: N=133 (BDI and BDII)		Q600 mg: −16.1 L: −13.6 P: −11.8 Difference vs P: Q300 mg: 3.6 Q600 mg: 4.3 L: 1.8	70% Q600 mg: 70% L: 63% P: 55%			P: 3% EPS: Q300 mg: 5% Q600 mg: 8% L: 8% P: 4% Sedation, somnolence, dry mouth, dizziness, constipation more common in both QTP groups
McElroy et al. (2010) Quetiapine 300 mg/d: N=229 Quetiapine 600 mg/d: N=232 Paroxetine 20 mg/d: N=118 Placebo: N=121 (BDI and BDII)	8 wk	Baseline: Q300 mg: 27.1 Q600 mg: 26.5 PAR: 27.3 P: 27.2 Change during treatment: Q300 mg: −16.2 Q600 mg: −16.3 PAR: −13.8 P: −12.6 Difference vs P: Q300 mg: 3.6 Q600 mg: 3.7 PAR: 1.2	Q300 mg: week 2 Q600 mg: week 2 PAR: did not separate	Response: Q300 mg: 67% Q600 mg: 67% PAR: 55% P: 53% Remission: Q300 mg: 65% Q600 mg: 69% PAR: 57% P: 55%	Q300 mg: 2% Q600 mg: 4% PAR: 11% P: 9%	Weight gain: Q300 mg: 1.1 kg Q600 mg: 1.7 kg PAR: −0.3 kg P: 0.5 kg Weight gain $\geq$ 7%: Q300 mg: 9% Q600 mg: 11% PAR: 3% P: 4% EPS: Q300 mg: 8% Q600 mg: 10% PAR: 4% P: 2% Sedation, somnolence, dry mouth, dizziness, constipation more common in both QTP groups.

(Continued Overleaf)

Table 10.4 (Continued)

Study	Study arms	Duration	MADRS scores	Separation from comparator	Response/ remission rates	Treatment- emergent mania	Side effects
Suppes *et al.* (2010)	Quetiapine XR 300 mg/d: N = 133 Placebo: N = 137 (BDI and BDII)	8 wk	Baseline: Q: 29.8 P: 30.1 Change during treatment: Q: −17.4 P: −11.9 Difference vs P: 5.5	Week 1	Response: Q: 65.4% P: 43.1% Remission: Q: 54.1% P: 39.4%	Q: 4.4% P: 6.4%	Weight gain: Q: 1.3 kg P: −0.2 kg Weight gain ≥ 7%: Q: 8.2% P: 0.8% EPS: Q: 4.4% P: 0.7% Dry mouth somnolence, sedation, increased appetite more common in QTP arm

primary and secondary outcomes showed no major differences between the two doses. The incidence of treatment-emergent mania or hypomania was lower with quetiapine treatment than placebo. Common adverse events included dry mouth, sedation, somnolence, dizziness, and constipation (Thase *et al.*, 2006).

Combined analysis of the BOLDER I and II trials supported the significant improvements in MADRS total score with both quetiapine doses compared with placebo (Weisler *et al.*, 2008) (Figure 10.3). A secondary analysis of BOLDER I and II focusing on measures of quality of life Quality of Life Enjoyment and Satisfaction Questionnaire – Short Form (Q-LES-Q SF), sleep (Pittsburgh Sleep Quality Index), and disability (Sheehan Disability Scale) showed that quetiapine monotherapy is also effective in improving these measures in addition to improving depressive symptoms (Endicott *et al.*, 2008). Another *post-hoc* analysis of these two studies confirmed the effectiveness of monotherapy with quetiapine for depressive episodes in bipolar I disorder when compared with placebo (Weisler *et al.*, 2008).

EMBOLDEN I compared quetiapine and lithium with placebo in 802 patients with bipolar depression, and EMBOLDEN II compared quetiapine and paroxetine with placebo in 740 patients, with acute assessment of efficacy at eight weeks. In EMBOLDEN I, quetiapine (300 or 600 mg/day) was significantly more effective than placebo on the primary efficacy measure of change in MADRS total score as well as response and remission rates, but lithium was not more effective than placebo (Young *et al.*, 2010). The mean serum lithium level in this study was only 0.6 mEq/l, which may not have been therapeutic for alleviating depressive symptoms; however, a *post hoc* analysis of

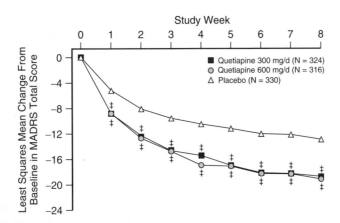

Figure 10.3 Quetiapine in the treatment of acute bipolar I and II depression. Combined analysis of two placebo-controlled monotherapy (BOLDER) studies, showing change from baseline in mean MADRS score over time. ‡p < 0.001 versus placebo.

From Weisler *et al.* (2008), with permission. Weisler, R.H., Calabrese, J.R., Thase, M.E., Arvekvist, R., Stening, G., Paulsson, B., and Suppes, T. Efficacy of quetiapine monotherapy for the treatment of depressive episodes in bipolar I disorder: a post hoc analysis of combined results from two double-blind, randomized, placebo-controlled studies. *J. Clin. Psychiatry*. 2008, **69**, 769–782.

the lithium treatment group, in which patients with median serum lithium concentrations ≥ 0.8 mEq/l were analyzed separately (n = 34; ITT population), revealed no difference from placebo in terms of the improvement in MADRS total score from baseline (difference of -2.76 points at week 8; P = 0.128).

In EMBOLDEN II, the improvements in MADRS score and response rate for quetiapine (both doses) were significantly greater than placebo, but paroxetine was not more effective than placebo (McElroy *et al.*, 2010). Remission rates were significantly greater with quetiapine 600 mg/day, but not for quetiapine 300 mg/day or paroxetine treatment, compared with placebo. It is unclear if a higher dose of paroxetine (greater than 20 mg/day) would have been effective, as patients in this study were treated with a fixed dose of 20 mg/day. Both trials also showed significant improvements in score on MADRS item 10 (suicidal thoughts) with quetiapine versus placebo.

Data from an eight-week randomized controlled trial assessing quetiapine XR monotherapy in 270 patients with bipolar I or bipolar II depression (Suppes *et al.*, 2010) showed significantly greater improvement in depressive symptoms from week 1 compared with placebo, which was maintained to study end.

10.4.1   BIPOLAR II DEPRESSION

The four previously cited randomized controlled trials included substantial numbers of patients with bipolar II depression: BOLDER I (n = 182) and II (n = 171) and EMBOLDEN I (n = 303) and II (n = 262). In patients with bipolar II depression in BOLDER I and EMBOLDEN I, improvements in MADRS total score in the quetiapine group were numerically but not statistically significantly greater at endpoint (week 8), although they were significant at various weekly visits. In contrast, in the BOLDER II and EMBOLDEN II trials, the quetiapine group showed significant benefits in patients with bipolar II depression relative to the placebo group. In addition, a post hoc pooled analysis of the patients with bipolar II depression from both BOLDER trials (n = 351) found that both doses of quetiapine demonstrated significant benefits as early as week 1, which were sustained throughout the eight weeks (Suppes *et al.*, 2008). Two sub-analyses of the BOLDER I data showed that, among patients with bipolar II depression, quetiapine was effective in patients with rapid cycling (Vieta *et al.*, 2007), but anxiety scores (Hamilton Rating Scale for Anxiety; HAM-A) were not significantly improved (Hirschfeld *et al.*, 2006). However, in the pooled analysis of BOLDER I and II, the changes in HAM-D, HAM-A, and CGI were significantly greater for both quetiapine groups versus placebo, and quetiapine 600 mg/day was effective in both rapid and non-rapid cycling depression (Suppes *et al.*, 2008). Although quetiapine is recommended as a first-line option for the acute treatment of bipolar II depression (Yatham *et al.*, 2009), extensive long-term data are not yet available. In a pooled analysis from the EMBOLDEN I and EMBOLDEN II trials for the maintenance treatment of bipolar II depression, quetiapine at 300 and 600 mg/day significantly reduced the risk of recurrence of any mood event (hazard ratio 0.47 and 0.18, respectively) or a depressive event (0.35 and 0.21, respectively) compared with placebo (p $\leq$ 0.05) (Young, Calabrese, and Gustafsson, 2009b).

10.5 QUETIAPINE IN THE MAINTENANCE TREATMENT OF BIPOLAR DISORDER

Five recent randomized controlled trials have demonstrated the efficacy of quetiapine alone or in combination with lithium/divalproex for maintenance therapy in bipolar disorder (Young *et al.*, 2008; McElroy *et al.*, 2008; Nolen *et al.*, 2009; Vieta *et al.*, 2008; Suppes *et al.*, 2009; Brecher, Anderson, and Paulsson, 2008) (see Table 10.5). In these studies, patients in remission after acute quetiapine treatment were randomized to continue quetiapine or switch to placebo maintenance therapy with the primary endpoint being the time to recurrence of any mood event.

10.5.1 MONOTHERAPY STUDIES

Two studies, EMBOLDEN I and II, assessed quetiapine monotherapy in patients in remission after eight weeks of double-blind treatment for acute bipolar depression. Pooled and individually, the EMBOLDEN studies demonstrated that the acute efficacy of quetiapine in bipolar depression was maintained in continuation treatment for 26–52 weeks compared with placebo (Olausson, Young, and McElroy, 2008; Young *et al.*, 2008; McElroy *et al.*, 2008). In the pooled analysis, recurrence of a mood event was observed in 24.5% (71/290) of patients in the quetiapine group and 40.5% (119/294) of patients in the placebo group. The risk of recurrence of any mood event (hazard ratio 0.51, $p < 0.001$) or a depression event (hazard ratio 0.43, $p < 0.001$) was significantly lower with quetiapine than placebo. Time to recurrence of a mania/hypomania event did not reach significance (hazard ratio 0.75) (Olausson, Young, and McElroy, 2008).

A recent 104-week randomized controlled trial compared the efficacy of quetiapine, lithium, or placebo monotherapy in patients who were stable for at least four weeks following up to 24 weeks of quetiapine therapy. The study was stopped after a planned interim analysis (~56 weeks) revealed statistically significant benefits. Quetiapine was significantly more effective than placebo in reducing the risk of any mood event (hazard ratio 0.29), including both manic (hazard ratio 0.29) and depressive episodes (hazard ratio 0.30) or any episode ($p < 0.001$) (Nolen *et al.*, 2009). The significant effect of quetiapine was observed independently of the pole of the index episode. Lithium was also more effective than placebo on all three measures. In addition, quetiapine was more effective than lithium for prevention of any event or depressive events, but the two therapies were similar for prevention of manic events. However, the mean serum lithium level in the study group was only 0.6 mEq/l.

10.5.2 ADJUNCTIVE THERAPY STUDIES

Two randomized controlled trials have assessed the efficacy of adjunctive quetiapine maintenance therapy (Trials 126 and 127: Vieta *et al.*, 2008; Suppes *et al.*, 2009). Patients were randomized to quetiapine or placebo added to mood stabilizing treatment with lithium or divalproex after achieving at least 12 weeks remission with open-label quetiapine plus lithium or divalproex (Vieta *et al.*, 2008; Suppes *et al.*, 2009). Individually and pooled, these studies demonstrated that quetiapine in combination with lithium or

Table 10.5 Randomized controlled trials of quetiapine in the maintenance treatment of bipolar disorder.

Study	Study arms	Design	Sample	% with relapse	% discontinuing trial for any reason	Median time to discontinuation	Side effects
Nolen et al. (2009)	Quetiapine: N = 404 Dose range: 300–800 mg/d Mean median dose: 546 mg/d Lithium: N = 364 Dose range: 600–1800 mg/d Mean median serum level: 0.63 mEq/l Placebo: N = 404	104 wk	Patients in remission (YMRS ≤ 12 and MADRS ≤ 12 for at least 4 wk) from a recent manic, mixed, or depressed episode that was treated with open-label quetiapine 300–800 mg/d	Hazard ratio: Any mood episode: Q vs P: 0.29 L vs P: 0.46 Q vs L: 0.66 Manic episode: Q vs P: 0.29 L vs P: 0.37 Q vs L: 0.78 Depressive episode: Q vs P: 0.30 L vs P: 0.59 Q vs L: 0.54 NB-only hazard ratios, and not percentages experiencing relapse, were reported	N/R	N/R	Weight gain: Q: 1.7 kg (open-label phase) Q: 0.6 kg (double-blind phase) L: −0.9 kg (double-blind phase) P: −1.5 kg (double-blind phase) Weight gain ≥ 7%: Q: 17% (open-label phase) Q: 11% (double-blind phase) L: 5% (double-blind phase) P: 3% (double-blind phase) EPS: Q: 9% (open-label phase) Q: 4% (double-blind phase) L: 9% (double-blind phase)

Study	Intervention	Duration	Inclusion criteria	Outcome			Adverse effects
							P: 5% (double-blind phase) Somnolence more common with QTP Headache, nausea, tremor, vomiting more common with Li
Vieta *et al.* (2008)	Quetiapine+ mood stabilizer: Dose range: 400–800 mg/d N = 336 Mean median dose: 497 mg/d Placebo+ mood stabilizer: N = 367	104 wk	Patients in remission (YMRS ≤ 12 and MADRS ≤ 12 for at least 12 wk) from a recent manic, mixed or depressed episode that was treated with open-label quetiapine 400–800 mg/d and lithium or divalproex for ≥ 12 wk	Any mood episode: Q: 19% P: 49% Manic episode: Q: 11% P: 26% Depressive episode: Q: 8% P: 23%	Q: 62% P: 80%	N/R	Weight gain: Q: 2.9 kg (open-label phase) Q: 0.5 kg (double-blind phase) P: −1.9 kg (double-blind phase) Weight gain ≥ 7%: Q: 24% (open-label phase) Q: 7% (double-blind phase) P: 2% (double-blind phase) EPS: Q: 11% (open-label phase) Q: 5% (double-blind phase) P: 5% (double-blind phase) Somnolence more common with QTP

(Continued Overleaf)

Table 10.5 (Continued)

Study	Study arms	Design	Sample	% with relapse	% discontinuing trial for any reason	Median time to discontinuation	Side effects
Suppes et al. (2009)	Quetiapine + mood stabilizer: N=310 Dose range: 400–800 mg/d Mean median dose: 519 mg/d Placebo + mood stabilizer: N=313	104 wk	Patients in remission (YMRS ≤ 12 and MADRS ≤ 12 for at least 12 wk) from a recent manic, mixed, or depressed episode that was treated with open-label quetiapine 400–800 mg/d and lithium or divalproex for ≥ 12 wk	Any mood episode: Q: 20% P: 52% Manic episode: Q: 7% P: 19% Depressive episode: Q: 13% P: 33%	Q: 81% P: 86%	N/R	Weight gain: Q: 3.1 kg (open-label phase): Q: 0.5 kg (double-blind phase) P: −2.0 kg (double-blind phase) Weight gain ≥ 7%: Q: 23% (open-label phase) Q: 12% (double-blind phase) P: 4% (double-blind phase) EPS: Q: 16% (open-label phase) Q: 11% (double-blind phase) P: 10% (double-blind phase) Somnolence and hypothyroidism more common with QTP

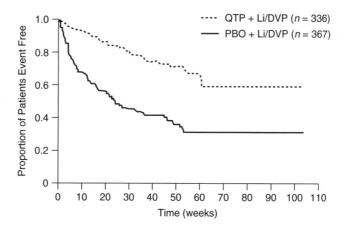

Figure 10.4 Adjunctive quetiapine in the maintenance treatment of bipolar I and II disorder. Time to recurrence of a mood event in Trial 126 (Kaplan-Meier curves). QTP, quetiapine; Li, lithium; DVP, divalproex.

From Vieta *et al.* (2008), with permission. Vieta E, Suppes T, Eggens I, *et al.* Efficacy and safety of quetiapine in combination with lithium or divalproex for maintenance of patients with bipolar I disorder (international trial 126). *J Affect Disord* 2008, **109**, 251–263.

divalproex was significantly more effective than lithium or divalproex alone in the prevention of both manic and depressive mood episodes during continuation treatment for up to 104 weeks (Figure 10.4). The significant effect of quetiapine was observed independent of the pole of the index episode (Brecher, Anderson, and Paulsson, 2008; Vieta *et al.*, 2008; Suppes *et al.*, 2009), with rates of relapse for any mood episode being 19 and 20% for quetiapine and 49 and 52% for placebo.

10.6   SAFETY AND TOLERABILITY OF QUETIAPINE

Quetiapine demonstrates a consistent safety and tolerability profile in adult studies of bipolar mania and bipolar depression. The most commonly reported adverse effects associated with quetiapine and quetiapine XR in these studies include somnolence, dry mouth, constipation, headache, and dizziness (as summarized in the U.S. Seroquel Prescribing Information, 2010, which also includes warnings and precautions relating to the use of quetiapine).

A review of the studies in acute mania concluded that quetiapine is well tolerated, with most adverse events mild to moderate in intensity (Adler *et al.*, 2007). In the acute monotherapy studies of up to 12 weeks' duration (to 800 mg/day), rates of adverse event-related discontinuations were 5.7% in the pooled quetiapine group versus 5.1% with placebo (Vieta, Mullen, and Brecher, 2005). Rates of EPS associated with quetiapine and placebo were 12.9 and 13.1%, respectively (Vieta, Mullen, and Brecher, 2005). In the three-week study of quetiapine XR (400–800 mg/day), rates of adverse event-related discontinuations in the quetiapine and placebo groups were 2.6 and 7.5%, respectively, while EPS rates were 6.6% versus 3.8% (Cutler *et al.*, 2008).

Quetiapine offers a large evidence base for the evaluation of safety and tolerability in bipolar depression (Bogart and Chavez, 2009). In the eight-week studies of quetiapine monotherapy (pooled BOLDER and EMBOLDEN data), discontinuations due to treatment-emergent adverse events were 10.8 and 15.5% in quetiapine 300 mg/day and 600 mg/day-treated patients, respectively, compared to 6.3% with placebo (Young et al., 2009a). Rates of EPS-related events were 8.8 and 9.8% in patients treated with quetiapine 300 and 600 mg, respectively, versus 4.5% with placebo. With quetiapine XR (300 mg/day), adverse event-related discontinuations were 12.1% versus 1.7% with placebo, and EPS rates were 4.4% versus 0.7% (Suppes et al., 2009).

The maintenance studies of quetiapine (as monotherapy or combined with a mood stabilizer) included treatment periods of up to 104 weeks following stabilization on acute treatment (Olausson, Young, and McElroy, 2008; Nolen et al., 2009; Vieta et al., 2008; Suppes et al., 2010). The pattern of treatment-emergent adverse events in the continuation phases of maintenance monotherapy studies was generally in line with that observed in the acute phases. In pooled analyses of the EMBOLDEN studies of bipolar depression, overall rates of discontinuation due to adverse events were 4.3% with quetiapine 300 mg/day, 4.0% with quetiapine 600 mg/day, and 1.7% with placebo (Olausson, Young, and McElroy, 2008). The incidence of treatment-emergent events potentially related to EPS was 2.1, 3.3, and 2.0% for quetiapine 300 mg/day, quetiapine 600 mg/day, and placebo, respectively. In the quetiapine monotherapy study including both patients with bipolar mania and bipolar depression, adverse events led to discontinuation in 3.5% of the quetiapine group versus 3.2% with placebo (Nolen et al., 2009). EPS-related adverse event rates were at 4.0 and 4.5% in the quetiapine and placebo groups, respectively. In the adjunctive studies of quetiapine for maintenance therapy in bipolar I disorder (Vieta et al., 2008; Suppes et al., 2009), a pooled analysis reported that rates of discontinuation associated with adverse events were 4.5% in the quetiapine plus lithium or divalproex group versus 2.6% in the placebo plus lithium or divalproex group during the randomized treatment phase (Brecher, Anderson, and Paulsson, 2008). Adverse events potentially associated with EPS were reported by 7.9% of patients receiving quetiapine plus lithium or divalproex and by 6.9% receiving lithium or divalproex alone.

As noted in the CANMAT guidelines (Yatham et al., 2009), risks for metabolic effects associated with individual agents remain, in general, poorly defined. A number of analyses have been published for quetiapine. Pooled analysis of the acute quetiapine studies identified a mean weight gain of 1.8 kg for quetiapine monotherapy versus 0.1 kg for placebo in mania, and a mean weight gain of 1.2 kg versus no weight change in bipolar depression (Newcomer et al., 2009). In long-term studies, quetiapine was associated with a mean weight gain of 0.5 kg, compared with a loss of 1.6 kg with placebo from the point of randomization (Newcomer et al., 2009). Pooled analyses of metabolic parameters in acute quetiapine studies across indications (~10 000 patients) identified differences in glucose regulation parameters between quetiapine and placebo of 1.39 mg/dl for glucose and 0.04% units for HbA_{1C}. The overall difference in total cholesterol was 5.48 mg/dl, with differences in high- and low-density lipoprotein (HDL and LDL) cholesterol of -0.62 and 1.69 mg/dl, respectively. The difference in change in triglycerides was 22.62 mg/dl (Newcomer et al., 2009).

In conclusion, acute and long-term studies demonstrate that quetiapine and quetiapine XR are generally well tolerated, with a well-characterized safety and tolerability profile in patients with bipolar mania and bipolar depression.

10.7 SUMMARY

The available data from randomized controlled trials demonstrate that quetiapine is clearly superior to placebo in the treatment of all phases of bipolar disorder. Evidence indicates that quetiapine, either as a monotherapy or in combination with mood stabilizer, is effective in the treatment of bipolar mania, with the combination more effective than a mood stabilizer alone in the management of manic episodes. Meta-analyses evaluating different treatments for acute mania suggest that quetiapine has similar efficacy to that of mood stabilizing medications and other antipsychotics. Quetiapine has the largest evidence base for efficacy in bipolar depression, where evidence for other treatments is mixed. Quetiapine is the only agent with evidence in bipolar I and bipolar II patient sub-groups and is the only atypical antipsychotic indicated in monotherapy for the treatment of bipolar depression. Long-term efficacy data for most atypicals is limited to patients with a manic/mixed index episode, whereas quetiapine has been shown to be effective at preventing mood event recurrence (manic/depressed) in patients with bipolar disorder irrespective of index episode (manic/mixed/depressed). Taken together, this evidence makes quetiapine one of the most versatile medications for the treatment of bipolar disorder.

References

Adler, C.M., Fleck, D.E., Brecher, M. *et al.* (2007) Safety and tolerability of quetiapine in the treatment of acute mania in bipolar disorder. *J. Affect. Disord.*, **100** (Suppl. 1), S15–S22.

Bogart, G.T. and Chavez, B. (2009) Safety and efficacy of quetiapine in bipolar depression. *Ann. Pharmacother.*, **43**, 1848–1856.

Bowden, C., Grunze, H., Mullen, J. *et al.* (2005) A randomized double blind placebo controlled efficacy and safety study of quetiapine or lithium as monotherapy for mania in bipolar disorder. *J. Clin. Psychiatry*, **66**, 111–121.

Brahm, N.C., Gutierres, S.L., and Carnahan, R.M. (2007) Quetiapine for acute mania in bipolar disorder. *Am. J. Health Syst. Pharm.*, **64**, 1045–1053.

Brecher, M., Anderson, R., and Paulsson, B. (2008) Quetiapine in the maintenance treatment of bipolar I disorder: combined data from two long-term, phase III studies (T126+127). *Int. J. Neuropsychopharmacol.*, **11** (Suppl. S1), 185–186.

Calabrese, J.R., Keck, P.E. Jr., Macfadden, W. *et al.* (2005) A randomized, double-blind, placebo-controlled trial of quetiapine in the treatment of bipolar I or II depression. *Am. J. Psychiatry*, **162**, 1351–1360.

Cutler, A., Earley, W., Datto, D. *et al.* (2008) Effectiveness of extended-release formulation of quetiapine as monotherapy for the treatment of acute bipolar mania (Trial D144CC00004) (Bipolar XR T004). *Int. J. Neuropsychopharmacol.*, **11** (Suppl. S1), 184–185.

Datto, C., Berggren, L., Patel, J.B. *et al.* (2009) Self-reported sedation profile of immediate-release quetiapine fumarate compared with extended-release quetiapine fumarate during dose initiation: a randomized, double-blind, crossover study in healthy adult subjects. *Clin. Ther.*, **31**, 492–502.

DelBello, M.P., Kowatch, R.A., Adler, C.M. *et al.* (2006) A double-blind randomized pilot study comparing quetiapine and divalproex for adolescent mania. *J. Am. Acad. Child Adolesc. Psychiatry*, **45**, 305–313.

DelBello, M., Schwiers, M., Rosenberg, H. *et al.* (2002) A double-blind, randomized, placebo-controlled study of quetiapine as adjunctive treatment for adolescent mania. *J. Am. Acad. Child Adolesc. Psychiatry*, **41**, 1216–1223.

DeVane, C.L. and Nemeroff, C.B. (2001) Clinical pharmacokinetics of quetiapine: an atypical antipsychotic. *Clin. Pharmacokinet.*, **40**, 509–522.

Endicott, J., Paulsson, B., Gustafsson, U. *et al.* (2008) Quetiapine monotherapy in the treatment of depressive episodes of bipolar I and II disorder: improvements in quality of life and quality of sleep. *J. Affect. Disord.*, **111**, 306–319.

Figueroa, C., Brecher, M., Hamer-Maansson, J. *et al.* (2009) Pharmacokinetic profiles of extended release quetiapine fumarate compared with quetiapine immediate release. *Prog. Neuropsychopharmacol. Biol. Psychiatry*, **33**, 199–204.

Hirschfeld, R.M., Weisler, R.H., Raines, S.R., *et al.* for the BOLDER Study Group (2006) Quetiapine in the treatment of anxiety in patients with bipolar I or II depression: a secondary analysis from a randomized, double-blind, placebo-controlled study. *J. Clin. Psychiatry*, **67**, 355–362.

Jensen, N.H., Rodriguiz, R.M., Caron, M.G. *et al.* (2008) N-Desalkylquetiapine, a potent norepinephrine reuptake inhibitor and partial 5-HT$_{1A}$ agonist, as a putative mediator of quetiapine's antidepressant activity. *Neuropsychopharmacology*, **33**, 2303–2312.

Judd, L.L., Akiskal, H.S., Schettler, P.J. *et al.* (2002) The long-term natural history of the weekly symptomatic status of bipolar I disorder. *Arch. Gen. Psychiatry*, **59**, 530–537.

Kapur, S., Zipursky, R., Jones, C. *et al.* (2000) A positron emission tomography study of quetiapine in schizophrenia: a preliminary finding of an antipsychotic effect with only transiently high dopamine D2 receptor occupancy. *Arch. Gen. Psychiatry*, **57**, 553–559.

Ketter, T.A., Jones, M., and Paulsson, B. (2007) Rates of remission/euthymia with quetiapine monotherapy compared with placebo in patients with acute mania. *J. Affect. Disord.*, **100** (Suppl. 1), S45–S53.

Li, K.Y., Li, X., Cheng, Z.N. *et al.* (2004) Multiple dose pharmacokinetics of quetiapine and some of its metabolites in Chinese suffering from schizophrenia. *Acta. Pharmacol. Sin.*, **25**, 390–394.

Mamo, D.C., Uchida, H., Vitcu, I. *et al.* (2008) Quetiapine extended-release versus immediate-release formulation: a positron emission tomography study. *J. Clin. Psychiatry*, **69**, 81–86.

McElroy, S.L., Olausson, B., Chang, W. *et al.* (2008) A double-blind, placebo-controlled study with acute and continuation phase of quetiapine in adults with bipolar depression (EMBOLDEN II). *Bipolar Disord.*, **10** (Suppl. 1), 59.

McElroy, S.L., Weisler, R.H., Chang, W., *et al.* for the EMBOLDEN II (Trial D1447C00134) Investigators (2010) A double-blind, placebo-controlled study of quetiapine and paroxetine as monotherapy in adults with bipolar depression (EMBOLDEN II). *J. Clin. Psychiatry*, **71**, 163–174.

McIntyre, R.S., Brecher, M., Paulsson, B. *et al.* (2005) Quetiapine or haloperidol as monotherapy for bipolar mania – a 12-week, double-blind, randomised, parallel-group, placebo-controlled trial. *Eur. Neuropsychopharmacol.*, **15**, 573–585.

McIntyre, R.S., Konarski, J.Z., Jones, M. *et al.* (2007) Quetiapine in the treatment of acute bipolar mania: efficacy across a broad range of symptoms. *J. Affect. Disord.*, **100** (Suppl. 1), S5–S14.

Miller, D.S., Yatham, L.N., and Lam, R.W. (2001) Comparative efficacy of typical and atypical antipsychotics as add-on therapy to mood stabilizers in the treatment of acute mania. *J. Clin. Psychiatry*, **62**, 975–980.

Newcomer, J., Ratner, R.E., Ala, H. *et al.* (2009) A review of metabolic parameters in quetiapine studies across diagnoses. *Eur. Psychiatry*, **24** (Suppl. 1), P03–P15.

Nolen, W.A., Weisler, R.H., Neijber, A. *et al.* (2009) Quetiapine or lithium versus placebo for maintenance treatment of bipolar I disorder after stabilization on quetiapine. *Eur. Psychiatry*, **24** (Suppl. 1), P01–207.

Nyberg, S., Takano, A., Jucaite, A. *et al.* (2008) PET-measured occupancy of the norepinephrine transporter by extended release quetiapine fumarate (quetiapine XR) in brains of healthy subjects. *Eur. Neuropsychopharmacol.*, **18** (Suppl. 4), S270 (Abstract P.1.e.019).

Olausson, B., Young, A.H., and McElroy, S.L. (2008) Quetiapine monotherapy up to 52 weeks in patients with bipolar depression: continuation phase data from the EMBOLDEN I and II studies (EMBOLDEN continuation). Poster presented at the Institute on Psychiatric Services, October 2, Chicago, IL.

Sachs, G., Chengappa, K., Suppes, T. *et al.* (2004) Quetiapine with lithium or divalproex for the treatment of bipolar mania: a randomized, double-blind, placebo-controlled study. *Bipolar Disord.*, **6**, 213–223.

Sajatovic, M., Calabrese, J.R., and Mullen, J. (2008) Quetiapine for the treatment of bipolar mania in older adults. *Bipolar Disord.*, **10**, 662–671.

Scherk, H., Pajonk, F.G., and Leucht, S. (2007) Second-generation antipsychotic agents in the treatment of acute mania: a systematic review and meta-analysis of randomized controlled trials. *Arch. Gen. Psychiatry*, **64**, 442–455.

Smith, L.A., Cornelius, V., Warnock, A. *et al.* (2007a) Pharmacological interventions for acute bipolar mania: a systematic review of randomized placebo controlled trials. *Bipolar Disord.*, **9**, 551–560.

Smith, L.A., Cornelius, V., Warnock, A. *et al.* (2007b) Acute bipolar mania: a systematic review and metaanalysis of co-therapy vs monotherapy. *Acta. Psychiatr. Scand.*, **115**, 12–20.

Suppes, T., Datto, C., Minkwitz, M. *et al.* (2010) Effectiveness of the extended release formulation of quetiapine as monotherapy for the treatment of acute bipolar depression. *J. Affect. Disord.*, **121**, 106–115.

Suppes, T., Hirschfeld, R.M., Vieta, E. *et al.* (2008) Quetiapine for the treatment of bipolar II depression: analysis of data from two randomized, double-blind, placebo-controlled studies. *World J. Biol. Psychiatry*, **9**, 198–211.

Suppes, T., Vieta, E., Liu, S. *et al.* (2009) Maintenance treatment for patients with bipolar I disorder: results from a North American study of quetiapine in combination with lithium or divalproex (trial 127). *Am. J. Psychiatry*, **166**, 476–488.

Sussman, N., Mullen, J., Paulsson, B. *et al.* (2007) Rates of remission/euthymia with quetiapine in combination with lithium/divalproex for the treatment of acute mania. *J. Affect. Disord.*, **100** (Suppl. 1), S55–S63.

Thase, M.E., Macfadden, W., Weisler, R.H. *et al.* (2006) Efficacy of quetiapine monotherapy in bipolar I and II depression: a double-blind, placebo-controlled study (the BOLDER II study). *J. Clin. Psychopharmacol.*, **26**, 600–609.

U.S. Seroquel Prescribing Information Available at http://www1.astrazeneca-us.com/pi/Seroquel.pdf and http://www1.astrazeneca-us.com/pi/seroquelxr.pdf (accessed 23 April 2010).

Vieta, E., Calabrese, J.R., Goikolea, J.M. *et al.* (2007) Quetiapine monotherapy in the treatment of patients with bipolar I or II depression and a rapidcycling disease course: a randomized, double-blind, placebo-controlled study. *Bipolar Disord.*, **9**, 413–425.

Vieta, E., Mullen, J., Brecher, M. *et al.* (2005) Quetiapine monotherapy for mania associated with bipolar disorder: combined analysis of two international, double-blind, randomised, placebo-controlled studies. *Curr. Med. Res. Opin.*, **21**, 923–934.

Vieta, E., Suppes, T., Eggens, I. *et al.* (2008) Efficacy and safety of quetiapine in combination with lithium or divalproex for maintenance of patients with bipolar I disorder (international trial 126). *J. Affect. Disord.*, **109**, 251–263.

Weisler, R.H., Calabrese, J.R., Thase, M.E. *et al.* (2008) Efficacy of quetiapine monotherapy for the treatment of depressive episodes in bipolar I disorder: a post hoc analysis of combined results from 2 double-blind, randomized, placebo-controlled studies. *J. Clin. Psychiatry*, **69**, 769–782.

Winter, H.R., Earley, W.R., Hamer-Maansson, J.E. *et al.* (2008) Steady-state pharmacokinetic, safety, and tolerability profiles of quetiapine, norquetiapine, and other quetiapine metabolites in pediatric and adult patients with psychotic disorders. *J. Child Adolesc. Psychopharmacol.*, **18**, 81–98.

Yatham, L.N. (2005) Atypical antipsychotics for bipolar disorder. *Psychiatr. Clin. N. Am.*, **28**, 325–347.

Yatham, L.N., Goldstein, J.M., Vieta, E. *et al.* (2005) Atypical antipsychotics in bipolar depression: potential mechanisms of action. *J. Clin. Psychiatry*, **66** (Suppl. 5), 40–48.

Yatham, L.N., Kennedy, S.H., Schaffer, A. *et al.* (2009) Canadian Network for Mood and Anxiety Treatments (CANMAT) and International Society for Bipolar Disorders (ISBD) collaborative update of CANMAT guidelines for the management of patients with bipolar disorder: update 2009. *Bipolar Disord.*, **11**, 225–255.

Yatham, L.N., Paulsson, B., Mullen, J. *et al.* (2004) Quetiapine versus placebo in combination with lithium or divalproex for the treatment of bipolar mania. *J. Clin. Psychopharmacol.*, **24**, 599–606.

Yatham, L.N., Vieta, E., and Young, A.H. (2007) A double blind, randomized, placebo-controlled trial of quetiapine as an add-on therapy to lithium or divalproex for the treatment of bipolar mania. *Int. Clin. Psychopharmacol.*, **22**, 212–220.

Young, A.H., Calabrese, J.R., Gustafsson, U. *et al.* (2009a) The efficacy of quetiapine monotherapy in bipolar depression: combined data from the BOLDER and EMBOLDEN studies. *Bipolar Disord.*, **11** (Suppl. 1), 14–95.

Young, A.H., Calabrese, J.R., and Gustafsson, U. (2009b) The efficacy of quetiapine monotherapy in bipolar II depression: combined data from the BOLDER and EMBOLDEN studies. Poster presented at the 162nd Annual Meeting of the American Psychiatric Association, May 16–21, San Francisco, CA.

Young, A.H., McElroy, S.L., Bauer, M. *et al.* (2010) A double-blind, placebo-controlled study of quetiapine and lithium monotherapy in adults in the acute phase of bipolar depression (EMBOLDEN I). *J. Clin. Psychiatry*, **71**, 150–162.

Young, A.H., McElroy, S.L., Chang, W. *et al.* (2008) A double-blind, placebo-controlled study with acute and continuation phase of quetiapine in adults with bipolar depression (EMBOLDEN I). *Bipolar Disord.*, **10** (Suppl. 1), 1–29.

11

Ziprasidone in the Treatment of Bipolar Disorder

Thomas L. Schwartz[1], Stephen M. Stahl[2,3], Elizabeth Pappadopulos[4,5] and Onur N. Karayal[5]

[1]Treatment Resistant Depression and Anxiety Disorders Program, SUNY Upstate Medical University, Syracuse, NY, USA
[2]Department of Psychiatry, University of California-San Diego, CA, USA
[3]Department of Psychiatry, University of Cambridge, UK
[4]Department of Psychiatry Research, Zucker Hillside Hospital, Glen Oaks, NY, USA
[5]Pfizer Inc., New York, NY, USA

11.1 INTRODUCTION

Ziprasidone is considered to be an *atypical antipsychotic*, or a *second generation antipsychotic* (SGA). As such, it shares the familiar SGA pharmacodynamic profile being an antagonist at dopamine D2 and serotonin 5HT2 receptors. Perhaps being labeled as an *antipsychotic* is a bit limiting as this agent is also approved for the treatment of certain bipolar disorder symptoms as well. Likewise, many of the SGAs are now known and approved for treating illness outside of schizophrenia. This paper will investigate the proposed mechanism of action of ziprasidone, its clinical indications, the evidence-base supporting its use, and finally how it is most effectively and safely used in treating the bipolar population.

11.2 ZIPRASIDONE AND ITS PROPOSED MECHANISM OF ACTION

Ziprasidone is a second generation antipsychotic (SGA), that is, a benzothiazolylpiperazine derivative, developed by Pfizer Inc. and was first approved by the US Food and Drug Administration (FDA) in 2001 for the treatment of schizophrenia, and subsequently for acute manic or mixed manic states, and as adjunctive maintenance treatment of bipolar disorder when added to lithium or valproate-treated patients. Finally an intramuscular preparation was approved for acute agitation in schizophrenia as well (Ziprasidone Package Insert, Pfizer Inc.).

Bipolar Psychopharmacotherapy: Caring for the patient, Second Edition. Edited by Hagop S. Akiskal and Mauricio Tohen.
© 2011 John Wiley & Sons, Ltd. Published 2011 by John Wiley & Sons, Ltd.

Ziprasidone's pharmacologic mechanism of action is unique among the SGAs due to complex receptor mediated actions and a pharmacodynamic profile that further distinguishes it from other SGAs (Stahl and Shayegan, 2003; Kim, Maneen, and Stahl, 2009). It is a dopamine (DA) D2 receptor antagonist similar to most other SGAs and all first generation *typical* antipsychotics (FGAs) (Stahl, 2008, 2009; Stahl and Mignon, 2010). Ziprasidone has a high affinity for blocking the D2 receptor (Ki = 4.8) (Ziprasidone Package Insert, Pfizer Inc; Schmidt *et al*., 2001; Stahl and Shayegan, 2003; Shayegan and Stahl, 2004), and this DA transmission dampening property lends itself to lowering manic symptoms. This is also the well-known mechanism for alleviating psychotic symptoms (Stahl, 2008). Further pharmacodynamic consideration would include ziprasidone's high affinity ability to block serotonin (5HT) 5-HT2A receptors (Ki = 0.4) (Ziprasidone Package Insert, Pfizer Inc; Stahl and Shayegan, 2003; Shayegan and Stahl, 2004). Classically this feature is thought to make the atypical drugs *atypical* in that they have remarkably lower extrapyramidal syndrome (EPS) adverse effect rates than the FGA class. The 5HT2A receptor antagonism allows for more selective anti-manic dampening of DA transmission in the mesolimbic system while allowing better DA transmission to progress through the nigrastriatal pathway and thus minimizes EPS. Ziprasidone's 5HT2A receptor antagonism may also dampen glutamate (GLU) cortical hyperactivity as a mechanism to lower manic symptoms as well (Stahl, 2008). These key mechanisms theoretically should allow for a clinical reduction in psychosis or mania and also help to diminish EPS rates. This dual mechanism is common to the SGA class (see Figure 11.1).

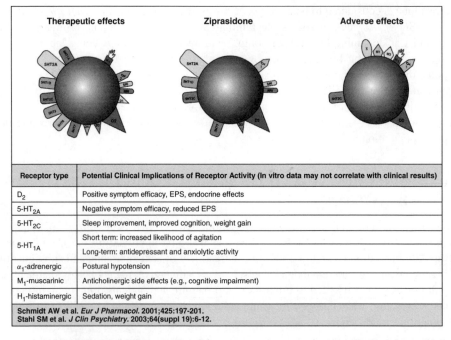

Receptor type	Potential Clinical Implications of Receptor Activity (In vitro data may not correlate with clinical results)
D_2	Positive symptom efficacy, EPS, endocrine effects
5-HT$_{2A}$	Negative symptom efficacy, reduced EPS
5-HT$_{2C}$	Sleep improvement, improved cognition, weight gain
5-HT$_{1A}$	Short term: increased likelihood of agitation
	Long-term: antidepressant and anxiolytic activity
α_1-adrenergic	Postural hypotension
M$_1$-muscarinic	Anticholinergic side effects (e.g., cognitive impairment)
H$_1$-histaminergic	Sedation, weight gain

Schmidt AW et al. *Eur J Pharmacol*. 2001;425:197-201.
Stahl SM et al. *J Clin Psychiatry*. 2003;64(suppl 19):6-12.

Figure 11.1 Schematic representation of the receptors involved in both the therapeutic and adverse effects of antipsychotics. Ziprasidone (middle) is shown for reference.

To look a bit further and more theoretically, ziprasidone has other noteworthy pharmacodynamic properties which lend to its unique clinical profile. It has little to no affinity for histamine H1 receptor blockade and has a low rate of sedation and weight gain as such (Ki = 47 nM: Ziprasidone Package Insert, Pfizer Inc; Schmidt _et al._, 2001; Stahl and Shayegan, 2003; Shayegan and Stahl, 2004). This may lend to the product's reputation for being a more metabolically friendly drug (Stahl, 2008). Outside of 5HT2A receptor antagonism, ziprasidone also blocks the 5HT2C receptor (Ki = 1.3 nM: Ziprasidone Package Insert, Pfizer Inc; Schmidt _et al._, 2001; Stahl and Shayegan, 2003; Shayegan and Stahl, 2004) and this property, in theory, may promote improved DA and norepinephrine (NE) transmission to the dorsolateral prefrontal cortex (DLPFC). The implications of this improved monoamine transmission might lend pro-cognitive and antidepressant activity to ziprasidone, but this has not been proven yet clinically. This drug has remarkable 5HT1D receptor antagonism (Ki = 2 nM) (Ziprasidone Package Insert, Pfizer Inc; Schmidt _et al._, 2001; Stahl and Shayegan, 2003; Shayegan and Stahl, 2004) which may be associated with antidepressant properties, as 5-HT1D blockade would be expected to increase serotonergic transmission (Stamford _et al._, 2000). Ziprasidone is furthermore a 5HT1A partial receptor agonist (Ki = 3.4 nM) (Ziprasidone Package Insert, Pfizer Inc; Schmidt _et al._, 2001; Stahl and Shayegan, 2003; Shayegan and Stahl, 2004), similar to the anxiolytic buspirone. Finally, this drug has some ability to block 5HT and NE transporter reuptake pumps in a manner similar to the antidepressant selective serotonin-norepinephrine reuptake inhibitors (SNRIs) lending support to potential clinical antidepressant and anxiolytic properties, neither of which have been proven via regulatory trials as of yet.

As far as adverse effects are concerned, the low H1 receptor antagonism predicts generally low amounts of sedation, and weak NE alpha1 receptor antagonism may promote some lightheadedness. Ziprasidone has no significant affinity for muscarinic cholinergic receptors and therefore is not known for anticholinergic effects such as dry mouth, blurred vision, constipation, and tachycardia (Ziprasidone Package Insert, Pfizer Inc). In summary, ziprasidone's pharmacodynamic properties are associated with proven ability to treat both psychosis and mania with the theoretical potential application to treat cognition, depression, and anxiety. From a tolerability standpoint, ziprasidone has relatively low EPS and very low metabolic syndrome rates, with mild risk of sedation and orthostasis. Adverse events are fully covered in Section 11.9 of this chapter.

11.3 ZIPRASIDONE IN TREATMENT GUIDELINES

Treatment guidelines are often compiled by a group of expert researchers, clinicians, and statisticians and are used to help steer clinicians toward more evidence based practices. The idea is to standardize care and provide clinicians and patients with bona fide, well tested treatment options. Some guidelines will also make reasonable pharmacologic treatment suggestions if there is a lack of data, or if off-label prescribing applications can be supported.

Ziprasidone fits clearly into treatment guidelines for schizophrenia and bipolar disorder.

Given that this chapter focuses on bipolar disorder, we will concentrate on guidelines for this disease state in particular.

The American Psychiatric Association (APA, 2002) has published a second edition set of guidelines regarding the treatment of bipolar patients which is now outdated. A third edition is due out in short order (Practice Guideline for the Treatment of Patients with Bipolar Disorder). This work group starts their guidelines with the clear mandate to make an accurate diagnosis, to develop rapport with the patient, and to provide for patient safety. Secondarily, the APA treatment guidelines for bipolar disorder suggest that acute management of mania or mixed features should take on a high clinical priority given morbidity and mortality risks. These guidelines were compiled and authored before an evidence base of ziprasidone data existed. The current APA treatment guidelines for bipolar disorder state:

- The first-line pharmacological treatment for more severe manic or mixed episodes is the initiation of either lithium plus an antipsychotic or valproate plus an antipsychotic.
- For less ill patients, monotherapy with lithium, valproate, or an antipsychotic such as olanzapine may be sufficient.
- Short-term adjunctive treatment with a benzodiazepine may also be helpful.
- For mixed episodes, valproate may be preferred over lithium.
- Atypical antipsychotics are preferred over typical antipsychotics because of their more benign side effect profile, with most of the evidence supporting the use of olanzapine or risperidone.
- Alternatives include carbamazepine or oxcarbazepine in lieu of lithium or valproate.
- Antidepressants should be tapered and discontinued if possible.
- If psychosocial therapy approaches are used, they should be combined with pharmacotherapy.
- For patients who, despite receiving maintenance medication treatment, experience a manic or mixed episode (that is, a "breakthrough" episode), the first-line intervention should be to optimize the medication dose.
- Introduction or resumption of an antipsychotic is sometimes necessary.
- Severely ill or agitated patients may also require short-term adjunctive treatment with a benzodiazepine.
- When first-line medication treatment at optimal doses fails to control symptoms, recommended treatment options include addition of another first-line medication.
- Alternative treatment options include adding carbamazepine or oxcarbazepine in lieu of an additional first line medication, adding an antipsychotic if not already prescribed, or changing from one antipsychotic to another.
- Clozapine may be particularly effective in the treatment of refractory illness.
- Electroconvulsive therapy (ECT) may also be considered for patients with severe or treatment-resistant mania . . .
- Manic or mixed episodes with psychotic features usually require treatment with an antipsychotic medication.

These guidelines are now considered out of date as much new evidence and several new drugs have been introduced in the past eight years since the latest APA treatment guidelines were published in 2002. Ziprasidone is mentioned seven times in its text. For acute mania, ziprasidone is listed in an *alternative* options section with less supporting evidence and suggests it could be used in lieu of another antipsychotic and carbamazepine or oxcarbazepine in lieu of lithium or valproate. At the time of these guidelines there was only one large regulatory study for ziprasidone and mania so its evidence base was considered reasonable, but weak compared to the already FDA approved olanzapine (Sachs, 2001). The guidelines placed ziprasidone also in the group of agents which are promising but would require further study. A similar set of guidelines, *Clinical Practice Guidelines for Bipolar Disorder from the Department of Veterans Affairs*, is also now outdated and was compiled before the SGAs were FDA approved and mention very little about SGA use overall (Bauer *et al.*, 1999).

In 2004, Keck *et al.* (2004) issued another set of guidelines. Here SGAs could be used as an alternative first line treatment for classic acute mania, mixed mania, or manic psychosis. Ziprasidone was clearly placed in the alternate category as it had just received its FDA approvals for bipolar mania. At the time of this publication, SGAs were limited to psychotic bipolar depression and none were noted to be warranted for nonpsychotic bipolar depression except for the olanzapine-fluoxetine combination as an alternative antidepressant strategy. However, the experts here ranked ziprasidone very highly for antidepressant potential compared to other SGAs. For long term maintenance, ziprasidone was also listed as an alternative due to an absence of data available at the time of this 2004 publication.

In 2006 the Royal Society of Psychiatry in the UK suggested guidelines where ziprasidone was noted to be well within the norm of clinical use (Ferrier *et al.*, 2006). They note that several atypical antipsychotics indicated superiority over placebo (aripiprazole, olanzapine, quetiapine, risperidone, ziprasidone) and equivalent efficacy to haloperidol (aripiprazole, olanzapine, quetiapine, risperidone, ziprasidone), lithium, and valproate in the treatment of mania. The addition of several atypical antipsychotics to either valproate or lithium in patients with partially treated mania has been shown also to be more effective than continuing treatment with valproate or lithium alone.

In 2009 the British Association for Psychopharmacology published their revised guidelines (Goodwin, 2009). They state that SGA should be used for moderate to severe acute mania or mixed mania due to their relatively benign acute side effect profile and their rapidity of onset of clinical action. Ziprasidone monotherapy is advocated positively in these guidelines for this situation. For bipolar depression, the SGAs should be added if psychosis is present but there is little mention of using SGA as antidepressant monotherapy.

The Canadian guidelines also were revised in 2009 (Yatham *et al.*, 2009). Ziprasidone is listed as a first line anti-manic agent, comparable to lithium, divalproex, and other SGAs. It is not listed as a bipolar depression treatment due to absence of data. Ziprasidone is also noted to be used in long term, adjunctive maintenance. In pediatric populations, the guidelines comment on a four week ziprasidone study and gave this data and use a moderate strength label comparable to olanzapine, quetiapine, risperidone, and aripiprazole. In bipolar II depressives, ziprasidone is listed as a clear third line agent given the lesser data available.

The World Federation of Societies of Biological Psychiatry (WFSBP) updated in 2009 their guidelines for the biological treatment of bipolar disorders as well (Grunze *et al.*, 2009). They comment on three ziprasidone trials showing antimanic effectiveness versus placebo, but also comment that an active comparator, haloperidol was more effective at times. Post hoc analyses suggested that ziprasidone was effective for dysphoric, mixed mania as well (Stahl *et al.*, 2009). Ziprasidone was shown to be effective on some secondary measures for long term adjunctive treatment to lithium or valproate as well. EPS syndromes were noted to be minimal with side effects of sedation and dizziness being prominent. QTc intervals were noted to increase 11 ms on average but never above 500 ms. Ziprasidone was noted to be weight and likely metabolically friendly compared to other SGAs.

11.4 OVERVIEW OF ZIPRASIDONE EFFICACY FROM CLINICAL TRIAL DATA

A number of clinical trials have examined the efficacy of ziprasidone as either monotherapy or an adjunctive therapy in the treatment of bipolar disorder.

The efficacy of ziprasidone as monotherapy in bipolar disorder has been established on the basis of two double-blind placebo-controlled trials and open-label extension studies. Initial demonstration of efficacy in bipolar mania stems from two paired studies in which ziprasidone, after an initial titration period, was administered for a three-week period (40–80 mg, twice daily with meals). Controls received placebo in the same dose regimen. Efficacy was assessed on the basis of decreases in the Mania Rating Scale (MRS) score from baseline. In the first of these studies (Keck *et al.*, 2003), ziprasidone was found to decrease MRS scores significantly as soon as two days after initiation of treatment, an effect which persisted throughout the treatment period. There were significant differences between ziprasidone and placebo groups in CGI-S and Positive and Negative Symptoms Scale (PANSS) scores from day 4 onwards and in Global Assessment of Functioning (GAF) from day 7 onwards.

The replication study (Potkin *et al.*, 2005), using a virtually identical protocol, found comparable decreases in MRS scores, again with separation between ziprasidone and placebo at two days. There were also significant differences at endpoint between ziprasidone and placebo groups on CGI S, CGI I, Montgomery-Asberg Depression Rating Scale (MADRS), Hamilton Rating Scale for Depression (HAM-D), and PANSS scores. A small eight-week open trial of ziprasidone effectiveness in pediatric bipolar disorder found ziprasidone treatment associated with clinically and statistically significant improvement in mean YMRS scores and CGI-I at endpoint (Biederman *et al.*, 2007).

A recent paper (Keck *et al.*, 2009) has addressed long-term efficacy in bipolar disorder. In this open extension trial, with ziprasidone dosing between 40 and 160 mg per day, improvements in efficacy measures (MRS and CGI) observed in the initial double-blind trial were sustained over the course of 52 weeks. When subdivided by diagnosis (manic or mixed presentation) or by the presence or absence of psychotic symptoms, there were no significant differences between groups.

Two more recent double-blind placebo-controlled studies have examined the efficacy of flexibly dosed ziprasidone against the symptoms of bipolar depression in bipolar disorder patients. Despite the duration of six weeks, neither study demonstrated significant efficacy against depressive symptoms, as measured on the MADRS scale (Lombardo *et al.*, 2010). Possible explanations included true inefficacy, rater inconsistency, and baseline score inflation.

A small number of studies have examined the effects of ziprasidone used as an adjunct therapy to mood stabilizers (valproate, lithium, lamotrigine) in the treatment of bipolar disorder. In one (Sachs *et al.*, 2010a), a six week double-blind placebo-controlled trial of adjunctive ziprasidone or placebo in addition to mood stabilizer in the treatment of bipolar depression failed to detect any significant difference on MADRS scores after six weeks. A second trial (Sachs *et al.*, 2010b), a three-week double-blind placebo-controlled trial of adjunctive ziprasidone in bipolar mania, also failed to detect differences between ziprasidone and placebo on YMRS scores at endpoint. In both cases, methodological considerations were thought to account for the trial failures. A more extensive and thorough discussion of these individual studies will occur in the next sections.

11.5 ACUTE MANIC/MIXED EPISODES

11.5.1 RANDOMIZED CLINICAL TRIALS OF ZIPRASIDONE MONOTHERAPY VERSUS PLACEBO IN MANIC/MIXED EPISODES

As mentioned above, ziprasidone monotherapy has been principally examined in two double-blind placebo-controlled trials and a single 12 week active comparator trial involving haloperidol (Vieta *et al.*, 2010) (See Figure 11.2).

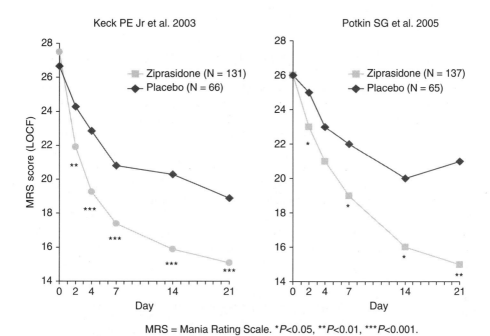

MRS = Mania Rating Scale. *$P<0.05$, **$P<0.01$, ***$P<0.001$.

Figure 11.2 Ziprasidone demonstrates significant efficacy vs placebo in acute mania by day 2, following early titration.

The first study recruited patients from 21 sites in the US and a further three in Brazil, resulting in a total patient cohort of 210 inpatients each with a primary diagnosis of bipolar I disorder and a current manic or mixed episode. Patients with comorbid schizophrenia or schizoaffective disorder were excluded from the trial, as were patients who presented with a depressed episode of bipolar disorder. The principal inclusion criteria was an MRS total score of >14, and a score of >2 on at least four sub-items. Patients were randomized to ziprasidone or placebo in a $2:1$ ratio. Efficacy was established on the basis of change in mean MRS scores and CGI scales.

Ziprasidone dosage averaged 139.1 mg per day in the first week after completion of titration, and 130.1 mg per day in the second week. A total of 36/70 patients in the placebo group and 87/140 in the ziprasidone group completed more than 14 days of treatment.

Ziprasidone produced a significantly greater reduction in MRS score (12.4 ± 12.0), compared with those who received placebo (7.8 ± 12.9). Separation between ziprasidone and placebo groups was detectable by day 2 and were sustained throughout the treatment period. Moreover there were more responders (defined as subjects in which MRS scores decreased by $\geq 50\%$ from baseline) in the ziprasidone arm (50%) than in the placebo group (35%, $P < 0.05$).

The second study (Potkin et al., 2005) followed essentially the same protocol, and recruited 202 patients on a two to one ziprasidone to placebo randomization. Comparable reductions in MRS score from baseline to endpoint (11.12 ± 11.46 and 5.62 ± 0.64: ziprasidone and placebo respectively) were observed. Again there were significantly more MRS responders in the ziprasidone group (46%) than in the placebo group (29%, $P < 0.05$).

Pooled analysis of these two studies was conducted to compare efficacy in patients presenting with either manic or mixed episodes. A second analysis compared efficacy in psychotic and nonpsychotic patients. In patients presenting with mixed episodes, ziprasidone significantly improved MRS scores relative to placebo with significant separation detectable as early as day 2 of treatment. These results were similar to those seen in manic episodes. Efficacy in psychotic and nonpsychotic patients showed some differences. In the nonpsychotic group ziprasidone subjects showed significantly greater improvement than placebo from day 2 onwards. In the psychotic group, separation between ziprasidone and placebo was significant only on days 4 and 14. The smaller number of psychotic patients analyzed (73) compared with nonpsychotic patients (324) may account in part for this.

A third study (Vieta et al., 2010) compared ziprasidone with placebo and haloperidol in the treatment of manic episodes of bipolar one disorder. The study lasted three weeks, after which all placebo patients were switched to ziprasidone. In this large study (438 patients), ziprasidone showed significantly greater reduction in MRS score at three weeks compared with placebo.

11.5.2   OTHER STUDIES ON ZIPRASIDONE TREATMENT IN MANIC/MIXED EPISODES

The Keck et al. (2003) study, following completion of the double-blind phase, was extended into a long-term (52-week) open-label extension phase which continued to monitor MRS and CGI scores. Reductions in MRS scores observed during the double-blind phase were sustained throughout the open-label period. Moreover there were significant reductions in MRS score in mixed, manic, psychotic, and nonpsychotic patients relative to baseline in the core study.

11.5.3 ZIPRASIDONE RANDOMIZED CLINICAL TRIALS OF ADJUNCT TREATMENT IN MANIC/MIXED EPISODES

Two recent Pfizer sponsored studies have examined the effects of ziprasidone as an adjunct treatment to mood stabilizers in subjects with bipolar disorder. The first of these examined effectiveness in acute mania. In this three week study ziprasidone was used at two dose levels as an adjunct therapy to lithium or divalproex. Control patients received placebo and their mood stabilizer. Of 680 subjects randomized, 656 were treated and 580 subjects completed the study. Discontinuations were highest in the high-dose ziprasidone group (26.7%) and lowest in the placebo group (17.1%). The study found no significant difference between the ziprasidone groups and placebo in YMRS change at three weeks, the primary outcome measure. Issues related to recruiting validity may have compromised the study (Sachs *et al.*, 2010b).

A second study in which ziprasidone was used as an adjunct to lithium, valproate, or lamotrigine treatment over six weeks in a randomized double blind multicenter controlled trial also evaluated bipolar I depression (discussed below).

11.6 ACUTE DEPRESSIVE EPISODES

11.6.1 RANDOMIZED CLINICAL TRIALS ON ZIPRASIDONE MONOTHERAPY AND DEPRESSIVE EPISODES

Two recent studies by Pfizer, both randomized, double-blind, placebo-controlled six-week studies, recently failed, indicating that either ziprasidone is ineffective in this patient cohort or that methodological issues confounded the result (Lombardo *et al.*, 2010).

Adult outpatients with bipolar depression, indicated by a total score on the HAM-D 17 scale of over 20, were randomized to receive either a low dose of ziprasidone, a higher dose, or placebo for six weeks. Outcomes were assessed on the MADRS scale. Both studies failed to demonstrate superiority of ziprasidone over placebo. High placebo responder rates were amongst the factors resulting in study failure (in terms of the primary endpoint – decreases in the MADRS score).

Stahl *et al.* (2009) examined the effectiveness of ziprasidone as monotherapy in dysphoric mania. Although there are no currently agreed and validated criteria for describing subdivisions of the bipolar spectrum, there has been an attempt to classify a subdivision of patients who present with subsyndromal depressive symptoms. Stahl *et al.* (2009) selected items from the HAM-D 17 scale to define dysphoric mania. These included dysphoric mood, worry, self-reproach, negative self-evaluation, discouragement, suicidal tendencies, feelings of fatigue, and loss of interest. They found a similar improvement in symptomatology (MRS) in dysphoric patients compared with the entire patient cohort which included manic and mixed states, suggesting that ziprasidone's efficacy is not confined to specific subgroups. The prevalence of adverse events were similar in the dysphoric patients.

11.6.2   OPEN STUDIES ON ZIPRASIDONE MONOTHERAPY IN DEPRESSIVE EPISODES

A small trial (30 patients completed the study: Liebowitz *et al.*, 2009) examined the use of ziprasidone in bipolar depression at low doses (Mean end of study dose was 58 mg/day) over an eight week open monotherapy trial in bipolar II patients suffering major depressive episodes (HAM-D $\geq$18 or greater). Nine (30%) and 18 (60%) patients were responders at weeks 1 and 8 respectively. Five (17%) and 13 (43%) were in remission at the same time points.

11.6.3   ZIPRASIDONE ADJUNCT THERAPY IN BIPOLAR DEPRESSION

Preliminary evidence is emerging that use of atypicals with mood stabilizers can help control the depressive phase of bipolar disorder (Bowden, 2005).

The efficacy and safety of adjunctive ziprasidone (mean daily dose 89.8 mg) in subjects with bipolar depression treated with lithium, lamotrigine or valproate was recently examined (Sachs *et al.*, 2010a) in a six week double-blind trial. Although ziprasidone was well tolerated, there were no significant improvements in MADRS (-13.2) over placebo (-12.9). Similarly, there was no effect on CGI-S.

11.7   LONG TERM MAINTENANCE TREATMENT OF BIPOLAR DISORDER

Ziprasidone is approved for the long term treatment of bipolar disorder as an adjunctive treatment. Most of the data available in the published literature is derived from open label continuation phases of much shorter double-blind trials. As relapse is common amongst bipolar patients, prevention of relapse is the target of continued maintenance therapy with atypical antipsychotics.

11.7.1   MONOTHERAPY

In an extension of the original three-week double-blind placebo-controlled trial of ziprasidone (Keck *et al.*, 2009), subjects who completed the trial (N = 65) were enrolled in a 52 week open label extension during which ziprasidone was flexibly dosed in the range of 40–160 mg per day. Effectiveness was measured by changes in MRS and CGI scores. Benefits obtained during the initial three-week period were sustained over the following 12 months. The mean reduction in MRS score was -23.5 from a baseline of 29.4. CGI

S scores decreased by 2.32 over the course of 12 months, compared to a baseline of 5.0. There were no differences between various subpopulations of patients (manic, mixed, psychotic or nonpsychotic). Responder rates ranged from 79% (mixed presentation) to 88% (manic) compared to the overall population responder rate of 86%. One caveat should be that it is difficult to draw definitive conclusions about the long-term efficacy of ziprasidone from these data, as the study was an open label design.

The principal adverse events noted were somnolence (42%), dizziness (23%), headache (19%), and akathisia (15%). Almost all adverse events reported (98%) were mild to moderate in severity. There was no significant difference in the adverse event profile over this one year extension period in patients who had been on placebo or on ziprasidone in the original double-blind acute phase.

11.7.2   ADJUNCTIVE THERAPY

Augmentation therapy with the atypical antipsychotics is effective in long-term maintenance treatment of bipolar disorder (Bowden, 2005). In an open label extension of a three-week double-blind placebo-controlled trial, ziprasidone (40–160 mg per day) was used in combination with concomitant mood stabilizers and/or antidepressants for 52 weeks. MRS scores continued to improve throughout the study period and remained significantly better than the baseline scores throughout. There were also significant improvements in CGI and HAM-D Scores. Tolerability was good with 12.4% of subjects discontinuing due to adverse events. The most frequent adverse events were somnolence (55%), abnormal vision (24%), tremor (23%), extrapyramidal symptoms (21%), and dizziness (20%).

A more recent study (Bowden *et al.*, 2010) compared the effects of ziprasidone versus placebo, each as an adjunct to a mood stabilizer, in a phase 3, randomized, six-month, double-blind trial in subjects with bipolar disorder. The principal study objective was to examine the time to intervention for a mood episode exacerbation in subjects receiving either adjunctive ziprasidone or placebo. The time to intervention for a mood episode was significantly longer in the adjunctive ziprasidone group compared to placebo. During the six months of the study in the 19.7% of the ziprasidone subjects required intervention compared to 32.4% of the placebo subjects. Moreover 33.9% of the ziprasidone subjects discontinued for any reason while 51.4% of the placebo subjects discontinued (Bowden *et al.*, 2010).

11.8   PRACTICAL GUIDANCE ON THE USE OF ZIPRASIDONE IN BIPOLAR DISORDER

11.8.1   PHARMACOECONOMICS

Bipolar disorder, being a chronic behavioral health condition, can significantly impact quality of life and productivity. Despite the cost of patient care being a factor in treatment and policy decisions, there is limited information available in the literature for ziprasidone specifically. In one review (Fleurence, Dixon, and Revicki, 2006), limited data on olanzapine, quetiapine, and risperidone was found with no significant differences in cost between the three agents. A recent publication examined medical care costs in patients taking ziprasidone, olanzapine, risperidone, quetiapine, and aripiprazole and adjusted medical care costs over 12 months for patients with bipolar disorder were significantly lower with ziprasidone compared to quetiapine and comparable with the other atypical antipsychotics (Mychaskiw *et al.*, 2009). Although assessed in terms of schizophrenia, Sorensen *et al.* (2008) found that the 10-year average cost per individual of treatment with olanzapine, quetiapine, risperidone, or ziprasidone, when assessed in terms of the burden of treatment, relapse, adverse events, and diabetes management, was more than 20% higher with olanzapine than with ziprasidone.

11.8.2   METABOLIC EFFECTS

Newcomer, Pappadopulos, and Kulluri (2010) have recently organized a compendium of metabolic data and ziprasidone use. Other reviews of this topic also exist (Stahl, 2008; Stahl, *et al.*, 2009). It appears that the atypical antipsychotics have afforded a safer side effect profile in that we see much less tardive dyskinesia and extrapyramidal symptoms. However it is now apparent that at least for some SGA, this safety profile of less tardive dyskinesia and EPS has been traded apparently for an increased risk of developing metabolic syndromes such as hyperlipidemia, hypertension, hyperglycemia, weight gain, and increased abdominal girth. As antipsychotics were once divided into those that were high potency in delivering more extrapyramidal symptoms versus low potency with less, the atypicals now probably should be divided into those that are more metabolically friendly versus those that are more deleterious (Stahl, Migon, and Meyer, 2009). In the literature, and in clinical practice (Reynolds and Kirk, 2010), it is typically felt that the original four atypicals, clozapine, risperidone, olanzapine, and quetiapine are the most likely to cause metabolic issues, where ziprasidone and ariprazole may carry less risk. Newer agents, paliperidone, and asenapine, appear to have 52 week data showing a more favorable profile where iloperidone is too new to determine where it will fall in this continuum, but its short term studies also suggest an intermediate metabolic risk (Emsley *et al.*, 2008; Asenapine FDA Package Insert, Schering Corporation).

Regarding ziprasidone, Newcomer's review included 1605 adult subjects who were treated with ziprasidone and 677 with placebo who took medication over an average of 28 days. Weight difference between those treated with ziprasidone and those with placebo at 12, 24, 48 weeks was -0.9 kg (n = 138), 4.8 kg (n = 13), 4.5 kg (n = 12), and 0.7 kg. Serum glucose was 4.8 ± 1.3 mg/dl for ziprasidone (n = 32), versus -0.8 ± 2.6 for placebo (n = 8) at four weeks and 4.7 ± 1.3 mg/dl for ziprasidone versus -0.1 ± 2.3 for placebo at end point (Table 11.1). Serum triglyceride levels measured 9.8 ± 9.0 mg/dl for ziprasidone (n = 16), versus -8.5 ± 15.5 for placebo (n = 6) at end point. The results for total cholesterol showed a mean change from baseline between ziprasidone and placebo of 7.1, -7.8, and 1.2 mg/dl for subjects with ≥ 12 weeks of treatment, ≥ 24 weeks of treatment, and all subjects, respectively. Categorical data for total cholesterol showed that similar proportions of ziprasidone and placebo recipients shifted from <240 to ≥ 240 mg/dl or from <200 to ≥ 200 mg/dl. The author concludes that treatment

Table 11.1 Summary of statistical analyses of change from baseline weight, fasting glucose, fasting triglycerides, and total cholesterol from 15 placebo-controlled studies of ziprasidone in adult subjects.

Measure	Time	Ziprasidone LS mean ± SE (n)	Placebo LS mean ± SE (n)	LS mean difference (95% CI)
Weight	12 wk	-1.7 ± 0.7 (98)	-0.8 ± 0.8 (40)	-0.9 (-2.2 to 0.4)
	24 wk	-3.0 ± 1.2 (10)	-7.7 ± 2.0 (3)	4.8 (-0.2 to 9.7)
	48 wk	-5.5 ± 2.4 (11)	-10.0 ± 6.6 (1)	4.5 (-11.1 to 20.1)
	LOCF endpoint	0.22 ± 0.19 (1419)	-0.5 ± 0.23 (589)	0.7 (-11.1 to 20.1)
Glucose	4 wk	4.8 ± 1.3 (32)	-0.8 ± 2.6 (8)	5.5 (-0.3 to 11.4)
	LOCF endpoint	4.7 ± 1.3 (34)	0.1 ± 2.3 (10)	4.7 (0.6 to 10.0)
Fasting triglycerides	LOCF endpoint	9.8 ± 9.0 (16)	-8.5 ± 15.5 (6)	1.3 (-35.7 to 38.4)
Total cholesterol	All times	1.7 ± 2.1 (1045)	-2.9 ± 2.4 (429)	1.2 (-2.4 to 4.7)
	≥ 12 wk	-2.9 ± 15.5 (61)	-10.1 ± 18.1 (22)	7.1 (-15.2 to 29.5)
	≥ 24 wk	-9.2 ± 15.3 (11)	-1.4 ± 26.7 (2)	-7.8 (-58.2 to 42.6)

Pappadopulos, E. *et al.* (2009) Presented at the *48th Annual American College of Neuropsychopharmacology Meeting*, Hollywood, FL, December 6–10, 2009.

with ziprasidone in adults had no clinically relevant negative effects on mean changes for a range of metabolic parameters, namely: weight, total cholesterol, glucose, and triglycerides. Furthermore, the results were comparable for patients treated with either ziprasidone or placebo. In addition to Newcomer's review (submitted), other researchers have published data suggesting that ziprasidone is a metabolically friendly or neutral drug (Haupt, 2006; Newcomer and Haupt, 2006; De Nayer *et al.*, 2007; de Leon *et al.*, 2007; Newcomer, 2007; Meyer *et al.*, 2008). Certainly as with all atypicals, routine metabolic monitoring should occur as in any given patient, metabolic changes may occur.

11.8.3 METABOLISM AND DOSING

Ziprasidone is extensively metabolized after oral administration, with only a small amount excreted unchanged in the urine (<1%) or feces (<4%). This drug must be taken with food at each dose to achieve adequate absorption. Ziprasidone is metabolized by two major pathways: aldehyde oxidase and cytochrome P450 enzymes. Approximately two thirds of ziprasidone metabolism is mediated by aldehyde oxidase, which has no known clinically relevant inhibitors or inducers. Approximately one third of ziprasidone metabolism is mediated via CYP450-catalyzed oxidation through CYP3A4, with no inhibition or induction of CYP450 enzymes by ziprasidone. There are no clinically significant pharmacokinetic drug-drug interactions with a variety of concomitantly administered medications (Prakash *et al.*, 1997; Beedham, Miceli, and Obach, 2003). Figure 11.3 shows the metabolic sequence.

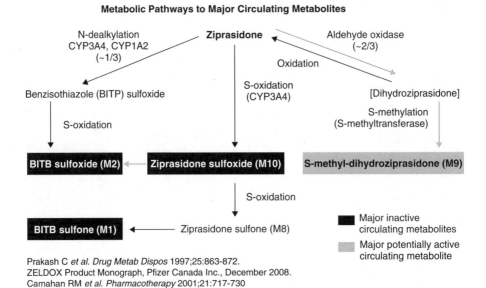

Figure 11.3 Ziprasidone metabolic pathway – primary route of metabolism limits drug-drug interactions.

Ziprasidone has some standard dosing guidelines based upon regulatory studies and indication being treated. For example, the FDA package insert states the following.

Ziprasidone should be administered for schizophrenia at an initial daily dose of 20 mg twice daily with food. Dosing with food is essential for absorption otherwise clinical effectiveness may be impaired. Maximum use up to 80 mg twice daily is allowed. Dosage adjustments, if indicated, should generally occur at intervals of not less than two days, as steady-state is achieved within one to three days. Efficacy in schizophrenia was demonstrated in a dose range of 20–100 mg twice daily in short-term, placebo-controlled clinical trials. Consistent efficacy was noted at doses 60 mg twice daily and above. There were trends toward dose response within the range of 20–80 mg twice daily, but results were not consistent. An increase to a dose greater than 80 mg twice daily is not generally recommended as the safety of doses above 100 mg twice daily have not been systematically evaluated in regulatory trials. However, a supra FDA dosing trial suggested reasonable safety compared to haloperidol at doses of 320 mg/day. QTc intervals increased on both agents and none elevated above the clinically relevant cut off of 450 ms (Miceli *et al.*, 2010). This chapter did not investigate the effectiveness of high dose ziprasidone. Citrome *et al.* performed a NY state hospital review of patients treated with ziprasidone and found it clinically being used above the FDA maximum (160 mg/day) approximately 50% of the time. He suggests this could be due to perceived dose-response curve or the fact that if the drug was taken without food, higher doses may have been needed for better absorption (Citrome, Jaffe, and Levine, 2007).

In the acute treatment of manic or mixed episodes, oral ziprasidone should be administered at an initial daily dose of 40 mg twice daily with food (Ziprasidone Package

Insert). This is higher than the usual starting dose noted above for schizophrenia. The dose may then be increased to 60 or 80 mg twice daily on the second day of treatment and subsequently adjusted on the basis of tolerance and efficacy within the range of 40–80 mg twice daily. Schizophrenia treatment usually starts at 20 mg twice daily, but similar to other atypical antipsychotics when used for mania, ziprasidone is used in a loading strategy where the starting dose is 40 mg twice daily with rapid escalation up to 80 mg twice daily. Efficacy tends to occur at the 60 mg twice daily or higher doses.

In using ziprasidone for the maintenance treatment (as an adjunct to lithium or valproate) of bipolar disorder, dosing should continue at the same dose on which the patient was initially stabilized, within the range of 40–80 mg twice daily with food.

Outside of the regulatory guidelines, some authors and clinicians might suggest dosing strategies that enhance tolerability and compliance (Cutler, Ball, and Stahl, 2008). Cutler *et al.* suggest that early in trials of ziprasidone, doses as low as 40 mg/day (20 mg BID) would be effective, but after several years on the market, the minimum effective dose in clinical practice is considered to be about 120 mg/day (60 mg twice daily). The average dose is likely 120–320 mg/day, with an average of 160 mg/day in schizophrenia. Doses of ziprasidone higher than the maximum label recommendation of 160 mg/day may improve efficacy, but this is anecdotal and not yet confirmed in fully controlled trials. This is considered an off-label practice, but in certain, refractory treatment situations the risk/benefit analysis may favor the more aggressive dosing.

The authors suggest that some clinicians have reported success with once-daily ziprasidone, but only when taken consistently with food and only in some individuals, that is, those taking >160 mg/day. There is, as of yet, little guidance as to which individuals may respond positively to once-daily ziprasidone. There is some evidence for the use of low-dose ziprasidone in other mood disorders. In reality, higher doses of ziprasidone are needed for DA-2 receptor blockade to treat schizophrenia or mania (doses > 120 mg/day). Ziprasidone is sometimes dosed lower for the depressed phase of bipolar disorder or for unipolar depression augmentation, perhaps more often at doses of 20–40 mg twice daily (Stahl and Shayegan, 2003; Stahl, 2008, 2009). It is possible that at lower doses, ziprasidone's pharmacodynamic profile of serotonin-2 receptor antagonism, serotonin-1a receptor agonism, NE reuptake inhibition, and serotonin reuptake inhibition may lend to clinical antidepressant effects. An average 58 mg/day dose was effective in a small open label bipolar depression trial and 80–160 mg doses were effective in a non-randomized pilot and a randomized open label trail in unipolar depression and in treatment resistant depression (Papakostas *et al.*, 2004; Dunner *et al.*, 2007; Liebowitz *et al.*, 2009). These findings suggest the possibility of theoretical and actual clinical antidepressant effectiveness. Double blind studies that are more stringent are warranted.

11.8.4 SWITCHING TO ZIPRASIDONE

In clinical practice, it is often necessary to switch from an initial psychotropic to another due to inefficacy or poor tolerability. In regards to ziprasidone, there is a minimum of evidence which focuses more so on switching to ziprasidone when previous agents have been problematic. One of the most recent switch studies (Alptekin *et al.*, 2009) looked at schizophrenia and schizoaffective disorder and found that patients switched from haloperidol, risperidone, or olanzapine experienced statistically significant improvements from baseline in positive symptoms, negative symptoms, and global functioning. Switching from haloperidol or risperidone was associated with statistically significant improvements in extrapyramidal symptoms, and from olanzapine in a significant reduction in body weight. Ziprasidone typically displayed a neutral effect on metabolic parameters, and in many patients, concomitant anti-Parkinsonian medication use either remained unchanged, or dosage was reduced. In this study, clinicians preferred an immediate switch to ziprasidone strategy with the most common dose being 120 mg/day.

Several other switches to ziprasidone studies predate the Alptekin *et al.* study above. Again, most observed similar changes, but were noted in non-bipolar patients. Often comparable, or improved efficacy and tolerability were the result. Varied improvements in metabolics and even cognition have been noted throughout (Garman *et al.*, 2003; Weiden *et al.*, 2003, 2006, 2008; Harvey *et al.*, 2004; Bartko *et al.*, 2006; Montes *et al.*, 2007; Lublin *et al.*, 2009; Rossi *et al.*, 2008).

11.9 SAFETY AND TOLERABILITY

11.9.1 ADVERSE EVENTS IN CLINICAL TRIALS

The safety and tolerability of ziprasidone shares general similarities with the class of atypical antipsychotics in that the most commonly recorded adverse events are somnolence, headache, nausea, and dizziness (see Table 11.2).

For instance in the two short-term studies of ziprasidone, somnolence was noted in 31% of patients on ziprasidone compared with 12% on placebo. Headache was as common in placebo patients (17%) as in those on ziprasidone (18%). Nausea (10% of ziprasidone patients) was only slightly more prevalent than in the placebo group (7%) while dizziness

Table 11.2 Common adverse events in short-term clinical trials of ziprasidone in schizophrenia and bipolar disorder.

	Schizophrenia		Bipolar disorder	
	% of patients reporting a reaction		% of patients reporting a reaction	
	Ziprasidone	Placebo	Ziprasidone	Placebo
Nausea	10	7	10	7
Diarrhea	5	4	5	4
Dry mouth	4	2	5	4
Extrapyramidal symptoms	14	8	31	12
Somnolence	14	7	31	12
Akathisia	8	7	10	5
Dizziness	8	6	16	7
Abnormal vision	3	2	6	3
Asthenia	5	3	6	2

occurred in 16% of ziprasidone patients and 7% of placebo patients. Short-term studies of ziprasidone in bipolar disorder typically report the above adverse events, usually rated mild or moderate in severity. Over the course of three weeks, 6.5% of ziprasidone treated patients discontinued the study due to an adverse drug reaction. The comparable placebo group value was 3.7%. The most commonly cited adverse events necessitating patient withdrawal from trials were akathisia, anxiety, depression, dizziness, dystonia, rash, and vomiting.

In a separate haloperidol-referenced study, somnolence, headache, and dizziness were observed in 10.7, 9.6, and 2.2% of ziprasidone treated subjects in the double-blind phase of the trial and in 14.0, 11.8, and 2.2% during the nine weeks open label extension phase, 3.9% of ziprasidone treated subjects and 2.3% of subjects on placebo discontinued during the first three weeks of the trial.

In a recent six-month double-blind placebo-controlled trial of adjunctive Ziprasidone, 62.2% of subjects in the ziprasidone group and 57.1% of subjects in the placebo group reported adverse events. (Following an open label period of 10–16 weeks, the most common adverse events reported for patients in the double-blind period were tremor (6.3 and 3.6% in the ziprasidone and placebo groups respectively), and insomnia (5.5 and 10.7% ziprasidone and placebo groups respectively); (Bowden *et al.*, 2010).

11.9.2   QTc INTERVAL

Although the effect is mild to modest, ziprasidone lengthens the cardiac QTc interval and has a bolded warning in the US. Lengthening of the QTc interval is associated with torsade de pointes and the risk of sudden cardiac death. Although there has been no clear incidents of torsade de pointes following administration of ziprasidone, ziprasidone typically lengthens the QTc interval by around 10 ms. In a Keck *et al.* study, there was a mean prolongation of the QTc interval of 11 ms versus baseline values. A comparable increase of 11.8 ms was observed in the Weisler *et al.* study of ziprasidone in combination with lithium. There was an increase in QTc interval of 6.1 ms in the placebo group comparatively. In neither study did any patient have a QTc interval value greater than 500 ms. Nonetheless, ziprasidone should not be used in patients with Congenital Long QT Syndrome or in combination with drugs that are themselves known to increase the QT duration, or drugs that may have a pharmacokinetic/pharmacodynamic interaction with ziprasidone. Ziprasidone should also not be used in combination with class I and III antiarrhythmic drugs. QTc prolongation data is shown in Figure 11.4.

Although there is an association between ziprasidone treatment and QTc prolongation, and an association between QTc prolongation and death from torsade de pointes, there is no clearly shown association between ziprasidone treatment and sudden death. Occasional incidences of sudden death have been reported with ziprasidone, as with the other atypical antipsychotics.

In a large simple trial of ziprasidone versus olanzapine, albeit in schizophrenia rather than bipolar disorder, there was no significant difference in sudden death outcomes between the two antipsychotics, even when readjudicated by an independent panel. (Kane *et al.*, 2010).

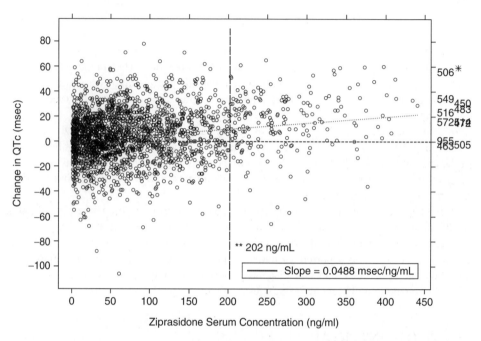

Figure 11.4 QTc change versus serum ziprasidone exposure (Data from 25 clinical trials representing 1486 subjects and 2687 pairs of QTc intervals. Samples collected within 1 hour of an ECG measurement). *Ziprasidone concentrations that exceed 450 ng/ml are marked by their levels at a vertical position marking their relative change in QTc from Baseline.**Vertical line indicates the mean Cmax observed (202 ng/ml) following administration of 80 mg BID (Study 128-043). Pfizer (data on file).

11.10   TREATMENT OF SPECIAL POPULATIONS

There is very little data in regards to special treatment populations. There are case reports about the use of ziprasidone in the geriatric and pediatric bipolar populations, but no large scale controlled studies. A MEDLINE search offered no clear findings in regards to pharmacogenetics studies in determining which patients might preferentially respond to ziprasidone.

11.11   SUMMARY AND CONCLUSIONS

In conclusion, this chapter summarizes the science behind clinical application, and the data supporting these clinical applications themselves in regard to the use of ziprasidone in treating patients who suffer from bipolar disorder. The science is fairly rigorous in regard to the pharmacokinetic and pharmacodynamic profile of this drug. Randomized and controlled trials lend strength to the use of ziprasidone in treating acutely manic, or mixed manic patients, and also over the long term in regards to adjunctive clinical maintenance of a euthymic state (Bowden *et al.*, 2010). Data is either modest to weak, or even absent, in regard to treating bipolar depression, bipolar comorbidities, or treatment in populations outside of adults with bipolar illness.

ACKNOWLEDGMENTS

Pfizer authors would like to thank Jon Stamford, Ph.D. of PAREXEL, for editorial assistance received on their section of this manuscript. Mr. Stamford's work was funded by Pfizer Inc.

Drs Stahl and Schwartz report receiving research, consultation and speaking grants and funds from Pfizer.

None of these potential conflicts of interest have weighed on the reporting of information contained in this chapter. Data and references are clearly in the public domain and both positive and failed studies, on and off-label applications are clearly noted in this chapter.

References

Alptekin, K., Hafez, J., Brook, S. *et al.* (2009) Efficacy and tolerability of switching to ziprasidone from olanzapine, risperidone or haloperidol: an international, multicenter study. *Int. Clin. Psychopharmacol.*, **24** (5), 229–238.

American Psychiatric Association (2002) Practice guideline for the treatment of patients with bipolar disorder (revision). *Am. J. Psychiatry*, **159** (Suppl. 4), 1–50.

Bartko', G., Trixler, M., Bitter, I. *et al.* (2006) Switching patients with schizophrenia to ziprasidone from conventional or other atypical antipsychotics. *Neuropsychopharmacol. Hung*, **8**, 201–209.

Bauer, M.S., Callahan, A.M., Jampala, C., *et al.* (1999) Clinical practice guidelines for bipolar disorder from the department of veterans affairs. *J. Clin. Psychiatry*, **60**, 9–21.

Beedham, C., Miceli, J.J., and Obach, R.S. (2003) Ziprasidone metabolism, aldehyde oxidase, and clinical implications. *J. Clin. Psychopharmacol.*, **23**, 229–232.

Biederman, J., Mick, E., Spencer, T. *et al.* (2007) A prospective open-label treatment trial of ziprasidone monotherapy in children and adolescents with bipolar disorder. *Bipolar Disord.*, **9** (8), 888–894.

Bowden, C.L. (2005) Atypical antipsychotic augmentation of mood stabilizer therapy in bipolar disorder. *J. Clin. Psychiatry*, **66** (Suppl. 3), 12–19.

Bowden, C.L., Vieta, E., Ice, K.S. *et al.* (2010) Ziprasidone plus a mood stabilizer in subjects with bipolar I disorder: a 6-month, randomized, placebo-controlled, double-blind trial. *J. Clin. Psychiatry*, **71** (2), 130–137.

Citrome, L., Jaffe, A., and Levine, J. (2007) Datapoints: The ups and downs of dosing second-generation antipsychotics. *Psychiatr. Serv.*, **58** (1), 11.

Cutler, A., Ball, S., and Stahl, S.M. (2008) Expert review supplement dosing atypical antipsychotics. *CNS Spectr.*, **13** (5, Suppl. 9), 1–14.

De Nayer, A., De Hert, M., Scheen, A. *et al.* (2007) Conference report: Belgian consensus on metabolic problems associated with atypical antipsychotics. *Encephale*, **33** (2), 197–202.

Dunner, D.L., Amsterdam, J.D., Shelton, R.C. *et al.* (2007) Efficacy and tolerability of adjunctive ziprasidone in treatment-resistant depression: a randomized, open-label, pilot study. *J. Clin. Psychiatry*, **68** (7), 1071–1077.

Elbe, D., and Carandang, G. (2008 November) Focus on Ziprasidone: A review of its use in child and adolescent psychiatry. *J. Can. Acad. Child Adolesc. Psychiatry*, **17** (4), 220–229.

Emsley, R., Berwaerts, J., Eerdekens, M. *et al.* (2008) Efficacy and safety of oral paliperidone extended-release tablets in the treatment of acute schizophrenia: pooled data from three 52-week open-label studies. *Int. Clin. Psychopharmacol.*, **23** (6), 343–356.

Ferrier, N., Pilling, S., Bazire, S. *et al.* (2006) *Bipolar Disorder: The Management of Bipolar Disorder in Adults, Children and Adolescents, in Primary and Secondary Care*, National Clinical Practice Guideline Number 38, Alden Press, London.

Fleurence, R.L., Dixon, J.M., and Revicki, D.A. (2006) Economics of atypical antipsychotics in bipolar disorder: a review of the literature. *CNS Drugs*, **20** (7), 591–599.

Garman, P.M., Ried, L.D., Bengtson, M.A. *et al.* (2003) Effect on lipid profiles of switching from olanzapine to another second-generation antipsychotic agent in veterans with schizophrenia. *J. Am. Pharm. Assoc.*, **47**, 373–378.

Goodwin, G.M., Consensus Group of the British Association for Psychopharmacology (2009) Evidence-based guidelines for treating bipolar disorder: Recommendations from the British Association for psychopharmacology. *J. Psychopharmacol.*, **23** (4), 346–388.

Grunze, H., Vieta, E., Goodwin, G. *et al.* (2009) The World Federation of Societies of Biological Psychiatry (WFSBP) Guidelines for the Biological Treatment of Bipolar Disorders: update 2009 on the treatment of acute mania. *World J. Biol. Psychiatry*, **10**, 85–116.

Harvey, P.D., Meltzer, H., Simpson, G.M. *et al.* (2004) Improvement in cognitive function following a switch to ziprasidone from conventional antipsychotics, olanzapine, or risperidone in outpatients with schizophrenia. *Schizophr. Res.*, **66**, 101–113.

Haupt, D.W. (2006) Differential metabolic effects of antipsychotic treatments. *Eur. Neuropsychopharmacol.*, **16** (Suppl. 3), S149–S155.

Hirschfeld, R.M., Bowden, C.L., Gitlin, M.J. *et al.* (2002) Practice guideline for the treatment of patients with bipolar disorder (Revision. *Am. J. Psychiatry*, **159** (Suppl. 4), 1–10.

Kane, J., Strom, B., Eng, S. *et al.* (2010) Primary and readjudication mortality results from ZODIAC, a large simple trial of ziprasidone vs. olanzapine in patients with schizophrenia. *Schizophr. Res.*, **117** (2–3), 183–184.

Keck, P.E. Jr., Perlis, R.H., Otto, M.W. *et al.* (2004) The expert consensus guidelines®: treatment of bipolar disorder 2004. *Postgrad. Med. Spec. Rep.*, 1–120.

Keck, P.E. Jr., Versiani, M., Potkin, S. *et al.*, Ziprasidone in Mania Study Group (2003) ziprasidone in the treatment of acute bipolar mania: a three-week, placebo-controlled, double-blind, randomized trial. *Am. J. Psychiatry*, **160** (4), 741–748.

Keck, P.E. Jr., Versiani, M., Warrington, L. *et al.* (2009) Long-term safety and efficacy of ziprasidone in subpopulations of patients with bipolar mania. *J. Clin. Psychiatry*, **70** (6), 844–851.

Kim, D., Maneen, M., and Stahl, S.M. (2009) Building a better antipsychotic: receptor targets for the treatment of multiple symptom dimensions of schizophrenia. *Neurotherapeutics: J. Am. Soc. Exp. Neurotherapeutics*, **6**, 78–85.

de Leon, J., Susce, M.T., Johnson, M. *et al.* (2007) A clinical study of the association of antipsychotics with hyperlipidemia. *Schizophr. Res.*, **92** (1–3), 95–102.

Liebowitz, M.R., Salmán, E., Mech, A. *et al.* (2009) ziprasidone monotherapy in bipolar II depression: an open trial. *J. Affect. Disord.*, **118** (1–3), 205–208.

Lombardo, I., Sachs, G., Kolluri, S., and Kremer, C. (2010) Two 6-week, randomized, double-blind, placebo-controlled studies of ziprasidone in outpatients with bipolar I depression: did baseline characteristics impact trial outcome? *J. Clin. Psychiatry*, submitted.

Lublin, H., Haug, H.-J., Koponen, H. *et al.* (2009) Ziprasidone versus olanzapine, risperidone or quetiapine in patients with chronic schizophrenia: a 12-week open-label, multicentre clinical trial. *World J. Biol. Psychiatry*, **10** (4), 710–718.

Meyer, J.M., Davis, V.G., Goff, D.C. *et al.* (2008) Change in metabolic syndrome parameters with antipsychotic treatment in the CATIE Schizophrenia Trial: prospective data from phase 1. *Schizophr. Res.*, **101** (1–3), 273–286.

Miceli, J.J., Tensfeldt, T.G., Shiovitz, T. *et al.* (2010) Effects of oral Ziprasidone and oral Haloperidol on QTc interval in patients with schizophrenia or schizoaffective disorder. *Pharmacotherapy*, **30** (2), 127–135.

Montes, J.M., Rodriguez, J.L., Balbo, E. *et al.* (2007) Improvement in antipsychotic-related metabolic disturbances in patients with schizophrenia switched to ziprasidone. *Prog. Neuropsychopharmacol. Biol. Psychiatry*, **31**, 383–388.

Mychaskiw, M., Sanders, K., Alvir, J. *et al.* (2009) Association between antipsychotic treatment and clinical and economic outcomes in schizophrenia and bipolar disorder. *Eur. Neuropsychopharmacol.*, **19** (Supp 3), S544.

Newcomer, J.W. (2007) Metabolic considerations in the use of antipsychotic medications: a review of recent evidence. *J. Clin. Psychiatry*, **68** (Suppl. 1), 20–27.

Newcomer, J.W. and Haupt, D.W. (2006) The metabolic effects of antipsychotic medications. *Can. J. Psychiatry: Rev. Can. Psychiatr.*, **51** (8), 480–491.

Newcomer, J.W., Pappadopulos, E., and Kolluri, S. (2010) Changes in Weight, Plasma Lipids and Blood Glucose in Adults Treated with Ziprasidone: An Analysis of Randomised, Placebo-controlled Trials, manuscript in submission.

Papakostas, G.I., Petersen, T.J., Nierenberg, A.A. *et al.* (2004) Ziprasidone augmentation of selective serotonin reuptake inhibitors (SSRIs) for SSRI-resistant major depressive disorder. *J. Clin. Psychiatry*, **65** (2), 217–221.

Potkin, S.G., Keck, P.E. Jr., Segal, S. *et al.* (2005) ziprasidone in acute bipolar mania: a 21-day randomized, double-blind, placebo-controlled replication trial. *J. Clin. Psychopharmacol.*, **25** (4), 301–310.

Prakash, C., Kamel, A., Gummerus, J., and Wilner, K. (1997) Metabolism and excretion of a new antipsychotic drug, ziprasidone, in humans. *Drug Metab. Dispos.*, **25**, 863–872.

Reynolds, G.P. and Kirk, S.L. (2010) Metabolic side effects of antipsychotic drug treatment – pharmacological mechanisms. *Pharmacol. Ther.*, **125** (1), 169–179.

Rossi, A., Vita, A., Tiradritti, P., and Romeo, F. (2008) Assessment of clinical and metabolic status, and subjective well-being, in schizophrenic patients switched from typical and atypical antipsychotics to ziprasidone. *Int. Clin. Psychopharmacol.*, **23**, 216–222.

Sachs, G.S. (2001) Emerging data: atypical antipsychotics in bipolar disorder, *Program and Abstracts of the 52nd Institute on Psychiatric Services*, American Psychiatric Association, Washington, DC.

Sachs, G., Ice, K., Chappell, P. *et al.* (2010a) Efficacy and safety of adjunctive oral ziprasidone the treatment of depression in patients with bipolar 1 disorder. *J. Clin. Psychiatry*, submitted.

Sachs, G., Vanderburg, D., Karayal, O. *et al.* (2010b) Adjunct to the oral ziprasidone versus placebo in patients with acute mania treated with lithium or divalproex. *Bipolar Disord.*, submitted.

Schmidt, A.W., Lebel, L.A., Howard, H.R. Jr. *et al.* (2001) Ziprasidone: a novel antipsychotic agent with a unique human receptor binding profile. *Eur. J. Pharmacol.*, **425**, 197–201.

Shayegan, D.K. and Stahl, S.M. (2004) Atypical antipsychotics: matching receptor profile to individual patient's clinical profile. *CNS Spectr.*, **9** (10, Suppl. 11), 6–14.

Sorensen S.V., Nasrallah H., Cragin L.S. *et al.* (2008) Clinical and economic outcomes of atypical antipsychotics in schizophrenia. Poster presented at the Winter Workshop on Schizophrenia and Bipolar Disorder, Montreux, Switzerland, February 2–8, 2008.

Stahl, S.M. (2008) *Stahl's Essential Psychopharmacology: Neuroscientific Basis and Practical Applications*, 3rd edn, Cambridge University Press, New York.

Stahl, S.M. (2009) *Essential Psychopharmacology: The Prescriber's Guide*, 3rd edn, Cambridge University Press, Cambridge, New York.

Stahl, S.M., Lombardo, I., Loebel, A., and Mandel, F. (2009) Efficacy of ziprasidone in dysphoric mania: pooled analysis of 2 double blind studies. *J. Affect. Disord.*, **122**, 39–45.

Stahl, S.M. and Mignon, L. (2010) *Stahl's Illustrated Antipsychotics*, 2nd edn, Cambridge University Press, New York.

Stahl, S.M., Mignon, L., and Meyer, J.M. (2009) What comes first: atypical antipsychotics or the metabolic syndrome. *Acta Psychiatr. Scand.*, **119**, 171–179.

Stahl, S.M. and Shayegan, D. (2003) The psychopharmacology of ziprasidone: receptor-binding properties and real-world psychiatric practice. *J. Clin. Psychiatry*, **64** (Suppl. 19), 6–12.

Stamford, J.A., Davidson, C., McLaughlin, D.P., and Hopwood, S.E. (2000) Control of dorsal raphé 5-HT function by multiple 5-HT(1) autoreceptors: parallel purposes or pointless plurality? *Trends Neurosci.*, **23** (10), 459–465.

Vieta, E., Ramey, T., Keller, D. *et al.* (2010) Ziprasidone in the treatment of acute mania: a 12-week, placebo-controlled, haloperidol-referenced study. *J. Psychopharmacol.*, **24** (4), 547–558.

Weiden, P.J., Daniel, D.G., Simpson, G., and Romano, S.J. (2006) Improvement in indices of health status in outpatients with schizophrenia switched to ziprasidone. *J. Clin. Psychopharmacol.*, **23**, 595–600.

Weiden, P.J., Newcomer, J.W., Loebel, A.D. *et al.* (2008) Long-term changes in weight and plasma lipids during maintenance treatment with ziprasidone. *Neuropsychopharmacology*, **33**, 985–994.

Weiden, P.J., Simpson, G.M., Potkin, S.G., and O'Sullivan, R.L. (2003) Effectiveness of switching to ziprasidone for stable but symptomatic outpatients with schizophrenia. *J. Clin. Psychiatry*, **64**, 580–588.

Yatham, L.N., Kennedy, S.H., Schaffer, A. *et al.* (2009) Canadian Network for Mood and Anxiety Treatments (CANMAT) and International Society for Bipolar Disorders (ISBD) collaborative update of CANMAT guidelines for the management of patients with bipolar disorder: update 2009. *Bipolar Disord.*, **11** (3), 225–255.

12

Aripiprazole in Bipolar Disorder

Alessandra Nivoli and Eduard Vieta

Clinical Institute of Neuroscience, Hospital Clinic, University of
Barcelona, IDIBAPS, CIBERSAM, Catalonia, Spain

12.1 ARIPIPRAZOLE AND ITS MODE OF ACTION

Aripiprazole is a second generation antipsychotic (SGA) that belongs to the quinoli-
none class, developed by Otsuka Ltd in Tokyo, Japan, and first approved by the Food
and Drug Administration of the United States (US' FDA) in 2002 for the treatment of
schizophrenia. In 2004 it received FDA approval for the treatment of acute manic and
mixed episode in patients with bipolar I disorder and for the maintenance treatment of
bipolar patients with a recent manic or mixed episode and this indication has also been
recognized by the European and other countries' regulators. It is also approved in America as an adjunctive agent for the treatment of major depression (Fountoulakis and Vieta,
2009). Aripiprazole's pharmacologic mechanism of action is unique among the atypical
antipsychotics due to a complex receptor profile with a pharmacodynamic profile that
distinguishes it from other SGAs. It is a *dopamine D2 partial and selective agonist* rather
than a D2 antagonist. Although similar in many ways to other SGAs, its profile of partial
agonist action at several G-protein coupled receptors: postsynaptic dopamine (D2), presynaptic dopamine autoreceptors, 5-hydroxtryptamine (5-HT1A) and antagonism at others
(5-HT2A) marks aripiprazole as the first functionally selective atypical antipsychotic. It
acts as a partial agonist at dopamine D2, D3, and serotonine 5-HT1A receptors, and as
an antagonist at 5-HT2a receptors. It can enhance as well as inhibit dopamine release
in specific regions of the brain: it exhibits typical antagonism at D2 receptors in the
mesolimbic pathway, as well as having unique partial agonist activity at D2 receptors
in the mesocortical pathway (Burris *et al.*, 2002). It acts as a presynaptic D2 agonist
and simultaneously has an antagonistic effect at the postsynaptic D2 receptors (Ozdemir,
Fourie, and Ozdener, 2002), increasing dopamine activity in the frontal cortex (Li *et al.*,
2004). It most likely exerts antimanic efficacy by way of *partial* dopamine D2 receptor agonist activity, thus lowering intrinsic and excessive dopamine neurotransmission.
Aripiprazole (ARP) is also a partial agonist at the 5-HT1A receptor (Jordan *et al.*, 2002;
Marona-Lewicka and Nichols, 2004), and an antagonist at the 5-HT2A receptor (Stark
et al., 2007). It occupied 70–80% of striatal dopamine receptors in healthy subjects at
doses of 2 mg/day, with dopamine occupancy at 95% when the dose was increased
to 30 mg/day while EPS was not observed (Muzina, 2009). A pure antagonist would

Bipolar Psychopharmacotherapy: Caring for the patient, Second Edition. Edited by Hagop S. Akiskal and Mauricio Tohen.
© 2011 John Wiley & Sons, Ltd. Published 2011 by John Wiley & Sons, Ltd.

likely induce extrapyramidal symptoms (EPS) at such high dopamine receptor occupancy levels. It has moderate affinity for histamine and α-adrenergic receptors and for the serotonin transporter, and no significant affinity for cholinergic muscarinic receptors (Davies, Sheffler, and Roth, 2004), which may explain the excellent tolerability of the drug in terms of sedation, heart rate, and weight gain. Aripiprazole is rapidly absorbed and demonstrates linear pharmacokinetics with a mean elimination half-life of 75 hours, allowing for single daily dosing. Elimination of aripiprazole occurs chiefly through hepatic metabolism via cytochrome P450-2D6 and 3A4. Clinically significant alterations in aripiprazole plasma levels may occur when co-administered with 3A4 inducers (that is, carbamazepine), inhibitors (that is fluvoxamine, ketoconazole), or substrates (that is, nefazodone, haloperidol), but has safely been co-administered with valproic acid and lithium.

Aripiprazole is recommended for the treatment of acute manic or mixed episodes of bipolar disorder in adults, as monotherapy or adjunctive therapy to either lithium or valproate. Aripiprazole monotherapy is also indicated for maintenance treatment of manic and mixed episodes associated with bipolar I disorder, and in the acute treatment of agitation associated with manic or mixed states, with more robust relapse prevention against manic than depressive episodes. There is also evidence to suggest that aripiprazole monotherapy is effective in the prevention of relapse among patients with rapid cycling, which may represent a more refractory form of bipolar disorder with greater morbidity than nonrapid cycling illness.

The data on the effectiveness of aripiprazole against acute manic/mixed episodes are strong, and so are the data concerning the prophylaxis against these episodes in patients who experienced predominantly manic episodes who responded to aripiprazole treatment. The data against acute bipolar depression are negative on the eight-week primary outcome, but it might work at lower dosages as suggested by secondary analyses from pivotal trials or as trigger of antidepressant response. There are also some open data supporting the usefulness of aripiprazole as adjunctive therapy to lithium or valproate in refractory bipolar depressive patients.

In the following paragraphs the efficacy and effectiveness of aripiprazole will be reviewed by summarizing recommendations from the most recently updated treatment guidelines, evidence-data derived from randomized controlled trials (RCTs) and results from recent literature (open and observational studies, systematic reviews, and meta-analysis).

12.2   ARIPIPRAZOLE IN TREATMENT GUIDELINES

A treatment guideline represents a synthesis of current scientific knowledge regarding a specific topic which integrates the evidence-based data (from randomized clinical studies, RCTs) with the rational clinical practice and experience. Existing data regarding the treatment of bipolar disorder are ranked according to *levels (or categories) of evidence (CE)*, depending on the methodology of study design, on number of positive trials and on absence or presence of negative evidence. *Clinical recommendations (RG* or Recommendation Grade) are then derived for every specific compound by integrating additional clinical aspects of safety, tolerability, and effectiveness.

Generally, all guidelines recommend the use of aripiprazole in the treatment of acute mania, considering a broad spectrum of action which includes mixed and dysphoric mania, as well as rapid cycling. Almost all guidelines do not suggest aripiprazole monotherapy in the treatment of acute depressive episode in bipolar disorder. In long-term treatment, aripiprazole is recommended for preventing manic and mixed episodes and, even with little evidence, depressive episodes too (see Table 12.1).

The *World Federation of Societies of Biological Psychiatry (WFSBP)* updated in 2009 their guidelines for the biological treatment of bipolar disorders both for acute mania (Grunze *et al.*, 2009) and for acute bipolar depression (Grunze *et al.*, 2010). Evidence data did not support the use of aripiprazole in acute bipolar depression as first line treatment (CE "E") because two negative controlled studies have been reported: although aripiprazole seemed to enhance improvement during first weeks, efficacy did not last over time (Thase *et al.*, 2008). On the other hand, for antimanic efficacy aripiprazole fulfills CE "A," with a good tolerability profile (RG "1"), Subanalyses confirm the broad spectrum of efficacy of aripiprazole across subtypes of mania, such as in dysphoric/mixed states and psychotic mania.

The *Canadian Network for Mood and Anxiety Treatments (CANMAT) and International Society for Bipolar Disorders (ISBD)* Guidelines (Yatham *et al.*, 2009) confirm recommendations against using aripiprazole monotherapy for the acute management of bipolar depression, while substantial data support the efficacy of aripiprazole monotherapy for the treatment of acute mania as first-line choice (Level 1). The authors highlight a positive effect of adjunctive aripiprazole in patients with bipolar depression, and the use of intramuscular (IM) aripiprazole as a first choice in the treatment of acute agitation (Level 2). Aripiprazole monotherapy is recommended as first-line option for maintenance treatment in preventing manic episodes.

The *Consensus Group of the British Association for Psychopharmacology* reviewed the Evidence-based guidelines for treating bipolar disorder (Goodwin, 2009). Aripiprazole is recommended in monotherapy for the treatment of acute mania. In patients already taking lithium or valproate, adjunctive aripiprazole has been shown to be superior to lithium or valproate alone. It is suggested also in the acute treatment of mixed states and in preventions of manic relapses, with no effect on depression.

The *International Consensus Group on the Evidence-based Pharmacologic treatment of bipolar I and II depression* (Kasper *et al.*, 2008) do not provide clinical evidence to support the efficacy of aripiprazole for the treatment of bipolar I depression, that showed a rapid onset of action with this effect not lasting.

The *NICE Guidelines*, revised in 2009 by the *National Collaborating Centre of Mental Health*, makes evidence-based recommendations for the identification, treatment, and management of bipolar disorder. For the treatment of acute mania, the suggestion is to prescribe an antipsychotic, such as aripiprazole, if there are severe manic symptoms or marked behavioral disturbance. Monotherapy should be considered if less severe symptoms. If it proves ineffective, augmentation with valproate or lithium is suggested. No suggestion for using aripiprazole in depression is given. For long-term treatment aripiprazole monotherapy is suggested if recent mania or rapid cycling.

The *Texas Implementation of Medication Algorithms: Update to the Algorithm for Treatment of Bipolar I Disorder* (Suppes *et al.*, 2005) includes different monotherapy

Table 12.1 Clinical indication of the use of aripiprazole in the most recently updated treatment guidelines.

Clinical indication	World Federation of Societies of Biological Psychiatry WFSBP	Canadian Network for Mood and Anxiety Treatments and International Society for Bipolar Disorders CANMAT and ISBD	British Association For Psychopharmacology BAP	International consensus group on the evidence-based pharmacologic treatment of bipolar I and II depression	National Institute of Clinical Excellence 2009 NICE	Texas medication algorithm
	Grunze et al. (2010)	Yatham et al. (2009)	Goodwin et al. (2009)	Kasper et al. (2008)	Nice (2009)	Suppes et al. (2005)
Mania						
First line	Monotherapy: CE A, RG 1 With a broad spectrum of efficacy across subtypes of mania (dysphoric/mixed states and psychotic mania)	Monotherapy: Level I I.M. in acute agitation: Level II	Monotherapy also for mixed mania		Monotherapy If severe manic symptoms or marked behavioral disturbances	Monotherapy Euphoric, irritable, dysphotic pts, and in mixed mania
Second line	Combination with Li/VPA	Combination with Li/VPA	Combination with Li/VPA for pts already on treatment		Combination with Li/VPA	Combination with other AAPs
Not recommended						

Depression						
First line	Not better than PBO at eight weeks				No evidence	No evidence
Second line	Adjunctive: CE E	Adjunctive				
Not recommended		Monotherapy	Monotherapy			
Maintenance						
Firstline	Monotherapy: prevention of mania	Monotherapy: prevention of mania	Monotherapy: prevention of mania	No evidence	Monotherapy: in pts with recent mania and/or rapid cycling	Monotherapy: in pts with recent mania (level II) and/or rapid cycling
Second line						Monotherapy: in pts with recent depression (level IV)
Not recommended			Monotherapy prevention of depression			

Li, Lithium; VPA, Valproate; CE, Category of evidence; RG, Recommendation grade; AAPs, Atypical antipsychotics.

options for the treatment of manic/mixed episodes. For those patients presenting with euphoric, irritable, and dysphoric mania or hypomania, clinicians may choose aripiprazole monotherapy as first-line treatment. In maintenance treatment among patients with the most recent hypomanic/manic episode, aripiprazole is recommended at level II. When the most recent episode is depressive, aripiprazole is not recommended as a first-line option, but there is evidence supporting its use at level IV.

12.3 ARIPIPRAZOLE EFFICACY FROM CLINICAL TRIAL DATA

Evidence-based information on aripiprazole in bipolar disorder comes basically from RCTs performed to set the efficacy of the studied drug. Studies have been performed among bipolar patients in order to assess aripiprazole efficacy in acute mania, in acute depression, and in maintenance treatment, both in monotherapy and adjunctive treatment, with and without a placebo arm (for extensive review see Fountoulakis and Vieta (2009); Fountoulakis *et al.*, in press). According to the phase of the illness (acute mania, depression, and maintenance), besides RCTs, further data on aripiprazole from open and observational studies, reviews, and meta-analyses will be summarized in the following paragraphs (see Table 12.2).

12.3.1 ACUTE MANIC/MIXED EPISODES

Mania remains one of the most challenging manifestations of bipolar disorder. The manic/mixed phases of the bipolar illness, although shorter in duration than depressive ones, can be devastating to both the patient and the family. They are often medical emergencies that require hospitalization in order to rapidly address abnormal affective symptomatology, restore behavioral control and protect patients from the consequences related to their impulsive and often dangerous actions. The effectiveness of acute treatment during manic/mixed episodes requires an intervention to have both a sufficiently rapid onset of action (that is, in order to allow rapid reduction of symptoms and discharge from the hospital within the first weeks) but also a long-term efficacy and a good tolerability profile (in order to facilitate compliance to chronic treatment) (Vieta *et al.*, 2005; Sachs *et al.*, 2006; Keck *et al.*, 2009). The efficacy of aripiprazole against acute mania is strongly supported by a number of RCTs, which also provide some support for its efficacy against mixed episodes and rapid cycling. Five RCTs involving a placebo arm (Sachs *et al.*, 2006; Keck *et al.*, 2003, 2009; Young *et al.*, 2009; El Mallakh *et al.*, 2010), one study without a placebo arm in monotherapy versus haloperidol (Vieta *et al.*, 2005), one study as adjunctive treatment (Vieta *et al.*, 2008), and one study on intramuscular (I.M.) treatment (Zimbroff *et al.*, 2007) will be summarized in the following paragraphs. Further data have been extracted from *post hoc* studies (Sachs *et al.*, 2007), meta-analyses, and reviews (Smith *et al.*, 2007; Cipriani, Rendell, and Geddes, 2006; Perlis *et al.*, 2006). One recently published study gave negative results vs. placebo in hospitalized patients (El Mallakh *et al.*, 2010). Practical recommendations for the management of aripiprazole in acute mania will be briefly mentioned (Aitchison *et al.*, 2009).

Table 12.2 Studies on aripiprazole in the treatment of bipolar disorder.

Clinical indication	Reference and study design		Review, meta-analysis, open studies	
	Randomized controlled study and post hoc analysis			
	Publication	Comments	Publication	Comments
Mania				
Monotherapy	Keck et al. Am. J. Psychiatry 2003	ARP > PBO	Sanford et al. CNS Drugs 2008	i.m. ARP > PBO in ↓ PANSS-exited
	Sachs et al. J Psychopharmacol 2006	ARP > PBO	Currier et al. J. Psychiatr. Pract. 2007	i.m. ARP > PBO in ↓ PANSS-exited
	Keck et al. J. Affect. Disord. 2009	ARP = Li > PBO	Smith et al. Bipolar Disord. 2007	ARP > PBO in ↓ YMRS
	Young et al. Br. J. Psychiatry 2009	ARP = Hal > PBO	Cipriani et al. Cochr Database Syst. Rev. 2006	ARP > Hal in ↓ manic symptoms
	Vieta et al. Br. J. Psychiatry 2005	ARP > Hal	Perlis et al. J. Clin. Psychiatry 2006	ARP = other AAPs in efficacy
	Unpublished (CN139-077/ NCT00046384)[a]	No results	Barzman et al. J. Child Adolesc. Psychopharmacol. 2004[1]	RESP: 67%;
	Sachs et al. J. Clin. Psychiatry 2007	ARP > PBO in ↓ manic sympt. and agitation	Biederman et al. CNS Spectr. 2007	Positive results
	Suppes et al. J. Affect. Disord. 2008	ARP > PBO in ↓ manic sympt	Tramontina et al. CNS Spectr. 2007	Positive results
			Biederman et al. CNS Spectr. 2005	RESP: 71% in ↓ manic symptoms
Adjunctive	Zimbroff et al. (2007)	i.m. ARP + Lor > PBO in agitation	Cipriani et al. Cochr Database Syst. Rev. 2006	ARP > Hal in ↓ manic symptoms
	Vieta et al. Am. J. Psychiatry 2008	ARP + Li/VPA > PBO	Perlis et al. J. Clin. Psychiatry 2006	ARP

(Continued Overleaf)

Table 12.2 (Continued)

Clinical indication	Reference and study design				
	Randomized controlled study and post hoc analysis		Review, meta-analysis, open studies		
	Publication	Comments	Publication	Comments	
Depression					
Monotherapy	Thase et al. J. Clin. Psychopharmacol. 2008	ARP = PBO (negative results)	Dunn et al. J. Affect. Disord. 2008	RESP: 44%	
			McElroy et al. J. Affect. Disord. 2007	RESP: 42%; REM: 35%	
			Mazza et al. Exp. Opin. Pharmacother. 2008	RESP: 65% ; REM: 37.5%	
Adjunctive			Ketter et al. Ann. Clin. Psychiatry 2006	RESP:27% ; REM: 13%	
			Sajatovic et al. J. Clin. Psychiatry 2008	↓ YMRS, ↓ MADRS	
			Ketter, J. Clin. Psychiatry 2008	Positive results	
			Sokolsky et al. Ann. Pharmacother. 2007	RESP: 70%	

			RESP: 33%
	Kemp et al. Prog. Neuropsychopharmacol. Biol. Psychiatry 2007		
	Schienberg, Hum. Psychopharmacol. 2009		ARP > LMT

Maintenance

Monotherapy	Keck et al. J. Clin. Psychiatry 2006	ARP > PBO
	Keck et al. J. Clin. Psychiatry 2007	ARP = COMP > PBO
	Keck et al. J. Affect. Disord. 2009	ARP = Li
	Vieta et al. Br. J. Psychiatry 2005	No results
	Muzina et al. Int. J. Clin. Pract. 2008	ARP > PBO
Adjunctive	Findling et al., (2009)	Positive results

---

[a]Study in bipolar children and adolescents.
Hal, Haloperidol; ARP, aripiprazole; PBO, placebo; COMP, Comparator; Li, lithium; VPA, valproic acid; RESP, response rate; REM, remission rate; i.m., intramuscular. PANSS: Positive and Negative Syndrome Scale; HAM-D: Hamilton Depression Rating Scale.

12.3.1.1 Aripiprazole Monotherapy in Manic/Mixed Episodes

12.3.1.1.1 RCTs on Aripiprazole Monotherapy vs Placebo in Manic/Mixed Episodes

The first study involving a placebo arm on the efficacy and safety of aripiprazole monotherapy in patients with acute bipolar mania, published in 2003 (Keck *et al.*, 2003) showed that aripiprazole had significantly greater efficacy than placebo for the treatment of acute and mixed episode in bipolar disorder, being safe, and well tolerated too. This placebo-controlled, double-blind, multicenter, three-weeks study, randomized 262 bipolar patients with a manic/mixed episode to aripiprazole, started at 30 mg/day and adjusted to between 15 and 30 mg/day after day 4 (mean dose at endpoint 27.9 mg daily) or placebo (1 : 1). The primary *efficacy* measure was mean change form baseline in total score on the Young Mania Rating Scale (YMRS). Aripiprazole significantly reduced the YMRS score (defined as a decrease in score of $>50\%$) in comparison to placebo (-8.2 vs -3.4, p $= 0.002$) and the Clinical Global Impression (CGI) score for mania (-1.0 vs -0.4, p $= 0.001$), depression (-0.2 vs $+ 0.1.4$, $p = 0.03$), and overall bipolar illness (-1.0 vs -0.4, p $= 0.001$). The response rate was significantly higher in the aripiprazole group in comparison to placebo at endpoint with a rapid onset of activity (by Day 4).

A second study, published in 2006 (Sachs *et al.*, 2006) confirmed the efficacy, safety, and tolerability of aripiprazole in the treatment of acute mania. This placebo-controlled, double-blind, multicenter, three-weeks study randomized 272 bipolar I patients with a manic/mixed episode to aripiprazole with the same flexible dosage of previous study (mean dose at endpoint 27.7 mg daily) or placebo (1 : 1). Aripiprazole significantly reduced the YMRS score in comparison to placebo (-12.5 vs -7.2, $P < 0.001$) and other measures (CGI score for mania, depression, and overall bipolar illness). A significantly higher response rate was observed in the aripiprazole group at endpoint (53% vs 32%) with a rapid onset of activity (by Day 4). The separate analysis of patients with rapid cycling suggested that aripiprazole significantly reduced the YMRS score in this group (-15.27 vs -5.45, $P = 0.002$) but not the Montgomery Åsberg Depression Rating Scale (MADRS) score. In addition, aripiprazole was also effective in significantly reducing PANSS Hostility Subscale Score.

The third study, published in 2009 (Keck *et al.*, 2009), comparing aripiprazole or lithium vs placebo, showed a significant improvement of acute mania compared to placebo and similar with lithium. It included 480 bipolar type I patients with a manic or mixed episode, involved in a randomized, double-blind placebo-, and lithium-controlled study (1 : 1 : 1), comparing aripiprazole (23.2 mg daily) to lithium and placebo for three weeks and aripiprazole and lithium for an additional nine weeks. The completion rate was similar for all study groups (placebo 47%, aripiprazole 47%, lithium 49%). Aripiprazole and lithium significantly reduced the YMRS score by more in comparison to placebo at week 3 (-12.6 and -12.0, respectively vs -9.0 for placebo, $P < 0.001$) and this effect was maintained at week 12 (-14.5 and -12.7, respectively). There was a significant change in the CGI score for mania ($P < 0.01$ between placebo and aripiprazole), but not in the MADRS change. There were some differences in the PANSS subscores between aripiprazole and placebo (total PANSS, cognitive, and hostility subscales). The response rate was significantly higher in the aripiprazole and lithium group in comparison to placebo at week 3 (46.8% vs 45.8% vs 34.4%, respectively) and at week 12 there was a slight superiority for aripiprazole in comparison to lithium (56.5% vs 49%, respectively). The remission rates followed a similar pattern both at week 3 (40.3% vs 40.0% vs 28.2%, respectively) and at week 12 there was again superiority for aripiprazole in comparison to lithium (49.4 vs 39.4%, respectively).

The fourth study (Young *et al.*, 2009) compared aripiprazole or haloperidol vs placebo, and showed a clinical improvement for ARP and a good tolerability. It was a 12-week randomized placebo- and haloperidol- controlled study, that included 485 patients with a manic or mixed episode, randomized 1 : 1 : 1 to aripiprazole (mean dosage 23.6 mg daily) haloperidol or placebo for 3 weeks and those on placebo were afterwards put blindly on aripiprazole. Overall, 356 (73.4%) completed the three-week trial duration and the completion rate was similar for all study groups. Aripiprazole and haloperidol significantly reduced the YMRS score by more in comparison to placebo at week 3 ($P < 0.05$) and this effect was maintained at week 12. There was a significant change in the CGI score for mania ($P < 0.05$). There were no differences in the MADRS change among groups, while there were some differences in the PANSS subscores between aripiprazole and placebo (total PANSS, positive, cognitive, and hostility subscales). The response rate was significantly higher in the aripiprazole and haloperidol group in comparison to placebo at three weeks (47% vs 49.7% vs 38.2%, respectively) and at 12 weeks there was a similar rate of response for aripiprazole and haloperidol (72.3% vs 73.9%, respectively). The remission rates followed a similar pattern both at 3 weeks and at 12 weeks there was again a similarity of rates between aripiprazole and haloperidol.

An additional three-week, placebo-controlled, fixed-dose trial showed that the primary outcome measurement in the aripiprazole-treated group was not different from that in the placebo group due to a higher than usual placebo response (El Mallakh *et al.*, 2010) This third trial was considered a failed trial. One recently published study evaluated the efficacy and safety of two fixed doses of aripiprazole (15 mg/day and 30 mg/day) compared with placebo in acutely manic or mixed bipolar I hospitalized patients. Aripiprazole was not significantly more effective than placebo in the treatment of bipolar I disorder acute mania at endpoint (Week 3), even if taking into account that a high placebo response rate may have accounted for the lack of separation between treatment groups.

12.3.1.1.2 RCTs on Aripiprazole Monotherapy without a Placebo in Manic/Mixed Episodes

Comparison with other active compounds support comparative efficacy of aripiprazole. Among RCTs without a placebo arm, the one study which compared aripiprazole vs haloperidol in acute mania demonstrated that aripiprazole offers superior effectiveness (not efficacy) to haloperidol in the treatment of patients for up to 12 weeks (Vieta *et al.*, 2005). This was a double-blind, multicenter, randomized, comparative 12-week trial, where 347 patients with bipolar I disorder experiencing acute manic/mixed episodes were randomized 1 : 1 to aripiprazole (starting dose 15 mg/day with option to increase to 30 mg/day, average daily dosage, 21.6 mg) and haloperidol (average daily dosage, 11.6 mg). Overall, 134 patients receiving aripiprazole and 95 receiving haloperidol completed the first three weeks of treatment; with 89 and 50 at the week 12. The response rate was 49.7% in the aripiprazole group and 28.4% in the haloperidol group ($P < 0.001$). The proportion of patients in remission at week 12 was significantly higher in the aripiprazole group than in the haloperidol group (50% vs. 27%; $P = 0.001$), with a high rate of drop-out in the haloperidol group due to extrapyramidal effect sides. Significantly more patients completing the study demonstrated a 50% or greater decrease in MADRS total score from baseline with aripiprazole than with haloperidol at week 12 (51% vs. 33%; $P = 0.001$) and aripiprazole treatment produced greater numerical reductions in depressive symptoms compared with haloperidol, as measured by the mean change in MADRS total score at endpoint. Fewer patients on aripiprazole switched to depression than patients with haloperidol (11.0% vs 17.7%). However, the study design favored aripiprazole to some extent because anticholinergic drugs were not allowed and the definition of response requested to complete the study.

A *post hoc* analysis of the two three-week acute mania RCTs (Sachs *et al.*, 2006; Keck *et al.*, 2003) was performed by Suppes and collaborators (2008) to assess the efficacy and safety of aripiprazole compared with placebo in subpopulations of type I bipolar patients with manic/mixed acute episodes. The results of this analysis suggest that aripiprazole may be effective and safe in a broad spectrum of patients subtypes experiencing manic or mixed episodes, including different levels of co-occurring depressive symptoms, rapid cycling, and psychotic symptoms.

Another *post hoc* analysis of these same RCTs suggested that aripiprazole was superior to placebo in reducing the severity of both mania and agitation in highly agitated patients with bipolar I disorder, and showed significant antimanic activity in patients with low levels of agitation without increasing agitation. These findings suggest that aripiprazole's antimanic effect is specific and not limited to control of agitation through sedation (Sachs *et al.*, 2007; Frye *et al.*, 2008).

12.3.1.1.3 Other Studies on Aripiprazole Treatment in Manic/Mixed Episodes

A systematic review and meta-analysis by Smith *et al.* (2007) of 13 randomized, placebo-controlled trials (involving 3089 subjects) in acute bipolar mania, which included two aripiprazole studies, suggested a response to treatment (at least 50% reduction in YMRS scores) more than 1.7 times higher in comparison to placebo (relative risk (RR) $= 1.74$, 95% confidence interval (CI) 1.54–1.96). Another meta-analysis on 15 RCTs and 2022 patients suggests that aripiprazole is more effective than haloperidol at reducing manic symptoms, both as monotherapy and as adjunctive treatment to lithium or valproate (Cipriani, Rendell, and Geddes, 2006). Perlis and collaborators (2006) in another systematic review and meta-analysis from 12 placebo-controlled monotherapy and 6 placebo-controlled adjunctive therapy trials involving a total of 4304 subjects of atypical antipsychotics for acute bipolar mania report that aripiprazole and others antipsychotics, demonstrated significant efficacy in monotherapy without any significant differences in efficacy among all antipsychotics.

12.3.1.2 Aripiprazole Adjunctive Treatment in Manic/Mixed Episodes

12.3.1.2.1 RCTs on Adjunctive Aripiprazole in Manic/Mixed Episodes

Comparison of aripiprazole versus placebo in combination with lithium/valproate furnished positive results for aripiprazole. In the one study of adjunctive aripiprazole with a placebo arm, to either valproate or lithium the authors (Vieta *et al.*, 2008) showed a significant improvement in bipolar patients with mania, partially nonresponsive to valproate/lithium monotherapy and demonstrated a tolerability profile similar to that of monotherapy studies. It was a multicenter, randomized, placebo-controlled, six-week trial. A total sample of 384 patients was randomly assigned in a 2:1 ratio to adjunctive aripiprazole (mean dosage, 19.0 mg/day) or placebo. Double-blind treatment was completed by 85 and 79% of patients randomly assigned to placebo and aripiprazole, respectively. Discontinuation rates due to adverse events were higher for patients in the aripiprazole group than for patients in the placebo group (9% vs 5%). As *efficacy* measures, adjunctive aripiprazole showed significantly greater improvements from baseline in YMRS total score than placebo ($P < 0.0$) but this was due to the valproate but not the lithium group. At endpoint the remission rate was 66.0% for aripiprazole and 50.8% for placebo ($P < 0.01$, number needed to treat (NNT = 7). The improvement over placebo in MADRS was not statistically significant at endpoint, however the proportion of patients with emergent depression was significantly lower in the aripiprazole arm than the placebo arm (7.7% vs 16.9%; $P < 0.01$).

Specifically concerning the effectiveness of aripiprazole against agitation, a placebo-controlled RCT showed that I.M. aripiprazole is an effective and well-tolerated therapy in the treatment of acute agitation in patients with bipolar I disorder, manic or mixed episodes (Zimbroff *et al.*, 2007). The mean improvements in PANSS-Excited component score at 2 hours were significantly greater with aripiprazole (-8.7 for the 9.75 mg group and -8.7 for the 15 mg group) and lorazepam (-9.6) versus placebo (-5.8), with $P < 0.001$.

12.3.1.3 Practical Guidance of the Use of Aripiprazole in Mania

Practical guidance for prescribe aripiprazole in bipolar mania (dose selection, for the switching strategies and for the management of side-effects) is needed in order to assist clinicians in using aripiprazole for the treatment of bipolar mania in real-world practice, since the limited generalizability of RCTs to routine clinical practice (Aitchison *et al.*, 2008). The appropriate choice of dose and formulation should take into account factors such as: speed of onset, reliability of delivery, efficacy, incidence of adverse events, interactions with other medications, specific antimanic activity independent of sedation, patient preference, therapeutic alliance, likelihood of treatment adherence, and current medication regimen. Where possible and appropriate, it is good clinical practice that the patient should participate in choosing medication. Whether aripiprazole is being initiated in a patient not currently receiving any other antipsychotic medication or switching from another one, it can be initiated at an oral starting dose of 15 mg/day, with a range of doses around 5–20 mg/day. Some patients may need to start at a lower dose (5 or 10 mg/day). If there is an urgent need for symptom control, a dose at the higher end of the range should be selected (that is, 30 mg/day), while if less urgent, a dose at the lower end of the spectrum should be used. If necessary, adjunctive medication should be used in early treatment to manage side effects or agitation. Where necessary, concomitant medications, for example, benzodiazepines, may be considered, as required, but should be short term if possible. Over the first few days and weeks of treatment, the patient's status should be monitored and the dose of aripiprazole adjusted until the minimum effective dose is reached, usually between 15 and 30 mg/day, depending on response.

Switching from an antipsychotic to another one is common in clinical practice, due to lack of response or induced side effects, and can result in clinical benefits to patients (Mir *et al.*, 2008). A switch should be considered for patients with a good response but with an intolerable level of side effects (that is, excessive sedation, dysphoria, weight gain, hyperprolactinaemia, dyslipidaemia, or metabolic syndrome), or for patients who are partially treatment refractory, are in acute relapse because their symptoms not controlled or discontinued their prior medication due to efficacy/tolerability issues. When switching patients from previous antipsychotic medication to aripiprazole, it is essential to ensure three to four weeks of coverage of aripiprazole starting dose (5 mg/day) with previous medication and that aripiprazole is titrated to its minimum effective dose before tapering down the previous agent. Adjust it to between 10 and 30 mg/day depending on tolerability and response, reach effective dose of aripiprazole and gradually reduce previous medication (may need to be done over more than two to four weeks and sometimes longer than that), consider maintaining full dose of previous medication for up to two weeks, if necessary. When switching only for tolerability reasons, it is suggested that a starting dose of 5 mg/day should be used, to be increased slowly over at least three to four weeks. It is essential that the cross-titration period is longer than five half-lives of aripiprazole to allow time for the serum level of aripiprazole to reach steady-state. Once the aripiprazole dose is established, the other medication can be tapered out gradually over at least two weeks, depending on its half-life. On the other hand, when switching for reason of inefficacy or partial efficacy and where there is a risk of relapse, a starting dose of 15 mg/day is suggested. The dose of current treatment regimen should be maintained whilst titrating up aripiprazole over at least three to four weeks, until a response is achieved. The previous medication should then be gradually reduced, aiming to withdraw it completely, if possible. When switching in an acute relapse, usually in the inpatient setting, it was recommended to start aripiprazole at 20 mg/day, while continuing the current treatment regimen. After at least three to four weeks, the previous medication should be gradually reduced, aiming to withdraw it completely. In all cases, a significant overlap with previous medication when carrying out a switch to aripiprazole is recommended because all other antipsychotics have a contrasting pharmacological profile.

Combination therapy with an antipsychotic plus lithium or valproate is a recommended approach for mania, and may arise because of the failure of monotherapy, the presence of psychotic symptoms or the need to use lithium or valproate as part of subsequent maintenance treatment. Several pharmacokinetic studies have demonstrated that co-administration of lithium or divalproex sodium with aripiprazole had no clinically significant effect on the steady-state pharmacokinetics of aripiprazole and vice versa and consequently, no dose adjustments are required when aripiprazole and lithium/valproate are administered concurrently. It is recommended to double the aripiprazole dose in combination therapy with carbamazepine, a CYP3A4 inducer. Dosage adjustments for aripiprazole are recommended during co-administration of fluoxetine and paroxetine, and antihistamines such as promethazine, inhibitors of CYP2D6.

12.3.2   ACUTE DEPRESSIVE EPISODES

Although depressive episodes occur most frequently in bipolar disorder and account for a significant amount of the morbidity and mortality of bipolar disorder, the majority of treatment research focus on mania, so that data are scarce and treating options limited (Judd *et al.*, 2002) . Increasing evidence suggests that atypical antipsychotics, having both antimanic and antidepressant effects could represent a novel treatment option for patients with bipolar depression (Thase *et al.*, 2008). Several lines of evidence suggested that aripiprazole might also be a useful treatment for acute bipolar depression (McElroy *et al.*, 2007). First, as a partial D2 and D3 receptor agonist, aripiprazole is thought to enhance dopamine activity in hypodopaminergic conditions, and bipolar depression may be associated with deficient dopamine function. Second, 5HT2A antagonism of aripiprazole, thought to be serotonin 5HT2A down-regulation, has been hypothesized to account in part for the efficacy of antipsychotics in acute bipolar depression (Keck and McElroy, 2003; Nemeroff, 2005). Third, aripiprazole has been reported to have antidepressant properties in adults and children with bipolar disorder in adults with treatment-resistant bipolar depression (Ketter *et al.*, 2006), and those with treatment-resistant unipolar depression (Worthington *et al.*, 2005; Arbaizar *et al.*, 2009). There are only two identical RCTs on aripiprazole monotherapy in bipolar I depression and they are both negative on the primary outcome, but some of the positive secondary outcomes deserve some discussion (Thase *et al.*, 2008). There are other open studies, both in acute bipolar depression (Dunn *et al.*, 2008) and in bipolar treatment-resistant depression (McElroy *et al.*, 2007; Mazza *et al.*, 2008).

12.3.2.1   Aripiprazole Monotherapy in Acute Depressive Episodes

12.3.2.1.1   RCTs on Aripiprazole Monotherapy in Depressive Episodes
The two identical negative studies on aripiprazole monotherapy in bipolar I depression (Thase *et al.*, 2008) are two multicenter, double-blind, placebo-controlled, eight-week trials on efficacy and safety of aripiprazole in monotherapy. They included 374 and 375 patients respectively, randomly assigned to placebo and aripiprazole (mean dose at endpoint 17.6 mg daily and 15.5 mg daily). The results suggest that in weeks 1–6 there is a significant reduction in the MADRS scores in the aripiprazole group in comparison to placebo, but at week 7 this difference disappears and the active agent is no better than placebo. The drug is therefore not formally indicated in bipolar depression even if some data support the importance of dose optimization in order to reduce the burden of side-effects. It could still work, hence, as a trigger of antidepressant response or even as an antidepressant at lower doses, given that most drop outs were due to dose-related side-effects.

12.3.2.1.2   Open Studies on Aripiprazole Monotherapy in Depressive Episodes
There are a number of open trials assessing the potential use of aripiprazole in bipolar disorder, especially in refractory depression. Open trials have methodological limitations, but may open new avenues for clinical research. A six-week prospective, non-randomized, open-label study in 20 bipolar depressed outpatients (type I, type II, and NOS) reported

a significant improvement in depressive symptoms, measured by MADRS (Dunn et al., 2008). Aripiprazole was dosed flexibility up to a maximum of 30 mg daily. The response rate was of 44% in patients who completed at least one week of treatment and a drop-out rate of 35%. The authors highlighted an improvement in the core symptoms, such as sadness, suicidal thoughts, anhedonia, and psychomotor slowing, especially in type II bipolar disorder and rapid cycling.

Aripiprazole monotherapy was tested amongst refractory bipolar depressive patients in two open studies. In the first one, aripiprazole response was prospectively assessed for eight weeks in 31 bipolar patients with acute bipolar depression. The results suggested that 42% of patients responded and 35% remitted (McElroy et al., 2007), with a high discontinuation rate primarily due to side effects. In the second study, aripiprazole response was prospectively assessed for 16 weeks in 85 acutely depressed bipolar patients. Only 3.5% of patients discontinued the study for side effects while 21.2% of patients experienced akathisia. The trial was completed by 94.1% of patients with a response rate of 65% and the remission rate of 37.5% (Mazza et al., 2008).

12.3.2.2 Aripiprazole Adjunctive Treatment in Bipolar Depression

12.3.2.2.1 Open Studies on Aripiprazole Adjunctive Treatment in Depressive Episodes

Adjunctive aripiprazole was studied in an open clinical trial of 30 outpatients with treatment-resistant bipolar depression (type I, type II, and NOS) by Ketter and collaborators (2006). Patients received aripiprazole for a mean duration of 84 ± 69 days, (mean dose 15.3 mg/day at endpoint). Aripiprazole yielded improvement in Clinical Global Impression–Severity (CGI–S) $(4.4 \pm 1.1–3.8 \pm 1.2,\ p < 0.01)$, with 27% of patients responding (CGI–S improvement $> = 2$). Authors also showed improvement in Global Assessment of Function, depressed mood, and suicidal ideation ratings. Aripiprazole was generally well tolerated, with no significant change in mean adverse effect ratings or mean weight.

In an open-label study aripiprazole was co-administered at 10 mg/day for three days, 20 mg/day for three days, then 30 mg/day for eight days, with lamotrigine in 18 bipolar patients. The results suggest aripiprazole has no meaningful effect on lamotrigine steady-state pharmacokinetics in patients with bipolar I disorder (Schieber et al., 2009).

12.3.3 MAINTENANCE PHASE

Since the chronic and persistent nature of bipolar illness, the majority of patients expect a lifelong course of recurrent acute episodes in addition to residual symptoms in the intervening periods. Recurrence rates can reach up to 49% within two years of recovery from an initial episode (Thase et al., 2008). The goals of treatment of bipolar disorder include, after resolution of acute symptoms, the prevention of recurrent mood symptoms to allow patients to achieve their optimal pre-morbid level of psychosocial functioning and quality of life (Suppes et al., 2005). In the US aripiprazole and olanzapine are the only atypical antipsychotics approved as monotherapy for the maintenance therapy of bipolar disorder, while quetiapine and ziprasidone are approved as combination therapy with lithium and/or valproate. Data from the first controlled 26-week study on maintenance in recently manic- or mixed-patients (Keck *et al.*, 2006), including one 76-week extension phase represented by studies by Keck *et al.* (2007, 2009) and a *post hoc* analysis by Muzina *et al.* (2008) will be resumed in the followings.

12.3.3.1 Aripiprazole Monotherapy in Maintenance

12.3.3.1.1 RCTs on Aripiprazole Monotherapy in Maintenance
The first study that investigated the efficacy and safety of aripiprazole monotherapy in the maintenance amongst bipolar I disorders, published in 2006, showed that aripiprazole was superior to placebo in preventing any mood episode in recently manic/mixed patients (Keck *et al.*, 2006). This randomized, double-blind, placebo-controlled, multicenter study enrolled 633 patients into a stablization phase (from 6 to 18 weeks), 161 patients who achieved 6 consecutive weeks of stabilization where randomized to a 1 : 1 ratio to aripiprazole (mean dosage 24.3 mg/day at the double-blind phase endpoint) or placebo for an additional 26 weeks, after a period of stabilization (from 6 to 18 weeks). The primary *efficacy* outcome was time to relapse for a mood episode. A total of 39 patients (50%) on aripiprazole and 28 (34%) on placebo completed the 26 weeks of the trial. The time to relapse was significantly longer for aripiprazole ($P = 0.02$). This was due to a prolongation in the time to relapse to a manic ($P = 0.01$) but not to a depressive episode. At the end of the study 49% of the placebo group and 72% of the aripiprazole group had not experienced a relapse to a mood episode. The difference was significant only concerning manic relapses (23% vs 8%; $P = 0.009$). The same was true for the final YMRS score while there was no difference concerning the MADRS score. There was also a superiority of aripiprazole in comparison to placebo concerning the CGI and the PANSS scores.

The study by Keck and colleagues (2007) included a 74-week placebo-controlled extension phase of the 26-week timepoint, which does not allow a conclusion to be reached, because of its high discontinuation rate, due to lack of efficacy, side effects (very low percentage) and most importantly the very design and structure of the study. During the 74-week, double-blind, extension phase, all but one of the discontinuations due to "other reasons" (n = 10 for PBO and n = 14 for ARP) occurred because the study was closed by the sponsor when the prespecified number of relapses had been attained. This study employed an enriched design, with patients first completing a stabilization treatment phase which included aripiprazole as therapy for an acute manic or mixed episode. Time to relapse for any mood episode was significantly longer for aripiprazole than placebo (p = 0.001; hazard ratio: 0.53; CI: 0.32–0.87). The only difference concerned manic relapses.

A *post hoc* subgroup analysis (Muzina *et al.*, 2008) of 28 patients (14 on placebo and 14 on aripiprazole) with rapid-cycling bipolar I disorder from the previous maintenance study suggested that aripiprazole was more effective than placebo in the prophylaxis of rapid cycling patients against manic/mixed episodes. The time to relapse was significantly longer with aripiprazole vs placebo treatment at both 26 weeks ($P = 0.033$; HR $= 0.21$) and 100 weeks ($P = 0.017$; HR $= 0.18$). The median survival time in the placebo group was 118 days at which time approximately 45% of patients had not yet relapsed. The median survival time for the aripiprazole group was not evaluable. At the time of the last relapse event in the study period, which occurred at day 101, 81% of aripiprazole-treated subjects with rapid-cycling bipolar disorder had not yet relapsed. The YMRS total scores increased in both groups and this increase was numerically smaller with aripiprazole vs placebo from at least week 26. The same for the MADRS total scores, which increased in both treatment groups with no statistically significant difference with aripiprazole versus placebo at end-point.

The extension of the acute phase trial by El-Mallakh and colleagues (2010) for an additional 40 weeks (52 weeks in total) comparing aripiprazole to lithium without a placebo arm suggested that aripiprazole is equal to lithium in maintenance against manic episodes. Of the original 480 patients during the acute phase, 94 entered the 40-week extension. For both treatment groups, the improvement that was observed at the end of 12-week double-blind treatment phase was maintained throughout the extension phase.

12.4 ARIPIPRAZOLE SAFETY AND TOLERABILITY

12.4.1 ADVERSE EVENTS IN CLINICAL TRIALS

Since the majority of bipolar patients require long-term treatment, the tolerability of the specific drug is a crucial point for clinicians to consider, in terms of safety and medication compliance. The overall safety and tolerability of aripiprazole is favorable compared to other atypical antipsychotics across the approved indications, probably reflecting its novel mechanism of action (dopamine-serotonin system stabilizer). In general, aripiprazole shows a minimal propensity for clinically significant weight gain and metabolic disruption. However, extrapyramidal side effects, such as akathisia, are reported and may limit its clinical use in some cases. The most common side effects during aripiprazole treatment include akathisia, tremor, headache, dizziness, somnolence, sedation fatigue, nausea, vomiting, dyspepsia, constipation, light-headedness, insomnia, restlessness, sleepiness, anxiety, hypersalivation, and blurred vision. The uncommon side effects, and those whose frequency is not precisely known, include uncontrollable twitching or jerking movements, seizures, weight gain, orthostatic hypotension or tachycardia, allergic reaction (such as swelling in the mouth or throat, itching, rash), speech disorder, agitation, fainting, transaminasaemia, pancreatitis, muscle pain, stiffness, or cramps, and very rarely neuroleptic malignant syndrome and tardive dyskinaesia. Sedation is less preeminent with aripiprazole than with other antipsychotics (Fountoulakis and Vieta, 2009).

Evidence based data resulting from treatment of acute manic/mixed episodes in bipolar patients highlight that during acute aripiprazole monotherapy is more frequently associated with nausea than placebo (23.3−15.8% vs 22.7−10%), dyspepsia (22−15.4% vs 6.8−10%), somnolence (20% vs 10−5%), anxiety (18% vs 10%), vomiting (16−11% vs 5−7.5%), insomnia (15% vs 9%), light-headedness (14% vs 8%), constipation (13% vs 5.3−6%), accidental injury (11.8−12% vs 2%), and akathisia (17.6−11% vs 2−4.5%) (Sachs et al., 2006; Keck et al., 2003, 2009). When used in combination (Vieta *et al.*, 2008) the most frequently reported adverse event is akathisia (aripiprazole: 18.6% vs placebo: 5.4%), tremor (placebo: 6.2% vs aripiprazole: 9.1%), EPS (placebo: 0.8% vs aripiprazole: 4.7%), hypertonia (placebo: 0% vs aripiprazole: 0.4%), hypokinaesia (placebo: 0% vs aripiprazole: 0.4%), muscle spasms (placebo: 0.8% vs aripiprazole: 2.0%), dyskinaesia (placebo: 0.8% vs aripiprazole: 0.4%), and muscle twitching (placebo: 0% vs aripiprazole: 0.4%). It is not significantly associated with change in body weight, elevated serum prolactin or QTc prolongation and electrocardiogram (ECG). Evidence based data resulting from treatment of acute depressive episodes in bipolar patients (Thase *et al.*, 2008) show that the most frequent adverse events are akathisia (21.4–27.5% vs 2.8–4.8% in PBO), insomnia (16.3–18.3% vs 4.8–11.0% in PBO), nausea (14.3–15.2% vs 5.4–7.7% in PBO), restlessness (10.1–12.1% vs 2.8–5.4% in PBO), fatigue (10.7–12.6% vs 4.3–7.7% in PBO), back pain (4.8–7.9% vs 1.6–2.8% in PBO), dry mouth (7.9–12.1% vs 2.7–8.8% in PBO), increased appetite (4.4–6.7% vs 1.7–2.2% in PBO), vomiting (6.2–4.9% vs 1.7–2.2% in PBO), anxiety (5.6–9.3% vs 2.8% in PBO), and sedation (5.1–5.5% vs 2.2% in PBO). The incidence of Serious AEs has been reported low both for aripiprazole and placebo (2.2% vs 1.3–1.3%). The incidence of suicidality (ideation and attempts) was reported to be low and comparable between aripiprazole and placebo. During maintenance therapy the most frequent adverse event are reported to be anxiety (16.9% in Aripiprazole vs 14.5% PBO), insomnia (15.6% vs 19.3%), depression (11.7% vs 14.5%), nervousness (10.4% vs 6.0%), tremor (9.1% vs 1.2%), nausea (9.1% vs 4.8%), agitation (7.8% vs 10.8%), akathisia 6.5% vs 1.2%), headache (7.8% vs 16.9%). No clinically relevant trends were reported in laboratory, vital sign, or ECG results during long-term treatment of aripiprazole (Keck *et al.*, 2007, 2009). Patients and their families should be continuously educated about the recurrent and sometimes chronic nature of bipolar disorder and the need for long-term medication and safety monitoring. Sustained weight increases can directly increase insulin resistance and the risk of type II diabetes (Scheen and De Hert, 2007). In addition, more direct effects of weight gain on lipid metabolism may arise early in treatment (Newcomer, 2005). The apparently low-risk metabolic profile of aripiprazole becomes a relevant factor in comparison with other drugs. Finally, potential prolactin elevation, even if relatively uncommon compared to D2 antagonists, can suppress the gonadal hormone axis, and this can lead to sexual dysfunction in men and women and an increased risk of osteopenia and fractures in women (Maguire 2002; Mir *et al.*, 2008). Suggested management strategies for adverse events have been proposed. If activation, use benzodiazepine or antihistamine, more in inpatient setting and with caution in the outpatient setting; psychosocial measures may also be valuable. If akathisia, then reduce the dose, use a benzodiazepine, beta-blockers, anticholinergics, or propranolol. If nausea or vomiting it is possible to wait, as usually is transient; if persist then reduce the dose and later return to the target dose, otherwise use conventional antiemetic medications. If present restlessness/agitation, use benzodiazepine or antihistamine, psychosocial, and psychoeducational measures. Ideally, aripiprazole should be administered in the morning to reduce the risk of insomnia. If insomnia is present, then check if patient is taking medication no later than mid-day; if yes, use benzodiazepine or non-benzodiazepine hypnotics.

12.4.2 SAFETY AND TOLERABILITY ISSUES AND SWITCHING STRATEGIES

In clinical practice, switching from an antipsychotic to another one is common, due to lack of response or induced side effects. Despite it, only recently the analysis of the best switching strategy between antipsychotics has received attention (Pae *et al.*, 2009a). Up until recently, no consensus was achieved and actual evidence is not univocal, especially for the new antipsychotic aripirazole. Clinical experience suggests that immediate switch to aripiprazole may worsen the positive symptomatology, possibly due to the specific mechanism of action of aripiprazole and to the relative increase in dopamine transmission mediated by its agonistic activity. Surprisingly in a previous study by Casey and collaborators (2003) no significant difference was found between different switch strategies, and a meta-analysis confirmed the nonsuperiority of a particular switching strategy (Remington *et al.*, 2005). Despite this evidence, some recent clinical guidelines for the treatment of schizophrenia recommend that prior antipsychotic should remain stable for several weeks after aripiprazole is introduced (Cassano *et al.*, 2007), and a recent study suggests that a clinically meaningful difference does exist between patients administered with abrupt discontinuation of a previous antipsychotic drug that showed a worsening of symptoms within the first two weeks of treatment, while patients administered with tapering off constantly improved over time (Pae *et al.*, 2009b). Over the long period, abrupt discontinuation or alternatively tapering off previous antipsychotic medication and contemporary initiation of aripiprazole may be similar in terms of efficacy and safety, but a significant advantage of the second strategy is suggested within the first weeks, protecting against drop-out and premature interruption of treatment. When switching to aripiprazole, the therapeutic dose of current treatment should be maintained while adding aripiprazole and titrating to 15 mg/day (5–20 mg/day). Only once an effective dose of aripiprazole is reached should previous medication be reduced.

12.5 TREATMENT OF SPECIAL POPULATIONS

12.5.1 PEDIATRIC BIPOLAR DISORDER

Aripiprazole was approved by US FDA for the treatment of bipolar disorder in pediatric patients (children aged 10–17 years). In their randomized, double-blind, placebo-controlled study, Findling and colleagues demonstrated the efficacy and good tolerability of aripiprazole (daily dose 10 or 30 mg) in the acute treatment of 296 paediatric bipolar I patients, recently manic or mixed, with or without psychotic symptoms. The response (>50% of reduction in YMRS total score) at week 4 was achieved in aripiprazole group significantly more than placebo. In a review by Greenaway and Elbe (2009) it is highlighted that aripiprazole may represent an important alternative for some children and adolescents who have experienced poor efficacy or significant metabolic adverse effects with their current antipsychotic treatment. In a RCT with a four-week acute phase and a 26-week continuation phase demonstrated the acute and long-term efficacy of aripiprazole in 296 pediatric patients with Bipolar Disorder Type I (BD I) (Level 2)

(Findling *et al.*, 2009). Aripiprazole 10 and 30 mg groups were significantly better than placebo in improving manic symptoms; response rates at week 4 were 45, 64, and 26%, and at week 30 were 50, 56, and 27%, respectively. In addition, aripiprazole monotherapy was associated with significant improvements in YMRS scores versus baseline in a small, eight-week, open-label trial (Biederman *et al.*, 2007). There was no statistically significant increase in body weight, but aripiprazole was associated with two dropouts due to extrapyramidal symptoms. Aripiprazole was effective in a six-week open trial in 10 pediatric patients with BD and comorbid ADHD, significantly improving both manic and ADHD symptoms (Tramontina *et al.*, 2007). Response to treatment with aripiprazole was studied in bipolar children in comorbidity with ADHD by the same authors (Tramontina *et al.*, 2009), finding that aripiprazole was effective in reducing manic symptoms and improving global functioning without severe adverse effects and weight gain.

12.5.2 ELDER BIPOLAR DISORDER

Few data are available on assessing BD pharmacotherapy in older patients. A 12-week open trial of aripiprazole in 20 older patients with BD suboptimally responsive to traditional mood stabilizers, found significant reductions in depression Hamilton Rating Scale for Depression (HAM-D) and mania Young Mania Rating Scale (YMRS) scores, and significant improvement in functional status (Sajatovic *et al.*, 2008). It appears to be well tolerated. Coley and collaborators retrospectively examined 52 elderly patients over three years with most of patients receiving aripiprazole 10–15 mg/day. They found that aripiprazole is well tolerated at doses lower than those recommended in the product labelling, with agitation/activation the most commonly reported side effect (Coley *et al.*, 2009).

12.6 PHARMACOGENETICS OF ARIPIPRAZOLE

The response to a specific treatment in clinical practice seems to vary significantly across different patients. The majority of significant studies focuses on schizophrenic and schizoaffective patients. Specifically for aripiprazole, patients exhibit a diverse clinical response (Known *et al.*, 2008). This variation in the clinical response prompted pharmacogenetic research of aripiprazole. Previous studies suggested that DRD2 Taq1A polymorphism status may be associated with the clinical response to aripiprazole in patients with schizophrenia (Kim *et al.*, 2008) and with schizoaffective disorder (Kwon *et al.*, 1999). The possible influence of other genotypes in TAAR6 on clinical outcome and side effects has been found by Serretti and collaborators (2009), while an association with alleles and genotypes in FAT and the response to aripiprazole treatment has been excluded by the same group (Pae *et al.*, 2009c). Replications studies, more homogeneous and numerous samples, more specific genetic analyses and treatment phenotype definitions are required in order to highlight the biological and genetic basis of the response to aripiprazole in bipolar disorders.

References

Aitchison, K.J., Bienroth, M., Cookson, J. *et al.* (2008) A UK consensus on the administration of aripiprazole for the treatment of mania. *J. Psychopharmacol.*, **23** (3), 231–240 [Epub].

Aitchison, K.J., Bienroth, M., Cookson, J., *et al.* (2009) A UK consensus on the administration of aripiprazole for the treatment of mania. *J. Psychopharmacol.* **23** (3), 231–240.

Arbaizar, B., Dierssen-Sotos, T., and Gómez-Acebo Llorca, J. (2009) Aripiprazole in major depression and mania: meta-analyses of randomized placebo-controlled trials. *Gen. Hosp. Psychiatry*, **31**, 478–483.

Biederman, J., Mick, E., Spencer, T. *et al.* (2007) An open-label trial of aripiprazole monotherapy in children and adolescents with bipolar disorder. *CNS Spectr.*, **12**, 683–689.

Burris, K.D., Molski, T.F., Xu, C., *et al.* (2002) Aripiprazole, a novel antipsychotic, is a high-affinity partial agonist at human dopamine D2 receptors. *J. Pharmacol. Exp. Ther.*, **302** (1), 381–389.

Casey, D.E., Carson, W.H., Saha, A.R. *et al.* (2003) Aripiprazole Study Group Switching patients to aripiprazole from other antipsychotic agents: a multicenter randomized study. *Psychopharmacology (Berl.)*, **166** (4), 391–399.

Cassano, G.B., Fagiolini, A., Lattanzi, L. *et al.* (2007) Aripiprazole in the treatment of schizophrenia: a consensus report produced by schizophrenia experts in Italy. *Clin. Drug Investig.*, **27** (1), 1–13.

Cipriani, A., Rendell, J.M., and Geddes, J.R. (2006) Haloperidol alone or in combination for acute mania. *Cochrane Database Syst. Rev.*, **3** (Art. No: CD004362).

Coley, K.M., Scipio, T.M., Ruby, C. *et al.* (2009) Aripiprazole prescribing patterns and side effect in elderlu psychiatric inpatients. *J. Psychiatr. Pract.*, **15** (2), 150–153.

Davies, M.A., Sheffler, D.J., and Roth, B.L. (2004) Aripiprazole: a novel atypical antipsychotic drug with a uniquely robust pharmacology. *CNS Drug Rev.*, **10** (4), 317–336.

Dunn, R.T., Stan, V.A., Chriki, L.S. *et al.* (2008) A prospective, open-label study of aripiprazole mono- and adjunctive treatment in acute bipolar depression. *J. Affect. Disord.*, **110**, 70–74.

El Mallakh, R.S., Vieta, E., Rollin, L., Marcus, R., Carson, W.H., and McQuade, R. (2010) A comparison of two fixed doses of aripiprazole with placebo in acutely relapsed, hospitalized patients with bipolar disorder I (manic or mixed) in subpopulations (CN138-007). *Eur Neuropsychopharmacol.* **20** (11), 776–783.

Findling, R.L., Nyilas, M., Forbes, R.A., *et al.* (2009) Acute treatment of pediatric bipolar I disorder, manic or mixed episode, with aripiprazole: a randomized, double-blind, placebo-controlled study. *J. Clin. Psychiatry*, **70** (10), 1441–1451.

Goodwin, G.M. and Consensus Group of the British Association for Psychopharmacology. (2009) Evidence-based guidelines for treating bipolar disorder: revised second edition – recommendations from the British Association for Psychopharmacology. *J. Psychopharmacol.* **23**, 346–388.

Fountoulakis, K.N. and Vieta, E. (2009) Efficacy and safety of aripiprazole in the treatment of bipolar disorder: a systematic review. *Ann. Gen. Psychiatry*, **8**, 16.

Fountoulakis, K.N., Vieta, E., and Schmidt, F. Aripiprazole monotherapy in the treatment of bipolar disorder: A meta-analysis. *J. Affect. Disord.* (in press)·

Goodwin, G.M. (2009) Evidence-based guidelines for treating bipolar disorder: revised second edition – recommendations from the British Association for Psychopharmacology. *J. Psychopharmacol.*, **23** (4), 346–388.

Greenaway, M. and Elbe, D. (2009) Greenaway Masa'il, focus on aripiprazole: a review of its use in child and adolescent psychiatry. *Can. Acad. Child Adolesc. Psychiatry*, **18** (3), 250–260.

Grunze, H., Vieta, E., Goodwin, G. *et al.* (2009) The World Federation of Societies of Biological Psychiatry (WFSBP) guidelines for the biological treatment of bipolar disorders: update 2009 on the treatment of acute mania. *World J. Biol. Psychiatry*, **10**, 85–116.

Grunze, H., Vieta, E., Goodwin, G. *et al.* (2010) The World Federation of Societies of Biological Psychiatry (WFSBP) guidelines for the biological treatment of bipolar disorders: update 2009 on the treatment of bipolar depression. *World J. Biol. Psychiatry*, **11** (2), 81–109.

Jordan, S., Koprivica, V., Chen, R. *et al.* (2002) The antipsychotic aripiprazole is a potent, partial agonist at the human 5–HT1A receptor. *Eur. J. Pharmacol.*, **441** (3), 137–140.

Judd, L.L., Akiskal, H.S., Schettler, P.J. *et al.* (2002) The long-term natural history of the weekly symptomatic status of bipolar I disorder. *Arch. Gen. Psychiatry*, **59**, 530–537.

Kasper, S., Calabrese, J.R., Johnson, G. *et al.* (2008) International consensus group on the evidencebased pharmacological treatment of bipolar I and Ii depression. *J. Clin. Psychiatry*, **69**, 1632–1646.

Keck, P.E. Jr., Calabrese, J.R., McIntyre, R.S. *et al.* (2007) Aripiprazole monotherapy for maintenance therapy in bipolar I disorder: a 100-week, double-blind study versus placebo. *J. Clin. Psychiatry*, **68**, 1480–1491.

Keck, P.E. Jr., Calabrese, J.R., McQuade, R.D. *et al.* (2006) A randomized, double-blind, placebo-controlled 26-week trial of aripiprazole in recently manic patients with bipolar I disorder. *J. Clin. Psychiatry*, **67**, 626–637.

Keck, P., Marcus, R., Tourkodimitris, S. *et al.* (2003) A placebocontrolled, double-blind study of the efficacy and safety of aripiprazole in patients with acute bipolar mania. *Am. J. Psychiatry*, **160**, 1651–1658.

Keck, P.E. and McElroy, S.L. (2003) Bipolar disorder, obesity, and pharmacotherapy-associated weight gain. *J. Clin. Psychiatry*, **64** (12), 1426–1435.

Keck, P.E., Orsulak, P.J., Cutler, A.J. *et al.*, CN138-135 Study Group (2009) Aripiprazole monotherapy in the treatment of acute bipolar I mania: a randomized, double-blind, placebo- and lithium-controlled study. *J. Affect. Disord.*, **112** (1–3), 36–49.

Ketter, T.A., Wang, P.W., Chandler, R.A. *et al.* (2006) Adjunctive aripiprazole in treatment-resistant bipolar depression. *Ann. Clin. Psychiatry*, **18**, 169–172.

Kim, H.J., Kim, M.H., Choe, B.K. *et al.* (2008) Genetic association between 5'-upstream single-nucleotide polymorphisms of PDGFRB and schizophrenia in a Korean population. *Schizophr. Res.*, **103** (1–3), 201–208.

Kwon, J.S., Kim, E., Kang, D.H. *et al.* (1999) Interactions of the novel antipsychotic aripiprazole (OPC-14597) with dopamine and serotonin receptor subtypes. *Neuropsychopharmacology*, **20**, 612–627.

Known, J.S., Kim, E., Kang, D.H. *et al.* (2008) Taq1A polymorphism in the dopamine D2 receptor gene as a predictor of clinical response to aripiprazole. *Eur. Neuropsychopharmacol.*, **18**, 897–907.

Li, Z., Ichikawa, J., Dai, J., and Meltzer, H.Y. (2004) Aripiprazole, a novel antipsychotic drug, preferentially increases dopamine release in the prefrontal cortex and hippocampus in rat brain. *Eur. J. Pharmacol.*, **493**, 75–83.

Maguire, G. (2002) Prolactin elevation with antipsychotic medications: mechanisms of action and clinical consequences. *J. Clin. Psychiatry*, **63**, 56–62.

Marona-Lewicka, D. and Nichols, D.E. (2004) Aripiprazole (OPC-14597) fully substitutes for the 5-HT1A receptor agonist LY293284 in the drug discrimination assay in rats. *Psychopharmacology (Berl.)*, **172** (4), 415–421.

Mazza, M., Squillacioti, M.R., Pecora, R.D. *et al.* (2008) Beneficial acute antidepressant effects of aripiprazole as an adjunctive treatment or monotherapy in bipolar patients unresponsive to mood stabilizers: results from a 16-week open-label trial. *Expert. Opin. Pharmacother.*, **9** (18), 3145–3149.

McElroy S.L., Suppes, T., Frye, M.A. *et al.* (2007) Open-label aripiprazole in the treatment of acute bipolar depression: a prospective pilot trial. *J. Affect. Disord.*, **101**, 275–281.

Mir, A., Shivakumar, K., Williamson, R.J. *et al.* (2008) Change in sexual dysfunction with aripiprazole: a switching or add-on study. *J. Psychopharmacol.*, **22**, 323–329.

Muzina, D.J. (2009) Treatment and prevention of mania in bipolar I disorder: focus on aripiprazole. *Neuropsychiatr. Dis. Treat.*, **5**, 279–288.

Muzina, D.J., Momah, C., Eudicone, J.M. *et al.* (2008) Aripiprazole monotherapy in patients with rapid-cycling bipolar I disorder: an analysis from a long-term, double-blind, placebo-controlled study. *Int. J. Clin. Pract.*, **62** (5), 679–687.

Nemeroff, C.B. (2005) Use of atypical antipsychotics in refractory depression and anxiety. *J. Clin. Psychiatry*, **66** (Suppl. 8), 13–21.

Newcomer, J.W. (2005) Second-generation (atypical) antipsychotics and metabolic effects: a comprehensive literature review. *CNS Drugs*, **19**, 1–93.

NICE Clinical Guidelines. (2009) *Bipolar Disorder: The Management of Bipolar Disorder in Adults, Children and Adolescents, in Primary and Secondary Care*. National Institute for Health and Clinical Excellence.

Ozdemir, V., Fourie, J., and Ozdener, F. (2002) Aripiprazole (Otsuka Pharmaceutical Co). *Curr. Opin. Investig. Drugs*, **3**, 113–120.

Pae, C.U., Serretti, A., Chiesa, A., *et al.* (2009a) Immediate versus gradual suspension of previous treatments during switch to aripiprazole: results of a randomized, open label study. *Eur. Neuropsychopharmacol.*, **19** (8), 562–570.

Pae, C.U., Serretti, A., Chiesa, A. *et al.* (2009b) Immediate versus gradual suspension of previous treatments during switch to aripiprazole: results of a randomized, open label study. *Eur. Neuropsychopharmacol.*, **19** (8), 562–570, [Epub].

Pae, C.U., Chiesa, A., Mandelli, L. *et al.* (2009c) No influence of FAT polymorphisms in response to aripiprazole. *J. Hum. Genet.*, **55** (1), 32–36.

Perlis, R.H., Ostacher, M.J., Patel, J.K. *et al.* (2006) Predictors of recurrence in bipolar disorder: primary outcomes from the Systematic Treatment Enhancement Program for Bipolar Disorder (STEP-BD). *Am. J. Psychiatry*, **163** (2), 217–224.

Remington, G., Chue, P., Stip, E., Kopala, L., Girard, T., and Christensen, B. (2005) The crossover approach to switching antipsychotics: what is the evidence? *Schizophr. Res.*, **76** (2–3), 267–272.

Sachs, G.S., Gaulin, B.D., Gutierrez-Esteinou, R. *et al.* (2007) Antimanic response to aripiprazole in bipolar I disorder patients is independent of the agitation level at baseline. *J. Clin. Psychiatry*, **68**, 1377–1383.

Sachs, G., Sanchez, R., Marcus, R. *et al.* (2006) Aripiprazole in the treatment of acute manic or mixed episodes in patients with bipolar I disorder: a 3-week placebo-controlled study. *J. Psychopharmacol.*, **20**, 536–546.

Sajatovic, M., Coconcea, N., Ignacio, R.V. *et al.* (2008) Aripiprazole therapy in 20 older adults with bipolar disorder: a 12-week, open-label trial. *J. Clin. Psychiatry*, **69**, 41–46.

Scheen, A.J. and De Hert, M.A. (2007) Abnormal glucose metabolism in patients treated with antipsychotics. *Diabetes Metab.*, **33**, 169–175.

Schieber, F.C., Boulton, D.W., Balch, A.H. *et al.* (2009) A non-randomized study to investigate the effects of the atypical antipsychotic aripiprazole on the steady-state pharmacokinetics of lamotrigine in patients with bipolar I disorder. *Hum. Psychopharmacol.*, **24** (2), 145–152.

Serretti, A., Pae, C.U., Chiesa, A. *et al.* (2009) Influence of TAAR6 polymorphisms on response to aripiprazole. *Prog. Neuropsychopharmacol. Biol. Psychiatry 1*, **33** (5), 822–826.

Smith, L.A., Cornelius, V., Warnock, A. *et al.* (2007) Pharmacological interventions for acute bipolar mania: a systematic review of randomized placebocontrolled trials. *Bipolar Disord.*, **9**, 551–560.

Stark, A.D., Jordan, S., Allers, K.A. *et al.* (2007) Interaction of the novel antipsychotic aripiprazole with 5-HT1A and 5-HT 2A receptors: functional receptor-binding and in vivo electrophysiological studies. *Psychopharmacology (Berl.)*, **190** (3), 373–382.

Suppes, T., Dennehy, E.B., Hirschfeld, R.M. *et al.* (2005) Texas consensus conference panel on medication treatment of bipolar disorder. The Texas implementation of medication algorithms: update to the algorithms for treatment of bipolar I disorder. *J. Clin. Psychiatry*, **66** (7), 870–886.

Suppes, T., Eudicone, J., McQuade, R. *et al.* (2008) Efficacy and safety of aripiprazole in sub-populations with acute manic or mixed episodes of bipolar I disorder. *J. Affect. Disord.*, **107**, 145–154.

Thase, M.E., Jonas, A., Khan, A. *et al.* (2008) Aripiprazole monotherapy in nonpsychotic bipolar I depression: results of 2 randomized, placebo-controlled studies. *J. Clin. Psychopharmacol.*, **28**, 13–20.

Tramontina, S., Zeni, C.P., Ketzer, C.R. *et al.* (2009) Aripiprazole in children and adolescents with bipolar disorder comorbid with attention-deficit/hyperactivity disorder: a pilot randomized clinical trial. *J. Clin. Psychiatry*, **70** (5), 756–764.

Tramontina, S., Zeni, C.P., Pheula, G.F. *et al.* (2007) Aripiprazole in juvenile bipolar disorder comorbid with attention-deficit/hyperactivity disorder: an open clinical trial. *CNS Spectr.*, **12**, 758–762.

Vieta, E., Bourin, M., Sanchez, R. *et al.*, (2005) Effectiveness of aripiprazole v. haloperidol in acute bipolar mania: double-blind, randomised, comparative 12-week trial. *Br. J. Psychiatry*, **187**, 235–242.

Vieta, E., T'joen, C., McQuade, R.D. *et al.* (2008) Efficacy of adjunctive aripiprazole to either valproate or lithium in bipolar mania patients partially nonresponsive to valproate/lithium monotherapy: a placebo-controlled study. *Am. J. Psychiatry*, **165**, 1316–1325.

Worthington, J.J. III, Kinrys, G., Wygant, L.E., and Pollack, M.H. (2005) Aripiprazole as an augmentor of selective serotonin reuptake inhibitors in depression and anxiety disorder patients. *Int. Clin. Psychopharmacol.*, **20** (1), 9–11.

Yatham, L.N., Kennedy, S.H., Schaffer, A. *et al.* (2009) Canadian Network for Mood and Anxiety Treatments (CANMAT) and International Society for Bipolar Disorders (ISBD) collaborative update of CANMAT guidelines for the management of patients with bipolar disorder: update 2009. *Bipolar Disord.*, **11**, 225–255.

Young, A.H., Oren, D.A., Lowy, A. *et al.* (2009) Aripiprazole monotherapy in acute mania: 12-week randomised placebo- and haloperidol-controlled study. *Br. J. Psychiatry*, **194** (1), 40–48.

Zimbroff, D.L., Marcus, R.N., Manos, G. *et al.* (2007) Management of acute agitation in patients with bipolar disorder: efficacy and safety of intramuscular aripiprazole. *J. Clin. Psychopharmacol.*, **27**, 171–176.

13

Asenapine in Bipolar Disorder

Roger S. McIntyre[1,2,3,4]

[1]Department of Psychiatry, University of Toronto, ON, Canada
[2]Department of Pharmacology, University of Toronto, ON, Canada
[3]Mood Disorders Psychopharmacology Unit, University Health Network,
Toronto, ON, Canada
[4]Institute of Medical Science, University of Toronto, ON, Canada

13.1 INTRODUCTION

During the past decade, intensified efforts have evaluated the therapeutic index of several atypical antipsychotics across various phases of bipolar disorder (McIntyre and Konarski, 2005; Ng *et al.*, 2009; Perlis *et al.*, 2006a). These endeavors have provided practitioners and patients with alternative therapeutic avenues for symptom control and functional recovery. Notwithstanding these developments, the majority of individuals with bipolar disorder do not fully recover from their index manic episode with currently approved agents (Tohen *et al.*, 2006; Perlis *et al.*, 2006b). Moreover, treatment emergent adverse events, as well as safety concerns, often belie the acceptability of atypical antipsychotics (McIntyre and Konarski, 2005; Newcomer, Nasrallah, and Loebel, 2004; McIntyre, McCann, and Kennedy, 2001).

Asenapine was approved August 2009 by the US FDA for the acute treatment of adults with manic or mixed episodes associated with bipolar I disorder with or without psychotic features (and in the acute treatment of adults with schizophrenia). Asenapine was the first antipsychotic agent to receive contemporaneous FDA approval for both bipolar and schizophrenia indications. Asenapine is a dibenzo-oxepino pyrrole, a new chemical class of atypical antipsychotics and is the first antipsychotic to be available as a sublingual rapidly absorbed agent (Tarazi and Shahid, 2009). This review will focus on registration trials that evaluated the efficacy, tolerability, and safety of asenapine in adults with acute mania and mixed states.

13.2 PHARMACOLOGY

Asenapine maleate (trans-5-chloro-2,3,3a,12b-tetrahydro-2-methyl-1H-dibenz [2,3:6,7] oxepino [4,5-c] pyrrole) is a novel second-generation antipsychotic agent. Asenapine's affinity for neuroreceptors, transporters, ion channels as well as its electrophysiological

Bipolar Psychopharmacotherapy: Caring for the patient, Second Edition. Edited by Hagop S. Akiskal and Mauricio Tohen.
© 2011 John Wiley & Sons, Ltd. Published 2011 by John Wiley & Sons, Ltd.

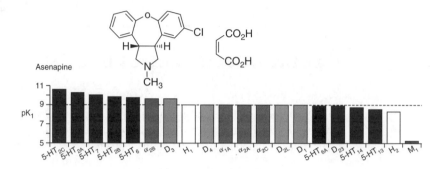

Figure 13.1 The in vitro receptor binding affinity for asenapine. Higher pK_1 indicates greater binding affinity.

Adapted from (Tarazi and Shahid, 2009).

and behavioral effects have been evaluated in several preclinical studies. Asenapine's *in vivo* profile in humans, however, remains to be fully characterized (Figure 13.1). Results from in vitro studies with cloned human receptors indicate that asenapine exhibits high affinity for 5-HT_{2C}, 5-HT_{2A}, 5HT_7, 5HT_{2B}, 5HT_6, and receptor subtypes, α-1-a, α-2-a, α-2b, and α-2c adrenergic as well as D_3 and D_4 dopaminergic receptors. Asenapine exhibits potent antagonistic activity at D_2, 5-HT_{2A}, and α-2 receptors, agonist effects on somatodendritic 5-HT_{1A} autoreceptors and postsynaptic 5-HT_{1A} receptors in the hippocampus (Ghanbari *et al.*, 2009). Similar to other atypical antipsychotics, asenapine exhibits a higher affinity for 5HT-$_{2A}$ versus D_2 and 5HT-$_{2C}$ versus D_2 (Tarazi and Shahid, 2009; Bishara and Taylor, 2009; Tarazi *et al.*, 2009; Marston *et al.*, 2009). Asenapine exhibits minimal affinity for muscarinic receptors; asenapine exhibits high affinity for histaminergic H_1 and moderate affinity for H_2 receptors. Long-term administration of asenapine increases D_2 receptor binding in the medial prefrontal cortex, caudate, and putamen, as well as D_4 receptor binding in the nucleus accumbens, caudate, and putamen. Asenapine also facilitates D_2 and D_4 receptor binding in the hippocampus (Tarazi *et al.*, 2008). In addition to its effects on cell surface receptors, asenapine increases dopamine and noradrenaline neuronal firing as well as cortical noradrenaline, dopamine, and serotonin output in the cortex (Franberg *et al.*, 2009).

Electrophysiological studies indicate that systemic administration of asenapine increases the spontaneous firing rate of dopamine neurons in the ventral tegmental area by approximately 15% but does not alter the spontaneous firing rate of norepinephrine and serotonin neurons. Asenapine dose-dependently and potently reverses the inhibitory action of α-2 adrenergic, D_2, and 5-HT_2 agonists on the firing of catecholamine neurons. (Ghanbari *et al.*, 2009).

Continuous (i.e., four weeks) administration of asenapine significantly decreases binding of (3H)-K-801 to NMDA-MK-801 modulatory sites in nucleus accumbens, medial and lateral caudate, and putamen. Asenapine did not alter binding of (3H)-glycine to NMDA-glycine modulatory sites in any brain region (Tarazi *et al.*, 2009). Asenapine treatment significantly increases labeling of AMPA receptors in hippocampal CA1 and

CA3 regions. This latter observation may be unique to asenapine when compared to other conventional and atypical agents (Tarazi *et al.*, 2009).

Animal behavioral studies indicate that asenapine reduces the conditioned avoidance response, attenuates amphetamine-induced locomotor activity, and restores apomorphine-induced disruption of prepulse inhibition without inducing catalepsy (Tarazi and Shahid, 2009). Subacute asenapine administration (i.e., five weeks) reverses chronic mild stress-induced reduction in sucrose consumption suggestive of possible antidepressant effects. Asenapine also attenuates the deficit in reversal learning as well as object recognition memory associated with subchronic treatment with phencyclidine PCP (Tarazi and Shahid, 2009).

13.3 HUMAN PHARMACOKINETICS

Asenapine sublingual is absorbed within seconds through the oral mucosa, its bioavailability is much higher when administered sublingually (that is, 35%) when compared to the swallowed tablet (that is, less than 2%) as a result of extensive first-pass metabolism. Buccal administration leads to approximately 20% greater bioavailability than sublingual administration; supralingual administration results in similar exposure to the sublingual route.

The effect of drinking water following sublingual administration of a single dose of asenapine (10 mg) was evaluated at 2, 5, 10, and 30 minutes after dosing in 15 healthy male subjects. The exposure of asenapine 10 minutes after dosing was equivalent to that when water was administered 30 minutes after dosing. As a result, there are no restrictions for food or drink after 10 minutes. A 19% reduction in bioavailability was noted following water administration at 2 minutes and a 10% reduction noted when water was administered at 5 minutes. In the phase 3 clinical trials, patients were instructed to wait 10 minutes before eating/drinking. Concomitant smoking exhibited no significant effect on the absorption of asenapine. It is unknown however if cigarette smoking affects overall asenapine bioavailability via its effect on inducing phase 1 metabolism (for example, CYP1A2).

Asenapine is rapidly absorbed, has a large volume of distribution (approximately 20–25 l/kg) and is highly bound to circulating proteins (for example, albumin and α-1-acid glycoprotein). Asenapine is noted to have a maximal plasma concentration of 0.5–1.5 hours after oral administration and a biphasic elimination half-life of 4–6 and 24 hours (Bishara and Taylor, 2009). N-Glucoronide-asenapine and N-desmethylasenapine are the two primary human metabolites of asenapine; they are not known to possess clinically relevant pharmacodynamic effects (Tarazi and Shahid, 2009).

Steady-state concentrations of asenapine are reached within three days of BID dosing. Asenapine is a substrate for CYP1A2, UGT1A4 and to a lesser extent CYP3A4 and CYP2D6. Asenapine is a weak inhibitor of CYP2D6 and does not induce CYP1A2 or CYP3A4 (Bishara and Taylor, 2009; Choi *et al.*, 2010). The potential effects of concomitant medications on asenapine bioavailability were evaluated in healthy volunteers administered a single 5 mg dose of asenapine. Fluvoxamine, a CYP1A2 inhibitor, when administered at low dose (that is, 25 mg BID for eight days), increased asenapine maximum concentration (C_{max}) by 13% and increased area under the curve (AUC) by 29%.

Paroxetine 20 mg daily for nine days reduced C_{max} 13% and AUC 9%; imipramine as a 75 mg single dose increased C_{max} 17% and AUC 10%; cimetidine 800 mg BID for eight days reduced C_{max} 13% and increased AUC 1%; carbamazepine 400 mg BID for 15 days decreased C_{max} and AUC 16% respectively; while valproate 500 mg BID for nine days increased C_{max} 2% and decreased AUC 1%. It was concluded that no asenapine dose adjustments will be required when co-administering with these agents.

13.4 ASENAPINE: EFFICACY IN BIPOLAR MANIA AND MIXED STATES

Asenapine's efficacy in the acute treatment of bipolar mania and mixed states was evaluated in two similarly designed acute registration trials. Both studies were randomized, double-blind, placebo-controlled, multicentre, international, parallel group studies that randomly assigned subjects to flexible-dose sublingual asenapine (10 mg BID on day 1 and 5 or 10 mg BID thereafter), placebo, or oral olanzapine (15 mg QD on day 1 and 5–20 mg QD thereafter) (McIntyre et al., 2009a). Olanzapine was included for assay sensitivity; efficacy, tolerability, and safety analysis primarily compared asenapine to placebo.

All subjects were adults (≥ 18 years old) with a current Diagnostic and Statistical Manual of Mental Disorders Fourth Edition (DSM-IV) primary diagnosis of bipolar I disorder experiencing a manic or mixed episode with a Young Mania Rating Scale (YMRS) total score of ≥ 20 at screening and baseline, a current manic or mixed bipolar I episode that began ≤ 3 months before the screening visit, and a documented history of more than one previous moderate to severe mood episode with or without psychotic features. Individuals with a history of rapid cycling bipolar disorder in the past year were excluded.

In both studies, a single-blind placebo run-in period up to seven days preceded randomization. Participants remained in an inpatient treatment center for up to seven days for screening procedures and for at least seven days during treatment. Patients that were deemed suitable for discharge by the investigator could complete the trial as outpatients. Subjects however were not permitted to be discharged if they had a score of ≥ 2 on item, 7, 10, or 11 of the modified version of the InterSePT scale for suicidal thinking. Depot antipsychotics were required to be discontinued ≥ 1 dosing cycle before baseline. Other antipsychotic agents, mood stabilizers, antidepressants, and dopamine-antagonist antiemetics were not permitted. Medications employed for treating extrapyramidal side effects (EPS) (that is, anticholinergics, β-blockers) could be continued for the first seven days of treatment with tapering thereafter. Benzodiazepines (≤ 4 mg per day lorazepam for agitation, ≤ 30 mg/day temazepam for $\leq$three nights/week for insomnia or others with comparable half-lives) were allowed during screening and the first seven days following the baseline assessment, as were non-benzodiazepine sedative-hypnotics (10 mg/day zolpidem or 20 mg/day zaleplon for ≤ 3 nights/week for insomnia). Use of benzodiazepines and sedative-hypnotics was not permitted after day 7 and they were not administered within 4 hours of efficacy assessment during the first seven days of treatment.

After completing the run-in period, subjects were randomized to three weeks of double-blind, flexible-dose treatment with asenapine, placebo, or olanzapine in a ratio of $2:1:2$.

The drug administration was performed in a double-dummy fashion, using three film-coated tablets containing olanzapine or placebo and two sublingual fast-dissolving tablets containing asenapine or placebo. Sublingual asenapine treatment started at 10 mg BID on day 1, and was flexibly dosed (5–10 mg BID thereafter). Oral olanzapine was initiated at 15 mg daily and was flexibly dosed (5–20 mg QD thereafter).

The primary efficacy variable was the change from baseline to day 21 in YMRS total score. Secondary efficacy endpoints included change from baseline to day 21 in mania or mixed state severity as measured by the Clinical Global Impression for Bipolar Disorder (CGI-BP) scale, as well as the percentage of responders (≥50% decrease in YMRS total score from baseline to endpoint), and remitters (YMRS total score ≤12 at endpoint). Other secondary outcome measures (that is, Positive and Negative Syndrome Scale, Montgomery-Asberg Depression Rating Scale, Readiness to Discharge Questionnaire, a modified version of the InterSePT Scale for Suicide Thinking, CNS vital signs cognitive testing battery, Short Form-36 version 2.0 of the Health Outcomes Quality of Life Scale, and Treatment Satisfaction Questionnaire for Medication) were collected. Safety and tolerability were assessed in all patients who took ≥1 dose of study medication (that is, the all-treated (AT) population). The severity of abnormal movements was also assessed using the Simpson-Angus Scale (SAS), Barnes Akathisia Rating Scale (BARS), and Abnormal Involuntary Movement Scale (AIMS).

13.4.1 STATISTICAL ANALYSIS

Efficacy was assessed in patients who took ≥1 dose of study medication and completed ≥1 postbaseline YMRS assessment (that is, the intent-to-treat (ITT) population). A mixed model for repeated measures (MMRMs) was a prespecified secondary analysis in the protocol and was used when assessing efficacy. A fixed-effects analysis of covariance (ANCOVA), with baseline score as a covariate and the last observation carried forward (LOCF) for missing data, was the primary analysis. Comparisons between active treatment and placebo were made using the difference in least squares (LSs) means. Olanzapine was used as a positive control to assess assay sensitivity and was not compared directly to asenapine. The categorical variables, YMRS response, and remission, were analyzed using Pearson chi-square tests, with LOCF for missing values at study endpoint.

In the first study, 611 patients were screened, 488 were randomized (McIntyre *et al.*, 2010). Completion rates were 67% with asenapine, 58% with placebo, and 79% with olanzapine. Study discontinuations were attributable to adverse events (asenapine 9.2%; placebo 4.1%; olanzapine 3.4%), lack of efficacy (7.6; 14.3; 6.3%), withdrawal of consent (13.5; 13.3; 7.3%), lost to follow up (0.5; 4.1; 2.9%), and other reasons (2.2; 6.1; 1.5%).

The mean ± SD daily dose of asenapine and olanzapine were 18.4 ± 2.7 and 15.9 ± 2.5 mg respectively. More than 90% of asenapine-treated subjects maintained the original 10 mg BID dosage throughout the study, with the remainder maintained at 5 mg BID. Concomitant medication was utilized by 78.4, 78.6, and 78.0% of patients in the asenapine, placebo, and olanzapine groups respectively.

Baseline (mean ± SD) YMRS total scores were comparable across groups (asenapine 29.4 ± 6.7; placebo 28.3 ± 6.3; olanzapine 29.7 ± 6.6). The YMRS total score reduction (LOCF) were significantly greater with asenapine and olanzapine than with placebo. At day 21, the LS ± standard error (SE) changes from baseline were −11.5 ± 0.8 with ase-napine (p < 0.007 vs placebo), −7.8 ± 1.1 with placebo, and −14.6 ± 0.8 with olanzapine (p < 0.0001 vs. placebo) (Figure 13.2). Asenapine (−3.2 ± 0.4; p = 0.022 vs placebo) and olanzapine (−4.4 ± 0.4; p < 0.0001 vs. placebo) demonstrated superiority over placebo (−1.7 ± 0.5) on treatment day 2. Using MMRM analysis, YMRS total score reductions were −14.2 ± 0.9 with asenapine (p = 0.026 vs placebo), −10.8 ± 1.2 with placebo, and −16.1 ± 0.8 with olanzapine (p = 0.0003 vs placebo) at day 21 and −3.2 ± 0.4 with ase-napine (p = 0.020 vs placebo), −1.7 ± 0.6 with placebo, and −4.3 ± 0.4 with olanzapine (p = 0.0001 vs placebo) at day 2. The changes in YMRS total score from baseline to day 21 for olanzapine were significantly greater than those for asenapine with LOCF analysis (p = 0.004) but not with MMRM analysis.

The response rates and remission rates with asenapine (42.6, 35.5% respectively) did not significantly differ from placebo (34 and 30.9% respectively). Olanzapine was superior to placebo in rates of response (54.7%; p < 0.002) and remission (46.3%; p = 0.016). The mean ± SD CGI-BP mania score reductions were greater with asenapine and olanzapine compared with placebo at day 21 (−1.2 ± 0.1 with asenapine, p = 0.012 vs placebo; −0.8 ± 0.13 with placebo; and −1.5 ± 0.09 with olanzapine, p < 0.0001 vs placebo). Superiority over placebo was seen from day 14 with asenapine and from day 2 with olanzapine with both LOCF and MMRM analysis. Mean baseline scores on the MADRS were comparable across groups (asenapine 10.5 ± 6.9; placebo 11.1 ± 6.7; olanzapine 10.6 ± 6.8). Changes from baseline using LOCF analysis at day 7 and 21 were −3.5 ± 0.4

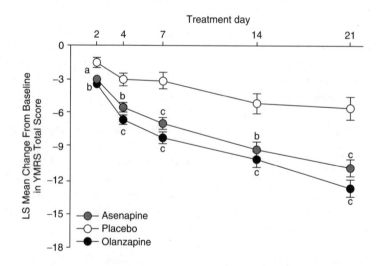

Figure 13.2 Changes in Young Mania Rating Scale (YMRS) total score from baseline with last observation carried forward (LOCF). The change in YMRS total score from baseline was determined in the intent to treat (ITT) population on treatment days 2, 4, 7, 14, and 21. LS = least squares. [a]p ≤ 0.01; [b]p ≤ 0.001; [c]p ≤ 0.0001, active treatment versus placebo.

(p = 0.011 vs placebo) and −3.0 ± 0.4 with asenapine (p = NS vs placebo) and −4.1 ± 0.4 (p < 0.003 vs placebo with olanzapine). There were no differences between asenapine and olanzapine from baseline to day 21 on MADRS total score. Shifts in MADRS scores from ≤8 to ≥16 at end point were reported in relatively few patients (asenapine 0%; placebo 4.4%; olanzapine 1.0%).

During the second trial, 654 patients were screened, 489 were randomized to treatment (McIntyre et al., 2009a). The trial was completed by 62.9, 61.5, and 79.6% of asenapine-, placebo-, and olanzapine-treated subjects. Reasons for discontinuation in the three groups were lack of efficacy (8.2; 16.3; 5.8%, respectively) treatment-emergent adverse events 10.3; 6.7; 4.2%, respectively), withdrawal of consent (14.4; 12.5; 8.4%, respectively), lost to follow up (2.6; 1.9; 1.0%, respectively), and other reasons (1.5; 1.0; 1.0% respectively). The mean daily dose of asenapine and olanzapine were 18.2 ± 3.1 and 15.8 ± 2.3 mg respectively. Similar to the first study, the majority of subjects (that is, ≥90%) treated with asenapine were maintained at the 10 mg BID dose. Concomitant medication use was reported by 85, 84, and 78% of asenapine-, placebo-, and olanzapine-treated patients respectively.

The mean ± SD YMRS total score at baseline was comparable between groups with asenapine (28.3 ± 5.5), placebo (29.0 ± 6.1), and olanzapine (28.6 ± 5.9) (Figure 13.3). With LOCF analysis, the change from baseline to day 21 was significantly greater with asenapine (−10.8 ± 0.8 and olanzapine (−12.6 ± 0.8) compared with placebo (−5.5 ± 10, p < 0.0001 vs. placebo for both). The change from baseline to day 2 was −3.0 ± 0.4 with asenapine, −3.4 ± 0.4 with olanzapine, and −1.5 ± 0.5 with placebo (p < 0.008 vs placebo for both). Using MMRM analysis, the change from YMRS baseline to day 21 was

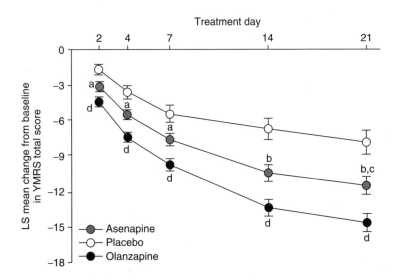

Figure 13.3 Changes in YMRS total score from baseline in the ITT population with LOCF. Data are presented as LS mean ± SEM. ITT, intent to treat; LOCF, last observation carried forward; LS, least squares; YMRS, Young Mania Rating Scale. [a]p ≤ 0.05; [b]p ≤ 0.01; [c]p < 0.01 vs olanzapine (based on post hoc analysis conducted at day 21 only); [d]p ≤ 0.0001 vs placebo.

significantly greater with asenapine and olanzapine than with placebo, as well as at day 2. In study two, a separate subgroup analysis was conducted evaluating asenapine efficacy in mania and mixed states. Superiority over placebo with asenapine and olanzapine at day 21 was apparent with LOCF (and MMRM) analysis. Superiority over placebo in patients with a diagnosis of mania was apparent at day 2 with olanzapine and day 4 with asenapine. In subjects with a mixed episode, the change from baseline to day 21 approached but did not reach significance with asenapine but was significantly greater with olanzapine than with placebo. Superiority over placebo was observed on treatment day 2 with asenapine and olanzapine. The results were similar with both LOCF and MMRM analysis.

Asenapine-treated subjects exhibited significantly greater response (42.3%) and remission (40.2%) rates compared with placebo (25.2 and 22.3% respectively, $p < 0.001$ for both). Using LOCF analysis, the mean change from baseline to day 21 on the CGI-BP were -1.2 ± 0.01 with asenapine ($p < 0.002$ vs placebo), -1.4 ± 0.01 with olanzapine ($p < 0.0001$ vs placebo), and 0.7 ± 0.1 with placebo. Superiority of asenapine and olanzapine over placebo was observed at treatment day 2 (as in the first study); the mean reduction in total MADRS was not significantly different between asenapine and placebo (but was for olanzapine) treatment emergent adverse events were not significantly different between groups in shifts in MADRS scores from ≤ 8 to ≥ 16 at study endpoint.

13.4.2 TOLERABILITY IN ACUTE MANIA

Treatment-emergent adverse events were reported by 75.7 and 55.1% in asenapine- and placebo-treated subjects respectively in study 1. A similar rate was reported in study 2 (that is, 73.7 and 60.8% for asenapine- and placebo-treated subjects respectively). In both studies, most adverse events were mild to moderate in intensity. In study 1, adverse events occurring in $\geq 5\%$ of patients and twice the placebo rate were somnolence, dizziness, sedation, increased weight, and vomiting. In study 2, the events included sedation, dizziness, somnolence, fatigue, and oral hypoesthesia. The incidence of subjects reporting one or more EPS as an adverse event was 10.3% with asenapine, 3.1% with placebo, and 6.8% with olanzapine. In study 2, the comparable rates were 7.2, 2.9, and 7.9% respectively. There were no significant differences between groups in both studies in change on the AIMS, BARS, and SAS scores.

In study 1, mean $\pm$ SD weight change from baseline to endpoint was 0.9 ± 3.0 kg with asenapine, 0.1 ± 2.0 with placebo, and 2.6 ± 3.6 with olanzapine. For study 2, the comparable changes were 1.6 ± 2.9 kg, 0.3 ± 2.0, and 1.9 ± 3.2 respectively. In study 1, the incidence of clinically significant weight gain ($\geq 7\%$ increase from baseline) was 7.2% with asenapine, 1.2% with placebo, and 19.0% with olanzapine. In study 2, the comparable rates were 1.8, 2.3, and 1.2% respectively.

No statistically significant changes were noted between asenapine and placebo in change from baseline in fasting glucose, triglycerides, and total cholesterol in both studies. In both studies, oral adverse reactions (that is, oral hypoesthesia and dysgeusia), were evaluated. Spontaneously reported incidence of oral hypoesthesia was 4% in the acute mania trials; the rate of discontinuation due to oral hypoesthesia was 0.27%. Dysgeusia was reported at 3% in the acute bipolar mania trials; no patients discontinued treatment due to dysgeusia in either the short-term or long-term trials.

13.5 ASENAPINE: EFFICACY AND TOLERABILITY DURING EXTENSION TREATMENT

A multicentre, nine-week noninferiority double-blind extension of the three-week double-blind trials in patients with acute mania or mixed episodes as part bipolar I disorder was completed (McIntyre *et al.*, 2009b). This nine-week extension did not include a placebo arm and instead was a direct comparison of asenapine versus olanzapine. The nine-week extension study began at the end of the three-week acute trials without breaking the blind occurring at week 12. There was no re-randomization at the beginning of the extension study and no identification of patients who had received active treatment versus placebo during the three-week trial. In the extension study, patients who had received acute treatment with asenapine or olanzapine continued the same regimen and were evaluated at the end of week 12 for efficacy and safety. Patients who received placebo during the acute treatment were blindly switched to asenapine 10 mg BID on day one with flexible dosing thereafter and included in the safety analysis only.

A total of 504 patients were enrolled in the extension study (McIntyre *et al.*, 2009b). At day 84, the mean change from baseline in YMRS total score was -24.4 (8.7) for asenapine and -23.9 (7.9) for olanzapine (Figure 13.4). Noninferiority statistical analysis indicated no significant difference between asenapine and olanzapine. The incidence of EPS of any type was 10% with placebo/asenapine, 15% with asenapine, and 13% with olanzapine treatment. The percentage of patients with clinically significant weight gain was greater with olanzapine (31%) than asenapine (19%). Similar to the acute trials, there were no clinically significant changes in laboratory measures, metabolic parameters or vital signs.

Subjects completing the extension phase (that is, 12-week study) were eligible for a 40-week extension double-blind study. Subjects enrolled in the 40-week extension study were maintained on the treatment regimen established during the 3-week efficacy trials and the 9-week extension, with the blind maintained for all patients and investigators. The "placebo/asenapine" group comprised patients who received placebo during the three-week efficacy trials and were switched to asenapine in the nine-week extension study (10 mg BID on day 1, with flexible dosing at 5 or 10 mg BID thereafter) with the blind unbroken. These patients were maintained on this regimen in the 40-week extension study and were included in the safety analyses only. Concomitant medications were allowed provided patients followed protocol guidelines established during the three-week efficacy trials.

Of the 308 patients who completed the nine-week extension (placebo/asenapine, n = 50; asenapine, n = 112; olanzapine, n = 146), 218 enrolled in the 40-week extension and received ≥ 1 dose of study medication (treated population). A total of 133 (61.0%) completed the 40-week extension (placebo/asenapine, n = 13 (40.6%); asenapine, n = 52 (65.8%); olanzapine, n = 68 (63.6%)). Discontinuation rates due to AEs were highest in the placebo/asenapine group (n = 5, 15.6%) but were comparable in the asenapine

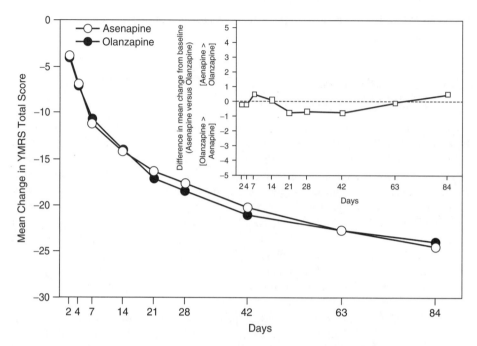

Figure 13.4 Mean change in Young Mania Rating Scale (YMRS) total score from baseline of the acute mania trials to day 84 in the per protocol population using observed case data. Inset: Difference (asenapine – olanzapine) in mean changes from baseline. Positive values indicate that the mean change with asenapine exceeded that of olanzapine; negative values indicate that the mean change with olanzapine exceeded that of asenapine.

(n = 7, 8.9%) and olanzapine (n = 9, 8.4%) groups. The discontinuation rate due to AEs among all patients who received asenapine (79 patients in the asenapine group plus 32 patients in the placebo/asenapine group) was 10.8% (12 of 111). Discontinuation rates due to lack of efficacy were 3.1% with placebo/asenapine (n = 1), 2.5% with asenapine (n = 2), and 2.8% with olanzapine (n = 3); the rate of discontinuation for lack of efficacy among all patients treated with asenapine was 2.7% (3 of 111). The mean ± SD treatment duration was 250 ± 101 days in the placebo/asenapine group, 313 ± 88 days in the asenapine group and 300 ± 98 days in the olanzapine group. The mean ± SED total daily dose was 15.7 ± 4.1 mg in the placebo/asenapine group, 16.3 ± 3.7 mg in the asenapine group, and 15.4 ± 4.0 mg in the olanzapine group. Concomitant medications were used by 68.8, 73.4, and 71.0% OF patients in the three groups respectively.

The incidence of treatment emergent adverse events was 71.9, 86.1, and 79.4% in the three groups respectively. Two deaths were reported during the study, one in the asenapine group which was considered possibly related to study medication and one in the olanzapine group that was considered to be unlikely related to the medication. The most common treatment-emergent adverse events associated with asenapine and occurring at a rate of ≥10% and occurring at least twice as often as the olanzapine group were depression, dizziness, nausea, parkinsonism, tremor, and constipation. Mean changes from baseline on the AIMS, BARS, and SAS were no different across groups. During the study, the percentage of patients shifting from AIMS global scores >2 and SAS mean total scores >0.3 were higher in the placebo/asenapine and the asenapine group than in the olanzapine group.

The mean ± SD increase in weight from baseline to study endpoint was 1.7 ± 6.0, 3.5 ± 6.7, and 6.0 ± 6.6 kg in the placebo/asenapine, asenapine, olanzapine groups. Clinically significant weight gain occurred in 21.9, 39.2, and 55.1% of patients in the placebo/asenapine, asenapine, and olanzapine groups respectively. Shifts from low or normal fasting blood glucose levels to high levels were observed in 10% of placebo/asenapine, 26.0% of asenapine, and 22.2% of olanzapine patients.

As with the acute clinical trials, there were no clinically significant changes in electro-cardiographic or prolactin measures. The mean ± SD in YMRS total score from baseline in the ITT population at week 52 was −28.6 ± 8.1 for asenapine vs 28.2 ± 6.8 for olanzapine. Rates of response and remission at week 52 were similar (97.8 and 98.4% respectively) with no between-group differences. The mean ± SD change from baseline in CGI-BP was −3.6 ± 1.1 with asenapine vs −3.5 ± 0.9 with olanzapine at week 52. There was no evidence of worsening of depression as measured by MADRS scores.

13.6 SUMMARY AND CONCLUSION

Asenapine is a sublingual atypical antipsychotic with proven efficacy in the treatment of manic and mixed states associated with adult bipolar I disorder. Asenapine's benefits were seen at the pre-specified day 21 as well as at day 2, indicating rapid onset of efficacy. Asenapine treatment is also superior to placebo on many secondary outcome measures at both endpoint and day 2. Asenapine exhibits minimal propensity for acute EPS as well as sedation/somnolence. Moreover, weight gain associated with this treatment is modest relative to olanzapine and placebo. Asenapine does not exhibit a propensity to alter laboratory parameters, prolactin levels or changes in the electrocardiogram.

Taken together, asenapine represents a treatment alternative for individuals with bipolar disorder. Asenapine is the first rapidly absorbed sublingual atypical antipsychotic agent available. It remains unknown whether the rapid absorption of asenapine results in a faster onset of action of this agent when compared to other atypical antipsychotics and antimanic agents. The advantage of this formulation is axiomatic in individuals with swallowing difficulties and difficulties with medication absorption. Anecdotally, some patients have reported an unpleasant taste in the mouth after using asenapine on some occasions. It is highly recommended however, that oral rinsing and/or consumption of food and/or beverage not occur for a minimum of 10 minutes, as it may adversely affect bioavailability. Recently, the FDA has approved a black cherry flavored formulation of asenapine that appears to be associated with considerably less unpleasant taste. This instruction was emphasized during the clinical trial development program for asenapine, and as predicted, there were many occasions where this was not followed by protocol. It is not known however, if this protocol deviation will predictably diminish asenapine's efficacy (it did not seem to alter efficacy in the clinical trials, albeit that issue was not specifically evaluated). Notwithstanding, it seems a reasonable and testable hypothesis that in some cases, therapeutic effectiveness might be compromised if patients do not exhibit fidelity to the administration recommendations.

During the last decade there has been appropriate and increasing concern related to the safety and tolerability of atypical antipsychotic agents. The major categories are CNS (for example, sedation/somnolence), body composition (for example, weight gain), metabolic disruption (for example, glucose-lipid alterations), cardiotoxicity, hormonal (for example, prolactin elevation), and neurological toxicity (for example, EPS). On each of these categories, asenapine is either without clinically significant risk and/or exhibits minimal risk (for example, weight gain). Taken together, this therapeutic index represents an advance over other agents in the treatment of bipolar disorder. Future trials will evaluate asenapine's efficacy in acute bipolar (and major) depression as well as recurrence prevention in bipolar samples. Moreover, the sponsor has completed a combination study in acute mania wherein asenapine was compared to placebo as an adjunct to lithium or divalproex. The results of this study were not publicly available at the time of writing this chapter. The results from studies evaluating asenapine's efficacy and safety in bipolar depression (bipolar I/II disorder), as well as recurrence prevention should be available in the near future.

References

Bishara, D. and Taylor, D. (2009) Asenapine monotherapy in the acute treatment of both schizophrenia and bipolar I disorder. *Neuropsychiatr. Dis. Treat.*, **5**, 483–490.

Choi, Y.K., Wong, E.H., Henry, B., Shahid, M. and Tarazi, F.I. (2010) Repeated effects of asenapine on adrenergic and cholinergic muscarine receptors. *Int. J. Neuropsychopharmacol.*, **13** (3), 405–410.

Franberg, O., Marcus, M.M., Ivanov, V. *et al.* (2009) Asenapine elevates cortical dopamine, noradrenaline and serotonin release. Evidence for activation of cortical and subcortical dopamine systems by different mechanisms. *Psychopharmacology (Berl.)*, **204** (2), 251–264.

Ghanbari, R., EI Manssari, M., Shahid, M., and Blier, P. (2009) Electrophysiological characterization of the effects of asenapine at 5-HT(1A), 5-HT(2A), alpha(2)-adrenergic and D(2) receptors in the rat brain. *Eur. Neuropsychopharmacol.*, **19** (3), 177–187.

Marston, H.M., Young, J.W., Martin, F.D. *et al.* (2009) Asenapine effects in animal models of psychosis and cognitive function. *Psychopharmacology (Berl.)*, **206** (4), 699–714.

McIntyre, R.S., Cohen, M., Zhao, J. *et al.* (2009a) A 3-week, randomized, placebo-controlled trial of asenapine in the treatment of acute mania in bipolar mania and mixed states. *Bipolar Disord.*, **11** (7), 673–686.

McIntyre, R.S., Cohen, M., Zhao, J. *et al.* (2009b) Asenapine versus olanzapine in acute mania: a double-blind extension study. *Bipolar Disord.* **11** (8), 815–826.

McIntyre, R.S., Cohen, M., Zhao, J. *et al.* (2010) Asenapine in the treatment of acute mania in bipolar I disorder: A randomized, double-blind, placebo-controlled trial. *.J Affect. Disord.*, **122** (1–2), 27–38.

McIntyre, R.S. and Konarski, J.Z. (2005) Tolerability profiles of atypical antipsychotics in the treatment of bipolar disorder. *J. Clin. Psychiatry*, **66** (Suppl. 3), 28–36.

McIntyre, R.S., McCann, S.M., and Kennedy, S.H. (2001) Antipsychotic metabolic effects: weight gain, diabetes mellitus, and lipid abnormalities. *Can. J. Psychiatry*, **46** (3), 273–281.

Newcomer, J.W., Nasrallah, H.A., and Loebel, A.D. (2004) The atypical antipsychotic therapy and metabolic issues national survey: practice patterns and knowledge of psychiatrists. *J. Clin. Psychopharmacol.*, **24** (Suppl. 1), (5), S1–S6.

Ng, F., Mammen, O.K., Wilting, I. *et al.* (2009) The International Society for Bipolar Disorders (ISBD) consensus guidelines for the safety monitoring of bipolar disorder treatments. *Bipolar Disord.*, **11** (6), 559–595.

Perlis, R.H., Ostacher, M.J., Patel, J.K. *et al.* (2006b) Predictors of recurrence in bipolar disorder: primary outcomes from the systematic treatment enhancement program for bipolar disorder (STEP-BD). *Am. J. Psychiatry*, **163** (2), 217–224.

Perlis, R.H., Welge, J.A., Vornik, L.A. *et al.* (2006a) Atypical antipsychotics in the treatment of mania: a meta-analysis of randomized, placebo-controlled trials. *J. Clin. Psychiatry*, **67** (4), 509–516.

Tarazi, F.I., Choi, Y.K., Gardner, M. *et al.* (2009) Asenapine exerts distinctive regional effects on ionotropic glutamate receptor subtypes in rat brain. *Synapse*, **63** (5), 413–420.

Tarazi, F.I., Moran-Gates, T., Wong, E.H. *et al.* (2008) Differential regional and dose-related effects of asenapine on dopamine receptor subtypes. *Psychopharmacology (Berl.)*, **198** (1), 103–111.

Tarazi, F.I. and Shahid, M. (2009) Asenapine maleate: a new drug for the treatment of schizophrenia and bipolar mania. *Drugs Today (Barc.)*, **45** (12), 865–876.

Tohen, M., Bowden, C.L., Calabrese, J.R. *et al.* (2006) Influence of sub-syndromal symptoms after remission from manic or mixed episodes. *Br. J. Psychiatry*, **189**, 515–519.

14

Complex Combination Therapy for Long-Term Stability in Bipolar Disorder

Robert M. Post

Bipolar Collaborative Network, Bethesda, MD, USA

14.1 INTRODUCTION

The evidence that complex combination therapy is required for effective long-term treatment of a large proportion of patients with bipolar illness is substantial and growing. Yet there are a dearth of clinically relevant systematic studies to delineate the best combinations for which types of patients, and the best sequence of treatments.

In this chapter we focus on the rationale for complex combination therapy, general principles that may be useful in the development of treatment strategies for individual patients, and suggestions about the use of specific drug combinations and how individual drugs may best be added to inadequately effective regimens. However, given the relative lack of a systematic clinical trials database available to guide this type of therapeutics, the specific treatment suggestions in this chapter must be taken as highly provisional and subject to rapid revision as further evidence becomes available.

14.2 RATIONALE FOR COMPLEX COMBINATION THERAPY IN BIPOLAR ILLNESS

Treatment-resistance in bipolar illness has been vastly underestimated, and a substantial portion of patients remains symptomatic despite the use of multiple drugs in combination in naturalistic treatment (Post *et al.*, 2003, 2010a; Nolen *et al.*, 2004; Judd *et al.*, 2002) (Figure 14.1). A few controlled studies in the literature are particularly revealing. For example, Calabrese *et al.* found that less than 20% of the intent-to-treat population of bipolar patients with rapid cycling stabilized enough for a short period of time to be randomized to either lithium or valproate monotherapy (Calabrese *et al.*, 2005). Upon such randomization, about 50% of the patients relapsed on either monotherapy, revealing that only some 10–12% of these patients were able to sustain a good long-term effect on either of two of the most widely used monotherapies in the U.S. – lithium or valproate.

Bipolar Psychopharmacotherapy: Caring for the patient, Second Edition. Edited by Hagop S. Akiskal and Mauricio Tohen.
© 2011 John Wiley & Sons, Ltd. Published 2011 by John Wiley & Sons, Ltd.

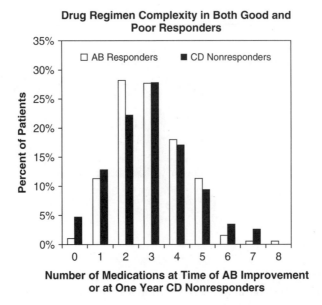

Figure 14.1 An average of three medications was needed for the Responders, and was also used at any one time in the Nonresponders.

The data of Kemp *et al.* (2009) in those with substance use comorbidity revealed similar difficulties in achieving even acute stabilization with the combination of lithium and valproate. The findings of Findling and colleagues (2006) similarly indicate that childhood-onset bipolar illness very often requires the lithium/valproate combination, since two-thirds of the patients who initially stabilized on the combination then relapsed during treatment with either monotherapy, but the majority rapidly re-stabilized when the combination was again initiated. Moreover, the bulk of the patients also required adjunctive psychomotor stimulants for ADHD and, in a small number of instances, atypical antipsychotics.

Similarly, very low long-term response rates were observed in outpatients with bipolar illness after a year of double-blind treatment with lithium or carbamazepine monotherapy, and some 50% of patients remained inadequately responsive during a third year on the combination of lithium and carbamazepine (Denicoff *et al.*, 1997a, 1997b). In many of these studies, response consists not always of "very much improved" on the CGI-BP, or an essential remission, but sometimes "much improved," meaning only partial symptom amelioration. A clinical response involving only partial improvement is a particular problem because multiple studies have indicated that patients with incomplete remission and residual symptomatology are at higher risk for relapse than those with a sustained complete response (Judd *et al.*, 2008; Nierenberg *et al.*, 2009).

In most formal randomized clinical trials (RCTs) aimed at drug registration, response rates are typically the focus of consideration, and sustained remission end-points are rarely utilized, even in the evaluation of long-term prophylaxis. Thus, one gets a rosy view about the efficacy of drugs acutely and in long-term prophylaxis from the RCT literature, especially since those with major or multiple comorbidities are often excluded from clinical trials, as are severely ill patients with suicidality. Such complicated patients form a substantial portion of clinical practice, especially since some 40% of bipolar patients in many clinical settings have a comorbid alcohol or substance abuse problem, and 40% have a comorbid anxiety disorder (McElroy *et al.*, 2001).

Thus, if our goal is to sustain long-term remission in real world complicated patients, clinical treatment approaches necessarily must rapidly exceed FDA single-drug or dual-drug approval status, as well as the majority of treatment guidelines, which laud themselves for largely relying on an RCT literature that is virtually nonexistent for more complicated patients and rarely goes beyond recommendations of dual combination therapy.

Another perhaps counter-intuitive rationale for complex combination therapy is the avoidance of side effects. The literature is filled with statements that the use of greater numbers of medications is associated with greater numbers of side effects, but such observations are not based on data in which doses are carefully titrated on an individual basis so that maximum tolerability is achieved. Attempting to maximize doses of a single agent (such as lithium) in order to achieve more complete therapeutic efficacy is known to be associated with a greater number of side effects (Gelenberg *et al.*, 1989). If lithium is used below its side-effects threshold, and other drugs with other mechanisms of action are utilized, there is, in fact, a better chance for a more tolerable regimen and potentially even greater therapeutic success because of additional alternative pharmacodynamic mechanisms being brought into play.

14.3 PRINCIPLES OF BUILDING AN EFFECTIVE THERAPEUTIC REGIMEN

We have already mentioned the need for careful dose titration for side-effects avoidance, and it is also highly recommended that one attempt to add only a single new treatment agent at a time (Table 14.1). In this fashion, one is able to evaluate the degree of added therapeutic efficacy achieved by the latest adjunct. While single prolonged monotherapy trials have some academic support, the low incidence in which they achieve a complete response (as noted above), and the potential long time required for such repeated individual drug evaluations in prophylaxis make such an approach clinically impractical and, in some instances, inhumane.

Rather, we suggest the utility of evaluating the new drug initially as an add-on in a combination regimen. This is particularly true in instances when there is an inadequate or incomplete response to the new combination regimen, such that the next set of treatment options can be explored more rapidly. This strategy avoids the case in which a patient must experience two separate and failed sequential monotherapy trials, followed by a combination trial, before moving on to the next treatment step.

Table 14.1 Principles of rational polypsychopharmacotherapy.

Add one drug at a time (to evaluate effectiveness and side effects of new agent)

Augmentation saves time over substitution

Consider predominant affective target (mania, depression, mixed state) and comorbidities in initial choice of a mood stabilizer

Equally consider the long term side-effects profile and overall tolerability of drug for its use in combination strategies

Add drugs with different mechanisms of action (and from different classes)

Titrate each drug to optimal effectiveness and to a dose below its side-effects threshold (not to conventional dose/blood levels)

Consider the presence of a positive family history of affective and anxiety disorders and family history of specific drug response

Emphasize lithium and psychotherapy for management of suicidality

Simplify dosage regimen to enhance compliance (i.e., only H.S. or A.M. dosing, if possible)

Anticipate and manage predicted pharmacokinetic interactions

In presence of side effects, decrease dose of drug most likely implicated

Watch literature for efficacy and availability of new treatment modalities such as rTMS and VNS

Follow emerging literature on clinical, neurochemical, and genetic predictors of individual drug response

Have patient (or a family member) daily chart medications, mood, sleep, comorbid symptoms, and side effects to help optimize pharmacotherapy; consense about early warning signs and symptoms (EWS) of an impending episode, and agree on appropriate course of action

Monitor side effects (cognition/sedation/unsteadiness, etc.) and comorbid conditions as carefully as mood

In the face of a good response, be conservative and maintain full-dose treatment into continuation and prophylaxis (in absence of side effects)

In the absence of a good response, consider major changes in the core treatment strategies and then more experimental approaches as required until effectiveness is achieved

---

Involving the patient as a collaborator and co-investigator in this carefully monitored and evolving therapeutic process is of critical importance. We suggest that patients systematically chart their mood, medications, sleep, side effects, and residual comorbid symptoms on an ongoing daily basis in order to guide a more systematic evaluation of the effectiveness of individual agents for their own particular illness and symptoms (Post and Leverich, 2008; Leverich and Post, 1998). Such careful monitoring also provides timely information about the early emergence of side effects so that drug doses can be efficiently titrated toward their peak efficacy in the absence of side effects. Without such careful clinical response and side-effects information from the patient, the treating physician is essentially "flying blind" in attempting to safely reach the desired destination of long-term stability for the patient.

The analogy to careful monitoring of blood sugar by patients with diabetes in order to regulate their diet, exercise, and insulin doses is an apt one, particularly since such careful monitoring and glucose regulation has resulted in many years of extended well being and a marked delay in mortality arising from the complications of diabetes. In bipolar illness, the years of life expectancy lost compared with the general population is catastrophically large (Newcomer and Hennekens, 2007). It is some 13 years in Virginia and 25–30 years in some Western states in the U.S. in patients with severe mental disorders compared with nonmentally ill patients in the same states and regions of the country (Colton and Manderscheid, 2006). While the excess medical mortality is largely due to cardiovascular disease, almost every primary medical condition is more prone to occur and/or more difficult to control if a patient is depressed.

Another critical element in long-term management is a component of a good working relationship in the development of an early warning system (EWS), such that when a patient begins to experience breakthrough symptoms, appropriate therapeutic measures can be taken in a timely fashion. The attempt is not only to rapidly treat these symptoms, but also ward off the likelihood that these will be the precursor to a more full-blown syndromic relapse. Setting specific thresholds and parameters for adjunctive use of PRN medicine or direct contact with the physician should be worked out and stipulated as part of the EWS, so that if, for example, a patient loses more than two hours of sleep for two consecutive nights, there are clear directives as to how they should proceed.

In developing an optimal therapeutic regimen, it is important to assess any residual symptoms and comorbidities that remain unresolved by the initial therapeutic maneuvers. This should lead to further attempts at a judicious targeting of this symptomatology with additional medications that would be most likely to achieve the desired therapeutic efficacy goals in the absence of side effects.

Thus, whatever complexity of treatment regimen is required in order to achieve the maximum degree of mood stability in bipolar illness, in those with comorbid medical illnesses or at high risk for the metabolic syndrome and other medical complications, the regimens typically must be that much more complex in order to address these added difficulties. If the patient with bipolar illness does not have good access to an internist or other primary care physician, the psychiatrist should begin to deal with the multiple vulnerability factors for cardiovascular disease and other problems linked to the metabolic syndrome and other risk factors. Blood pressure, cholesterol, weight, waist circumference, blood glucose, and hemoglobin A1C levels need to be monitored by a specified clinician and appropriate treatment administered accordingly. Patients with bipolar illness smoke cigarettes at a rate in great excess to smokers in the general population, and efforts at smoking cessation are required in attempting to reduce the array of medical comorbidities with which smoking is associated.

While monotherapy is widely recommended and many patients deserve a clinical trial on monotherapy in the initiation of their long-term prophylaxis, some groups of patients should be started on combination treatment from the outset. This recommendation is made not only on the basis of the low response rates to monotherapy in patients in many academic centers and, in particular, in those with either rapid cycling or comorbid substance abuse (as noted above), but also in patients otherwise at high risk for nonresponse to monotherapy or dual combination therapy. For example, these might include bipolar patients with a comorbid anxiety disorder or other complicating factors that suggest a low likelihood of complete response to lithium or any single agent considered for initiating prophylactic therapy.

This recommendation for combination therapy from the outset in selected patients is also supported by new data presented by Geddes *et al.* in the BALANCE study (Geddes *et al.*, 2010). In that study, patients with bipolar illness were randomized to two years of treatment with one of three treatments, lithium monotherapy, valproate monotherapy, or the combination of both drugs. The combination was vastly superior to valproate monotherapy and more minimally superior to lithium, that is, only on some outcome measures. However, lithium was substantially superior to valproate on virtually all treatment endpoints. Thus, I would endorse Geddes' conclusions that if one were to consider the use of valproate as a primary therapeutic modality, lithium should be given with it from the outset of prophylaxis. If lithium were to be the drug of first choice, one might be more circumspect before adding valproate or some other adjunctive treatment, because there is a greater likelihood of sustained long-term therapeutic response to lithium, at least as revealed in Geddes' European cohort.

However, this clinical investigator would add the caveat that lithium combined with other agents should be considered from the outset in the large number of instances in which a patient has a presentation that has previously been associated with a lower lithium response rate. These include those without a family history of affective illness in first-degree relatives; those with an anxiety disorder comorbidity; schizoaffective illness or mood incongruent delusions; rapid cycling presentation (particularly without a well interval); the presence of alcohol or substance abuse; the illness sequence of depression, mania, well interval (D-M-I) as opposed to M-D-I; a history of head trauma or other neurological insult; or a prior history of relative lithium intolerance (Post and Leverich, 2008).

When many of these poor-prognosis factors for lithium response are present, carbamazepine or valproate may be particularly effective. However, these agents should be used cautiously in women of child-bearing age. Valproate should be avoided, if possible, not only because of its increased incidence of *spina bifida* and other major malformations, but also the very substantial incidence of developmental delay and an average reduction in some nine I.Q. points compared with women with epilepsy treated with other agents (Nicolai, Vles, and Aldenkamp, 2008).

In this regard, lamotrigine appears to have a relatively good safety profile. When used in pregnant women in a case registry involving more than 1000 women, no major malformations were associated with the drug. In addition, potential predictors for a good response to lamotrigine monotherapy are a personal and positive family history of anxiety disorders as well as a more rapid cycling presentation (Grof, Angs, and Haines, 1974; Alda *et al.*, 2002; Duffy *et al.*, 2007).

None of these last three mood-stabilizing anticonvulsants has as strong a database as lithium for anti-suicide effects, and their record for likely neuroprotection to neurons and glia is also not as robust as that of lithium. Multiple studies have documented that lithium increases measures of neuronal integrity in humans measured on MRS as well as increases in gray matter in patients with bipolar illness, as revealed on MRI (Post and Leverich, 2008; Moore *et al.*, 2009; Manji, Moore and Chen, 2000; Schloesser *et al.*, 2008). Not only does lithium increase the anti-apoptotic factors Bcl-2 and BDNF, but it also reduces the pro-apoptotic factors BAX and p53. Still, valproate is a potent histone-deacetylase inhibitor (while carbamazepine is only a weak one, and lithium does not possess this effect). How this action might relate to a specific therapeutic profile of valproate compared with the other agents has not yet been adequately elucidated but is promising (Bredy and Barad, 2008).

Better antisuicide effects of clozapine over that of olanzapine have been demonstrated in schizophrenia but not yet studied in bipolar patients. The atypicals as a class appear to have major advantages over old typical neuroleptics in terms of their lower incidence of both acute extrapyramidal side effects and longer-term liability of tardive dyskinesia, and substantially improved efficacy in the depressive phase of the illness. The side-effects profiles of the atypicals vary considerably, with some agents being problematic for weight gain and the metabolic syndrome, while others are more benign or neutral on these indices (Tables 14.1 and 14.2). In this regard, on weight gain and metabolic indices, clozapine and olanzapine are most problematic; quetiapine and risperidone are intermediate, and aripiprazole and ziprasidone are the least problematic.

Quetiapine, consistent with its positive effects in monotherapy of both unipolar and bipolar depression, increases neurogenesis and BDNF in the hippocampus, and prevents stress from decreasing BDNF, the latter effect which is shared by ziprasidone, but

Table 14.2 Potential off-label approaches to substance comorbidities in bipolar disorder.

Alcohol Abstinence	Withdrawal	Cocaine	Nicotine	Food/bulimia
12 Step (I)A	Carbamazepine (I)A	N-Acetylcysteine (I)A	Buproprion (I)A	Topiramate (I)A
Valproate (I[a])A	Benzodiazepines (I)C	Topiramate (I)A	Nicotine Patch/ Gum (I)A	Zonisamide (I)A
Topiramate (I)A	Valproate (III)A	Modafinil (I)A	Varenicline (I)C	Sibutramine[b] (I)C
Gabapentin (I)A	Gabapentin (IV, V)B	12 Step (I)A	Rimonabant[b] (I)D	Rimonabant[b] (I)D
Naltrexone (I)B	—	Carbamazepine (II)A	—	—
Acamprosate (I)B	—	Disulfiram (I)C	—	—
Zonisamide (I)B	—	Baclofen (I)D	—	—
Carbamazepine (III)B	—	—	—	—
Disulfiram (I)C	—	—	—	—

First rating: level of evidence in primary disorder only:
(I) = Double blind clinical trial.
(II) = Large case experience.
(III) = Much open study.
(IV) = Few cases.
(V) = Ambiguous.
(VI) = Worsens.
[a]Studied in bipolar disorder; [b]No longer available.
Second rating: potential utility in bipolar disorder:
A = Very likely useful; high priority for consideration.
B = Likely useful; moderate priority.
C = Ambiguous data; low priority.
D = Should be avoided.

exacerbated by haloperidol (Post and Leverich, 2008; Park *et al.*, 2006, 2009; Post and Altshuler, 2009; Post, 2007). Olanzepine and clozapine may also increase BDNF, as does valproate, carbamazepine and lamotrigine.

All of the atypicals are acutely antimanic in monotherapy and most have additional adjunctive efficacy where used in combination with lithium or valproate. Most of the atypicals are approved for longer-term prophylaxis. Quetiapine is approved as an adjunct to lithium or valproate; however, evidence also indicates its efficacy in monotherapy prophylaxis as well (Brecher *et al.*, 2008; Young *et al.*, 2008).

Thus, as an overall therapeutic strategy, one would recommend initial choice of one or two agents for long-term prophylaxis that appear to most ideally target an individual patient's bipolar illness profile and ancillary comorbidities, and at the same time, have the best chance for long-term tolerability (Tables 14.2 and 14.3). In the absence of major discriminating features that would lead to clear choices among several agents for initial therapeutic use, this author would recommend a heavy reliance on long-term tolerability of a treatment approach as a major deciding factor. This recommendation is based not only on the increased likelihood of long-term compliance if an agent is well tolerated, but also the minimal exacerbation of medical indices and syndromes such as weight gain and other aspects of the metabolic syndrome. Medical comorbidities and potential years

Table 14.3 Potential adjunctive approaches to target anxiety disorder comorbidities.

Social phobia	Panic/agrophobia	PTSD	OCD
Gabapentin (I)A	Gabapentin (I)A	Atypical	Atypicals (I)A
Pregabalin (I) A	Pregabalin (I)A	Antipsychotics (I)A	Topiramate (I)A
Clonazepam (I)A	Clonazepam (I)A	Lamotrigine (II[a])A	N-Acetylcysteine (I)A
Antidepressants (I)B	Valproate (II)A	Topiramate (III)A	Lamotrigine (IV)A
—	Lamotrigine (II[a])A	Carbamazepine (III)A	Carbamazepine (IV)A
—	Carbamazepine (III)A	SSRIs (I)B	SSRI's (I)B
—	Antidepressants (I)B	Prazosin (I)B	Gabapentin (IV, V)B
		Benzodiazepines (V, VI)C	

First rating: level of evidence in primary disorder only:
(I) = Double blind clinical trial.
(II) = Large case experience.
(III) = Much open study.
(IV) = Few cases.
(V) = Ambiguous.
(VI) = Worsens.
[a] = Studied in bipolar disorder.
Second rating: potential utility in bipolar disorder:
A = Very likely useful; high priority for consideration.
B = Likely useful; moderate priority.
C = Ambiguous data; low priority.
D = Should be avoided.

of loss of life expectancy should be factored into the choice of prophylactic regimens, particularly in those at high risk or those already suffering medical problems.

14.3.1   SELECTED COMMENTS ON A FEW SPECIFIC DRUGS FOR TARGETING COMORBIDITIES

Although off label, a number of drugs have been shown in small placebo-controlled studies to be helpful in the instance of comorbid cocaine use (Table 14.2). These include modafinil and n-acetylcysteine, which have been shown to have positive effects in the primary symptoms of affective dysregulation as well. Even though topiramate is not an effective antimanic in monotherapy, it has positive effects on several of the comorbidities commonly associated with bipolar illness, such as alcohol and cocaine abuse, PTSD, bulimia, and migraine headaches. In contrast to these potentially useful options is baclofen, which has shown some success in controlled studies in cocaine abusers, but would not be recommended because of its role in exacerbating depressive symptomatology (Post and Leverich, 2008).

Approaches to bipolar patients with comorbid anxiety disorders are vastly understudied, but options again include the mood-stabilizing anticonvulsants and atypical antipsychotics (Table 14.3). These latter drugs should be used in the anxiety comorbidities, including posttraumatic stress disorder, perhaps in preference to the unimodal antidepressants, which are the typically chosen first-line agents in those without bipolar disorder.

Likewise, a number of FDA-approved options are available for those with primary alcoholism, but their effects in bipolar patients with comorbid alcoholism have not been systematically studied (Table 14.2). Topiramate is not FDA-approved for alcohol avoidance, but two large, positive, placebo-controlled clinical trials, and its general widespread use for other indications in bipolar patients, suggests its possible utility for this purpose. A recent trial also supports the use of N-acetylcysteine for this and many other addictions (Table 14.4). Similar indirect inferences from studies in nonbipolar patients suggest possible strategies for approaching comorbid cognitive dysfunction (Table 14.5) and ADHD (Table 14.6).

Quetiapine is an atypical of special interest because of its broad spectrum of efficacy across a variety of diagnoses from schizophrenia to mania and mixed states to bipolar and unipolar depression and generalized anxiety disorder. Remission rates in many of these syndromes approach 50%, and its optimal use in combination with other agents in those not adequately responsive or tolerant remains to be better explored. Ketter and associates found a substantial response rate to quetiapine and lamotrigine when used in combination in open studies of those nonresponsive to more traditional approaches (Ketter *et al.*, 2007).

14.4   CONCLUSIONS

The high incidence of comorbid disorders in bipolar illness practically demands complex combination treatment because these more complex presentations of the illness typically

Table 14.4 N-Acetylcysteine (NAC) – positive effects on mood, addictions, and compulsions[a].

I. Affective and cognitive symptoms	
A. Bipolar disorder, especially depression (over placebo at three and six months)[b]	Berk et al. (2008a)
B. Schizophrenia, especially negative symptoms[b]	Berk et al. (2008b)
C. Autism, irritability and stereotypy	Fung et al. (2010)
II. Addictions	
A. Cocaine craving	LaRowe et al. (2006)
B. Heroin craving	
C. Gambling urges	Grant et al. (2007)
D. Marijuana craving[a]	Gray (2010)
E. Nicotine craving	Knackstedt et al. (2009)
III. Compulsions	
A. Trichotillomania (after two months)	Grant et al. (2009)
B. OCD (adjunct to SSRI), especially obsessive symptoms	Lafleur et al. (2006)
C. Nail-biting[a]	Berk et al. (2009)

[a] All studies placebo-controlled except Nailbiting and Marijuana craving
[b] Usual dose; NAC 500 mg one cap BID for 1 week then two caps BID thereafter.

Table 14.5 A possible sequence of approaches to cognitive dysfunction in bipolar disorder.

	Strength of evidence	Utility for BP
1. Prevent as many affective episodes as possible	A	A
2. Reduce dose or discontinue drugs contributing to sedation/confusion	A	A
3. Optimize the treatment of comorbid residual depressive symptoms and anxiety disorders	A	A
4. Rule out (R/O):	A	A
a. Lithium induced hypothyroidism	—	—
b. VPA-induced hyperammoniaemia	—	—
c. CBZ/OXC hyponatremia	—	—
d. Lithium and LTG toxicity at convential doses	—	—
e. Topiramate-induced dysfunction	—	—
5. Augment lithium with T_3 even with normal thyroid indices	B	A
6. Potentiate with folate (to decrease homocysteine)	B	A
7. R/O cardiovascular risk factors	A	A
8. Consider adjunctive use of:	—	—
a. Modafinil 100 → 200 mg in AM → 300 mg in AM after one month (warn about serious rash)	A	A
b. Psychomotor stimulants (see Table 14.6)	B	B
c. Amantadine (dopaminergic, antiglutaminergic)	C	C
d. Nimodipine (increases somatostatin)	A/B	B
e. AntiAlzheimer's drugs[a]	A	B

[a] Acetylcholine esterase inhibitor and/or glutamate NMDA receptor antagonist memantine.

Table 14.6 ADHD comorbidity in bipolar disorder.

    I. ADHD comorbidity with bipolar disorder decreases with age

        a. Childhood-very common 40–80%
        b. Adolescent-infrequent 10–20%
        c. Adult-rare 5–10%

    II. Consider ADHD-like symptoms in a bipolar adult as residual symptoms of inadequately treated mania or depression until proven otherwise

    III. A suggested treatment sequence of ADHD-like symptoms in adults with bipolar disorder

        A. Optimize antimanic regime
        B. Optimize antidepressant/antianxiety regime
        C. Consider bupropion (especially if residual depression is present); avoid atomoxetime as an NE selective reuptake inhibitor
        D. Consider modafinil (100–200 mg in AM, to 300 mg in AM after one month if needed)
        E. Consider a psychomotor stimulant (in low doses)

---

require targeted and differential treatment compared with those without comorbidities. How one optimally deploys and sequences these treatments in the service of achieving and maintaining long-term remission is an art form that must be developed in each patient on the basis of individual responsiveness (Post and Leverich, 2008). While a minority of patients achieve optimal long-term stabilization with a given monotherapy, the good clinician must use all of his or her resources of clinical observation, awareness of the literature, inference, and intuition in order to optimally treat patients with bipolar disorder, particularly those in the U.S. who tend to have a variety of poor prognosis factors, including early onset, anxiety disorders, substance abuse comorbidity, and accumulation of greater number of prior episodes, compared to similarly recruited bipolar patients in several cities in the Netherlands and Germany (Post *et al.*, 2008b; Post et al., 2010c). The duration of the delay from illness onset to first treatment varies inversely with an earlier age of onset, and the time delay to first treatment is an independent predictor of a more difficult course of illness in adulthood, including more time depressed, greater severity of depression, less time euthymic, more episodes, and ultradian cycling (Post *et al.*, 2010b).

A paradigm shift toward earlier, more aggressive and consistent therapeutic approaches to this highly disabling and potentially lethal disorder is sorely needed. Sir William Osler said that the artful physician is skilled in the use of polytherapy. Employing complex combination therapy when needed is obviously meritorious, even in the absence of an adequate controlled clinical trials literature to reach definitive recommendations. This author would also very much endorse the use of widely studied and efficacious targeted psychotherapies and psychoeducational approaches as a necessary part of the therapeutic regimen in almost all patients with bipolar disorder (Miklowitz, 2008; Miklowitz *et al.*, 2008; Miklowitz and Scott, 2009).

References

Alda, M., Passmore, M., Garnham, J., *et al.* (2002) Clinical presentation of bipolar disorders responsive to lithium or lamotrigine. *Int. J. Neuropsychopharmacol.*, (5), S58.

Berk, M., Copolov, D.L., Dean, O., *et al.* (2008a) N-acetyl cysteine for depressive symptoms in bipolar disorder – a double-blind randomized placebo-controlled trial. *Biol. Psychiatry*, **64** (6), 468–475.

Berk, M., Copolov, D., Dean, O., *et al.* (2008b) N-acetyl cysteine as a glutathione precursor for schizophrenia – a double-blind, randomized, placebo-controlled trial. *Biol. Psychiatry*, **64** (5), 361–368.

Berk, M., Jeavons, S., Dean, O.M., *et al.* (2009) Nail-biting stuff? The effect of N-acetyl cysteine on nail-biting. *CNS Spectr.*, **14** (7), 357–360.

Brecher, M., Suppes, T., Vieta, E., Liu, S., and Paulsson, B. (2008) Quetiapine in the maintenance treatment of bipolar I disorder: combined data from two long-term, phase III studies. 161st Annual Meeting of the American Psychiatric Association, Washington, DC.

Bredy, T.W. and Barad, M. (2008) The histone deacetylase inhibitor valproic acid enhances acquisition, extinction, and reconsolidation of conditioned fear. *Learn Mem.*, **15** (1), 39–45.

Calabrese, J.R., Shelton, M.D., Rapport, D.J. *et al.* (2005) A 20-month, double-blind, maintenance trial of lithium versus divalproex in rapid-cycling bipolar disorder. *Am. J. Psychiatry*, **162** (11), 2152–2161.

Colton, C.W. and Manderscheid, R.W. (2006) Congruencies in increased mortality rates, years of potential life lost, and causes of death among public mental health clients in eight states. *Prev. Chronic Dis.*, **3** (2), A42.

Denicoff, K.D., Smith-Jackson, E.E., Bryan, A.L., Ali, S.O., and Post, R.M. *et al.* (1997a) Valproate prophylaxis in a prospective clinical trial of refractory bipolar disorder. *Am. J. Psychiatry*, **154** (10), 1456–1458.

Denicoff, K.D., Smith-Jackson, E.E., Disney, E.R., Ali, S.O., Leverich, G.S., and Post, R.M. *et al.* (1997b) Comparative prophylactic efficacy of lithium, carbamazepine, and the combination in bipolar disorder. *J. Clin. Psychiatry*, **58** (11), 470–478.

Duffy, A., Alda, M., Crawford, L., Milin, R., and Grof, P. *et al.* (2007) The early manifestations of bipolar disorder: a longitudinal prospective study of the offspring of bipolar parents. *Bipolar Disord.*, **9** (8), 828–838.

Findling, R.L., McNamara, N.K., Stansbrey, R. *et al.* (2006) Combination lithium and divalproex sodium in pediatric bipolar symptom re-stabilization. *J. Am. Acad. Child Adolesc. Psychiatry*, **45** (2), 142–148.

Fung, L.K., Libove, R., Hornbeak, K. *et al.* (2010) A Randomized, Placebo-Controlled, Double-Blind Trial of N-Acetylcysteine in Children with Autism. Scientific Proceeding AACAP 57th Annual Meeting, New York. Poster 1.20, p. 225.

Geddes, J.R., Goodwin, G.M., Rendell, J. *et al.* (2010) Lithium plus valproate combination therapy versus monotherapy for relapse prevention in bipolar I disorder (BALANCE): a randomised open trial. *Lancet* **375** (9712), 385–395.

Gelenberg, A.J., Kane, J.M., Keller, M.B., *et al.* (1989) Comparison of standard and low serum levels of lithium for maintenance treatment of bipolar disorder. *N. Engl. J. Med.*, **321** (22), 1489–1493.

Grant, J.E., Kim, S.W., and Odlaug, B.L. (2007) N-acetyl cysteine, a glutamate-modulating agent, in the treatment of pathological gambling: a pilot study. *Biol. Psychiatry*, **62** (6), 652–657.

Grant, J.E., Odlaug, B.L., and Kim, S.W. (2009) N-acetylcysteine, a glutamate modulator, in the treatment of trichotillomania: a double-blind, placebo-controlled study. *Arch. Gen. Psychiatry*, **66** (7), 756–763.

Gray, K.M., Watson, N.L., Carpenter, M.J., and Larowe, S.D. (2010) N-acetylcysteine (NAC) in young marijuana users: an open-label pilot study. *Am. J. Addict.*, **19** (2), 187–189.

Grof, P., Angst, J., and Haines, T. (1974) The clinical course of depression: practical issues, in *Classification and Prediction of Outcome of Depression* (ed. J. Angst) F.K. Schattauer Verlag, Stuttgart, pp. 141–148.

Judd, L.L., Akiskal, H.S., Schettler, P.J. *et al.* (2002) The long-term natural history of the weekly symptomatic status of bipolar I disorder. *Arch. Gen. Psychiatry*, **59** (6), 530–537.

Judd, L.L., Schettler, P.J., Akiskal, H.S. *et al.* (2008) Residual symptom recovery from major affective episodes in bipolar disorders and rapid episode relapse/recurrence. *Arch. Gen. Psychiatry*, **65** (4), 386–394.

Kemp, D.E., Gao, K., Ganocy, S.J. *et al.* (2009) A 6-month, double-blind, maintenance trial of lithium monotherapy versus the combination of lithium and divalproex for rapid-cycling bipolar disorder and Co-occurring substance abuse or dependence. *J. Clin. Psychiatry*, **70** (1), 113–121.

Ketter, T., Ahn, Y.M. Nam, J.Y., Culver, J.L., Marsh, W.K., and Bonner, J.C. (2007) Acute effectiveness of lamotrigine plus quetiapine therapy in bipolar disorder patients with syndromal or subsyndromal depression. 46th Annual Meeting of the American College of Neuropsychopharmacology, Boca Raton, FL.

Knackstedt, L.A., LaRowe, S., Mardikian, P. *et al.* (2009) The role of cystine-glutamate exchange in nicotine dependence in rats and humans. *Biol. Psychiatry*, **65** (10), 841–845.

Lafleur, D.L., Pittenger, C., Kelmendi, B. *et al.* (2006) N-acetylcysteine augmentation in serotonin reuptake inhibitor refractory obsessive-compulsive disorder. *Psychopharmacology (Berl)*, **184** (2), 254–256.

LaRowe, S.D., Mardikian, P., Malcolm, R. *et al.* (2006) Safety and tolerability of N-acetylcysteine in cocaine-dependent individuals. *Am. J. Addict.*, **15** (1), 105–110.

Leverich, G. and Post, R.M. (1998) Life charting of affective disorders. *CNS Spectr.*, **3**, 21–37.

Manji, H.K., Moore, G.J., and Chen, G. (2000) Clinical and preclinical evidence for the neurotrophic effects of mood stabilizers: implications for the pathophysiology and treatment of manic-depressive illness. *Biol. Psychiatry*, **48** (8), 740–754.

McElroy, S.L., Altshuler, L.L., Suppes, T. *et al.* (2001) Axis I psychiatric comorbidity and its relationship to historical illness variables in 288 patients with bipolar disorder. *Am. J. Psychiatry*, **158** (3), 420–426.

Miklowitz, D.J. (2008) Adjunctive psychotherapy for bipolar disorder: state of the evidence. *Am. J. Psychiatry*, **165** (11), 1408–1419.

Miklowitz, D.J. and Scott, J. (2009) Psychosocial treatments for bipolar disorder: cost-effectiveness, mediating mechanisms, and future directions. *Bipolar Disord.*, **11** (Suppl. 2), 110–122.

Miklowitz, D.J. Axelson, D.A., Birmaher, B. *et al.* (2008) Family-focused treatment for adolescents with bipolar disorder: results of a 2-year randomized trial. *Arch. Gen. Psychiatry*, **65** (9), 1053–1061.

Moore, G.J., Cortese, B.M., Glitz, D.A. *et al.* (2009) A longitudinal study of the effects of lithium treatment on prefrontal and subgenual prefrontal gray matter volume in treatment-responsive bipolar disorder patients. *J. Clin. Psychiatry*, **70** (5), 699–705.

Newcomer, J.W. and Hennekens, C.H. (2007) Severe mental illness and risk of cardiovascular disease. *J. Am. Med. Assoc.*, **298** (15), 1794–1796.

Nicolai, J., Vles, J.S. and Aldenkamp, A.P. (2008) Neurodevelopmental delay in children exposed to antiepileptic drugs in utero: a critical review directed at structural study-bias. *J. Neurol. Sci.*, **271** (1–2), 1–14.

Nierenberg, A.A., Husain, M.M., Trivedi, M.H. *et al.* (2009) Residual symptoms after remission of major depressive disorder with citalopram and risk of relapse: a STAR*D report. *Psychol. Med.*, **40**, 1–10.

Nolen, W.A., Luckenbaugh, D.A., Altshuler, L.L. *et al.* (2004) Correlates of 1-year prospective outcome in bipolar disorder: results from the Stanley Foundation Bipolar Network. *Am. J. Psychiatry*, **161** (8), 1447–1454.

Park, S.W., Lee, S.K., Kim, J.M., Yoon, J.S., and Kim, Y.H. (2006) Effects of quetiapine on the brain-derived neurotrophic factor expression in the hippocampus and neocortex of rats. *Neurosci. Lett.*, **402** (1–2), 25–29.

Park, S.W., Lee, S.H., Lee, J.G. *et al.* (2009) Differential effects of ziprasidone and haloperidol on immobilization stress-induced mRNA BDNF expression in the hippocampus and neocortex of rats. *J. Psychiatr. Res.*, **43** (3), 274–281.

Post, R.M. (2007) Role of BDNF in bipolar and unipolar disorder: clinical and theoretical implications. *J. Psychiatr. Res.*, **41** (12), 979–990.

Post, R.M. and Altshuler, L. (2009) Mood disorders: treatment of bipolar disorders, in *Comprehensive Textbook of Psychiatry* (eds B. Sadock, V., Sadock, and P., Ruiz), Lippincott Williams & Wilkins, Philadelphia, pp. 1743–1812.

Post, R.M. and Leverich, G.S. (2008) *Treatment of Bipolar Illness: A Casebook for Clinicians and Patients*, NY, W.W. Norton Press, pp. 1–666.

Post, R.M., Denicoff, K.D., Leverich, G.S. *et al.* (2003) Morbidity in 258 bipolar outpatients followed for 1 year with daily prospective ratings on the NIMH life chart method. *J. Clin. Psychiatry*, **64** (6), 680–690; quiz 738–739.

Post, R.M., Luckenbaugh, D.A., Leverich, G.S. *et al.* (2008) Incidence of childhood-onset bipolar illness in the USA and Europe. *Br. J. Psychiatry*, **192** (2), 150–151.

Post, R., Altshuler, L.L., Frye, M.A. *et al.* (2010a) Complexity of pharmacological treatment required for sustained improvement in outpatients with bipolar disorder. *J. Clin. Psychiatry*, in press.

Post, R., Leverich, G.S., Kupka, R.W. *et al.* (2010b) Early onset bipolar disorder and treatment delay are risk factors for poor outcome in adulthood. *J. Clin. Psychiatry*, in press.

Post, R., Leverich, G., Altshuler, L.L. *et al.* (2010c) Differential clinical characteristics, medication usage and treatment response in the U.S. versus the Netherlands and Germany. *Int. Clin. Psychopharmacol.* [Epub ahead of print]

Schloesser, R.J., Huang, J., Klein, P.S., and Manji, H.K. *et al.* (2008) Cellular plasticity cascades in the pathophysiology and treatment of bipolar disorder. *Neuropsychopharmacology*, **33** (1), 110–133.

Young, A., McElroy, S., Olausson, B., Chang, W., and Paulsson, B. *et al.* (2008) Quetiapine monotherapy up to 52 weeks in patients with bipolar depression: continuation phase data from the EMBOLDEN I and II studies. 60th Institute on Psychatric Services Conference, Chicago, IL.

15

The Role of Antidepressants in Bipolar Disorder

Boghos I. Yerevanian

Department of Psychiatry and Biobehavioral Sciences, David Geffen School of Medicine, University of California, Los Angeles, CA, USA

15.1 INTRODUCTION

The clinical use of antidepressants in bipolar disorder is a subject of controversy. The clinician treating bipolar disorder is often faced with compelling reasons to consider the use of antidepressants in bipolar depression as well as during the maintenance phase. In fact, antidepressants are used more commonly in bipolar disorder than any other mood stabilizer. Data from the Stanley Foundation Bipolar Network as well as from the National Institute of Mental Health Systematic Treatment Enhancement Program for Bipolar Disorder (NIMH STEP BD) program have shown that between 35 and 55% of diagnosed bipolar patients receive antidepressants at some point during their treatment (Post *et al.*, 2003; Simon *et al.*, 2004). Often antidepressants are prescribed *before* the onset of bipolarity in patients presenting with depression (Shi, Thiebaud, and McCombs, 2004). In a recent review Baldessarini *et al.* (2006) reported that in a group of 7760 bipolar patients, 50% were on antidepressants vs. 25% on mood stabilizers.

Mood stabilizers *are not* particularly good antidepressants with remission rates for acute bipolar depression rarely exceeding 50% for any of the available mood stabilizers Several broad reviews of the treatment of bipolar disorder have been published recently (for example, Goodwin and Jamison, 2007; Fountoulakis and Vieta, 2008; Ghaemi *et al.*, 2008) There are also several treatment guidelines for the treatment of bipolar disorder with various perspectives (APA, 2002; Sachs *et al.*, 2000; Grunze *et al.*, 2002; Goodwin, 2003; Yatham *et al.*, 2006). Most, particularly North American guidelines, recommend extreme caution in the use of antidepressants. The fact that the class of medications least recommended by experts for bipolar disorder is the most widely used by clinicians needs scrutiny.

Mood stabilizers are also not very effective in preventing relapses into mania and depression, despite their demonstrated superiority over placebo in controlled studies (Fountoulakis and Vieta, 2008). When one examines the survival curves from controlled studies, the clinician's dilemma becomes apparent: relapse rates and recurrences are still high for lithium, divalproex, and lamotrigine (Bowden *et al.*, 2000). The recently

Bipolar Psychopharmacotherapy: Caring for the patient, Second Edition. Edited by Hagop S. Akiskal and Mauricio Tohen.
© 2011 John Wiley & Sons, Ltd. Published 2011 by John Wiley & Sons, Ltd.

recruited mood stabilizers from the antipsychotic group including quetiapine, aripiprazole, olanzapine, and olanzapine and fluoxetine combination (OFC) also suffer from the limitation of inconsistent and low rates of relapse prevention.

Because of these efficacy and effectiveness limitations, as well as other problems such as side effects and nonacceptance by patients, mood stabilizers are often not enough and the clinician is under pressure to consider what both patients and apparently most clinicians expect might help in the treatment of bipolar depression: antidepressants medications. Perhaps the name *antidepressant* attracts many, but beyond semantics, clinicians do indeed notice benefits for their patients when adding antidepressants only to discover that adverse psychiatric events *also occur* during the course of such treatment (Altshuler *et al.*, 1995). Thus, sometimes it is not clear to patient and doctor, whether the treatment is helpful, harmful, or both at the same time (Moller and Grunze 2000; Ghaemi, Lenox and Baldessarini, 2001; Ghaemi *et al.*, 2003, 2008). This is a serious public health concern because the estimated 50 million bipolars worldwide spend the majority of their ill time in depression rather than mania (Judd *et al.*, 2002, 2003).

In this chapter, we will consider the following traditional antidepressants: Tricyclics, Selective Serotonin Reuptake Inhibitors, Sertonin Norepinephrine Reuptake Inhibitors, MAO inhibitors, and other antidepressants including bupropion. Within each group we will attempt to examine data for each individual antidepressant since there is no a priori reason to believe that all SSRIs or all TCAs behave similarly with respect to their effect on the treatment and course of bipolar disorder. This is a difficult task, because there are limitations on research contributions to the pressing questions of clinicians. These limitations are scientific, financial, ethical, and practical. For example, there is virtually no likelihood of funding by drug companies or other agencies to appropriately study the impact of individual tricyclics on suicidality, for obvious financial reasons. From an ethical perspective, it is difficult to conceive of a prospective controlled study with suicide as the specific end point. Therefore we lump the individual antidepressants as if they all worked the same way on the various components of the bipolar experience, mostly for convenience. The clinician however must choose a *specific* antidepressant for a *specific* patient without having adequate information.

Among the many considerations regarding the use of antidepressants three issues specific for each phase of the illness are important to address. In the case of the acute treatment of bipolar depression, they are: (i) efficacy, (ii) the switch process, and (iii) induction of suicidality. For maintenance treatment the issues are (i) relapse prevention as a measure of efficacy, (ii) cycle acceleration and induction of instability of mood, and (iii) suicide induction or prevention over the long term. These factors may be interrelated but may have independent biological as well as psychosocial determinants. For example, the influence of antidepressants on suicidal behavior may be independent of any mood state or it may be an integral part of it, as in the cases of dysphoric manias leading to suicide.

Suicide prevention and avoidance of suicide induction should be of primary concern to all clinicians. All antidepressants currently carry a black box warning of suicidality as a potential adverse outcome. These FDA warnings were initially for children and adolescents but were later extended to adults in 2004. This aspect of the treatment of bipolar disorder has not received adequate attention in research where the data is particularly thin.

15.2 TRICYCLIC ANTIDEPRESSANTS

15.2.1 EFFICACY

The role of antidepressant monotherapy in the treatment of bipolar depression has surprisingly not been studied adequately. There are very few studies of tricyclics in acute bipolar depression, none that are randomized double blind placebo controlled. Gijsman *et al.* (2004) in a recent review and analysis reported that only 1% of all depressed patients included in randomized placebo controlled studies are recognized bipolars. Most of what we know may be extrapolation from studies of TCAs in unipolar depression where response rate is in the range of 50–70%. Moller *et al.* (2001) in a retrospective study of 2032 patients admitted for the treatment of depression did not find a significant difference in response to TCAs between unipolar and bipolar depressives. In their recent meta-analysis of randomized controlled trials on the efficacy and safety of antidepressants in the short term treatment of bipolar depression, Gijsman *et al.* (2004) concluded that the effect size of antidepressants was similar for unipolar and bipolar depression and that tricyclics, although superior to placebo, were somewhat less effective than other antidepressants. In the 12 studies examined, few addressed monotherapy with tricyclic antidepressants. Only 4/12 were studies of antidepressants without concomitant use of mood stabilizers and of those four, only two studies included bipolar depressives exclusively. Such data will not provide answers to the question of the efficacy of TCA monotherapy in bipolar disorder. In most studies, patients were on some type of mood stabilizers. In the study Nemeroff *et al.* (2001) bipolar patients who were maintained on lithium were randomized to imipramine, paroxetine, or placebo. If lithium levels were therapeutic, (defined as 0.8 mEq/l or above) neither paroxetine nor imipramine added benefit to the lithium treatment.

In a randomized double blind parallel group study involving 156 bipolar depressives Silverstone (2001) compared moclebomide (reversible MAO I) to imipramine and found similar decrease in HAM-D and MADRS scores in both groups.

Tricyclics as add-on or combination therapy have been reported in several early randomized controlled studies. Thus imipramine has been compared with lithium and placebo, lithium outperforming imipramine in efficacy (Prien *et al.*, 1979), Lithium vs. Li + imipramine, or desipramine (Wehr and Goodwin, 1979; Quitkin *et al.*, 1981; Kane, Quitkin, and Rifkin, 1982), with the combination better than or equal to imipramine in efficacy. In almost all cases, better outcome with TCAs is offset by higher likelihood of manic switch. In a review of five separate early studies, Goodwin and Jamison (2007) assessed the response to TCA in bipolar disorder as "relatively poor." In the Sachs *et al.* study (2007) adjunctive antidepressants were no better than placebo in the treatment of bipolar disorder. By contrast, in a more recent meta-analysis of 12 randomized trials of antidepressants in bipolar disorder, Gijsman concluded that although somewhat less effective than other antidepressants, tricyclics were overall effective, with an average 46.9% of patients responding acutely vs. 55.6% for other antidepressants. In the recent meta-analysis of Ghaemi *et al.* (2008) of 12 long term studies, most of which used TCAs as the antidepressant, the relative risk for a new depression comparing antidepressants only to mood stabilizers only was 1.00 (95% CI 0.57–1.75) when compared to placebo, antidepressants – only had a relative risk of 0.46 (95% CI 0.27–0.80) suggesting some effectiveness in preventing depressive relapse. The problem was complicated by a high risk of relapse into mania with relative risk (RR) of 2.37 and 1.57 respectively.

15.2.2   SWITCH AND LONG TERM DESTABILIZATION

In the Gijsman metanalysis, the switch rate for TCAs was 10% vs. 3.2% for all other antidepressants combined.

In the more recent meta-analysis by Ghaemi *et al*. (2008) involving a carefully selected seven studies with at least six month treatment in randomized controlled trials, the relative risk of developing mania when antidepressants are used alone was higher than when used in mood stabilizer combination, with a relative risk of 1.72; (95% CI 1.23–2.41). That mood stabilizers may not be very protective against antidepressant induced switches was shown by the Post *et al*. study (2001), in which upto one-third of patients on mood stabilizers who were given antidepressants switched into mania/hypomania on follow up.

In a study of bipolar inpatients, Koszewska and Rybakowski (2009), found that about one-third of patients given antidepressants switched into mania/hypomania. In this group of 333 bipolars, a retrospective analysis showed that the highest risk was with tricyclics with the highest rate for amytriptilene (42% of treated episodes) closely followed by imipramine and clomipramine.

Taking into consideration the above newer reports, along with the extensive older literature reviewed by Goodwin and Jamison (2007) the consensus remains that tricyclics continue to be the group most likely to induce mania/hypomania as well as cycle acceleration in the long term. Attempts to explore whether *individual* tricyclics differ with respect to destabilizing bipolar course yielded no meaningful data. It is possible to speculate that differential properties of individual tricyclics, such as propensity to cause anticholinergic effects, or differential effects on other neurotransmitters and neurotrophic agents might allow some selectivity within the TCA group.

15.2.3   SUICIDALITY

Tricyclics, similar to other antidepressants carry FDA warnings against suicidality. After decades of mostly debate and little research, the role of antidepressants, in this case tricyclics, in inducing suicidality in bipolar disorder is not clear.

There are few studies looking into suicidal outcome as a result of institution of TCAs in bipolar depression. Most studies have looked at antidepressants as a class. The reports on TCA and suicide generally address the lethality of TCAs in suicidal overdoses, but I could not find articles addressing suicidal induction or protection from suicide by tricyclics in bipolar depression. Data from unipolar depressives suggest that in unipolar depression tricyclics may be protective against suicide (Yerevanian *et al*., 2004) but in bipolar disorder the situation may be the reverse with antidepressants in general (including tricyclics) may be associated with or contribute to suicidality. (McElroy *et al*., 2006; Yerevanian, Koek, and Mintz, 2007).

In the large meta-analysis of Ferguson *et al.* (2005) the odds ratio comparing TCAs to SSRIs for suicide attempts (0.88 CI 0.54–1.42) and for suicides (1.08 CI 0.28–4.09) indicates that there may not be a significant difference between TCAs and SSRIs in the study populations which was composed of patients registered in a large number of clinical trials for depression and anxiety disorder but NOT for bipolar disorders. However, given the large number of patients (87 650 adults in 702 trials) one has to wonder what percentage were actual unrecognized bipolars and how those may have influenced the outcome.

15.3 MAO INHIBITORS

15.3.1 EFFICACY

In a recent retrospective analysis comparing MAO inhibitors to paroxetine, Mallinger *et al.* (2009) found that 27% of paroxetine treated patients had a durable recovery compared to a 53% durable recovery rate for MAO inhibitors.

In the Himmelhoch *et al.* (1991) double blind study comparing imipramine to tranylcypramine in BIP I and II depressed patients, the response rate for tranylcypramine was 81% compared to 40% for imipramine at four weeks of treatment. Thase *et al.* (1992) in a crossover study comparing tranylcypramine to imipramine, found 9/12 patients crossed over from imipramine (IMI) to tranylcypromine (TRANYL) responded whereas crossing in the other direction resulted in 1/4 response. Taken together, these studies suggest that MAO inhibitors may be superior to tricyclics, especially if one considers the "anergic" features of bipolar depression.

Nolen *et al.* (2007), in a comparison of lamotrigine and tranylcypromine for treatment refractory bipolar depression, found a higher proportion of response to tranylcypramine (62.5%) than to lamotrigine (36.4%) when added to an existing mood stabilizer over a 10 week period. This was an open randomization study in this treatment refractory group of patients. Their conclusion was that tranylcypramine may have a place in the treatment of refractory bipolar depression.

15.3.2 SWITCH AND LONG TERM STABILITY

In the NIMH STEP BD study (Goldberg *et al.*, 2007), switching into mania hypomania occurred less frequently with MAOs and bupropion compared with tricyclics and other antidepressants as assessed by patient self reports. In the study Himmelhoch *et al.* (1991) the switch rate on MAO Is was reported at 21%.

When examined in a group composed exclusively of bipolar II disorders, Agosti and Stewart (2007) in a *post hoc* analysis of a double blind study comparing placebo, imipramine and phenelzine, found no differences between unipolar and bipolar depressives both in terms of response and switch into mania/hypomania which was not observed at all in this group. Some (Baker *et al.*, 2003) consider bipolar II patients at highest risk for switching and for suicide, but the issue is still not settled.

15.4 SSRIs

15.4.1 EFFICACY

The Selective Serotonin re-uptake inhibitors have become the cornerstone in the treatment of depression in its various forms but their place in bipolar depression is not well established and at best appears to be limited. Currently, no antidepressants are FDA approved for the treatment of bipolar depression except for fluoxetine and then only in combination with olanzapine.

Simpson and DePaulo (1991) in a study of pure bipolar II patients (n = 16) found that the majority of patients who continued on fluoxetine (10/13) did well on follow up.

Amsterdam, Garcia-Espana, and Fawcett (1998) found the efficacy of fluoxetine in a pure sample of bipolar II patients to be similar to rates in unipolar depression.

In a small randomized double blind study of a mixed group of bipolar I and II, Young *et al.* (2000), found that the addition of paroxetine to a mood stabilizer did not result in a better clinical outcome, although the combination paroxetine mood stabilizer was better tolerated than two mood stabilizers. Kupfer *et al.* (2001) in a similar bipolar group (n = 45) reported a 64% response rate when SSRIs were added to a mood stabilizer. Ghaemi *et al.* (2004) reported that in a group composed of both unipolar and bipolar patients, non response to SSRIs as well as relapse was more likely in the bipolar group than the unipolar group.

In a post hoc analysis of an eight week large double blind trial of bipolar I patients comparing olanzapine with OFC and placebo in mixed depression (Benazzi *et al.*, 2009) found that non mixed bipolars had consistently higher response than mixed ones across all categories. But within the mixed group, who had predominantly irritability, decreased need for sleep and racing thought and therefore were at more risk for switching with fluoxetine, the OFC group outperformed both placebo and olanzapine alone in response to treatment, and the switch rate, although numerically higher than olanzapine alone or placebo, (8.5% vs 6.8% vs 7.8%) was not statistically significantly different.

In another study from Puerto Rico, Tamayo *et al.* (2009) reported on a two phase study of OFC. Responders in acute treatment entered a second phase by randomization between continuing on olanzapine or continuing on OFC. Significantly more patients in the OFC group maintained response or remission. When switched to olanzapine, a lower percentage of OLZ patients maintained remission as compared to both OFC maintenance or acute response. To the authors, fluoxetine appears to be effective in both the acute phase of bipolar depression and in maintaining remission after response, when used with olanzapine. There was no fluoxetine arm alone.

In a recent report on the long term maintenance (six month) randomized double blind comparison of lamotrigine with OFC in bipolar I patients (Brown *et al.*, 2009), OFC outperformed lamotrigine on several of the scales for depression from week 5 through week 25 of the study. After the seven week acute phase, the two groups had similar rates of relapse as well as similar treatment emergent mania rates (Brown *et al.*, 2006).

In a recent report assessing the long term outcome of bipolar patients, Altshuler *et al.* (2009), 83 bipolar outpatients were treated acutely for 10 weeks with antidepressants as add-on to MS. Sixty-one out of eighty-three had good acute response, a rate higher than most reported, and 22/83 had a partial response. At one year follow up, 69% of acute responders maintained response and 53% achieved remission. Partial responders fared worse with only 27% achieving full treatment response by set criteria. The switch rate on the combined group was not higher than those reported for MS monotherapy. This appears to be a less sick and more treatment responsive group compared to most other studies.

Earlier studies by Altshuler *et al.* (2001, 2003) have indicated that in a group of bipolars who had remitted on a regimen of mood stabilizer and antidepressants, early discontinuation of antidepressants (within six months of remission), led to a higher rate of relapse into depression compared to those who continued. This occurred without increase in the rate of switching, suggesting that a subgroup may benefit from continued use of antidepressants and may indeed be more stable with than without them.

In a recent *post hoc* analysis of a previous study of OFC in bipolar I depression Vieta *et al.* (2009) reported that predominance of past manic episodes in men but not women predicted a better response to treatment compared with predominantly depressive history. Thus past polarity predicted acute response to treatment in bipolar I depression.

In a study of antidepressant as adjunctive therapy in 176 bipolars, Frye *et al.* (2009) reported that treatment emergent mania could be predicted in those with increased motor activity and speech and language or thought disorder while depressed.

In a 12 week randomized double blind study comparing lamotrigine to citalopram in a small group bipolar depressives maintained on mood stabilizers, Schaffer, Zuker, and Levitt (2006), no differences were found between the two groups. The overall response rate increased between 6 and 12 weeks of treatment but barely exceeded 50%. It appears that the choice for add-on between citalopram or lamotrigine should depend on considerations other than efficacy or switch rate. In another small open ended study (Fonseca *et al.*, 2006), escitalopram was found useful in decreasing depression scores in a group of bipolar I and II depressives maintained on mood stabilizers. The switch rate in this group was about 10%.

15.4.2   SWITCH AND LONG TERM DESTABILIZATION

That monotherapy with antidepressants may be more dangerous than in combination with mood stabilizers is suggested by the study of Gao *et al.* (2008). In a mix of 180 bipolar I and II patients, all rapid cyclers, 153 had at least one monotherapy period. About 49.3% of patients had treatment emergent mania/hypomania. Fluoxetine had an unusually high rate of 42.1%, By contrast, fluvoxamine and mirtazapine showed 0% but the numbers were small and the study was retrospective, subject to recall bias. Earlier, Vieta *et al.* (2002) in a study in which paroxetine was compared to venlafaxine found a switch rate of 3% compared to 13% for venlafaxine.

In a recent systemic review and meta-analysis of 13 studies comparing antidepressant use in bipolar one, bipolar II, and unipolar depressives Bond *et al.* (2008), the mean rates of antidepressant associated mood switch was 14.2% for bipolar I vs 7.1% of bipolar II in acute trials. Over the longer term, in maintenance studies, the comparison rates were 23.4% vs 13.9%. When comparing to unipolar depressives, bipolars had a fivefold increase in switch rates in short term studies (8.1% vs. 1.5%) and almost a threefold higher risk in maintenance studies (16.5% vs 6%). In addition, bipolar II patients developed mostly hypomania but no mania whereas bipolar I patients had an equal mix of manias and hypomanias. There are several important conclusions to be drawn from this study: while it may be comforting that the risk as well as the severity of switch is less in bipolar II than bipolar I patients it nowhere close to unipolars; therefore accurate diagnosis becomes paramount for any patient presenting with depression. Similarly, the choice of antidepressants and their effect on the switch process becomes important.

Some (Parker *et al.*, 2006) have even hypothesized that SSRIs may serve as a long term mood stabilizer. In a small sample of bipolar II patients (n = 10), these authors found a diminution of depression, days spent depressed and days disabled on SSRI compared with placebo. Although only speculative, there may be a subgroup of bipolar II patients who may never need a mood stabilizer, if they could be identified as such.

What is emerging from a comprehensive review of older studies (Goodwin and Jamison, 2007) and the more recent data is that SSRIs are less likely to induce switching into mania and probably less destabilizing over the long term, although they are capable of contributing to both. There are however unresolved pressing clinical and research issues. Thus, do the different subtypes of bipolar respond differently to SSRIs? Is it safe to use SSRIs in bipolar II but not bipolar I? Can SSRI induced dysphoric mixed states be predicted and prevented? (Rihmer and Akiskal, 2006). Further data is needed to answer these questions.

15.4.3   SUICIDALITY

Relative risk of SSRIs in preventing or inducing suicidality in bipolar patients, compared to other antidepressants is not known. In fact the whole issue of whether antidepressants as a class are associated with suicidality specifically in bipolar patients is an open one. There are only a few reports that have looked at this issue. (Bauer *et al.*, 2005, 2006; Bridge *et al.*, 2007)

A group of *unrecognized* bipolar patients in a community sample of depressives (who are often given antidepressants for depressive phase illness) were significantly more likely to attempt suicide (0.9%) than recognized bipolar patients (0.3%) or non-bipolar patients (0.2%)) (Shi, Thiebaud, and McCombs, 2004). In this large study of patients who received antidepressants in a Medicaid fee for service program, 47% of recognized bipolars received an antidepressant alone, and 77% of unrecognized bipolars received an antidepressant alone for initial therapy.

In a group of bipolar veterans followed for an average of three years, suicidal event rates were almost eight times higher during treatment with antidepressant monotherapy (25.92 events/100pt-years) compared with treatment with mood stabilizer monotherapy (3.48) and almost three times higher compared to mood stabilizer + antidepressant combination therapy (9.75). This was a detailed retrospective study, which did not control for severity and other potential confounding variables (Yerevanian, Koek, and Mintz, 2007).

A cross sectional analysis from the STEP-BD program found that suicidal ideation was more prevalent in patients taking antidepressants vs those not taking them (25% vs 14%). (Goldberg *et al.*, 2005).

In a study of 100 manic patients, suicidal ideation was present in 59% of mixed manic patients and was nearly four times more common in patients who had taken antidepressants in the *week* prior to admission compared to those who had not taken any antidepressants (Goldberg *et al.*, 1999). In other words, although all patients were at higher risk by virtue of being mixed, the presence of antidepressants increased the risk of suicidality (ideation in this study), even more.

In another recent study (Akiskal *et al.*, 2003) antidepressant associated hypomanic patients were twice as likely (43% vs 80%) to have been admitted with suicidal ideation than bipolar IIs with spontaneous hypomanias.

An earlier retrospective chart review, Stoll *et al.* (1994) found that antidepressant associated manic states, although clinically assessed as less severe compared to a group of spontaneous manics, nevertheless had similar degrees of suicidal ideation.

In a large cohort study from Denmark (Kessing *et al.*, 2005), lithium users (presumably mostly bipolars) who also purchased an antidepressant had a higher risk of completed suicide with a risk ratio of 6.07 (95% CI 5.10–7.21).

Although very few, there are some studies that looked into and did not find an association between antidepressant use and suicidality in bipolar patients. Bauer *et al.* (2006) in evaluating the first 425 patients in the NIMH STEP-BD program, did not find an association between new onset suicidality and either initiating or increasing the dose of antidepressants in this bipolar cohort. If one takes a longer term view, the studies of Jules Angst *et al.* (2005) show that over the long term medication treatment reduced mortality by suicide in both unipolar and bipolar groups, including in patients who were treated with antidepressants in combination with various mood stabilizers. Although not directly addressing suicide per se, Altshuler's studies (2003, 2006) have shown that early discontinuation of antidepressants in bipolar patients maintained on combination therapy, relapse, and morbidity are more than twice as common compared with those who continue antidepressants.

In the placebo controlled study of Tohen *et al.* (2003) comparing olanzapine, OFC, and placebo in bipolar I depression, there were no serious suicidal events in any of the three groups and there was a modest reduction on the MADRS suicidal thought item in all three groups. It is difficult to interpret the effect of fluoxetine alone or even in combination with an antipsychotic, in their carefully preselected group that excluded patients with a history of suicidal behavior within the past three months. Furthermore the study was only eight weeks, limiting the interpretation of any suicidality effect of fluoxetine in this bipolar group.

Recently in a case controlled prospective study, Marangell *et al.* (2008) reported on the suicidal events in a group of bipolar patients from the STEP-BD program. There were 270 suicide events (eight completed suicides, 262 attempts). These occurred in 182 of STEP-BD participants (cases). The findings were somewhat surprising in that in the lithium cohort, no suicide protective effects were noted, while antidepressants of the SSRI type were associated with increased suicidality. The authors did caution however about difficulties in ascribing a causal relationship between antidepressant use and suicidality in bipolar disorder. It is entirely possible that different antidepressants and mood stabilizers affect completed suicide differentially from attempted suicide which may have different neurobiological basis and may not reflect the same phenomenon.

Suicide and suicidal behaviors are complex phenomena and have multiple determinants: some are genetic, some environmental, and some have to do with the nature of the illness and its different phases. Severity, which is often difficult to define, is another factor. Suicidality is also impacted by comorbid conditions including alcoholism, drug addiction, anxiety disorders, psychotic disorders, all of which carry independent risks factors for suicidality. Under those conditions, it is an immense challenge to figure out if antidepressant use in bipolar patients increases, decreases or has no effects on suicidal behavior. The methodological hurdles do not appear to have been resolved. The main hurdle of course is that there are no randomized controlled prospective studies addressing the issue and so all the literature supporting a prosuicidal position for antidepressants in bipolar disorder must be tentative.

The central issue of "confounding by indication" is far from being resolved. As McElroy *et al.* (2006) have indicated in four out of five studies supporting the pro-suicidal position, the findings could potentially be explained by the fact that higher suicidality may actually have led to the choice of an antidepressant rather than the reverse. Such conclusions have recently been reached in studies of unipolar patients (Brent, 2007) based on numerous studies.

Much of the available data thus points to the possibility of heightened risk of suicidal behavior in antidepressant exposed bipolars. Whether SSRIs are different from other antidepressants in this regard is not known at this point.

The discrepancies between the prosuicidal and antisuicidal positions for antidepressants in bipolar disorder may force us to search for other explanations for this putative relationship. Finer suicide monitoring and predicting tools are necessary. Some bipolar patients will need antidepressants, will do well on it and will never be suicidal. Others may very quickly be activated and become suicidal very quickly. How can we distinguish between the two? General suicide risk considerations are not very useful for the individual patient and predicting which (especially newly diagnosed) bipolar patients should not be given antidepressants is really not well defined. At this time, although caution should be exercised with antidepressants in bipolar patients, a blanket statement that antidepressants cause suicidality in bipolar patients and should not be used in this group cannot be made. With adequate safeguards, there may yet be a place for antidepressants in bipolar disorder.

When it comes to iatrogenic suicidality, unipolar and bipolar disorders emerge as very different disorders. Findings for the effects of antidepressant on suicidality in unipolar disorders should not be extrapolated to bipolar disorders. Antidepressants may be protective in the first group and have the opposite effect in the second. In fact, the de novo development of suicidality after antidepressant introduction should raise one's index of suspicion of a bipolar diathesis and a bipolar course. There is some evidence for this statement in children and adolescents (Akiskal, 1995) whether this is true in at least a subgroup among adult bipolars is interesting heuristically and practically. In fact, one can posit that antidepressant induced suicidality may be an external validator or eventually an endophenotype of bipolar disorder.

There is also no a priori reason to lump all antidepressants into one category as far as suicidality is concerned. There are differences in the neurobiologic effects even among the group of SSRI medications. The neurotrophic effects of each drug may be different and such differences in the second messenger system and beyond may be important. As of yet, there is hardly any literature that has looked at INDIVIDUAL antidepressants and suicidal behavior as well as at subtypes of antidepressants and suicidal outcomes.

15.5   SNRIs: VENLAFAXINE, MIRTAZAPINE, DULOXETINE

15.5.1   EFFICACY REVIEW

Few have studied the efficacy and effectiveness of the dual acting novel antidepressants.

Post *et al.* (2006) reported a response rate of 51% for venlafaxine compared to 49% for bupropion and 53% for sertraline and remission rate of 34% compared to 41% for bupropion and 36% for sertraline.

Amsterdam *et al.* (2009, #38) reported on a comparison between lithium and venlafaxine as an initial treatment for bipolar depression in a randomized, parallel group open label trial. Of 43 patients receiving venlafaxine and 40 receiving lithium, about a third had a history of rapid cycling. Venlafaxine resulted in a higher proportion of responders and remitters compared to lithium and this effect was independent of rapid cycling status.

15.5.2   SWITCH AND LONG TERM STABILITY

In the study Post *et al.* (2006) switch rates occurred much more frequently in the venlafaxine group (29%) compared to 10% for bupropion and 9% for sertraline.

In the study Amsterdam *et al.* (2009) lithium and venlafaxine had similar rates of conversion into mania. The study however was under powered and there was a high dropout rate.

Goodnick (2007) in his review of randomized clinical trials of bipolar depression concluded that the greatest risk of destabilization over the long term was with venlafaxine.

In the Vieta *et al.* study (2002) venlafaxine had a higher switch rate of 13% as opposed to paroxetine (3%).

The majority of the data thus puts venlafaxine, somewhere between SSRIs and TCAs in terms of potential for switching and possibly in terms of long term stabilization.

15.5.3   SUICIDALITY

We could not find any studies examining the effect of venlafaxine either to prevent or to be associated with increased suicidality. That it may be involved in increased suicidality should be suspected on two bases: one is it's propensity to induce switches and mixed states (Leverich *et al.*, 2006) and mixed states carry a high risk profile (Akiskal *et al.*, 2005; Balázs *et al.*, 2006; Leverich *et al.*, 2006). The second basis is that in BIPOLAR disorder there is an association between antidepressant use, especially as monotherapy, and suicidal outcomes, mostly in the form of attempts or ideation (Yerevanian, Koek and Mintz, 2007).

15.6   BUPROPION

15.6.1   EFFICACY

Sachs *et al.* (1994) compared bupropion to desipramine in 15 bipolar depressives maintained on moodstabilizers. Two-third of both groups showed some evidence of response.

In the study Post *et al.* (2006) 49% of bipolar depressives responded acutely to bupropion and 41% remitted.

15.6.2   SWITCH AND LONG TERM

In the study Post *et al.* (2006), switch rates were 10% for bupropion, 9% for sertraline, and 23% for venlafaxine suggesting a relatively low switch for this interesting antidepressant which has become a popular one for bipolar depression riding on this reputation of causing low switch rates (Haykal and Akiskal, 1990).

15.6.3   SUICIDALITY

There are no studies of bupropion and suicidality specifically. At this time bupropion should be considered similar to other antidepressant pending reliable data in bipolar disorder. The fact that it causes less switch or mixed state may be a potential advantage in this regard.

15.7   CLINICAL AND RESEARCH IMPLICATIONS

It appears from this review that many of the core issues regarding the use of antidepressants in bipolar disorder continue to be unresolved. The debate of the relative merit of antidepressants in bipolar states continues between its proponents and opponents and may not be resolved easily for several reasons:

1.   At a technical level, large randomized controlled prospective studies examining efficacy, as well as negative outcomes like destabilization and suicidality will likely not occur with each *individual* antidepressant for various reasons. Short of such studies however, treating the whole gamut of antidepressants as a group or as categories based on putative modes of action, is fundamentally unsound. Two very recent meta-analyses found 'antidepressants' as a category to have either no efficacy in the acute treatment of bipolar depression (Sidor and Macqueen, 2010), or show no differential response between and unipolar and bipolar depressives (Vasquez, Tondo, and Baldessarini, 2010). Such studies, despite their methodological rigour and heuristic value, are unlikely to help the clinician.
2.   Randomized clinical trials continue recruiting selective patients thus sometimes ignoring clinical realities and limiting the usefulness and generalizeability of the data for the clinician. Naturalistic studies suffer from the lack of methodological rigor and thus are of limited scientific value.
3.   As long as the fundamental nature of response to treatment, relapse, and suicidality remains in the descriptive domain, the drug-behavior connection remains speculative.

4. A clearer emphasis is needed to identify not only general *clinical predictors of response*, relapse, and negative outcomes, but also biological predictors. The association of serotonin transporter polymorphism with the switch process (Mundo *et al.*, 2001) is one such example. It is hoped that research in this area will open new vistas for researchers and clinicians alike.

In the meantime, for the individual clinician treating an individual patient, the following are some reasonable assumptions:

1. There is no a priori reason to exclude antidepressants in the treatment of bipolar disorder. Given the paucity and unattractiveness of other choices and the frequent need to use multiple medications, antidepressants may be needed at least for certain periods of time. If treatment is initiated careful monitoring for destabilization and the emergence of suicidality is necessary.
2. At present, various treatment guidelines notwithstanding, the choice is not based on efficacy since there is no clear indication of superiority of any particular antidepressants within the group nor between mood stabilizers and particular antidepressants, except perhaps for mono amine inhibitors in anergic bipolar depressions. The choice of antidepressants is still determined by traditional considerations such as the potential for "side effects" including disease modifying ones, the medical condition of the patient, and potential drug interactions. However, the literature suggests that as general classes, the tricyclics are the most likely to induce a switch process and cycle acceleration with or without a mood stabilizer. Venlafaxine is intermediate in that effect. Looking for subtle clues of destabilization may help avoid a full blast relapse of depression or mania. For patients with a broadly defined mixed state or with many previous episodes, antidepressants should be avoided if possible or used for shorter periods of time. Under almost no circumstances however should antidepressants be stopped suddenly and without supervision because of the documented increased occurrences of rebound or withdrawal manias, depressions, and suicidality (Landry, 1997; Yerevanian *et al.*, 2004; Yerevanian, Koek, and Mintz, 2007; Valuck, Orton, and Libby, 2009).
3. The question of whether acute response to antidepressants predicts good prophylactic response to them is not resolved. The FDA approval process is confusing in that regard. Drugs approved for bipolar depression are not necessarily approved for maintenance treatment. No antidepressants are approved for both phases. If a response to antidepressants is convincing to the clinician, it is probably best to continue although there is no data that acute response and relapse prevention are mediated through the same neurobiological processes. If one continues on antidepressants, monitoring closely for treatment emergent problems and if present, tapering down over a reasonable time becomes necessary.
4. Finally, antidepressant treatment in bipolar disorder is only one, increasingly diminishing aspect of the total management of the bipolar patient. Antidepressants should be used within the broader aspect of the patients' medical, psychological, and social context. With these safeguards in mind, there is still a place for antidepressants in the management of the bipolar patient.

References

Agosti, V. and Stewart, J.W. (2007) Efficacy and safety of antidepressant monotherapy in the treatment of bipolar-II depression. *Int. Clin. Psychopharmacol.*, **22**, 309–311.

Akiskal, H.S. (1995) Developmental pathways to bipolarity: are juvenile-onset depressions prebipolar? *J. Am. Acad. Child Adolesc. Psychiatry*, **34**, 754–763.

Akiskal, H.S., Benazzi, F., Perugi, G., and Rihmer, Z. (2005) Agitated "unipolar" depression re-conceptualized as a depressive mixed state: implications for the antidepressant-suicide controversy. *J. Affect. Disord.*, **85**, 245–258.

Akiskal, H.S., Hantouche, E.G., Allilaire, J.F. *et al.* (2003) Validating antidepressant-associated hypomania (bipolar III): a systematic comparison with spontaneous hypomania (bipolar II). *J. Affect. Disord.*, **73**, 65–74.

Altshuler, L., Kiriakos, L., Calcagno, J. *et al.* (2001) The impact of antidepressant discontinuation versus antidepressant continuation on 1-year risk for relapse of bipolar depression: a retrospective chart review. *J. Clin. Psychiatry*, **62**, 612–616.

Altshuler, L., Post, R.M., Hellemann, G. *et al.* (2009) Impact of antidepressant continuation after acute positive or partial treatment response for bipolar depression: a blinded, randomized study. *J. Clin. Psychiatry*, **70**, 450–457.

Altshuler, L., Post, R.M., Leverich, G.S. *et al.* (1995) Antidepressant-induced mania and cycle acceleration: a controversy revisited. *Am. J. Psychiatry*, **152**, 1130–1138.

Altshuler, L., Suppes, T., Black, D. *et al.* (2003) Impact of antidepressant discontinuation after acute bipolar depression remission on rates of depressive relapse at 10 year follow-up. *Am. J. Psychiatry*, **160**, 1252–1262.

Altshuler, L., Suppes, T., Black, D. *et al.* (2006) Lower switch rate in depressed patients with bipolar II than bipolar I disorder treated adjunctively with second-generation antidepressants. *Am. J. Psychiatry*, **163**, 313–315.

Amsterdam, J., Garcia-Espana, F., and Fawcett, J. (1998) Efficacy and safety of fluoxetine in treating bipolar II major depressive episode. *J. Clin. Psychopharmacol.*, **8**, 435–440.

Amsterdam, J.D., Wang, C.H., Shwarz, M., and Shults, J. (2009) Venlafaxine versus lithium monotherapy of rapid and non-rapid cycling patients with bipolar II major depressive episode: a randomized, parallel group, open-label trial. *J. Affect. Disord*, **112** (1–3), 219–230.

Angst, J., Angst, F., Gerber-Werder, R., and Gamma, A. (2005) Suicide in 406 mood-disorders patients with and without long-term medication: a 40 to 44 years' follow-up. *Arch. Suicide Res.*, **9**, 279–300.

APA (2002) Practice guideline for the treatment of patients with bipolar disorder (revision). *Am. J. Psychiatry*, **159**, 1–50.

Baker, R.W., Tohen, M., Fawcett, J. *et al.* (2003) Acute dysphoric mania: treatment response to olanzapine versus placebo. *J. Clin. Psychiatry*, **23**, 132–137.

Balázs, J., Benazzi, F., Rihmer, Z. *et al.* (2006) The close link between suicide attempts and mixed (bipolar) depression: implications for suicide prevention. *J. Affect. Disord.*, **91**, 133–138.

Baldessarini, R.J., Tondo, L., Davis, P. *et al.* (2006) Decreased risk of suicides and attempts during long-term lithium treatment: a meta-analytic review. *Bipolar Disord.*, **8**, 625–639.

Bauer, M., Rasgon, N., Grof, P. *et al.* (2005) Mood changes related to antidepressants: a longitudinal study of patients with bipolar disorder in a naturalistic setting. *Psychiatry Res.*, **133**, 73–80.

Bauer, M., Wisniewski, S.R., Marangell, L.B. *et al.* (2006) Are antidepressants associated with new-onset suicidality in bipolar disorder? *J. Clin. Psychiatry*, **67**, 48–55.

Benazzi, F., Berk, M., Frye, M.A. *et al.* (2009) Olanzapine/fluoxetine combination for the treatment of mixed depression in bipolar I disorder: a post hoc analysis. *J. Clin. Psychiatry*, **70**, 1424–1431.

Bond, D.J., Noronha, M.M., Kauer-Sant'Anna, M. *et al.* (2008) Antidepressant-associated mood elevations in bipolar II disorder compared with bipolar I disorder and major depressive disorder: a systematic review and meta-analysis. *J. Clin. Psychiatry*, **69**, 1589–1601.

Bowden, C.L., Calbrese, J.R., McElroy, S.L. *et al.*, Divalproex Maintenance Study Group (2000) A randomized, placebo-controlled 12-month trial of divalproex and lithium in treatment of outpatients with bipolar I disorder. *Arch Gen. Psychiatry*, **57**, 481–489.

Brent, D. (2007) Antidepressants and suicidal behavior: cause or cure? *Am. J. Psychiatry*, **164**, 989–991.

Bridge, J., Iyengar, S., Salary, C. *et al.* (2007) Clinical response and risk for reported suicidal ideation and suicide attempts in pediatric antidepressant treatment. A meta-analysis of randomized controlled trials. *J. Am. Med. Assoc.*, **297**, 1683–1696.

Brown, E., Dunner, D.L., McElroy, S.L. *et al.* (2009) Olanzapine/fluoxetine combination vs. lamotrigine in the 6-month treatment of bipolar I depression. *Int. J. Neuropsychopharmacol.*, **12**, 773–782.

Brown, E.B., McElroy, S.L., Keck, P.E. Jr. *et al.* (2006) A 7-week, randomized, double-blind trial of olanzapine/fluoxetine combination versus lamotrigine in the treatment of bipolar I depression. *J. Clin. Psychiatry*, **67**, 1025–1033.

Fergusson, D., Doucette, S., Glass, K.C., *et al.*, (2005) Association between suicide attempts and selective serotonin reuptake inhibitors: systematic review of randomized controlled trials. *BMJ*, **330**, 396.

Fonseca, M., Soares, J.C., Hatch, J.P. *et al.* (2006) An open trial of adjunctive escitalopram in bipolar depression. *J. Clin. Psychiatry*, **67**, 81–86.

Fountoulakis, K.N. and Vieta, E. (2008) Treatment of bipolar disorder: a systematic review of available data and clinical perspectives. *Int. J. Neuropsychopharmacol.*, **11**, 999–1029.

Frye, M.A., Helleman, G., McElroy, S.L., *et al.*, (2009) Correlates of treatment-emergent mania associated with antidepressant treatment in bipolar depression. *Am. J. Psychiatry*, **166** (2), 164–172.

Gao, K., Kemp, D.E., Ganocy, S.J. *et al.* (2008) Treatment-emergent mania/hypomania during antidepressant monotherapy in patients with rapid cycling bipolar disorder. *Bipolar Disord.*, **10**, 907–915.

Ghaemi, S.N., Hsu, D.J., Soldani, F., and Goodwin, F.K. (2003) Antidepressants in bipolar depression: the case for caution. *Bipolar Disord.*, **5**, 421–433.

Ghaemi, S.N., Lenox, M.S., and Baldessarini, R.J. (2001) Effectiveness and safety of long-term antidepressant treatment in bipolar disorder. *J. Clin. Psychiatry*, **62**, 565–569.

Ghaemi, S.N., Rosenquist, Kj., Ko, J.Y. *et al.* (2004) Antidepressant treatment in bipolar versus unipolar depression. *Am. J. Psychiatry*, **161**, 163–165.

Ghaemi, S.N., Wingo, W.P., Filkowski, M.A., and Baqldessarini, R.J. (2008) Long-term antidepressant treatment in bipolar disorder: mata-analyses of benefits and risks. *Acta Psychiatr. Scand.*, **118**, 347–356.

Gijsman, H.J., Geddes, J.R., Rendell, J.M. *et al.* (2004) Antidepressants for bipolar depression: A systematic review of randomized, controlled trials. *Am. J. Psychiatry*, **161**, 1537–1547.

Goldberg, J.F., Allen, M.H., Miklowitz, D.A. *et al.*, (2005) Suicidal ideation and pharmacotherapy among STEP-BD patients. *Psych. Serv.*, **56** (12), 1534–1540.

Goldberg, J.F., Garno, J.L., Portera, L. *et al.* (1999) Correlates of suicidal ideation in dysphoric mania. *J. Affect. Disord.*, **56**, 75–81.

Goldberg, J.F., Perlis, R.H., Ghaemi, S.N. *et al.* (2007) Adjunctive antidepressant use and symptomatic recovery among bipolar depressed patients with concomitant manic symptoms: findings from the STEP-BD. *Am. J. Psychiatry*, **164**, 1348–1355.

Goodnick, P.J. (2007) Bipolar depression: a review of randomized clinical trials. *Expert. Opin. Pharmacother.*, **8**, 13–21.

Goodwin, G.M. (2003) Evidence-based guidelines for treating bipolar disorder: recommendations from the British Association for Psychopharmacology. *J. Psychopharmacol.*, **17**, 149–173; discussion 147.

Goodwin, F.K. and Jamison, K.R. (2007) *Manic-Depressive Illness; Bipolar Disorders and Recurrent Depression*, 2nd edn, Oxford University Press.

Grunze, H., Kasper, S., Goodwin, G. *et al.* (2002) World Federation of Societies of Biological Psychiatry (WFSBP) guidelines for biological treatment of bipolar disorders. Part I: treatment of bipolar depression. *World J. Biol. Psychiatry*, **3**, 115–124.

Haykal, R.F. and Akiskal, H.S. (1990) Bupropion as a promising approach to rapid-cycling bipolar II patients. *J. Clin. Psychiatry*, **51**, 450–455.

Himmelhoch, J.M., Thase, M.E., Mallinger, A.G., and Houck, P. (1991) Tranylcypromine versus imipramine in anergic bipolar depression. *Am. J. Psychiatry*, **148**, 910–916.

Judd, L.L., Akiskal, H.S., Schettler, P.J. *et al.*, (2002) The long-term natural history of the weekly symptomatic status of bipolar I disorder. *Arch. Gen. Psychiatry*, **59** (6), 530–537.

Judd, L.L., Schettler, P.J., Akiskal, H.S. *et al.* (2003) Long-term symptomatic status of bipolar I vs. bipolar II disorders. *Int. J. Neuropsychopharmacol.*, **6**, 127–137.

Kane, J.M., Quitkin, F.M., and Rifkin, A. (1982) Lithium carbonate and imipramine in the prophylaxis of unipolar and bipolar II illness: a prospective, placebo-controlled comparison. *Arch. Gen. Psychiatry*, **39**, 1065–1069.

Kessing, L.V., Søndergård, L., Kvist, K., and Anderson, P.K. (2005) Suicide risk in patients treated with lithium. *Arch Gen. Psychiatry*, **62**, 860–866.

Koszewska, I. and Rybakowski, J.K. (2009) Antidepressant-induced mood conversions in bipolar disorder: a retrospective study of tricyclic versus non-tricyclic antidepressant drugs. *Neuropsychobiology*, **59**, 12–16.

Kupfer, D.J., Chengappa, K.N., Gelenberg, A.J. *et al.* (2001) Citalopram as adjunctive therapy in bipolar depression. *J. Clin. Psychiatry*, **62**, 985–990.

Landry, P. (1997) Withdrawal hypomania associated with paroxetine. *J. Clin. Psychopharmacol.*, **17**, 60–61.

Leverich, G.S., Altshuler, L.L., Frye, M.A. *et al.* (2006) Risk of switch in mood polarity to hypomania or mania in patients with bipolar depression during acute and continuation trials of venlafaxine, sertraline, and bupropion as adjuncts to mood stabilizers. *Am. J. Psychiatry*, **163**, 232–239.

Mallinger, A.G., Frank, E., Thase, M.E. *et al.* (2009) Revisiting the effectiveness of standard antidepressants in bipolar disorder: are monoamine oxidase inhibitors superior? *Psychopharmacol. Bull.*, **42**, 64–74.

Marangell, L.B., Dennehy, F.B., Wisniewski, S.R. *et al.* (2008) Case-control analyses of the impact of pharmacotherapy on prospectively observed suicide attempts and completed suicides in bipolar disorder: findings from STEP-BD. *J. Clin. Psychiatry*, **69**, 916–922.

McElroy, S.L., Kotwal, R., Kaneria, R., and Keck, P.E. (2006) Antidepressants and suicidal behavior in bipolar disorder. *Bipolar Disord.*, **8**, 596–617.

Moller, H.J., Bottlender, R., Grunze, H. *et al.* (2001) Are antidepressants less effective in the acute treatment of bipolar I compared to unipolar depression? *J. Affect. Disord.*, **67**, 141–146.

Moller, H.J. and Grunze, H. (2000) Have some guidelines for the treatment of acute bipolar depression gone too far in the restriction of antidepressants? *Eur. Arch Psychiatry Clin. Neurosci.*, **250**, 57–68.

Mundo, E., Walker, M., Cate, T. *et al.* (2001) The role of serotonin transporter protein gene in antidepressant-induced mania in bipolar disorder: preliminary findings. *Arch Gen. Psychiatry*, **58**, 539–544.

Nemeroff, C.B., Evans, D.L., Gyulai, L. *et al.* (2001) Double-blind, placebo controlled comparison of imipramine and paroxetine in the treatment of bipolar depression. *Am. J. Psychiatry*, **158**, 906–912.

Nolen, W.A., Kupka, R.W., Hellemann, G. *et al.* (2007) Tranylcypromine vs. lamotrigine in the treatment of refractory bipolar depression: a failed but clinically useful study. *Acta Psychiatr. Scand.*, **11**, 360–365.

Parker, G., Tully, L., Olley, A., and Hadzi-Pavlovic, D. (2006) SSRIs as mood stabilizers for bipolar ii disorder? A proof of concept study. *J. Affect. Disord.*, **92**, 205–214.

Post, R.M., Altshuler, L.L., Frye, M.A. *et al.* (2001) Rate of switch in bipolar patients prospectively treated with second-generation antidepressants as augmentation to mood stabilizers. *Bipolar Disord.*, **3**, 259–265.

Post, R.M., Altshuler, L.L., Leverich, G.S. *et al.* (2006) Mood switch in bipolar depression: comparison of adjunctive velafaxine, bupropion, and sertraline. *Br. J. Psychiatry*, **189**, 124–131.

Post, R.M., Leverich, G.S., Nolen, W.A. *et al.* (2003) A re-evaluation of the role of antidepressants in the treatment of bipolar depression: data from the Stanley Foundation Bipolar Network. *Bipolar Disord.*, **5**, 396–406.

Prien, R.F., Klett, C.J., and Caffey, E.M. (1979) Lithium carbonate and imipramine in prevention of affective episodes. *Arch Gen. Psychiatry*, **29**, 420–425.

Quitkin, F.M., Kane, J., Rifkin, A. *et al.* (1981) Prophylactic lithium carbonate with and without imipramine for bipolar I patients. *Arch Gen. Psychiatry*, **38**, 902–907.

Rihmer, Z. and Akiskal, H. (2006) Do antidepressants t(h)reat(en) depressives? Toward a clinically judicious formulation of the antidepressant-suicidality FDA advisory in light of declining national suicide statistics from many countries. *J. Affect. Disord.*, **94**, 94–913.

Sachs, G.S., Nierenberg, A.A., Calabrese, J.R. *et al.* (2007) Effectiveness of adjunctive antidepressant treatment for bipolar depression. *N. Engl. J. Med.*, **356**, 1711–1722.

Sachs, G.S., Printz, D.J., Kahn, D.A. *et al.* (2000) The expert consensus guidelines series: medication treatment of bipolar disorder 2000. *Postgrad. Med.*, April, Spec No. 1–104.

Sachs, G.S., Thase, M.E., Otto, M.W. *et al.* (1994) A double-blind trial of buproprion versus desipramine for bipolar depression. *J. Clin. Psychiatry*, **55**, 391–393.

Schaffer, A., Zuker, P., and Levitt, A. (2006) Randomized, double-blind pilot trial comparing lamotrigine versus citalopram for the treatment of bipolar depression. *J. Affect. Disord.*, **96**, 95–99.

Shi, L., Thiebaud, P., and McCombs, J.S. (2004) The impact of unrecognized bipolar disorders for patients treated for depression with antidepressants in the fee-for-services California Medicaid (Medi-Cal) program. *J. Affect. Disord.*, **82**, 373–383.

Sidor, M.M., and Macqueen, G.M. (2010) Antidepressants for the acute treatment of bipolar depression: a systematic review and meta-analysis. *J. Clin. Psychiatry*. (Epub)

Silverstone, T. (2001) Moclobemide vs. imipramine in bipolar depression: a multicentre double-blind clinical trial. *Acta Psychiatr. Scand.*, **104**, 104–109.

Simon, N.M., Otto, M.W., Weiss, R.D. *et al.* (2004) Pharmacotherapy for bipolar disorder and comorbid conditions: baseline data from STEP-BD. *J. Clin. Psychopharmacol.*, **24**, 512–520.

Simpson, S.G. and DePaulo, J.R. (1991) Fluoxetine treatment of bipolar II depression. *J. Clin. Psychopharmacol.*, **11**, 52–54.

Stoll, A.L., Mayer, P.V., Kolbrener, M. *et al.*, (1994) Antidepressant-associated mania: a controlled comparison with spontaneous mania. *Am. J. Psychiatry*, **151** (11), 1642–1645.

Tamayo, J.M., Sutton, V.K., Mattei, M.A. *et al.* (2009) Effectiveness and safety of the combination of fluoxetine and olanzapine in outpatients with bipolar depression: an open-label, randomized, flexible-dose study in Puerto Rico. *J. Clin. Psychiatry*, **29** (4), 358–361.

Thase, M.E., Mallinger, A.G., McKnight, D., and Himmelhoch, J.M. (1992) Treatment of imipramine-resistant recurrent depression, IV: A double-blind crossover study of tranyl-cypromine for anergic bipolar depression. *Am. J. Psychiatry*, **149** (2), 195–198.

Tohen, M., Vieta, E., Calabrese, J. *et al.* (2003) Efficacy of olanzapine and olanzapine-fluoxetine combination in the treatment of bipolar I depression. *Arch Gen. Psychiatry*, **60**, 1079–1088.

Valuck, R.J., Orton, H.D., and Libby, A.M. (2009) Antidepressant discontinuation and risk of suicide attempt: a retrospective, nested case-control study. *J. Clin. Psychiatry*, **70**, 1069–1077.

Vasquez, G., Tondo, L., and Baldessarini, R.J. (2010) Comparison of antidepressant responses in patients with bipolar vs unipolar depression: a meta-analytic review. *Pharmacopsychiatry* (Epub).

Vieta, E., Berk, M., Wang, W. *et al.* (2009) Predominant previous polarity as an outcome predictor in a controlled treatment trial for depression in bipolar I disorder patients. *J. Affect. Disord.*, **119**, 22–27.

Vieta, E., Martinez-Aran, A., Goikolea, J.M. *et al.* (2002) A randomized trial comparing paroxetine and venlafaxine in the treatment of bipolar depressed patients taking mood-stabilizers. *J. Clin. Psychiatry*, **63**, 508–512.

Wehr, T.A. and Goodwin, F.K. (1979) Rapid cycling in manic-depressives induced by tricyclic antidepressants. *Arch Gen. Psychiatry*, **36**, 555–559.

Yatham, L.N., Kennedy, S.H., O'Donovan, C. *et al.* (2006) Canadian Network for Mood and Anxiety Treatments (CANMAT) guidelines for the management of patients with bipolar disorder: update 2007. *Bipolar Disord.*, **8**, 721–739.

Yerevanian, B.I., Koek, R.J., Feusner, J.D. *et al.* (2004) Antidepressants and suicidal behavior in unipolar depression. *Acta Psychiatr. Scand.*, **110**, 452–458.

Yerevanian, B.I., Koek, R.J., and Mintz, J. (2007) Bipolar pharmacotherapy and suicidal behavior: Part I: Lithium, divalproex, and carbamazepine. *J. Affect. Disord.*, **103**, 5–11.

Young, L.T., Joffe, R.T., Robb, J.C. *et al.* (2000) Double-blind comparison of addition of a second mood stabilizer versus an antidepressant to an initial mood stabilizer for treatment of patients with bipolar depression. *Am. J. Psychiatry*, **157**, 124–126.

16

Bipolarity in Women: Therapeutic Issues

Susan L. McElroy[1], Lesley M. Arnold[2] and Lori L. Altshuler[3]

[1]Lindner Center of HOPE, Mason and Department of Psychiatry and Behavioral Neuroscience, University of Cincinnati College of Medicine, OH, USA
[2]Department of Psychiatry and Behavioral Neuroscience, University of Cincinnati College of Medicine, OH, USA
[3]Department of Psychiatry and Behavioral Sciences, Veterans Affairs Greater Los Angeles Healthcare System, The David Geffen School of Medicine at UCLA, Los Angeles, CA, USA

16.1 INTRODUCTION

Although mania and hypomania are equally prevalent in women and men, bipolarity differs between the two genders in clinically important ways. This chapter reviews gender differences in the phenomenology, course, and comorbidity of the bipolar spectrum, discusses interactions between the female reproductive cycle and bipolar disorder, and highlights special issues regarding the treatment of women with bipolar disorder, particularly in pregnancy and the postpartum.

16.2 EPIDEMIOLOGY AND GENDER DISTRIBUTION OF THE BIPOLAR SPECTRUM

Epidemiologic studies have consistently shown that depressive disorders (both major depressive disorder and dysthymia) are more common in women, whereas bipolar I disorder is equally common in women and men (Kessler *et al.*, 1993, 1994; Merikangas *et al.*, 2007; Regier *et al.*, 1988; Szadoczky *et al.*, 1998; Weissman, Bruce, and Leaf, 1991). Bipolar II disorder was once thought to be more common in women, but growing epidemiologic data indicates it is also equally distributed between the genders (Merikangas *et al.*, 2007; Mitchell *et al.*, 2001; Szadoczky *et al.*, 1998). In the National Comorbidity Survey Replication, for example, no gender differences were found in the distribution of bipolar I disorder, bipolar II disorder, or subthreshold bipolar disorder (Merikangas *et al.*, 2007).

Bipolar Psychopharmacotherapy: Caring for the patient, Second Edition. Edited by Hagop S. Akiskal and Mauricio Tohen.
© 2011 John Wiley & Sons, Ltd. Published 2011 by John Wiley & Sons, Ltd.

16.3 GENDER DIFFERENCES IN PHENOMENOLOGY

16.3.1 IS FEMALE BIPOLARITY CHARACTERIZED BY A DEPRESSIVE DIATHESIS?

Depressive symptoms are more common than manic and hypomanic symptoms in both women and men with bipolar I and II disorders (Angst, 1978; Judd *et al.*, 2002, 2003; Kupka *et al.*, 2007). However, several lines of evidence suggest female bipolarity is even more likely than male bipolarity to be characterized by depressive symptoms (Leibenluft, 1996, 1997, 1999). Perhaps most important is that of the five prospective studies that evaluated mood as a function of gender reported in the literature, three found women experienced more depression than men (Altshuler *et al.*, 2010). In the first, Angst (1978) followed 95 patients over a 16-year period after an initial inpatient admission, and found that women had nearly twice the percentage of depressive episodes than men (60% versus 35.5%), and nearly a third less the percentage of manic episodes (13.6% versus 35.5%). Thus, women not only outnumbered men in the proportion of depressions, but also spent a greater portion of their ill time in the depressed (60%) versus manic (14%) phase than men, who showed no difference in ill time spent in the depressed (35.5%) versus manic (35.5%) phase. In a smaller study, Christensen *et al.* (2003) followed 56 bipolar subjects prospectively for up to three years with structured mood rating scales. Women spent a significantly greater proportion of time in depression than men (10% versus 5% of clinical visits), whereas men spent a significantly greater proportion of time in mania than women (13% versus 5% of clinical visits). In the third study, 711 subjects were evaluated in 13 191 visits over seven years (Altshuler *et al.*, 2010). The main outcome measures were the presence of depressive or hypomanic/manic symptoms, measured by the Inventory of Depressive Symptomatology and the Young Mania Rating Scale, respectively. The likelihood of having depressive symptoms during visits was significantly greater for women than men (36% of the visits for women vs. 29% for men; $p = 0.04$), even after controlling for the higher rate of rapid cycling in women (see below). This was true for both the bipolar I and bipolar II cohorts.

Another finding suggesting that female bipolarity is characterized by a predominance of depression is its frequent misdiagnosis as unipolar depression. In their registry of 2839 persons with bipolar disorder, Kupfer *et al.* (2002) found that bipolar women were more likely than bipolar men to receive diagnoses of depression. Similarly, in a study of 345 patients with DSM-IV bipolar I or II disorder, time from illness onset to maintenance lithium treatment was significantly longer for women (9.14 years, SD = 8.77) than men (7.02 years, SD = 7.32) (Baldessarini *et al.*, 1999). The authors' concluded that this delay in treatment might reflect differences in clinical presentation. Studies of temperament in mood disorder have found that women have high rates of antecedent depressive temperament (Perugi *et al.*, 1990), whereas men have high rates of hyperthymic temperament (Akiskal *et al.*, 1998).

Yet another finding supporting a depressive diathesis for female bipolarity is its relationship with suicidality as compared to women in the general population and men with bipolar disorder. In the U.S. general population, women attempt suicide two to three times more often than men, but men account for 65% of completed suicides (Goodwin and Jamison, 2007; Kornstein and Wojcik, 2002). In both the Epidemiological Catchment Area and National Comorbidity Studies, the lifetime rate of suicide attempts was higher in persons with bipolar disorder than in those with unipolar depression or any other Axis I disorder (Chen and Dilsaver, 1996; Kessler, Borges, and Walters, 1999). Like women and men in the general population, bipolar women were more likely to attempt suicide than bipolar men (Chen and Dilsaver, 1996; Kessler, Borges, and Walters, 1999). More-over, studies have not shown a clear predominance of males among persons with bipolar disorder who committed suicide (Goodwin and Jamison, 2007; Isometsa *et al.*, 1994; Tsai *et al.*, 2002). For example, in a study of all 31 suicide victims with DSM-IV bipolar I disorder in Finland within a one-year period, 13(42%) were female and 18(58%) were male (Isometsa *et al.*, 1994). Similarly, in a Chinese study of all 43 patients with DSM-IV bipolar I disorder who had committed suicide following admission after 1 January 1985 until 31 December 1996, 19 (44%) were female and 24 (56%) were male (Tsai *et al.*, 2002). Indeed, two recent studies of mortality in patients with hospital diagnoses of bipolar disorder found that bipolar women had higher standardized mortality ratios for suicide than bipolar men (20.3 versus 18.1 and 22.4 versus 15.0, respectively) (Hoyer, Mortensen, and Olesen, 2000; Osby *et al.*, 2001).

Finally, additional support for female bipolarity having a depressive diathesis is its association with mixed mania and rapid cycling – two affective states characterized by prominent depressive symptoms (McElroy *et al.*, 1992; Calabrese *et al.*, 2001) (see below).

16.3.2   IS FEMALE BIPOLARITY CHARACTERIZED BY MIXED STATES (MIXITY)?

Many clinical studies have found that mixed mania is more common in bipolar women than bipolar men (Arnold, McElroy, and Keck, 2000; Akiskal *et al.*, 1998; Cassidy and Carroll, 2001; McElroy *et al.*, 1992, 1995; Robb *et al.*, 1998). In a review of 17 studies of mixed mania, 5 of the 6 studies that provided information on gender distribution found that mixed mania was more common in women (McElroy *et al.*, 1992). A sub-sequent review evaluated 13 studies that reported on the gender distribution in mixed mania using broad, intermediate, and narrow definitions of mixed mania according to the amount of required depression (Arnold, McElroy, and Keck, 2000). Mixed mania was more common in women when defined narrowly (mania with syndromal major depression), but equally common in women and men when defined by lesser degrees of depression (mania with any depressive symptom or mania with several depressive symptoms). Akiskal *et al.* (1998) obtained a similar finding when they examined the gender distribution of 104 manic inpatients using a dimensional scheme to define pure versus dysphoric (mixed) mania. Specifically, they found significantly more women in the "definite" dysphoric mania category (presence of ≥ 3 depressive symptoms), but not the "probable" dysphoric mania category (presence of two depressive symptoms), compared with a combined group of patients with "pure" and "doubtful" dysphoric mania (absence of depressive symptoms and one depressive symptom, respectively) (91% versus 63% versus 58%).

Other mixed states may also be more common in bipolar women than bipolar men. Evaluating 908 patients prospectively over seven years in the Stanley Foundation Bipolar Treatment Network, Suppes *et al.* (2005) found that the likelihood of mixed hypomania, defined at a given visit as having both a Young Mania Rating Scale score $\geq$ 12 and an Inventory of Depressive Symptomatology – Clinical Rated Version score $\geq$ 15, was significantly greater for women (72%) than men (42%) (p < 0.001). Moreover, for women, the probability of mixed symptoms increased with the severity of hypomania and then decreased at the most severe levels of hypomania or mania. For men, a linear symptom-related increase in mixed symptoms was observed.

The few studies examining whether mixed depression (syndromal depression with hypomania or manic symptoms) is more common in women than men are inconsistent (Benazzi, 2003, 2008). Nonetheless, taken together, available clinical data suggest female bipolarity is characterized by mixity, or the co-occurrence of manic and depressive symptoms.

16.3.3 IS FEMALE BIPOLARITY CHARACTERIZED BY RAPID CYCLING (CYCLICITY)?

Rapid cycling, most commonly defined as four or more mood episodes in one year, has been reported to be more common in bipolar women than in bipolar men in numerous clinical studies (Coryell, Endicott, and Keller, 1992; Bauer, Whybrow, and Winokur, 1990; Bowden *et al.*, 1999; Calabrese and Delucchi, 1990; Coryell *et al.*, 2003; Dunner and Fieve, 1974; Dunner, Patrick, and Fieve, 1977; Kukopulos *et al.*, 1983, 1980; Maj *et al.*, 1999; Nurnberger *et al.*, 1988; Robb *et al.*, 1998; Wehr *et al.*, 1988). Two meta-analyses have supported an association between female bipolarity and rapid cycling. In the first, Tondo and Baldessarini (1998) analyzed 10 studies of 2057 bipolar patients and found that rapid cycling occurred in significantly more women (29.6%) than men (16.6%). In the second, Kupka *et al.* (2003) analyzed 20 studies of 3709 bipolar patients and similarly found that significantly more rapid cyclers were women (66%) than were nonrapid cyclers (53%). Indeed, of importance are studies showing that gender distribution in rapid cycling varied depending on how it was defined, with higher rates of women seen in definitions that waived duration criteria for mood episodes and required circularity of course (that is, were associated with more extreme mood instability or more frequent polarity shifts) (Maj *et al.*, 1999) or required ≥ 8 rather than ≥ 4 episodes per year (Kupka *et al.*, 2005). This observation also raises the issue that the rapid cycling definition of four mood episodes in one year does not completely overlap with the dimensional construct of cyclicity, or the alternation of manic or hypomanic and depressive symptoms or episodes. Thus, the higher rates of rapid cycling in women with bipolar disorder may reflect an association between female bipolarity and greater cyclicity (Kupka *et al.*, 2003).

16.3.4   IS FEMALE BIPOLARITY CHARACTERIZED BY ATYPICALITY?

A number of studies examining possible gender differences in the phenomenology of unipolar major depression have found that women are more likely than men to report atypical or reverse vegetative symptoms, particularly increased appetite and weight gain (Kornstein and Wojcik, 2002). Studies comparing the phenomenology of bipolar and unipolar depression have similarly suggested that bipolar depression is more likely to be associated with atypical features (Benazzi and Akiskal, 2003; Mitchell *et al.*, 2001). Very few studies, however, have specifically assessed whether there are gender differences in the phenomenology of bipolar depression. One study of 211 patients with bipolar I and II depression found women were more likely than men to report appetite and weight changes (Kawa *et al.*, 2005). Another study of bipolar II disorder found women were more likely than men to have an index episode of atypical depression (Benazzi, 2006). More research is needed to understand the relationships among bipolarity, atypicality, and gender.

16.4   GENDER DIFFERENCES IN COURSE AND OUTCOME

A number of gender differences beyond depressive episode frequency have been reported in the course and outcome of bipolar disorder. First, several studies have found that females have a later age of illness onset than males (Robb *et al.*, 1998; Viguera, Baldessarini, and Tondo, 2001; Yildiz and Sachs, 2003). Other studies, however, have not found gender differences in the age of onset of bipolar disorder (Bellivier *et al.*, 2001; Hendrick *et al.*, 2000; Suppes *et al.*, 2001; Winokur *et al.*, 1994). Indeed, the one epidemiologic study that reported age of onset for both genders found a nonsignificantly earlier illness onset of illness for females than males (17.9 years vs. 22.0 years) (Szadoczky *et al.*, 1998). Nonetheless, reports of women having a later illness onset are consistent with clinical findings that patients with prepubertal mania are more likely to be male (Geller *et al.*, 2002).

Second, several gender differences in episode pattern occurrence have been described in bipolar disorder. Thus, some studies (Kubacki, 1986; Szadoczky *et al.*, 1998), though not all (Abrams and Taylor, 1974), have reported that unipolar mania is more common in males than females. Some studies (Viguera, Baldessarini, and Tondo, 2001), though not all (Kukopulos *et al.*, 1980), have reported that bipolar women are more likely than bipolar men to have an episode pattern of depression followed by mania (sometimes called the DMI pattern), whereas bipolar men are either equally likely or more likely to have the episode pattern of mania followed by depression (the MDI pattern).

Third, some studies have reported gender differences in the impact and long-term outcome of bipolar disorder. Thus, even when euthymic, women with bipolar disorder have described their health and well-being as being poorer overall than that of men (Robb *et al.*, 1998). In a large community survey, Mood Disorder Questionnaire (MDQ)-positive women reported significantly more disruption in social/leisure life

(17.2% vs. 10.8%, p = 0.002) and family life (23.62% vs 15.8%, p = 0.001) in the 12 months prior to study participation compared with MDQ-positive men (Hirschfeld *et al.*, 2003). Specifically, MDQ-positive women reported significantly more symptom disruption as a result of irritability, increased confidence, talkativeness, distractibility, and spending money compared with MDQ-positive men.

By contrast, other data suggest women may have better functional outcomes than men. Loyd, Simpson, and Tsuang (1985) compared the outcome of women and men hospitalized for mania, and found a trend ($x^2 = 9.21$, df = 4, p < 0.06) for women to have more favorable outcomes, which he attributed to their having slightly better occupational and residential outcomes. In a prospective follow-up study of 73 manic patients 1.7 years after hospitalization, there was a minor trend for women to show more favorable overall functioning (p < 0.20) and a significant finding for women to show better work functioning (p < 0.01) (Harrow *et al.*, 1990). Similarly, in a prospective study of 75 inpatients with DSM-III bipolar disorder who had recovered from a manic episode, Tohen, Waternaux, and Tsuang (1990) found that male gender predicted poorer residential status at four-year follow-up.

Another gender difference in outcome is that bipolar men may be more likely than bipolar women to become involved with the legal system (Baldassano *et al.*, 2005). In the large community survey mentioned earlier, almost three times as many MDQ-positive men had been jailed, arrested, or convicted of a crime compared with MDQ-positive women (36.5% versus 13.1%, p < 0. 00001) (Calabrese *et al.*, 2003). Taken together, these findings raise the issue of whether some of the gender differences in bipolarity reflect gender differences in help seeking behavior or access to health care (Weissman and Olfson, 1995).

16.5 GENDER DIFFERENCES IN COMORBIDITY

Bipolarity is highly comorbid with other mental and general medical disorders (Angst, 1998; Angst and Sellaro, 2000; Boyd *et al.*, 1984; Calabrese *et al.*, 2003; Kessler *et al.*, 1997; Merikangas *et al.*, 2007), and these comorbid disorders may have adverse effects on the course, outcome, and treatment response of bipolar disorder (Black *et al.*, 1988a, 1988b; Frank *et al.*, 2002; McElroy *et al.*, 2001). Common co-occurring mental disorders include anxiety, substance use, eating, and impulse control disorders (Angst, 1998; Boyd *et al.*, 1984; Chen and Dilsaver, 1995; Kessler *et al.*, 1997). Some of these disorders (that is, anxiety and eating disorders) are more common in women in general, and are more common in women with bipolar disorder than in men with bipolar disorder (Baldassano *et al.*, 2005; Calabrese *et al.*, 2003; Frank *et al.*, 2002; Kawa *et al.*, 2005; Lewinsohn, Striegel-Moore, and Seeley, 2000; MacKinnon *et al.*, 2002; McElroy, Kotwal, and Keck, 2006). Substance use disorders, though more common in bipolar men than in bipolar women, are much more common in women with bipolar disorder than in women without bipolar disorder (Frye *et al.*, 2003; Hendrick *et al.*, 2000). Indeed, several studies have shown the association between bipolar disorder and substance use disorders is stronger for women than men. Based on data for 267 bipolar patients enrolled in the Stanley Foundation Bipolar Network, the risk of alcoholism was greater for women with bipolar disorder (odds ratio $= 7.35$) than for men with bipolar disorder (odds ratio $= 2.77$) as compared to the general population (Frye *et al.*, 2003). Also, in a study of 41 manic patients at first hospitalization, women had a higher rate of alcohol abuse or dependence than men (36.0% vs. 6.3%) (Strakowski *et al.*, 1992). Thus, substance abuse in a woman should be considered a marker for bipolarity.

General medical disorders that frequently co-occur with bipolar disorder include migraine (Breslau, Merikangas, and Bowden, 1994), thyroid disease (Hendrick, Altshuler, and Whybrow, 1998; Kupka *et al.*, 2002, 2003), and overweight and obesity (Simon *et al.*, 2006). Both migraine (Breslau, Merikangas, and Bowden, 1994) and thyroid disease (Tunbridge *et al.*, 1977; Vanderpump *et al.*, 1995) are more common in women than men in general, including in bipolar women than bipolar men (Baldassano *et al.*, 2005; Blehar *et al.*, 1998; Calabrese *et al.*, 2003). In one community study, the sex-specific prevalence of comorbid migraine in bipolar disorder was 35% for women versus 15% for men (McIntyre *et al.*, 2006). Both overt and subclinical thyroid disease has been hypothesized to contribute to the higher rates of rapid cycling and mixed states in women with bipolar disorder, as well as the depressive diathesis of female bipolarity (Kleiner *et al.*, 1999). Cole *et al.* (2002), for example, found that lower pretreatment thyroid function (that is, lower free thyroxine index (FTI) and higher thyroid stimulating hormone (TSH) values) was significantly associated with longer time to response in 65 patients with bipolar depression. Regarding obesity and bipolar disorder, one study of 644 patients from the United States and Europe found that women were more likely to be obese and extremely obese, whereas men were more likely to be overweight (McElroy *et al.*, 2001). Another study of 89 euthymic outpatients from New Zealand found that women and men had similar rates of obesity, but that women had higher rates of overweight (Elmslie *et al.*, 2000). Obesity has been associated with a higher rate of recurrence, particularly depressive recurrence, in lithium-treated bipolar patients (Fagiolini *et al.*, 2003).

Female patients with bipolar disorder are more likely to report a history of sexual abuse, but not physical abuse, than are male bipolar patients (Leverich *et al.*, 2002). A higher rate of post-traumatic stress disorder has also been reported in bipolar women than bipolar men (Baldassano *et al.*, 2005). A history of childhood or adolescent abuse has been associated with a worse course of bipolar disorder, including earlier age of onset, greater comorbidity, and a higher rate of suicide attempts (Leverich *et al.*, 2002).

Preliminary studies suggest comorbidity in general is either more common in mania at first hospitalization in women than men (Strakowski *et al.*, 1992) or equally common in women and men with bipolar disorder (Black *et al.*, 1988a, 1988b; Vieta *et al.*, 2001), but this issue needs more study. Possible gender differences in the effects of comorbidity on the presentation, course, outcome, and treatment response of bipolar disorder have not been systematically evaluated (Black *et al.*, 1988a, 1988b).

16.6 BIPOLAR DISORDER AND THE REPRODUCTIVE CYCLE

16.6.1 MENSTRUAL CYCLE

There have been reports of bipolar disorder worsening during the premenstrual (late luteal) phase in some women (Blehar *et al.*, 1998; Hendrick, Altshuler, and Burt, 1996;

Leibenluft, 1996, 1997). Ota, Mukai, and Gotoda (1954) described female bipolar patients whose manic relapses occurred regularly during the premenstrual phases of their cycles. Diamond et al. (1976) reported an increased rate of hospitalizations among women attending a lithium clinic during their luteal phase. D'Mello, Pinheiro, and Lalinec-Michaud (1993) described two women who experienced recurrent irritability, hyperactivity, and decreased need for sleep in the five days before their menses but who were euthymic for the remainder of their menstrual cycles. Their mood symptoms responded to maintenance lithium treatment. Kukopulos, Minnai, and Muller-Oerlinghausen (1985) and Conrad and Hamilton (1986) each described women with bipolar disorder who experienced late luteal symptomatic exacerbations with lithium level decreases. In one case, increasing the lithium dose one week prior to menses successfully maintained lithium levels and prevented the premenstrual deterioration over a two-year period (Conrad and Hamilton, 1986). Blehar et al. (1998) reported that 66% of 186 women with bipolar I disorder described regularly occurring premenstrual or menstrual (early follicular) mood changes. Similarly, in a prospective evaluation of 17 women with bipolar disorder who kept daily self-reported mood ratings, 11 (65%) reported a significant change in mean mood between the first seven days and the last seven days during at least one menstrual cycle, with 6 of the 11 reporting a significant mood change in more than one menstrual cycle (Rasgon et al., 2003). However, there was no clear pattern to the mood changes across the menstrual cycle. By contrast, in a sample of 41 outpatient bipolar women whose daily mood ratings were assessed with the National Institutes of Health Life Chart Method-p (NIMH-LCM-p), there was no significant relationship between phases of the menstrual cycle and changes in depression or mania (Shivakumar et al., 2008).

No studies, to our knowledge, have evaluated DSM-IV premenstrual dysphoric disorder (PMDD) in females with bipolar disorder. Roy-Byrne et al. (1985) found that 25% of 16 women with bipolar disorder met criteria for a premenstrual "depressive syndrome." Endicott et al. (1985) reported that females with bipolar II disorder (N = 66; 71%) were more likely to suffer from "premenstrual dysphoria" as compared to females with bipolar I disorder (N = 122; 44%) or unipolar depressive disorder (N = 104; 42%). Price and DiMarzio (1986) found that 15 (60%) of 25 women with rapid-cycling bipolar disorder reported "severe premenstrual tension syndrome." Interestingly, a consistent relationship between the menstrual cycle and rapid cycling has not been found (Diamond et al., 1976; Leibenluft et al., 1999; Price and DiMarzio, 1986; Wehr et al., 1988).

An increasing number of reports suggest that menstrual cycle dysfunction may be common in women with bipolar disorder. Thus, Rasgon et al. (2000) reported that 18 (82%) of 22 women taking lithium (N = 11), valproate (N = 10), or both (N = 2) had menstrual irregularities. In 14 (64%) women, the menstrual irregularities preceded the onset of the bipolar disorder. In a subsequent study by the same authors, 59% of 17 prospectively evaluated bipolar women, including those taking oral contraceptives, displayed long menstrual cycles (Rasgon et al., 2003). In a recent study of 295 women with bipolar disorder, 245 women with unipolar depression, and 619 healthy controls, bipolar women more commonly reported menstrual cycle dysfunction before onset of psychiatric illness (34%) as compared to unipolar women (24.5%, $p < 0.0001$), and early onset menstrual dysfunction as compared to healthy controls (22%, $p = 0.01$) (Joffe et al., 2006c). The menstrual abnormalities in women with bipolar disorder have been hypothesized to be due in part to the hypothalamic pituitary adrenal axis dysfunction associated with the illness. Some menstrual disturbances, however, can be induced by medication (see section on polycystic ovary syndrome).

16.6.2 PREGNANCY

Growing research indicates bipolar women who are pregnant experience mood episodes at rates similar to those who are not pregnant (Blehar *et al.*, 1998; Nonacs, Viguera, and Cohen, 2002; Viguera *et al.*, 2007b). For example, Viguera *et al.* (2000a) retrospectively compared recurrence rates for 101 women with DSM-IV bipolar disorder (68 bipolar I, 33 bipolar II) during pregnancy and the postpartum (N = 42) or during equivalent periods for age-matched, nonpregnant controls (N = 59) after either rapid (1–14 days) or gradual (15–30 days) discontinuation of stable lithium maintenance treatment. Recurrence rates after lithium discontinuation were similar for pregnant (52%) and nonpregnant women (58%), but had been much lower for both in the year before treatment was discontinued (21%). In addition, recurrence risk was greater after rapid than after gradual discontinuation (consistent with previous studies in broader groups of bipolar patients (Baldessarini *et al.*, 1997; Faedda *et al.*, 1993)).

In a subsequent prospective study, Viguera *et al.* (2007b) compared the risk of recurrence for 89 women with DSM-IV bipolar disorder (69% bipolar I, 31% bipolar II) who were euthymic at conception and continued mood stabilizer therapy, or discontinued pharmacotherapy within six months before or 12 weeks after conception. Most patients (71%) were taking more than one psychotropic agent, which usually included a mood stabilizer in combination with an antidepressant and/or antipsychotic. The overall risk of recurrence in pregnancy was 71%. Among women who discontinued versus continued treatment, recurrence risk was twofold greater, median time to first recurrence was more than fourfold shorter, and weeks ill during pregnancy was fivefold greater. The median latency period until recurrence was 11 times shorter after abrupt versus gradual discontinuation of the mood stabilizer. Most recurrences were depressed or mixed, and most occurred in the first trimester. Five or more years of illness, younger age of onset, and a bipolar II diagnosis were the top three illness related factors that predicted recurrence.

16.6.3 POSTPARTUM PERIOD

Extensive data show that the postpartum is a high risk period for mood and psychotic episodes for women in general (Miller, 1999). This is particularly true for women with bipolar disorder, who are at increased risk of experiencing first onset and recurrent depressive, manic, mixed, and psychotic episodes (Kendell, Chalmers, and Platz, 1987; Leibenluft, 1996).

For example, one study found that 13 (36%) of 36 consecutively hospitalized bipolar mothers reported onset of the disorder in the postpartum compared with none of eight bipolar fathers, with postpartum relapse rates of 25–40% after subsequent pregnancies (Hunt and Trevor, 1995). In another study, one third of women with bipolar disorder developed manic episodes temporally related to childbirth (Kubacki, 1986). A retrospective review of the impact of reproductive events on the course of bipolar disorder in

30 outpatient mothers showed that 67% had experienced postpartum mood episodes, and that the rate of recurrent postpartum episodes after subsequent pregnancies was 64% (Freeman *et al.*, 2002). In addition, the presence of mood symptoms during pregnancy was significantly associated with postpartum mood episodes. Similarly, in their study of 101 gravid and nongravid women with DSM-IV bipolar disorder who discontinued lithium maintenance treatment, Viguera *et al.* (2000a) found that, among the patients who remained stable over the first 40 weeks after lithium discontinuation and were subsequently followed from week 41 through week 64, postpartum recurrences were 2.9 times more frequent than recurrences in nonpregnant women (70% versus 24%, respectively).

Although women with bipolar disorder often have postpartum mood episodes, it is unknown how often postpartum depression represents bipolar disorder. Several studies, however, have found that postpartum depression is often characterized by bipolar features, including emotional lability, psychosis, disorientation, and elevated hypomania ratings (Dean and Kendall, 1981; Lane *et al.*, 1997). Some authorities now consider postpartum onset depression a marker for bipolarity.

By contrast, it is well documented that postpartum psychosis is more frequently associated with bipolar disorder than any other psychiatric disorder (Videbech and Gouliaev, 1995; Chaudron and Pies, 2003). The rate of postpartum psychosis in women with bipolar disorder has been reported to be between 20 and 30% (Jones and Craddock, 2001). Postpartum depression with filicide (child murder by the mother) is also associated with high rates of bipolar disorder (Kim, Choi, and Ha, 2008). Women who have had one postpartum psychotic episode are at a high risk of recurrent mood episodes (Jones and Craddock, 2001). Moreover, a vulnerability to postpartum episodes clusters in families (Forty *et al.*, 2006; Jones and Craddock, 2001). Preliminary evidence indicates that variation at the serotonin transporter gene influences susceptibility to postpartum episodes in women with bipolar disorder (Coyle *et al.*, 2000). A genome-wide significant linkage signal has been observed on chromosome 16 p 13, and a genome-wide suggestive linkage has been observed on chromosome 8q24 (Jones *et al.*, 2007). These findings have lead to the suggestion that bipolar postpartum psychosis is a genetically meaningful subtype of bipolar disorder (Jones *et al.*, 2007).

16.6.4 MENOPAUSAL TRANSITION AND MENOPAUSE

Growing data suggest that the menopausal transition may be a time of increased mood instability for women with bipolar disorder. In one study, 19% of 56 postmenopausal bipolar women reported worsening of mood symptoms after menopause (Blehar *et al.*, 1998). In a follow-up study of 68 women with rapid-cycling bipolar disorder, 28% were noted to begin rapid cycling during the perimenopausal age range (45–54 years) (Koukopoulos *et al.*, 2003). In another study, bipolar women who were not using hormone replacement therapy (HRT) during the perimenopause and menopause were significantly more likely to report worsening of mood symptoms, primarily depressive, than those not using HRT, suggesting HRT had a protective effect during this period (Freeman *et al.*, 2002). In a study of 47 bipolar women followed prospectively for a mean of 17 months, a significantly increased frequency of depressive episodes was seen in the perimenopause compared to that reported in the reproductive years (Marsh *et al.*, 2008).

Another prospective study by the same group found that menopausal transition age bipolar women experienced a greater proportion of clinic visits with depressive symptoms compared to similarly aged men, and younger women and men with bipolar disorder (Marsh, Ketter, and Rasgon, 2009).

The perimenopause may also be a time of increased risk in bipolar women with a history of postpartum psychosis. Robertson Blackmore *et al.* (2008) described five women with bipolar disorder and postpartum psychosis who subsequently developed perimenopausal mood episodes. Four of the five women had remained well in the time between childbirth and perimenopause.

16.7   TREATMENT OF BIPOLAR DISORDER IN FEMALES

16.7.1   GENDER AND RESPONSE TO MOOD STABILIZERS

Though limited, available data suggest gender does not affect pharmacodynamic response of bipolarity to lithium. Viguera, Tondo, and Baldessarini (2000b) systematically reviewed 17 studies of 1043 lithium-treated subjects with major mood disorders that allowed determination of separate response rates for men and women. Response rates were similar for women and men for major mood disorder (63.5% versus 59.9%) and for bipolar disorder (63.5% versus 59.9%). Similarly, in a retrospective study of lithium prophylaxis in bipolar disorder, gender did not impact overall morbidity (Berghofer, Kossmann, and Muller-Oerlinghausen, 1996). In a study of the effectiveness of restarting lithium treatment after its discontinuation in patients with bipolar I and II disorders, both the response to lithium discontinuation and its re-institution did not differ in women and men (Tondo *et al.*, 1997). More recently, Viguera, Baldessarini, and Tondo (2001) evaluated 360 men and women with DSM-IV bipolar disorder before and during lithium maintenance monotherapy. Although women started lithium maintenance treatment at an older age, women did not differ from men regarding treatment response when defined by episodes per year, hospitalizations per year, or percent of time ill. Indeed, a survival analysis of time to first recurrence during lithium maintenance treatment showed significantly earlier recurrence in men than women. Of note, women required or tolerated slightly (but significantly) lower serum concentrations of lithium than men (mean serum lithium (mEq/l): 0.60 ± 0.13 versus 0.64 ± 0.14) (Viguera, Baldessarini, and Tondo, 2001).

Possible gender differences in the pharmacodynamic response of bipolar disorder to valproate, lamotrigine, carbamazepine, and second generation antipsychotics have been less systematically evaluated. No data exist, however, to suggest clinically relevant gender differences in response to these agents. For example, a reanalysis of pooled data from two double-blind, placebo-controlled trials of olanzapine in acute bipolar mania showed that women and men responded equally well to the drug (Baldessarini *et al.*, 2003). However, one retrospective study found that the mean dose of first generation antipsychotic medication was higher in a group of bipolar women who were older than 40 years compared with a younger group. The finding was hypothesized to be due to the older women's declining estrogen levels and subsequent loss of estrogen's putative antidopaminergic effects (D'Mello and McNeil, 1990).

16.7.2 GENDER AND SIDE EFFECTS TO MOOD STABILIZERS

There may be gender differences in side effects to mood stabilizers. Women may be more likely to develop lithium-associated hypothyroidism and weight gain, whereas men may be more likely to develop tremor (Henry, 2002; Johnston and Eagles, 1999). It is unknown if the increased rate of hypothyroidism in lithium-treated bipolar women represents the increased rate of thyroid disease in women than men in general, if women are more vulnerable than men to lithium's thyrotoxic effects, or a combination of these factors. In one study, the only factor predictive of hypothyroidism with lithium treatment (beyond female gender) was weight gain during the first year of treatment (Henry, 2002). In another study of 226 bipolar outpatients, thyroid autoimmunity, defined as the presence of thyroperoxidase antibodies, was found to be equally and highly prevalent in women and men with bipolar disorder; thyroid autoimmunity tended to be associated with hypothyroidism; lithium exposure was associated with hypothyroidism but not thyroid autoimmunity; and women were more likely than men to develop hypothyroidism (Kupka et al., 2002). Thus, thyroid autoimmunity and lithium exposure were independent, but cumulative, risk factors for hypothyroidism, especially in bipolar women.

16.7.3 HYPERPROLACTINEMIA

First generation antipsychotic medications and the second generation antipsychotics risperidone and paliperidone are associated with hyperprolactinemia. Hyperprolactinemia may cause galactorrhea, amenorrhea and menstrual cycle irregularities, anovulation, infertility, and sexual dysfunction, as well as anxiety, depression, and hostility (Byerly et al., 2007). Whether the degree of prolactin level elevation associated with these drugs is different between women and men remains controversial (Aichhorn et al., 2006). Antipsychotic-associated hyperprolactinemia can be managed by (i) switching to a prolactin-sparing antipsychotic (that is, olanzapine, quetiapine, or clozapine); (ii) lowering the dose of the antipsychotic; or (iii) adding a dopamine agonist, such as bromocriptine.

16.7.4 POLYCYSTIC OVARY SYNDROME

Growing research suggests there may be a relationship between polycystic ovarian syndrome (PCOS; an endocrine disorder characterized by menstrual irregularities and hyperandrogenism) and valproate exposure in females with bipolar disorder, as has been observed in females with epilepsy (Akdeniz et al., 2003; O'Donovan et al., 2002; Rasgon et al., 2005, 2000; Reynolds, Sisk, and Rasgon, 2007). Joffe et al. (2006c) evaluated 230 women with bipolar disorder 18–45 years of age for PCOS, and found women receiving valproate developed a significantly higher rate of oligomenorrhea with hyperandrogenism (10.5%) than women receiving lithium or a nonvalproate anticonvulsant (1.4%). Follow-up (mean 17 months) of 14 women showed most who discontinued valproate had improved menstrual cycle function despite static body weight (Joffe et al., 2006a). Interestingly, Jiang, Kenna, and Rasgon (2009) have hypothesized that bipolar disorder and PCOS may share a common pathophysiologic platform, because of the relatively high prevalence of PCOS in bipolar females and metabolic abnormalities shared by both conditions, including obesity, insulin resistance, and hyperglycemia. Reproductive aged-aged females with bipolar disorder treated with valproate should be monitored for menstrual irregularities and hyperandrogenism (Joffe and Hayes, 2008).

16.7.5   GENDER AND RESPONSE TO ANTIDEPRESSANTS

The treatment of bipolarity with antidepressants in general is controversial because of inadequate data regarding their short and long-term efficacy in bipolar depression (McElroy *et al.*, 2010; Sachs *et al.*, 2007; Tohen *et al.*, 2003) and inconsistencies in available data regarding their ability to induce hypomania, mania, mixed states, and rapid cycling (Akiskal *et al.*, 2003; Altshuler *et al.*, 1995; Calabrese *et al.*, 1999; Coryell *et al.*, 2003). Nonetheless, clinical studies suggest that some patients with bipolar I and II disorder destabilize upon antidepressant exposure (Benazzi, 1997), whereas others require acute and even maintenance treatment with antidepressants (typically in combination with mood stabilizers) for optimal response (Altshuler *et al.*, 2003). Moreover, there may be gender differences in the pharmacodynamic and pharmacokinetic response of patients with major depressive disorder to antidepressants (Gorman, 2006; Kornstein and Wojcik, 2002; Yonkers *et al.*, 1992). These include findings that women with major depression may respond better to selective serotonin reuptake inhibitors (SSRIs) than to tricyclics (which does not appear to be true for men) (Kornstein *et al.*, 2000), and that women may respond better than men to the SSRI citalopram (Young *et al.*, 2009) and to augmentation strategies with triiodothyonine (Altshuler *et al.*, 2001; Coppen *et al.*, 1972; Whybrow, 1995), lithium (Dallal *et al.*, 1990), and stimulants (Askinazi, Weintraub, and Karamouz, 1986). Relatively few gender differences in the response of bipolar depression to antidepressants have been reported but this area has received very little systematic attention. One study observed that women were more likely than men to develop rapid cycling upon antidepressant exposure (Yildiz and Sachs, 2003). A prospective evaluation of 26 bipolar patients who received an antidepressant for a depressive episode and 56 who did not found that female gender and past antidepressant-related manic switch predicted development of dysphoria, irritability, and middle insomnia (El-Mallakh *et al.*, 2008). Two other studies, however, suggested there may not be gender differences in rates of development of antidepressant-associated manic switch (Frye *et al.*, 2009; Truman *et al.*, 2007). Further research into possible gender differences in the response of bipolar depression to antidepressants is greatly needed.

16.7.6   PHARMACOTHERAPY OF BIPOLARITY DURING PREGNANCY

When deciding whether or not to use pharmacotherapy for women with bipolar disorder who wish to conceive or who already are pregnant, the risk that a psychotropic medication may harm the fetus must be balanced with the risk that untreated bipolar disorder may harm both the pregnant woman and the fetus (ACOG Committee on

Practice Bulletins – Obstetrics, 2008; Altshuler *et al.*, 1996; Arnold, 2003; Cohen and Rosenbaum, 1998; Freeman *et al.*, 2002; Nguyen, Sharma, and McIntyre, 2009; Viguera and Cohen, 1998; Yonkers *et al.*, 2004). Specific risks to the offspring from prenatal exposure to psychotropic drugs include major and minor congenital malformations, neonatal syndromes, and neurobehavioral toxicity (see below). Conversely, psychopathology during pregnancy may be associated with adverse effects on offspring. Maternal depressive symptoms during pregnancy have been associated with preterm delivery, low birth weight, and developmental delay, though findings are inconsistent (Yonkers *et al.*, 2009). Thus, active bipolarity during pregnancy may have long-term deleterious effects on the infant. Indeed, community data show women with bipolar disorder have an increased risk of low birth weight, preterm, and small-for-gestational age birth outcomes than women without mental illness (Lee and Lin, 2010).

As reviewed earlier, discontinuation of stable maintenance mood stabilizer regimens increases the risk of relapse in pregnant women with bipolar I and II disorder, and the risk of relapse is even higher in women who discontinue such regimens abruptly (that is, in less than two weeks) and in women with certain illness factors (that is, four or more prior mood episodes, duration of illness ≥ 5 years, early age of onset, and bipolar II subtype) (Viguera *et al.*, 2000a, 2007b). In other words, lithium and mood stabilizers in general have been shown to be effective in preventing mood episodes in bipolar women who are pregnant. In addition, a small study found continuing lamotrigine was more effective than discontinuing all mood stabilizer therapy for preventing new episodes during pregnancy (Newport *et al.*, 2008). As lamotrigine might not be associated with increased teratogenic risks (see below), this agent is a viable option to discontinuation of all medications. Finally, repeated mood episodes, including those associated with discontinuation of stable maintenance mood stabilizer regimens, may lead to chronicity, treatment resistance, and suicide in the mother (Post *et al.*, 1992; Maj, 2000; Tondo, Baldessarini, and Floris, 2001). Thus, for those women with more severe forms of bipolar disorder, discontinuing effective mood stabilizer therapy for reasons related to pregnancy may not be a viable option.

16.7.7   TERATOGENESIS OF ANTIBIPOLAR AGENTS

Initial retrospective data suggested that fetal exposure to lithium was associated with a 400-fold increase in congenital heart disease, particularly Ebstein's anomaly (ACOG Committee on Practice Bulletins - Obstetrics, 2008). However, a subsequent meta-analysis estimated the risk ratio for cardiac malformations to be 1.2–7.7 and the risk ratio for overall congenital malformations to be 1.5–3 (Cohen *et al.*, 1994). Moreover, the absolute risk with lithium exposure remains low (one in 1000 births or 0.1%) (Altshuler *et al.*, 1996; Cohen *et al.*, 1994).

Prenatal exposure to valproate is associated with a 1–3.8% risk of neural tube defects, with a corresponding dose-response relationship (ACOG Committee on Practice Bulletins – Obstetrics, 2008). Other congenital malformations associated with valproate exposure include craniofacial, limb, and cardiovascular anomalies. A "fetal valproate syndrome" has also been described, characterized by inhibited fetal growth, facial dysmorphology, and limb and heart defects (DiLiberti *et al.*, 1984).

It is unclear whether prenatal exposure to carbamazepine increases the risk of neural tube defects or other major congenital malformations (ACOG Committee on Practice Bulletins - Obstetrics, 2008). In a large prospective study of 3607 pregnant women with epilepsy, carbamazepine monotherapy was associated with the lowest risk of major congenital malformations (2.2%) (Morrow *et al.*, 2006).

A committee assembled by the American Academy of Neurology and the American Epilepsy Society recently reassessed the evidence of antiepileptic drug teratogenicity, restricting their analysis to studies that accounted for confounding by maternal age and socioeconomic status (Harden *et al.*, 2009a). Women taking antiepileptics for conditions other than epilepsy, however, were not included. This committee concluded that: (i) it was highly probable that first-trimester intrauterine exposure to valproate had a higher risk of major congenital malformations compared to carbamazepine and (ii) it was probable that valproate as part of polytherapy and possible as monotherapy contributed to the development of major congenital malformations (page 1237).

It is not established that lamotrigine increases the risk for major congenital malformations above the baseline rate, except possibly at doses above 200 mg/day (Morrow *et al.*, 2006). The pooled risk of reported major fetal anomalies following first trimester exposure to lamotrigine was recently estimated to be 2.6% (Newport *et al.*, 2008). Malformations associated with gestational exposure to lamotrigine include oral cleft (that is, cleft lip, cleft palate), hypospadias, and gastrointestinal defects (Morrow *et al.*, 2006).

To date, no definitive association has been found between the use of first or second generation antipsychotics during pregnancy and an increased risk of major malformations (Coppola *et al.*, 2007; Einarson and Boskovic, 2009; Ernst and Goldberg, 2002; McKenna *et al.*, 2005). However, the general paucity of information and lack of large, well designed prospective trials warrants further investigation into the reproductive safety of these agents.

16.7.8 NEONATAL SYNDROMES

The most recognized neonatal syndrome associated with in utero lithium exposure is "floppy baby syndrome," characterized by hypotonicity, cyanosis, and lethargy (Schou and Amdisen, 1975; Woody, London, and Wilbanks, 1971). Fetal and neonatal hypothyroidism, nontoxic goiter, nephrogenic diabetes insipidus, hypoglycemia, cardiac murmurs, arrhythmias, polyhydramnios, and respiratory distress have also been reported with late gestational lithium exposure (ACOG Committee on Practice Bulletins - Obstetrics, 2008; Arnold, 2003). An analysis of 32 cases in which maternal lithium was administered throughout delivery found lower Apgar scores, longer hospital stays, and higher rates of central nervous system (CNS) and neuromuscular complications in infants with higher lithium concentrations at delivery (>0.064 meq/l) (Newport *et al.*, 2005). It is therefore recommended that lithium therapy be suspended 24–48 hours before a scheduled Cesarean section or at the onset of labor and reinstated as soon as the patient is medically stabilized post delivery.

Neonatal toxicity associated with valproate includes heart rate decelerations; withdrawal symptoms of irritability, feeding difficulties, and abnormal tone; liver toxicity;

coagulopathies; and hypoglycemia (ACOG Committee on Practice Bulletins - Obstetrics, 2008; Yonkers *et al.*, 2004). Carbamazepine has been associated with transient hepatotoxicity (Yonkers *et al.*, 2004). The American Academy of Neurology and the American Epilepsy Society concluded that neonates of women with epilepsy taking antiepileptics have an increased risk of being small for gestational age and possibly have an increased risk of a 1-minute Apgar score of <7, which is about twice the risk of normal (Harden *et al.*, 2009a).

In a prospective observational study of 54 pregnant women, significant differences in the placental passage rates of four antipsychotics were found, with olanzapine the highest, quetiapine the lowest, and haloperidol and risperidone intermediate (Newport *et al.*, 2007). There were tendencies toward higher rates of lower birth weight (38%) and neonatal intensive care unit admissions among neonates exposed to olanzapine. Clozapine has been associated with floppy infant syndrome and neonatal seizures (DiMichele, Ramenghi, and Sabatino, 1996; Stoner *et al.*, 1997). Self-limited extrapyramidal effects and a withdrawal syndrome of tremor, jitteriness, irritability, feeding problems, and somnolence has been reported with risperidone (Coppola *et al.*, 2007).

16.7.9   NEUROBEHAVIORAL DEFICITS

Lithium has not yet been associated with any reports of significant postnatal behavioral sequelae. In one study, 60 infants who were exposed to lithium in utero and born without malformations "had gone through a normal development, both physically and mentally" at a rate comparable to that of 57 unexposed siblings (Schou, 1976). In contrast, growing evidence indicates gestational exposure to valproate is associated with neurobehavioral toxicity (Nguyen, Sharma, and McIntyre, 2009). Children exposed to valproate in utero are more likely to show verbal IQ deficits (Adab *et al.*, 2004; Gaily *et al.*, 2004) and require special education (Adab *et al.*, 2001). There have also been reports linking prenatal valproate exposure with features of autism spectrum disorder (Rasalam *et al.*, 2005; Williams and Hersh, 1997). Data regarding developmental delay for carbamazepine are mixed. While several studies evaluating school children exposed in utero to carbamazepine did not identify a significant increase in neurobehavioral deficits when compared with the control group, two separate independent investigations found that fetal carbamazepine exposure was associated with a variable degree of development delay (Holmes *et al.*, 2005; Jones *et al.*, 1989). The American Academy of Neurology and the American Epilepsy Society recently concluded that in the gestationally exposed offspring of women with epilepsy, valproate was probably associated with poor cognitive outcomes compared with unexposed controls while carbamazepine was not (Harden *et al.*, 2009a).

16.7.10   TERATOGENESIS FOR OTHER TREATMENTS

The safety of antidepressants in pregnancy is described in detail elsewhere (Gorman, 2006; Yonkers *et al.*, 2009). On the whole, use of tricyclics and SSRIs in early pregnancy is not associated with an increased risk of structural malformations. However, associations between gestational SSRI use and craniosynostosis, omphalocele, and heart defects have been reported, though the absolute risks are small (Louik *et al.*, 2007). Neurobehavioral deficits have rarely been reported in studies of in-utero exposure to SSRIs (Gentile, 2010). Teratogenic effects unique to the combination of olanzapine and fluoxetine, which is indicated for acute bipolar depression, have not yet been described (Nguyen, Sharma, and McIntyre, 2009).

Electroconvulsive therapy (ECT), which is highly effective for bipolar manic, depressive, and mixed states, has not consistently been associated with deleterious effects in pregnant women or neonates (Ferrill, Kehoe, and Jacisin, 1992; Miller, 1994; Yonkers *et al.*, 2004). Although more data are needed, ECT should presently be viewed as a safe and effective treatment for bipolarity during pregnancy, especially for severe or life-threatening mood and psychotic episodes.

16.7.11   GENERAL GUIDELINES

Pregnancy and medication risks should be discussed with all females with bipolar disorder of child bearing potential regardless of their immediate plans for pregnancy. Based on the particular features of a woman's bipolarity, an individualized treatment plan can be developed that promotes the woman's health and minimizes fetal exposure to potential teratogens (Altshuler *et al.*, 1996; Arnold, 2003; Cohen and Rosenbaum, 1998; Freeman *et al.*, 2002; Viguera and Cohen, 1998; Yonkers *et al.*, 2004). Thus, women with mild bipolarity (for example, one past hypomanic or manic episode and long periods of affective stability) may elect to gradually taper and discontinue medication prior to conception because of their relatively low risk of relapse (Tohen, Waternaux, and Tsuang, 1990). Women with moderate bipolarity (for example, two to three episodes of hypomania, mania, or depression, and relative interepisode euthymia) may also choose to taper and discontinue medication(s) prior to conception. However, as the risk of relapse is greater in these women, they may elect to continue pharmacotherapy until early confirmation of pregnancy, prolonging the time of prophylaxis. Once a woman is pregnant, a medication can be tapered in the two weeks prior to the establishment of the placental-fetal circulation, before the fetus is vulnerable to teratogens (Arnold, 2003; Viguera and Cohen, 1998). Because this strategy requires a more rapid medication taper it increases the risk of relapse. However, pharmacotherapy can be instituted for any recurrence of clinically significant symptoms. Women with severe or unstable bipolarity (for example, illness duration ≥5 years, 4 or more mood episodes, and/or clinically significant subsyndromal symptoms) have a high rate of relapse, and the risks to the mother and fetus from the disorder may exceed the risks of psychotropic exposure to the fetus. Many of these women may not be able to safely discontinue pharmacotherapy during pregnancy.

If pharmacotherapy during pregnancy is to be pursued, several general steps may reduce risk to the fetus. Using the lowest effective dose of any medication and limiting the number of medications decreases fetal exposure. Folate supplementation before and during pregnancy has been shown to reduce the risk of neural tube defects (MRC Vitamin Study Research Group, 1991). Although folate has not been proven to prevent neural tube defects or other major congenital malformations in women receiving anticonvulsants, it is often recommended that women who elect to continue anticonvulsants during pregnancy take folate (at least 0.4 mg/day) starting at least four weeks before conception (if they are not already doing so) and continue through week 12 of pregnancy (Altshuler et al., 1996; Ernst and Goldberg, 2002; Harden et al., 2009b; Yonkers et al., 2004). Women who have taken mood stabilizers during the first trimester have the option of receiving a high resolution ultrasound and fetal echocardiogram at 18–20 weeks gestation to detect cardiac abnormalities, and an ultrasound at 16–19 weeks gestation to detect neural tube defects, followed, if necessary, by amniocentesis for detection of spina bifida (Altshuler et al., 1996; Arnold, 2003; Cohen et al., 1994; Ernst and Goldberg, 2002; Viguera and Cohen, 1998).

Mood stabilizers should be monitored when taken during pregnancy. Lithium levels may fall because of enhanced renal clearance. Lamotrigine and carbamazine levels may fall because of increased metabolic clearance (Harden et al., 2009b).

16.7.12 PHARMACOTHERAPY OF BIPOLARITY DURING THE POSTPARTUM AND LACTATION

Prophylactic treatment with lithium has been shown to substantially reduce the risk of recurrence of mood and psychotic episodes during the postpartum (Austin, 1992; Chaudron and Pies, 2003; Cohen et al., 1995; Stewart et al., 1991). (A single-blind, nonrandomized trial, however, found divalproex plus symptom monitoring was not superior to monitoring without drug for preventing postpartum mood episodes in 26 bipolar women (Wisner et al., 2004)). Because of the extremely high risk for relapse during the postpartum, prophylaxis with mood stabilizers thought to be effective for the individual patient is generally recommended for the postpartum woman with bipolar disorder.

When weighing the risks and benefits of breast-feeding in women with bipolar disorder, the most important consideration is the health of the mother and infant (Arnold, 2003; Yonkers et al., 2004). Maternal postpartum illness has an adverse effect on both mother and developing infant. Although breast-feeding has many benefits for the infant and is encouraged by the American Academy of Pediatrics, no psychotropic drugs are known to be absolutely safe for the breast-feeding infant, and the sleep loss associated with breast feeding can be detrimental to the bipolar mother (Arnold, 2003; Llewellyn and Stowe, 1998; Suri et al., 1999). Bottle-feeding with formula is an obvious alternative.

There are limited data about the use of antibipolar agents while breast-feeding (Burt and Rasgon, 2004; Stowe, 2007). The concentration of lithium in the serum of nursing infants is approximately one-tenth to one-half the mother's serum concentration (Schou and Amdisen, 1973; Sykes, Quarrie, and Alexander, 1976). A recent study of 10 nursing mother-infant pairs found that infant serum contained about one-quarter the concentration of lithium in maternal serum (Viguera et al., 2007a). Because of reports of high lithium levels and symptoms of toxicity in some, but not all, nursing infants (Sykes, Quarrie, and Alexander, 1976; Tunnessen and Hertz, 1972), the American Academy of Pediatrics Committee on Drugs (2001), which had once stated lithium was contraindicated during breast feeding, now recommends that it "should be given to nursing mothers with caution." Laboratory monitoring should include assays of infant serum lithium and TSH, blood urea nitrogen, and creatinine levels (Stowe, 2007; Viguera *et al.*, 2007a).

Valproate serum concentrations in nurslings have ranged from 0.9 to 40% of maternal serum concentrations (Wisner and Perel, 1998). Valproate has not yet been associated with adverse effects in nursing infants, but data are limited and hepatotoxicity is a theoretical risk (Piontek *et al.*, 2000; Suri *et al.*, 1999). Carbamazepine serum concentrations in nursing infants have ranged from 15 to 65% of maternal serum concentrations (Wisner and Perel, 1998). Carbamazepine has been associated with cholestatic hepatitis (Frey, Schubiger, and Musy, 1990), and elevated gamma-glutamyltransferase (GGT) and direct bilirubin levels in nursing infants (Merlob, Mor, and Litwin, 1992). The American Academy of Pediatrics Committee on Drugs (2001) considers both valproate and carbamazepine as "usually compatible" with breast-feeding. In addition, the American Academy of Neurology and the American Epilepsy Society recently concluded that valproate and carbamazepine probably were not transferred into breast milk in clinically important amounts (Harden *et al.*, 2009b).

Serum levels of lamotrigine in nurslings have ranged from 18 to 30% of maternal serum concentrations (Newport *et al.*, 2008; Ohman, Vitols, and Tomson, 2000; Stowe, 2007). In a study of 30 lamotrigine-treated women and their breastfed infants, mild thrombocytosis was present in seven of eight infants at the time of serum sampling, and no other adverse events were reported or observed (Newport *et al.*, 2008). A review of 16 other mother/nursling pairs found no adverse events (Stowe, 2007). It has been suggested that lamotrigine-exposed nurslings be monitored for rash and liver enzyme elevations (Stowe, 2007)

Information is also limited about use of antipsychotics and antidepressants during breast feeding. Of 20 reports of nurslings exposed to olanzapine, 4 described adverse events. These included jaundice, sedation, cardiomegaly, and a heart murmur; shaking, poor suckling, and lethargy; protruding tongue; and rash, diarrhea, and a sleeping disorder (Ernst and Goldberg, 2002). In a recent review of 27 mother/infant pairs exposed to olanzapine ($N = 16$), quetiapine ($N = 7$), or risperidone ($N = 4$), no adverse events were reported (Stowe, 2007). Regarding typical antipsychotics, one nursling exposed to chlorpromazine was drowsy and lethargic for an unspecified amount of time, whereas nine others had no adverse effects (Suri *et al.*, 1999). Adverse effects reported in nurslings exposed to antidepressants have been reviewed elsewhere (Lanza di Scalea and Wisner, 2009; Weissman *et al.*, 2004). The American Academy of Pediatrics Committee on Drugs (2001) has classified antidepressants as "drugs whose effects on nursing infants is unknown but may be of concern."

Currently, there are no formal guidelines for monitoring of the nursing infant exposed to antibipolar agents (Stowe, 2007). Because of the limited information about the risks of exposure to psychotropics in general through breast milk, careful monitoring of the infant is required and nursing should be discontinued immediately if an adverse event is suspected in the infant. The nursling's drug exposure might be minimized by the mother limiting the number of medications, using the lowest effective dose, and by taking her medication just after she has breast-fed and before the infant has a lengthy sleep period (American Academy of Pediatrics Committee on Drugs, 2001).

16.7.13   USE OF HORMONAL AGENTS IN WOMEN WITH BIPOLAR DISORDER

Very few controlled data regarding the use of hormonal treatments in women with bipolar disorder are available. Several small placebo-controlled trials suggest the estrogen receptor antagonist tamoxifen is effective in bipolar mania (Kulkarni *et al.*, 2006; Yildiz *et al.*, 2008; Zarate *et al.*, 2007). Estrogen has been found effective for depressive disorders in perimenopausal women (Soares *et al.*, 2001). The induction of mania (Zohar *et al.*, 1985) and rapid cycling (Oppenheim, 1984) have been reported with the use of exogenous estrogen, further supporting the possibility that estrogen may have an antidepressant effect in some women. Moreover, as mentioned earlier, one retrospective study suggested HRT in menopausal bipolar women might protect against depressive symptoms (Freeman *et al.*, 2002). However, there are three case reports of mood stabilization with a combination of estrogen and progesterone in women with bipolar disorder; one of these cases was for treatment-refracting post-partum mania (Chouinard, Steinberg, and Steiner, 1987; Huang, Wang, and Chan, 2008).

Available data on oral contraceptives in female bipolarity are equivocal. In a retrospective review of 33 bipolar women who had used oral contraceptives, 22 (67%) reported either not having (N = 17) or not recalling mood changes (N = 5), 4(12%) reported improved mood symptoms, and 7 (21%) reported worsened mood symptoms associated with oral contraceptive use (Freeman *et al.*, 2002). In a prospective study of menstrual cycle related mood changes in 17 bipolar women, women taking oral contraceptives (N = 6) did not have significant mood changes across the menstrual cycle while those not taking oral contraceptives (N = 11) did (Rasgon *et al.*, 2003). Of note, progesterone was ineffective in the treatment of postpartum mania in one woman (Meakin and Brockington, 1990).

Interactions of antibipolar agents with oral contraceptives are a major concern for the bipolar woman of childbearing age. Carbamazepine strongly induces the metabolism of oral contraceptives via the hepatic cytochrome P450 (CYP) 3A4 enzyme system, hence lowering the efficacy of this method of birth control and increasing the risk of contraceptive failure (Spina, Pisani, and Perucca, 1996; Sabers, 2008). Lithium, valproate, lamotrigine, and second generation antipsychotics generally do not interfere with the metabolism or effectiveness of oral contraceptives (Elwes and Binnie, 1996; Shenfield, 1993). However, estrogen-containing oral contraceptives may reduce the plasma levels and effects of antiepileptic drugs cleared by glucuronidation, such as lamotrigine and valproate (Christensen *et al.*, 2007; Sabers, 2008).

16.7.14   EVALUATION OF WOMEN FOR AND WITH BIPOLARITY

A complete assessment of bipolarity in females includes a psychiatric and medical history, family and social history, and mental status exam with a focus on mood, psychotic, anxiety, substance use, and eating disorder signs, and symptoms (Arnold, 2003). Because female bipolarity frequently presents as depression, comorbid Axis I disorders, Axis II personality disorders, behavioral dysregulation (including hypersexuality), or general medical disorders (for example, migraine or other types of pain, overweight, or obesity), it is important to carefully evaluate for a history of hypomania or mania, including subthreshold hypomanic symptoms, in females with these presentations (Benazzi, 2001; Benazzi and Akiskal, 2003). Because patients often have difficulty identifying or recognizing hypomania, the use of structured clinical interviews, such as the Structured Clinical Interview for DSM-IV (SCID) (First *et al.*, 2001), and screening instruments, such as the MDQ (Hirschfeld *et al.*, 2000) or the Hypomania Symptom Checklist (Angst *et al.*, 2003), in combination with consultation of a significant other (with the patient's permission), will improve the identification of bipolarity, particularly "soft" or "occult" forms.

When indicated, the medical evaluation of female bipolarity includes a physical examination, weight and vital signs, various laboratory tests (for example, thyroid function tests, glucose and lipid screening profiles), and toxicology screen. General medical disorders to be considered include endocrine disorders (for example, thyroid disease, PCOS), neurological disorders (for example, multiple sclerosis, stroke), immunological diseases (for example, systemic lupus erythematosis), infectious diseases (e.g., HIV/AIDS), and metabolic disorders (for example, porphyurias, vitamin deficiencies). Medications that may cause or worsen mood symptoms in females include antidepressants, stimulants, drugs of abuse, corticosteroids, oral contraceptives and other hormonal agents, antihypertensives, and benzodiazepines. Menstrual and reproductive history should be reviewed, and a history of any menstrual, pregnancy, postpartum, or menopausal-related psychiatric symptoms should be determined. History of hormonal treatments and their effects on mood should also be assessed. Finally, a discussion of plans about contraception and pregnancy is critical in reproductive-aged females, especially since evidence suggests women treated for bipolar disorder may use contraceptive methods suboptimally (Magalhaes, Kapczinski, and Kauer-Sant'Anna, 1999). Careful family planning should be advised as planned pregnancies maximize treatment options.

16.8 SUMMARY

Although mania and hypomania are equally prevalent in women and men, female bipolarity differs from male bipolarity in several important ways. Considerable evidence suggests women with bipolar disorder experience depressive symptoms, suicide attempts, mixed states, and rapid cycling more often than men with bipolar disorder. Although less well studied, bipolar women may be more likely than bipolar men to have atypical depression. Comorbidity with certain psychiatric and general medical disorders, especially anxiety disorders, eating disorders, migraine, and thyroid disease, may be more common in women than men, and this comorbidity may adversely affect the course of bipolar disorder in women. While substance use disorders are more common in bipolar men than bipolar women, women with bipolar disorder are at higher risk for alcohol use disorders than are men with bipolar disorder. Thus, in addition to a depressive diathesis, female bipolarity may be characterized by mixity, cyclicity, atypicality, and psychiatric and medical comorbidity.

Although women may be susceptible to delayed diagnosis and treatment, there is no evidence that gender affects response to mood stabilizers. Gender differences in response of bipolar disorder to antidepressants have not been evaluated except for the observation that women may be more likely to develop rapid cycling. Pregnancy neither worsens nor exacerbates bipolar disorder, but the postpartum is a period of high risk for onset and recurrence of bipolar disorder in women. Bipolar mood symptoms may also worsen in relation to the menstrual cycle and the perimenopause and menopause in some women. Treatment of bipolarity in women during pregnancy and lactation is challenging because available mood stabilizers pose potential risks to the developing fetus and infant. Individualized risk/benefit assessments of pregnant and postpartum women with bipolar disorder are required to promote the health of the woman and fetus and limit exposure of the fetus or infant to potential adverse effects of medication.

References

Abrams, R. and Taylor, M.A. (1974) Unipolar mania: a preliminary report. *Arch. Gen. Psychiatry*, **30**, 441–443.

ACOG Committee on Practice Bulletins – Obstetrics (2008) ACOG Practice Bulletin: Clinical management guidelines for obstetrician-gynecologists number 92, April 2008 (replaces practice bulletin number 87, November 2007). Use of psychiatric medications during pregnancy and lactation. *Obstet. Gynecol.*, **111**, 1001–1020.

Adab, N., Jacoby, A., Smith, D., and Chadwick, D. (2001) Additional educational needs in children born to mothers with epilepsy. *J. Neurol. Neurosurg. Psychiatr.*, **70**, 15–21.

Adab, N., Kini, U., Vinten, J. *et al.* (2004) The longer term outcome of children born to mothers with epilepsy. *J. Neurol. Neurosurg. Psychiatr.*, **75**, 1575–1583.

Aichhorn, W., Whitworth, A.B., Weiss, E.M., and Marksteiner, J. (2006) Second-generation antipsychotics: is there evidence for sex differences in pharmacokinetic and adverse effect profiles? *Drug Saf.*, **29**, 587–598.

Akdeniz, F., Taneli, F., Noyan, A. *et al.* (2003) Valproate-associated reproductive and metabolic abnormalities: are epileptic women at greater risk than bipolar women? *Prog. Neuropsychopharmacol. Biol. Psychiatry*, **27**, 115–121.

Akiskal, H.S., Hantouche, E.G., Allilaire, J.F. *et al.* (2003) Validating antidepressant-associated hypomania (bipolar III): a systematic comparison with spontaneous hypomania (bipolar II). *J. Affect. Disord.*, **73**, 65–74.

Akiskal, H.S., Hantouche, E.G., Bourgeois, M.L. *et al.* (1998) Gender, temperament, and the clinical picture in dysphoric mixed mania: findings from a French national study (EPIMAN). *J. Affect. Disord.*, **50**, 175–186.

Altshuler, L.L., Bauer, M., Frye, M.A. *et al.* (2001) Does thyroid supplementation accelerate tricyclic antidepressant response? A review and meta-analysis of the literature. *Am. J. Psychiatry*, **158**, 1617–1622.

Altshuler, L.L., Cohen, L., Szuba, M.P. *et al.* (1996) Pharmacologic management of psychiatric illness during pregnancy: dilemmas and guidelines. *Am. J. Psychiatry*, **153**, 592–606.

Altshuler, L.L., Kupka, R.W., Helleman, G. *et al.* (2010) Gender and depressive symptoms in 711 patients with bipolar disorder evaluated prospectively in the Stanley Foundation Bipolar Treatment Network. *Psychiatry*, **167**, 708–715.

Altshuler, L.L., Post, R.M., Leverich, G.S. *et al.* (1995) Antidepressant-induced mania and cycle acceleration: a controversy revisited. *Am. J. Psychiatry*, **152**, 1130–1138.

Altshuler, L., Suppes, T., Black, D. *et al.* (2003) Impact of antidepressant discontinuation after acute bipolar depression remission on rates of depressive relapse at 1-year follow-up. *Am. J. Psychiatry*, **160**, 1252–1262.

American Academy of Pediatrics Committee on Drugs (2001) Transfer of drugs and other chemicals into human milk. *Pediatrics*, **108**, 776–789.

Angst, J. (1978) The course of affective disorders. II. Typology of bipolar manic-depressive illness. *Arch. Psychiatr. Nervenkr.*, **226**, 65–73.

Angst, J. (1998) The emerging epidemiology of hypomania and bipolar II disorder. *J. Affect. Disord.*, **50**, 143–151.

Angst, J., Gamma, A., Benazzi, F. *et al.* (2003) Toward a re-definition of subthreshold bipolarity: epidemiology and proposed criteria for bipolar-II, minor bipolar disorders and hypomania. *J. Affect. Disord.*, **73**, 133–146.

Angst, J. and Sellaro, R. (2000) Historical perspectives and natural history of bipolar disorder. *Biol. Psychiatry*, **48**, 445–457.

Arnold, L.M. (2003) Gender differences in bipolar disorder. *Psychiatr. Clin. North Am.*, **26**, 595–620.

Arnold, L.M., McElroy, S.L., and Keck, P.E. Jr. (2000) The role of gender in mixed mania. *Compr. Psychiatry*, **41**, 83–87.

Askinazi, C., Weintraub, R.J., and Karamouz, N. (1986) Elderly depressed females as a possible subgroup of patients responsive to methylphenidate. *J. Clin. Psychiatry*, **47**, 467–469.

Austin, M.P. (1992) Puerperal affective psychosis: is there a case for lithium prophylaxis? *Br. J. Psychiatry*, **161**, 692–694.

Baldassano, C.F., Marangell, L.B., Gyulai, L. *et al.* (2005) Gender differences in bipolar disorder: retrospective data from the first 500 STEP-BD participants. *Bipolar Disord.*, **7**, 465–470.

Baldessarini, R.J., Hennen, J., Wilson, M. *et al.* (2003) Olanzapine versus placebo in acute mania: treatment responses in subgroups. *J. Clin. Psychopharmacol.*, **23**, 370–376.

Baldessarini, R.J., Tondo, L., and Hennen, J. (1999) Treatment delays in bipolar disorders. *Am. J. Psychiatry*, **156**, 811–812.

Baldessarini, R.J., Tondo, L., Floris, G., and Rudas, N. (1997) Reduced morbidity after gradual discontinuation of lithium treatment for bipolar I and II disorders: a replication study. *Am. J. Psychiatry*, **154**, 551–553.

Bauer, M.S., Whybrow, P.C., and Winokur, A. (1990) Rapid cycling bipolar affective disorder. I. Association with grade I hypothyroidism. *Arch. Gen. Psychiatry*, **47**, 427–432.

Bellivier, F., Golmard, J.L., Henry, C. *et al.* (2001) Admixture analysis of age at onset in bipolar I affective disorder. *Arch. Gen. Psychiatry*, **58**, 510–512.

Benazzi, F. (1997) Antidepressant-associated hypomania in outpatient depression: a 203-case study in private practice. *J. Affect. Disord.*, **46**, 73–77.

Benazzi, F. (2001) Sensitivity and specificity of clinical markers for the diagnosis of bipolar II disorder. *Compr. Psychiatry*, **42**, 461–465.

Benazzi, F. (2003) The role of gender in depressive mixed state. *Psychopathology*, **36**, 213–217.

Benazzi, F. (2006) Gender differences in bipolar-II disorder. *Eur. Arch. Psychiatry Clin. Neurosci.*, **256**, 67–71.

Benazzi, F. (2008) Reviewing the diagnostic validity and utility of mixed depression (depressive mixed states). *Eur. Psychiatry*, **23**, 40–48.

Benazzi, F. and Akiskal, H.S. (2003) Refining the evaluation of bipolar II: beyond the strict SCID-CV guidelines for hypomania. *J. Affect. Disord.*, **73**, 33–38.

Berghofer, A., Kossmann, B., and Muller-Oerlinghausen, B. (1996) Course of illness and pattern of recurrences in patients with affective disorders during long-term lithium prophylaxis: a retrospective analysis over 15 years. *Acta Psychiatr. Scand.*, **93**, 349–354.

Black, D.W., Winokur, G., Bell, S. *et al.* (1988a) Complicated mania. Comorbidity and immediate outcome in the treatment of mania. *Arch. Gen. Psychiatry*, **45**, 232–236.

Black, D.W., Winokur, G., Hulbert, J., and Nasrallah, A. (1988b) Predictors of immediate response in the treatment of mania: the importance of comorbidity. *Biol. Psychiatry*, **24**, 191–198.

Blehar, M.C., DePaulo, J.R. Jr., Gershon E.S. *et al.* (1998) Women with bipolar disorder: findings from the NIMH Genetics Initiative sample. *Psychopharmacol. Bull.*, **34**, 239–243.

Bowden, C.L., Calabrese, J.R., McElroy, S.L. *et al.* (1999) The efficacy of lamotrigine in rapid cycling and non-rapid cycling patients with bipolar disorder. *Biol. Psychiatry*, **45**, 953–958.

Boyd, J.H., Burke, J.D. Jr., Gruenberg, E. *et al.* (1984) Exclusion criteria of DSM-III. A study of co-occurrence of hierarchy-free syndromes. *Arch. Gen. Psychiatry*, **41**, 983–989.

Breslau, N., Merikangas, K., and Bowden, C.L. (1994) Comorbidity of migraine and major affective disorders. *Neurology*, **44**, S17–S22.

Burt, V.K. and Rasgon, N. (2004) Special considerations in treating bipolar disorder in women. *Bipolar Disord.*, **6**, 2–13 (Review).

Byerly, M., Suppes, T., Tran, Q.V., and Baker, R.A. (2007) Clinical implications of antipsychotic-induced hyperprolactinemia in patients with schizophrenia spectrum or bipolar spectrum disorders: recent developments and current perspectives. *J. Clin. Psychopharmacol.*, **27**, 639–661.

Calabrese, J.R. and Delucchi, G.A. (1990) Spectrum of efficacy of valproate in 55 patients with rapid-cycling bipolar disorder. *Am. J. Psychiatry*, **147**, 431–434.

Calabrese, J.R., Hirschfeld, R.M., Reed, M. *et al.* (2003) Impact of bipolar disorder on a U.S. community sample. *J. Clin. Psychiatry*, **64**, 425–432.

Calabrese, J.R., Rapport, D.J., Kimmel, S.E., and Shelton, M.D. (1999) Controlled trials in bipolar I depression: focus on switch rates and efficacy. *Eur. Neuropsychopharmacol.*, **9** (Suppl. 4), S109–S112.

Calabrese, J.R., Shelton, M.D., Bowden, C.L. *et al.* (2001) Bipolar rapid cycling: focus on depression as its hallmark. *J. Clin. Psychiatry*, **62** (Suppl. 14), 34–41.

Cassidy, F. and Carroll, B.J. (2001) The clinical epidemiology of pure and mixed manic episodes. *Bipolar Disord.*, **3**, 35–40.

Chaudron, L.H. and Pies, R.W. (2003) The relationship between postpartum psychosis and bipolar disorder: a review. *J. Clin. Psychiatry*, **64**, 1284–1292.

Chen, Y.W. and Dilsaver, S.C. (1995) Comorbidity of panic disorder in bipolar illness: evidence from the Epidemiologic Catchment Area Survey. *Am. J. Psychiatry*, **152**, 280–282.

Chen, Y.W. and Dilsaver, S.C. (1996) Lifetime rates of suicide attempts among subjects with bipolar and unipolar disorders relative to subjects with other Axis I disorders. *Biol. Psychiatry*, **39**, 896–899.

Chouinard, G., Steinberg, S., and Steiner, W. (1987) Estrogen-progesterone combination: another mood stabilizer? *Am. J. Psychiatry*, **144**, 826.

Christensen, E.M., Gjerris, A., Larsen, J.K. *et al.* (2003) Life events and onset of a new phase in bipolar affective disorder. *Bipolar Disord.*, **5**, 356–361.

Christensen, J., Petrenaite, V., Atterman, J. *et al.* (2007) Oral contraceptives induce lamotrigine metabolism: evidence from a double-blind, placebo-controlled trial. *Epilepsia*, **48**, 484–489.

Cohen, L.S., Friedman, J.M., Jefferson, J.W. *et al.* (1994) A reevaluation of risk of in utero exposure to lithium. *J. Am. Med. Assoc.*, **271**, 146–150.

Cohen, L.S. and Rosenbaum, J.F. (1998) Psychotropic drug use during pregnancy: weighing the risks. *J. Clin. Psychiatry*, **59** (Suppl. 2), 18–28.

Cohen, L.S., Sichel, D.A., Robertson, L.M. *et al.* (1995) Postpartum prophylaxis for women with bipolar disorder. *Am. J. Psychiatry*, **152**, 1641–1645.

Cole, D.P., Thase, M.E., Mallinger, A.G. *et al.* (2002) Slower treatment response in bipolar depression predicted by lower pretreatment thyroid function. *Am. J. Psychiatry*, **159**, 116–121.

Conrad, C.D. and Hamilton, J.A. (1986) Recurrent premenstrual decline in serum lithium concentration: clinical correlates and treatment implications. *J. Am. Acad. Child Psychiatry*, **25**, 852–853.

Coppen, A., Whybrow, P.C., Noguera, R. *et al.* (1972) The comparative antidepressant value of L-tryptophan and imipramine with and without attempted potentiation by liothyronine. *Arch. Gen. Psychiatry*, **26**, 234–241.

Coppola, D., Russo, L.J., Kwarta, R.F. Jr. *et al.* (2007) Evaluating the postmarketing experience of risperidone use during pregnancy: pregnancy and neonatal outcomes. *Drug Saf.*, **30**, 247–264.

Coryell, W., Endicott, J. and Keller, M. (1992) Rapidly cycling affective disorder. Demographics, diagnosis, family history, and course. *Arch. Gen. Psychiatry*, **49**, 126–131.

Coryell, W., Solomon, D., Turvey, C. *et al.* (2003) The long-term course of rapid-cycling bipolar disorder. *Arch. Gen. Psychiatry*, **60**, 914–920.

Coyle, N., Jones, I., Robertson, E. *et al.* (2000) Variation at the serotonin transporter gene influences susceptibility to bipolar affective puerperal psychosis. *Lancet*, **356**, 1490–1491.

D'Mello, D.A. and McNeil, J.A. (1990) Sex differences in bipolar affective disorder: neuroleptic dosage variance. *Compr. Psychiatry*, **31**, 80–83.

D'Mello, D.A., Pinheiro, A.L., and Lalinec-Michaud, M. (1993) Premenstrual mania: two case reports. *J. Nerv. Ment. Dis.*, **181**, 330–331.

Dallal, A., Fontaine, R., Ontiveros, A., and Elie, R. (1990) Lithium carbonate augmentation of desipramine in refractory depression. *Can. J. Psychiatry*, **35**, 608–611.

Dean, C. and Kendall, R.E. (1981) The symptomatology of puerperal illness. *Br. J. Psychiatry*, **139**, 128–133.

Diamond, S.B., Rubinstein, A.A., Dunner, D.L., and Fieve, R.R. (1976) Menstrual problems in women with primary affective illness. *Compr. Psychiatry*, **17**, 541–548.

DiLiberti, J.H., Farndon, P.A., Dennis, N.R., and Curry, C.J. (1984) The fetal valproate syndrome. *Am. J. Med. Genet.*, **19**, 473–481.

DiMichele, V., Ramenghi, L.A., and Sabatino, G. (1996) Clozapine and lorazepam administration in pregnancy (letter). *Eur. Psychiatry*, **11**, 214.

Dunner, D.L. and Fieve, R.R. (1974) Clinical factors in lithium carbonate prophylaxis failure. *Arch. Gen. Psychiatry*, **30**, 229–233.

Dunner, D.L., Patrick, V., and Fieve, R.R. (1977) Rapid cycling manic depressive patients. *Compr. Psychiatry*, **18**, 561–566.

Einarson, A. and Boskovic, R. (2009) Use and safety of antipsychotic drugs during pregnancy. *J. Psychiatr. Pract.*, **15**, 183–192.

El-Mallakh, R.S., Ghaemi, S.N., Sagduyu, K. *et al.* (2008) Antidepressant-associated chronic irritable dysphoria (ACID) in STEP-BD patients. *J. Affect. Disord.*, **111**, 372–377.

Elmslie, J.L., Silverstone, J.T., Mann, J.I. *et al.* (2000) Prevalence of overweight and obesity in bipolar patients. *J. Clin. Psychiatry*, **61**, 179–184.

Elwes, R.D. and Binnie, C.D. (1996) Clinical pharmacokinetics of newer antiepileptic drugs. Lamotrigine, vigabatrin, gabapentin and oxcarbazepine. *Clin. Pharmacokinet.*, **30**, 403–415.

Endicott, J., Nee, J., Andreasen, N. *et al.* (1985) Bipolar II. Combine or keep separate? *J. Affect. Disord.*, **8**, 17–28.

Ernst, C.L. and Goldberg, J.F. (2002) The reproductive safety profile of mood stabilizers, atypical antipsychotics, and broad-spectrum psychotropics. *J. Clin. Psychiatry*, **63** (Suppl. 4), 42–55.

Faedda, G.L., Tondo, L., Baldessarini, R.J. *et al.* (1993) Outcome after rapid vs gradual discontinuation of lithium treatment in bipolar disorders. *Arch. Gen. Psychiatry*, **50**, 448–455.

Fagiolini, A., Kupfer, D.J., Houck, P.R. *et al.* (2003) Obesity as a correlate of outcome in patients with bipolar I disorder. *Am. J. Psychiatry*, **160**, 112–117.

Ferrill, M.J., Kehoe, W.A., and Jacisin, J.J. (1992) ECT during pregnancy: physiologic and pharmacologic considerations. *Convuls. Ther.*, **8**, 186–200.

First, M.B., Spitzer, R.L., Gibbon, M., and Williams, J.B. (2001) *Structured Clinical Interview for DSM-IV-TR Axis I Disorders, Research Version, Patient Edition (SCID-I/P)*, Biometrics Research Department, New York State Psychiatric Institute, New York.

Forty, L., Jones, L., Macgregor, S. *et al.* (2006) Familiality of postpartum depression in unipolar disorder: results of a family study. *Am. J. Psychiatry*, **163**, 1549–1553.

Frank, E., Cyranowski, J.M., Rucci, P. *et al.* (2002) Clinical significance of lifetime panic spectrum symptoms in the treatment of patients with bipolar I disorder. *Arch. Gen. Psychiatry*, **59**, 905–911.

Freeman, M.P., Smith, K.W., Freeman, S.A. *et al.* (2002) The impact of reproductive events on the course of bipolar disorder in women. *J. Clin. Psychiatry*, **63**, 284–287.

Frey, B., Schubiger, G., and Musy, J.P. (1990) Transient cholestatic hepatitis in a neonate associated with carbamazepine exposure during pregnancy and breast-feeding. *Eur. J. Pediatr.*, **150**, 136–138.

Frye, M.A., Altshuler, L.L., McElroy, S.L. *et al.* (2003) Gender differences in prevalence, risk, and clinical correlates of alcoholism comorbidity in bipolar disorder. *Am. J. Psychiatry*, **160**, 883–889.

Frye, M.A., Helleman, G., McElroy, S.L. *et al.* (2009) Correlates of treatment-emergent mania associated with antidepressant treatment in bipolar depression. *Am. J. Psychiatry*, **166**, 164–172.

Gaily, E., Kantola-Sorsa, E., Hiilesmaa, V. *et al.* (2004) Normal intelligence in children with prenatal exposure to carbamazepine. *Neurology*, **62**, 28–32.

Geller, B., Craney, J.L., Bolhofner, K. *et al.* (2002) Two-year prospective follow-up of children with a prepubertal and early adolescent bipolar disorder phenotype. *Am. J. Psychiatry*, **159**, 927–933.

Gentile, S. (2010) Neurodevelopmental effects of prenatal exposure to psychotropic medications. *Depress. Anxiety*, **27**, 675–686 (Review).

Goodwin, F.K. and Jamison, K.R. (2007) *Manic Depressive Illness: Bipolar Disorders and Recurrent Depression*, Oxford University Press, New York.

Gorman, J.M. (2006) Gender differences in depression and response to psychotropic medication. *Gend. Med.*, **3**, 93–109.

Harden, C.L., Meador, K.J., Pennell, P.B. *et al.* (2009a) Management issues for women with epilepsy-Focus on pregnancy (an evidence-based review): II. Teratogenesis and perinatal outcomes: Report of the Quality Standards Subcommittee and Therapeutics and Technology Subcommittee of the American Academy of Neurology and the American Epilepsy Society. *Epilepsia*, **50**, 1237–1246.

Harden, C.L., Pennell, P.B., Koppel, B.S. *et al.* (2009b) Management issues for women with epilepsy – focus on pregnancy (an evidence-based review): III. Vitamin K, folic acid, blood levels, and breast-feeding: Report of the Quality Standards Subcommittee and Therapeutics and Technology Assessment Subcommitte of the American Academy of Neurology and the American Epilepsy Society. *Epilepsia*, **50**, 1247–1255.

Harrow, M., Goldberg, J.F., Grossman, L.S., and Meltzer, H.Y. (1990) Outcome in manic disorders. A naturalistic follow-up study. *Arch. Gen. Psychiatry*, **47**, 665–671.

Hendrick, V., Altshuler, L.L., and Burt, V.K. (1996) Course of psychiatric disorders across the menstrual cycle. *Harv. Rev. Psychiatry*, **4**, 200–207.

Hendrick, V., Altshuler, L.L., Gitlin, M.J. *et al.* (2000) Gender and bipolar illness. *J. Clin. Psychiatry*, **61**, 393–396; quiz 397.

Hendrick, V., Altshuler, L., and Whybrow, P. (1998) Psychoneuroendocrinology of mood disorders. The hypothalamic-pituitary-thyroid axis. *Psychiatr. Clin. N. Am.*, **21**, 277–292.

Henry, C. (2002) Lithium side-effects and predictors of hypothyroidism in patients with bipolar disorder: sex differences. *J. Psychiatry Neurosci.*, **27**, 104–107.

Hirschfeld, R.M., Calabrese, J.R., Weissman, M.M. *et al.* (2003) Screening for bipolar disorder in the community. *J. Clin. Psychiatry*, **64**, 53–59.

Hirschfeld, R.M., Williams, J.B., Spitzer, R.L. *et al.* (2000) Development and validation of a screening instrument for bipolar spectrum disorder: the Mood Disorder Questionnaire. *Am. J. Psychiatry*, **157**, 1873–1875.

Holmes, L.B., Coull, B.A., Dorfman, J., and Rosenberger, P.B. (2005) The correlation of deficits in IQ with midface and digit hypoplasia in children exposed in utero to anticonvulsant drugs. *J. Pediatr.*, **146**, 118–122.

Hoyer, E.H., Mortensen, P.B., and Olesen, A.V. (2000) Mortality and causes of death in a total national sample of patients with affective disorders admitted for the first time between 1973 and 1993. *Br. J. Psychiatry*, **176**, 76–82.

Huang, M.C., Wang, Y.B., and Chan, C.H. (2008) Estrogen-progesterone combination for treatment-refractory post-partum mania. *Psychiatry Clin. Neurosci.*, **62**, 126.

Hunt, N. and Trevor, S. (1995) Does puerperal illness distinguish a subgroup of bipolar patients? *J. Affect. Disord.*, **34**, 101–107.

Isometsa, E.T., Henriksson, M.M., Aro, H.M., and Lonnqvist, J.K. (1994) Suicide in bipolar disorder in Finland. *Am. J. Psychiatry*, **151**, 1020–1024.

Jiang, B., Kenna, H.A., and Rasgon, N.L. (2009) Genetic overlap between polycystic ovary syndrome and bipolar disorder: the endophenotype hypothesis. *Med. Hypotheses*, **73**, 996–1004.

Joffe, H., Cohen, L.S., Suppes, T. *et al.* (2006a) Longitudinal follow-up of reproductive and metabolic features of valproate-associated polycystic ovarian syndrome features: a preliminary report. *Biol. Psychiatry*, **60**, 1378–1381.

Joffe, H., Cohen, L.S., Suppes, T. *et al.* (2006b) Valproate is associated with new-onset oligoamenorrhea with hyperandrogenism in women with bipolar disorder. *Biol. Psychiatry*, **59**, 1078–1086.

Joffe, H., Kim, D.R., Foris, J.M. *et al.* (2006c) Menstrual dysfunction prior to onset of psychiatric illness is reported more commonly by women with bipolar disorder than by women with unipolar depression and healthy controls. *J. Clin. Psychiatry*, **67**, 297–304.

Joffe, H. and Hayes, F.J. (2008) Menstrual cycle dysfunction associated with neurologic and psychiatric disorders: their treatment in adolescents. *Ann. N. Y. Acad. Sci.*, **1135**, 219–229.

Johnston, A.M. and Eagles, J.M. (1999) Lithium-associated clinical hypothyroidism. Prevalence and risk factors. *Br. J. Psychiatry*, **175**, 336–339.

Jones, I. and Craddock, N. (2001) Familiality of the puerperal trigger in bipolar disorder: results of a family study. *Am. J. Psychiatry*, **158**, 913–917.

Jones, I., Hamshere, M., Nangle, J.M. *et al.* (2007) Bipolar affective puerperal psychosis: genome-wide significant evidence for linkage to chromosome 16. *Am. J. Psychiatry*, **164**, 1099–1104.

Jones, K.L., Lacro, R.V., Johnson, K.A., and Adams, J. (1989) Pattern of malformations in the children of women treated with carbamazepine during pregnancy. *N. Engl. J. Med.*, **320**, 1661–1666.

Judd, L.L., Akiskal, H.S., Schettler, P.J. *et al.* (2002) The long-term natural history of the weekly symptomatic status of bipolar I disorder. *Arch. Gen. Psychiatry*, **59**, 530–537.

Judd, L.L., Schettler, P.J., Akiskal, H.S. *et al.* (2003) Long-term symptomatic status of bipolar I vs. bipolar II disorders. *Int. J. Neuropsychopharmacol.*, **6**, 127–137.

Kawa, I., Carter, J.D., Joyce, P.R. *et al.* (2005) Gender differences in bipolar disorder: age of onset, course, comorbidity, and symptom presentation. *Bipolar Disord.*, **7**, 119–125.

Kendell, R.E., Chalmers, J.C., and Platz, C. (1987) Epidemiology of puerperal psychoses. *Br. J. Psychiatry*, **150**, 662–673.

Kessler, R.C., Borges, G. and Walters, E.E. (1999) Prevalence of and risk factors for lifetime suicide attempts in the National Comorbidity Survey. *Arch. Gen. Psychiatry*, **56**, 617–626.

Kessler, R.C., McGonagle, K.A., Swartz, M. *et al.* (1993) Sex and depression in the National Comorbidity Survey. I: lifetime prevalence, chronicity and recurrence. *J. Affect. Disord.*, **29**, 85–96.

Kessler, R.C., McGonagle, K.A., Zhao, S. *et al.* (1994) Lifetime and 12-month prevalence of DSM-III-R psychiatric disorders in the United States. Results from the National Comorbidity Survey. *Arch. Gen. Psychiatry*, **51**, 8–19.

Kessler, R.C., Rubinow, D.R., Holmes, C. *et al.* (1997) The epidemiology of DSM-III-R bipolar I disorder in a general population survey. *Psychol. Med.*, **27**, 1079–1089.

Kim, J.H., Choi, S.S., and Ha, K. (2008) A closer look at depression in mothers who kill their children: is it unipolar or bipolar depression? *J. Clin. Psychiatry*, **69**, 1625–1631.

Kleiner, J., Altshuler, L., Hendrick, V., and Hershman, J.M. (1999) Lithium-induced subclinical hypothyroidism: review of the literature and guidelines for treatment. *J. Clin. Psychiatry*, **60**, 249–255.

Kornstein, S.G., Schatzberg, A.F., Thase, M.E. *et al.* (2000) Gender differences in treatment response to sertraline versus imipramine in chronic depression. *Am. J. Psychiatry*, **157**, 1445–1452.

Kornstein, S.G. and Wojcik, B.A. (2002) Depression, in *Women's Mental Health A Comprehensive Textbook* (eds S.G. Kornstein and A.H. Clayton), The Guilford Press, New York, pp. 147–165.

Koukopoulos, A., Sani, G., Koukopoulos, A.E. *et al.* (2003) Duration and stability of the rapid-cycling course: a long-term personal follow-up of 109 patients. *J. Affect. Disord.*, **73**, 75–85.

Kubacki, A. (1986) Male and female mania. *Can. J. Psychiatry*, **31**, 70–72.

Kukopulos, A., Caliari, B., Tundo, A. *et al.* (1983) Rapid cyclers, temperament, and antidepressants. *Compr. Psychiatry*, **24**, 249–258.

Kukopulos, A., Minnai, G., and Muller-Oerlinghausen, B. (1985) The Influence of mania and depression on the pharmacokinetics of lithium. *J. Affect. Disord.*, **8**, 159–166.

Kukopulos, A., Reginaldi, D., Laddomada, P. *et al.* (1980) Course of the manic-depressive cycle and changes caused by treatment. *Pharmakopsychiatr. Neuropsychopharmakol.*, **13**, 156–167.

Kulkarni, J., Garland, K.A., Scaffidi, A. *et al.* (2006) A pilot study of hormone modulation as a new treatment for mania in women with bipolar affective disorder. *Psychoneuroendocrinology*, **31**, 543–547.

Kupfer, D.J., Frank, E., Grochocinski, V.J. *et al.* (2002) Demographic and clinical characteristics of individuals in a bipolar disorder case registry. *J. Clin. Psychiatry*, **63**, 120–125.

Kupka, R.W., Altshuler, L.L., Nolen, W.A. *et al.* (2007) Three times more days depressed than manic or hypomanic in both bipolar I and bipolar II disorder. *Bipolar Disord.*, **9**, 531–535.

Kupka, R.W., Luckenbaugh, D.A., Post, R.M. *et al.* (2003) Rapid and non-rapid cycling bipolar disorder: a meta-analysis of clinical studies. *J. Clin. Psychiatry*, **64**, 1483–1494.

Kupka, R.W., Luckenbaugh, D.A., Post, R.M. *et al.* (2005) Comparison of rapid-cycling and non-rapid-cycling bipolar disorder based on prospective mood ratings in 539 outpatients. *Am. J. Psychiatry*, **162**, 1273–1280.

Kupka, R.W., Nolen, W.A., Post, R.M. *et al.* (2002) High rate of autoimmune thyroiditis in bipolar disorder: lack of association with lithium exposure. *Biol. Psychiatry*, **51**, 305–311.

Lane, A., Keville, R., Morris, M. *et al.* (1997) Postnatal depression and elation among mothers and their partners: prevalence and predictors. *Br. J. Psychiatry*, **171**, 550–555.

Lanza di Scalea, T. and Wisner, K.L. (2009) Antidepressant medication use during breastfeeding. *Clin. Obstet. Gynecol.*, **52**, 483–497.

Lee, H.C. and Lin, H.C. (2010) Maternal bipolar disorder increased low birthweight and preterm births: a nationwide population-based study. *J. Affect. Disord.*, **121**, 100–105.

Leibenluft, E. (1996) Women with bipolar illness: clinical and research issues. *Am. J. Psychiatry*, **153**, 163–173.

Leibenluft, E. (1997) Issues in the treatment of women with bipolar illness. *J. Clin. Psychiatry*, **58** (Suppl. 15), 5–11.

Leibenluft, E. (1999) Gender differences in major depressive disorder and bipolar disorder. *CNS Spectr.*, **4**, 25–33.

Leibenluft, E., Ashman, S.B., Feldman-Naim, S., and Yonkers, K.A. (1999) Lack of relationship between menstrual cycle phase and mood in a sample of women with rapid cycling bipolar disorder. *Biol. Psychiatry*, **46**, 577–580.

Leverich, G.S., McElroy, S.L., Suppes, T. *et al.* (2002) Early physical and sexual abuse associated with an adverse course of bipolar illness. *Biol. Psychiatry*, **51**, 288–297.

Lewinsohn, P.M., Striegel-Moore, R.H., and Seeley, J.R. (2000) Epidemiology and natural course of eating disorders in young women from adolescence to young adulthood. *J. Am. Acad. Child Adolesc. Psychiatry*, **39**, 1284–1292.

Llewellyn, A. and Stowe, Z.N. (1998) Psychotropic medications in lactation. *J. Clin. Psychiatry*, **59** (Suppl. 2), 41–52.

Louik, C., Lin, A.E., Werler, M.M. *et al.* (2007) First-trimester use of selective serotonin-reuptake inhibitors and the risk of birth defects. *N. Engl. J. Med.*, **356**, 2675–2683.

Loyd, D., Simpson, J.C., and Tsuang, M.T. (1985) Are there sex differences in the long-term outcome of schizophrenia? Comparisons with mania, depression, and surgical controls. *J. Nerv. Ment. Dis.*, **173**, 643–649.

MacKinnon, D.F., Zandi, P.P., Cooper, J. *et al.* (2002) Comorbid bipolar disorder and panic disorder in families with a high prevalence of bipolar disorder. *Am. J. Psychiatry*, **159**, 30–35.

Magalhaes, P.V., Kapczinski, F., and Kauer-Sant'Anna, M. (2009) Use of contraceptive methods among women treated for bipolar disorder. *Arch. Womens Ment. Health*, **12**, 183–185.

Maj, M. (2000) The impact of lithium prophylaxis on the course of bipolar disorder: a review of the research evidence. *Bipolar Disord.*, **2**, 93–101.

Maj, M., Pirozzi, R., Formicola, A.M., and Tortorella, A. (1999) Reliability and validity of four alternative definitions of rapid-cycling bipolar disorder. *Am. J. Psychiatry*, **156**, 1421–1424.

Marsh, W.K., Ketter, T.A., and Rasgon, N.L. (2009) Increased depressive symptoms in menopausal age women with bipolar disorder: age and gender comparison. *J. Psychiatr. Res.*, **43**, 798–802.

Marsh, W.K., Templeton, A., Ketter, T.A., and Rasgon, N.L. (2008) Increased frequency of depressive episodes during the menopausal transition in women with bipolar disorder: preliminary report. *J. Psychiatr. Res.*, **42**, 247–251.

McElroy, S.L., Altshuler, L.L., Suppes, T. *et al.* (2001) Axis I psychiatric comorbidity and its relationship to historical illness variables in 288 patients with bipolar disorder. *Am. J. Psychiatry*, **158**, 420–426.

McElroy, S.L., Keck, P.E. Jr., Pope, H.G. *et al.* (1992) Clinical and research implications of the diagnosis of dysphoric or mixed mania or hypomania. *Am. J. Psychiatry*, **149**, 1633–1644.

McElroy, S.L., Kotwal, R., and Keck, P.E. Jr. (2006) Comorbidity of eating disorders with bipolar disorder and treatment implications. *Bipolar Disord.*, **8**, 686–695.

McElroy, S.L., Strakowski, S.M., Keck, P.E. Jr. *et al.* (1995) Differences and similarities in mixed and pure mania. *Compr. Psychiatry*, **36**, 187–194.

McElroy, S.L., Weisler, R.H., Chang, W. *et al.* (2010) A double-blind, placebo-controlled study of quetiapine and paroxetine as monotherapy in adults with bipolar depression (EMBOLDEN II). *J. Clin. Psychiatry*, **71**, 163–174.

McIntyre, R.S., Konarski, J.Z., Wilkins, K. *et al.* (2006) The prevalence and impact of migraine headache in bipolar disorder: results from the Canadian Community Health Survey. *Headache*, **46**, 973–982.

McKenna, K., Koren, G., Tetelbaum, M. *et al.* (2005) Pregnancy outcome of women using atypical antipsychotic drugs: a prospective comparative study. *J. Clin. Psychiatry*, **66**, 444–449; quiz 546.

Meakin, C. and Brockington, I.F. (1990) Failure of progesterone treatment in puerperal mania. *Br. J. Psychiatry*, **156**, 910.

Merikangas, K.R., Akiskal, H.S., Angst, J. *et al.* (2007) Lifetime and 12-month prevalence of bipolar spectrum disorder in the National Comorbidity Survey replication. *Arch. Gen. Psychiatry*, **64**, 543–552.

Merlob, P., Mor, N., and Litwin, A. (1992) Transient hepatic dysfunction in an infant of an epileptic mother treated with carbamazepine during pregnancy and breastfeeding. *Ann. Pharmacother.*, **26**, 1563–1565.

Miller, L.J. (1994) Use of electroconvulsive therapy during pregnancy. *Hosp. Community Psychiatry*, **45**, 444–450.

Miller, L.J. (1999) *Postpartum Mood Disorders*, American Psychiatric Press, Washington, DC.

Mitchell, P.B., Wilhelm, K., Parker, G. *et al.* (2001) The clinical features of bipolar depression: a comparison with matched major depressive disorder patients. *J. Clin. Psychiatry*, **62**, 212–216; quiz 217.

Morrow, J., Russell, A., Guthrie, E. *et al.* (2006) Malformation risks of antiepileptic drugs in pregnancy: a prospective study from the UK Epilepsy and Pregnancy Register. *J. Neurol. Neurosurg. Psychiatry*, **77**, 193–198.

MRC Vitamin Study Research Group (1991) Prevention of neural tube defects: results of the Medical Research Council Vitamin Study. *Lancet*, **338**, 131–137.

Newport, D.J., Calamaras, M.R., DeVane, C.L. *et al.* (2007) Atypical antipsychotic administration during late pregnancy: placental passage and obstetrical outcomes. *Am. J. Psychiatry*, **164**, 1214–1220.

Newport, D.J., Pennell, P.B., Calamaras, M.R. *et al.* (2008) Lamotrigine in breast milk and nursing infants: determination of exposure. *Pediatrics*, **122**, e223–e231.

Newport, D.J., Viguera, A.C., Beach, A.J. *et al.* (2005) Lithium placental passage and obstetrical outcome: implications for clinical management during late pregnancy. *Am. J. Psychiatry*, **162**, 2162–2170.

Nguyen, H.T., Sharma, V., and McIntyre, R.S. (2009) Teratogenesis associated with antibipolar agents. *Adv. Ther.*, **26**, 281–294.

Nonacs, R., Viguera, A., and Cohen, L.S. (2002) Psychiatric aspects of pregnancy, in *Women's Mental Health. A Comprehensive Textbook* (eds S.G. Kornstein and A.H. Clayton), The Guilford Press, New York, pp. 70–90.

Nurnberger, J. Jr., Guroff, J.J., Hamovit, J. *et al.* (1988) A family study of rapid-cycling bipolar illness. *J. Affect. Disord.*, **15**, 87–91.

O'Donovan, C., Kusumakar, V., Graves, G.R., and Bird, D.C. (2002) Menstrual abnormalities and polycystic ovary syndrome in women taking valproate for bipolar mood disorder. *J. Clin. Psychiatry*, **63**, 322–330.

Ohman, I., Vitols, S., and Tomson, T. (2000) Lamotrigine in pregnancy: pharmacokinetics during delivery, in the neonate, and during lactation. *Epilepsia*, **41**, 709–713.

Oppenheim, G. (1984) A case of rapid mood cycling with estrogen: implications for therapy. *J. Clin. Psychiatry*, **45**, 34–35.

Osby, U., Brandt, L., Correia, N. *et al.* (2001) Excess mortality in bipolar and unipolar disorder in Sweden. *Arch. Gen. Psychiatry*, **58**, 844–850.

Ota, Y., Mukai, T. and Gotoda, K. (1954) Studies on the relationship between psychotic symptoms and sexual cycle. *Folia Psychiatr. Neurol. Jpn.*, **8**, 207–217.

Perugi, G., Musetti, L., Simonini, E. *et al.* (1990) Gender-mediated clinical features of depressive illness. The importance of temperamental differences. *Br. J. Psychiatry*, **157**, 835–841.

Piontek, C.M., Baab, S., Peindl, K.S., and Wisner, K.L. (2000) Serum valproate levels in 6 breast-feeding mother-infant pairs. *J. Clin. Psychiatry*, **61**, 170–172.

Post, R.M., Leverich, G.S., Altshuler, L., and Mikalauskas, K. (1992) Lithium-discontinuation-induced refractoriness: preliminary observations. *Am. J. Psychiatry*, **149**, 1727–1729.

Price, W.A. and DiMarzio, L. (1986) Premenstrual tension syndrome in rapid-cycling bipolar affective disorder. *J. Clin. Psychiatry*, **47**, 415–417.

Rasalam, A.D., Hailey, H., Williams, J.H. *et al.* (2005) Characteristics of fetal anticonvulsant syndrome associated autistic disorder. *Dev. Med. Child Neurol.*, **47**, 551–555.

Rasgon, N.L., Altshuler, L.L., Fairbanks, L. *et al.* (2005) Reproductive function and risk for PCOS in women treated for bipolar disorder. *Bipolar Disord.*, **7**, 246–259.

Rasgon, N.L., Altshuler, L.L., Gudeman, D. *et al.* (2000) Medication status and polycystic ovary syndrome in women with bipolar disorder: a preliminary report. *J. Clin. Psychiatry*, **61**, 173–178.

Rasgon, N., Bauer, M., Glenn, T. *et al.* (2003) Menstrual cycle related mood changes in women with bipolar disorder. *Bipolar Disord.*, **5**, 48–52.

Regier, D.A., Boyd, J.H., Burke, J.D. Jr. *et al.* (1988) One-month prevalence of mental disorders in the United States: based on five epidemiologic catchment area sites. *Arch. Gen. Psychiatry*, **45**, 977–986.

Reynolds, M.F., Sisk, E.C., and Rasgon, N.L. (2007) Valproate and neuroendocrine changes in relation to women treated for epilepsy and bipolar disorder: a review. *Curr. Med. Chem.*, **14**, 2799–2812.

Robb, J.C., Young, L.T., Cooke, R.G., and Joffe, R.T. (1998) Gender differences in patients with bipolar disorder influence outcome in the medical outcomes survey (SF-20) subscale scores. *J. Affect. Disord.*, **49**, 189–193.

Robertson Blackmore, E., Craddock, N., Walters, J., and Jones, I. (2008) Is the perimenopause a time of increased risk of recurrence in women with a history of bipolar affective postpartum psychosis? A case series. *Arch. Womens Ment. Health*, **11**, 75–78.

Roy-Byrne, P., Post, R.M., Uhde, T.W. *et al.* (1985) The longitudinal course of recurrent affective illness: life chart data from research patients at the NIMH. *Acta Psychiatr. Scand. Suppl.*, **317**, 1–34.

Sabers, A. (2008) Pharmacokinetic interactions between contraceptives and antiepileptic drugs. *Seizure*, **17**, 141–144.

Sachs, G.S., Nierenberg, A.A., Calabrese, J.R. *et al.* (2007) Effectiveness of adjunctive antidepressant treatment for bipolar depression. *N. Engl. J. Med.*, **356**, 1711–1722.

Schou, M. (1976) What happened to the lithium babies? A follow-up study of children born without malformations. *Acta Psychiatr. Scand.*, **54**, 193–197.

Schou, M. and Amdisen, A. (1973) Lithium and pregnancy. 3. Lithium ingestion by children breast-fed by women on lithium treatment. *Br. Med. J.*, **2**, 138.

Schou, M. and Amdisen, A. (1975) Letter: Lithium and the placenta. *Am. J. Obstet. Gynecol*, **122**, 541.

Shenfield, G.M. (1993) Oral contraceptives. Are drug interactions of clinical significance? *Drug Saf.*, **9**, 21–37.

Shivakumar, G., Bernstein, I.H., Suppes, T. *et al.* (2008) Are bipolar mood symptoms affected by the phase of the menstrual cycle? *J. Womens Health (Larchmt)*, **17**, 473–478.

Simon, G.E., Von Korff, M., Saunders, K. *et al.* (2006) Association between obesity and psychiatric disorders in the US adult population. *Arch. Gen. Psychiatry*, **63**, 824–830.

Soares, C.N., Almeida, O.P., Joffe, H., and Cohen, L.S. (2001) Efficacy of estradiol for the treatment of depressive disorders in perimenopausal women: a double-blind, randomized, placebo-controlled trial. *Arch. Gen. Psychiatry*, **58**, 529–534.

Spina, E., Pisani, F., and Perucca, E. (1996) Clinically significant pharmacokinetic drug interactions with carbamazepine. An update. *Clin. Pharmacokinet.*, **31**, 198–214.

Stewart, D.E., Klompenhouwer, J.L., Kendell, R.E., and van Hulst, A.M. (1991) Prophylactic lithium in puerperal psychosis. The experience of three centres. *Br. J. Psychiatry*, **158**, 393–397.

Stoner, S.C., Sommi, R.W. Jr., Marken, P.A. *et al.* (1997) Clozapine use in two full-term pregnancies. *J. Clin. Psychiatry*, **58**, 364–365.

Stowe, Z.N. (2007) The use of mood stabilizers during breastfeeding. *J. Clin. Psychiatry*, **68**, 22–28 (Review).

Strakowski, S.M., Tohen, M., Stoll, A.L. *et al.* (1992) Comorbidity in mania at first hospitalization. *Am. J. Psychiatry*, **149**, 554–556.

Suppes, T., Leverich, G.S., Keck, P.E. *et al.* (2001) The Stanley Foundation Bipolar Treatment Outcome Network. II. Demographics and illness characteristics of the first 261 patients. *J. Affect. Disord.*, **67**, 45–59.

Suppes, T., Mintz, J., McElroy, S.L. *et al.* (2005) Mixed hypomania in 908 patients with bipolar disorder evaluated prospectively in the Stanley Foundation Bipolar Treatment Network: a sex-specific phenomenon. *Arch. Gen. Psychiatry*, **62**, 1089–1096.

Suri, R.A., Altshuler, L.L., Burt, V.K., and Hendrick, V.C. (1999) Managing psychiatric medications in the breast-feeding woman. *Medscape Med.*, **1**, 1–10.

Sykes, P.A., Quarrie, J., and Alexander, F.W. (1976) Lithium carbonate and breast-feeding. *Br. Med. J.*, **2**, 1299.

Szadoczky, E., Papp, Z., Vitrai, J. *et al.* (1998) The prevalence of major depressive and bipolar disorders in Hungary. Results from a national epidemiologic survey. *J. Affect. Disord.*, **50**, 153–162.

Tohen, M., Vieta, E., Calabrese, J. *et al.* (2003) Efficacy of olanzapine and olanzapine-fluoxetine combination in the treatment of bipolar I depression. *Arch. Gen. Psychiatry*, **60**, 1079–1088.

Tohen, M., Waternaux, C.M., and Tsuang, M.T. (1990) Outcome in mania. A 4-year prospective follow-up of 75 patients utilizing survival analysis. *Arch. Gen. Psychiatry*, **47**, 1106–1111.

Tondo, L. and Baldessarini, R.J. (1998) Rapid cycling in women and men with bipolar manic-depressive disorders. *Am. J. Psychiatry*, **155**, 1434–1436.

Tondo, L., Baldessarini, R.J. and Floris, G. (2001) Long-term clinical effectiveness of lithium maintenance treatment in types I and II bipolar disorders. *Br. J. Psychiatry*, **178**, S184–S190.

Tondo, L., Baldessarini, R.J., Floris, G., and Rudas, N. (1997) Effectiveness of restarting lithium treatment after its discontinuation in bipolar I and bipolar II disorders. *Am. J. Psychiatry*, **154**, 548–550.

Truman, C.J., Goldberg, J.F., Ghaemi, S.N. *et al.* (2007) Self-reported history of manic/hypomanic switch associated with antidepressant use: data from the Systematic Treatment Enhancement Program for Bipolar Disorder (STEP-BD). *J. Clin. Psychiatry*, **68**, 1472–1479.

Tsai, S.Y., Kuo, C.J., Chen, C.C., and Lee, H.C. (2002) Risk factors for completed suicide in bipolar disorder. *J. Clin. Psychiatry*, **63**, 469–476.

Tunbridge, W.M., Evered, D.C., Hall, R. *et al.* (1977) The spectrum of thyroid disease in a community: the Whickham survey. *Clin. Endocrinol. (Oxf)*, **7**, 481–493.

Tunnessen, W.W. Jr. and Hertz, C.G. (1972) Toxic effects of lithium in newborn infants: a commentary. *J. Pediatr.*, **81**, 804–807.

Vanderpump, M.P., Tunbridge, W.M., French, J.M. *et al.* (1995) The incidence of thyroid disorders in the community: a twenty-year follow-up of the Whickham Survey. *Clin. Endocrinol. (Oxf)*, **43**, 55–68.

Videbech, P. and Gouliaev, G. (1995) First admission with puerperal psychosis: 7-14 years of follow-up. *Acta Psychiatr. Scand.*, **91**, 167–173.

Vieta, E., Colom, F., Corbella, B. *et al.* (2001) Clinical correlates of psychiatric comorbidity in bipolar I patients. *Bipolar Disord.*, **3**, 253–258.

Viguera, A.C., Baldessarini, R.J., and Tondo, L. (2001) Response to lithium maintenance treatment in bipolar disorders: comparison of women and men. *Bipolar Disord.*, **3**, 245–252.

Viguera, A.C. and Cohen, L.S. (1998) The course and management of bipolar disorder during pregnancy. *Psychopharmacol. Bull.*, **34**, 339–346.

Viguera, A.C., Newport, D.J., Ritchie, J. *et al.* (2007a) Lithium in breast milk and nursing infants: clinical implications. *Am. J. Psychiatry*, **164**, 342–345.

Viguera, A.C., Nonacs, R., Cohen, L.S. *et al.* (2000a) Risk of recurrence of bipolar disorder in pregnant and nonpregnant women after discontinuing lithium maintenance. *Am. J. Psychiatry*, **157**, 179–184.

Viguera, A.C., Tondo, L., and Baldessarini, R.J. (2000b) Sex differences in response to lithium treatment. *Am. J. Psychiatry*, **157**, 1509–1511.

Viguera, A.C., Whitfield, T., Baldessarini, R.J. *et al.* (2007b) Risk of recurrence in women with bipolar disorder during pregnancy: prospective study of mood stabilizer discontinuation. *Am. J. Psychiatry*, **164**, 1817–1824; quiz 1923.

Wehr, T.A., Sack, D.A., Rosenthal, N.E., and Cowdry, R.W. (1988) Rapid cycling affective disorder: contributing factors and treatment responses in 51 patients. *Am. J. Psychiatry*, **145**, 179–184.

Weissman, M.M., Bruce, M.L., and Leaf, P.J. (1991) Affective disorders, in *Psychiatry Disorders in America* (eds C.N. Robins and D.A. Regier), The Free Press, New York, pp. 53–80.

Weissman, A.M., Levy, B.T., Hartz, A.J. *et al.* (2004) Pooled analysis of antidepressant levels in lactating mothers, breast milk, and nursing infants. *Am. J. Psychiatry*, **161**, 1066–1078.

Weissman, M.M. and Olfson, M. (1995) Depression in women: implications for health care research. *Science*, **269**, 799–801.

Whybrow, P. (1995) Sex differences in thyroid axis dysfunction: relevance to affective disorder and its treatment. *Depression*, **3**, 33–42.

Williams, P.G. and Hersh, J.H. (1997) A male with fetal valproate syndrome and autism. *Dev. Med. Child Neurol.*, **39**, 632–634.

Winokur, G., Coryell, W., Akiskal, H.S. *et al.* (1994) Manic-depressive (bipolar) disorder: the course in light of a prospective ten-year follow-up of 131 patients. *Acta Psychiatr. Scand.*, **89**, 102–110.

Wisner, K.L. and Perel, J.M. (1998) Serum levels of valproate and carbamazepine in breastfeeding mother-infant pairs. *J. Clin. Psychopharmacol*, **18**, 167–169.

Wisner, K.L., Perel, J.M., Peindl, K.S. *et al.* (2004) Prevention of postpartum depression: a pilot randomized clinical trial. *Am. J. Psychiatry*, **161**, 1290–1292.

Woody, J.N., London, W.L., and Wilbanks, G.D. Jr. (1971) Lithium toxicity in a newborn. *Pediatrics*, **47**, 94–96.

Yildiz, A., Guleryuz, S., Ankerst, D.P. *et al.* (2008) Protein kinase C inhibition in the treatment of mania: a double-blind, placebo-controlled trial of tamoxifen. *Arch. Gen. Psychiatry*, **65**, 255–263.

Yildiz, A. and Sachs, G.S. (2003) Age onset of psychotic versus non-psychotic bipolar illness in men and in women. *J. Affect. Disord*, **74**, 197–201.

Yonkers, K.A., Kando, J.C., Cole, J.O., and Blumenthal, S. (1992) Gender differences in pharmacokinetics and pharmacodynamics of psychotropic medication. *Am. J. Psychiatry*, **149**, 587–595.

Yonkers, K.A., Wisner, K.L., Stewart, D.E. *et al.* (2009) The management of depression during pregnancy: a report from the American Psychiatric Association and the American College of Obstetricians and Gynecologists. *Gen. Hosp. Psychiatry*, **31**, 403–413.

Yonkers, K.A., Wisner, K.L., Stowe, Z. *et al.* (2004) Management of bipolar disorder during pregnancy and the postpartum period. *Am. J. Psychiatry*, **161**, 608–620.

Young, E.A., Kornstein, S.G., Marcus, S.M. *et al.* (2009) Sex differences in response to citalopram: a STAR*D report. *J. Psychiatr. Res.*, **43**, 503–511.

Zarate, C.A., Singh, J.B., Carlson, P.J. *et al.* (2007) Efficacy of a protein kinase C inhibitor (tamoxifen) in the treatment of acute mania: a pilot study. *Bipolar Disord.*, **9**, 561–570.

Zohar, J., Shapira, B., Oppenheim, G. *et al.* (1985) Addition of estrogen to imipramine in female-resistant depressives. *Psychopharmacol. Bull.*, **21**, 705–706.

17

Pediatric Bipolar Disorder: the Promise of Psychopharmacotherapy

Tiffany Thomas and Robert L. Findling

Division of Child and Adolescent Psychiatry, University Hospitals
Case Medical Center, Cleveland, OH, USA

17.1 INTRODUCTION

Pediatric bipolar disorder (PBD) is a serious and chronic illness that can have debilitating effects on the lives of children and adolescents suffering from this disorder. Studies show that children with PBD have significantly higher rates of morbidity and mortality than otherwise healthy children, including impaired psychosocial functioning impacting family and peer relationships; impaired academic performance with higher rates of school failure and dropout; increased levels of substance abuse; increased rates of suicide attempts and completion; greater legal difficulties; and more frequent hospitalizations (Danielyan and Kowatch, 2005). It is clear that adequate treatment of PBD is important to optimize functioning and decrease morbidity and mortality for children and adolescents with this disorder.

Pharmacological therapy is a mainstay in the management of pediatric bipolar disorder. In the past, the paucity of evidence-based studies in the pediatric population with bipolar disorder led practitioners to extrapolate findings from adult bipolar disorder treatment studies and treat PBD in much the same way as adults. However, when compared to what is known in adults, the efficacy and safety profiles of psychotropic medications are frequently different in children and adolescents (Wiznitzer and Findling, 2003). More recently, clinical trials in PBD have been conducted and new data are emerging. However, much less is known about the pharmacotherapy of bipolar disorder (BP) in youths when compared to what is known in adults. In addition, some medications that have been shown to be effective in adult BD remain unstudied in children. Therefore, further methodologically stringent clinical trials are needed to improve the evidence-based treatment of PBD.

In addition, the choice of medication for the treatment of PBD remains complex. In deciding on a medication for treatment, several factors should be considered including: (i) evidence of efficacy, (ii) the phase of illness, (iii) the presence of confounding presentations (such as psychotic symptoms or rapid cycling), (iv) the medication's side effect and safety profile, (v) the patient's history of past medication response, (vi) a history of

Bipolar Psychopharmacotherapy: Caring for the patient, Second Edition. Edited by Hagop S. Akiskal and Mauricio Tohen.
© 2011 John Wiley & Sons, Ltd. Published 2011 by John Wiley & Sons, Ltd.

treatment response in parents, (vii) the presence of comorbid conditions (such as substance abuse), and (viii) the preferences of the patient and his or her family (McClellan, Kowatch, and Findling, 2007). The target goals of treating PBD should include a reduction in acute symptoms, prevention of relapse, reduction in long-term morbidity, and promotion of normal development (Madaan and Chang, 2007).

Finally, it is evident that the treatment of pediatric bipolar disorder requires a multidisciplinary approach consisting of pharmacotherapy, psychotherapy, and psychosocial and educational interventions. However, the purpose of this chapter is to review available data regarding the pharmacological management of PBD. Particular emphasis will be placed on the most methodologically stringent clinical trials. There is an unfortunate paucity of data regarding intervention in juvenile BD's psychiatric comorbidities and intervention studies in symptomatic genetically at-risk youth. Most experts in the field of child psychiatry agree that when treating PBD, the initial goal is to stabilize the mood symptoms and then treat any associated comorbidities (McClellan, Kowatch, and Findling, 2007). Thus, this summary will focus on what is known about the acute and long-term treatment of manic, depressive, and mixed states in this patient population.

17.2 LITHIUM

Lithium was the first treatment approved by the United States Food and Drug Administration (FDA) for use in adolescents aged 12 and older with bipolar disorder. However, it should be noted that while a relatively large number of publications have considered the treatment of PBD with lithium, only a small number of studies were prospective clinical trials (Findling and Pavuluri, 2008). Please refer to Table 17.1 for a summary of selected studies of lithium in the treatment of pediatric bipolar disorder.

Dosing is a key consideration for lithium as it has been shown to have a narrow therapeutic window (0.6–1.2 mEq/l). In the absence of data specifically considering this topic, it has been assumed that therapeutic levels of lithium in children and adolescents are the same as in adults. As a result of this assumption, one possible strategy is to initiate lithium at a dose of 20 mg/kg/day, or 900 mg/day (whichever is less) divided into two or three daily doses. The initial dose is then gradually increased to achieve a target blood level of 0.6–1.2 mEq/l. Doses are generally not increased if: (i) blood levels of the drug exceed 1.2 mEq/l, (ii) side effects preclude dose increases, or (iii) adequate symptom reduction has already occurred (Findling and Pavuluri, 2008).

Due to lithium's narrow therapeutic window, monitoring of serum lithium levels is important to reduce the risk of toxicity. Early signs of lithium toxicity include ataxia, dysarthria, and reduced motor coordination. At levels substantially above the therapeutic window, severe toxicity can include seizures, coma, or even death. Lithium levels are generally measured 12 hours after the last administered dose. It is typically recommended that lithium levels be monitored frequently while adjustments in dosing are being made. Once lithium doses are stable with adequate therapeutic levels for three consecutive months, lithium levels may generally be checked every three months (Findling and Pavuluri, 2008).

As far as safety is concerned, the side effects that can occur in adults treated with lithium may also occur in children and adolescents who are administered this

Table 17.1 Findings from selected studies of lithium in the treatment of pediatric bipolar disorder.

Author (year)	Type of study	Sample size (number receiving study drug)	Age range (yr)	Patient diagnosis	Dosing	Study duration (wk)	Side effects	Outcome
Kowatch et al. (2007)	RCT	153 (66)	7–17	Bipolar I, mixed or manic stated	Initial = 20 mg/kg, Week 1 = 30 mg/kg (target levels: 0.8–1.2 mEq/l)	8	—	Although there was a trend toward efficacy, lithium did not separate from placebo
Patel et al. (2006)	OL	27 (27)	12–18	Bipolar I, depressed episode	30 mg/kg (twice daily dosing), target levels (1.0–1.2 mEq/l)	6	Headache and GI upset	Lithium found to be effective and well tolerated for bipolar depression
Kafantaris et al. (2003)	OL	100 (100)	12–18	Bipolar I, mixed or manic stated	Initial = 600 mg, target levels (0.6–1.2 mEq/l)	4	Weight gain, polydipsia, GI side effects	Lithium appears beneficial for acute stabilization of symptoms
Findling et al. (2003)	OL	90 (90)	5–17	Bipolar I or II disorder	Target dosing of Li (20 mg/kg/day) and serum levels (0.6–1.2 mEq/l)	Up to 20 wk, mean time 11.3 wk	GI side effects, enuresis, tremor, polydipsia	Combination lithium and divalproex showed statistically significant improvements in symptoms

GI, gastrointestinal; Li, lithium; OL, open label; RCT, randomized control trial.

agent. Although it has been asserted that younger children may be more vulnerable to lithium-related side effects than older adolescents, this assertion has yet to be definitively confirmed (Campbell *et al.*, 1991; Hagino, Weller, and Weller, 1995). The common side effects associated with lithium use include nausea, abdominal pain, sedation, diarrhea, polyuria, polydipsia, tremor, acne, hypothyroidism, and weight gain. Long-term treatment may also result in nephrogenic diabetes insipidus. Baseline laboratory monitoring including serum electrolytes, renal function tests, thyroid function tests, and complete blood counts is recommended. In addition, because lithium may adversely affect renal tubular function secondary to a deficit in urine concentrating ability, renal function tests should be checked every two to three months in the first six months of treatment and every six months thereafter. Thyroid function should be monitored every six months. It is also recommended that an electrocardiogram and a pregnancy test be checked before initiating treatment with lithium (Madaan and Chang, 2007).

In regards to effectiveness, lithium has been reported to be associated with reductions in symptomatology as a drug monotherapy in multiple open-label trials pertaining to its use in young people suffering from manic or mixed states. However, it has been repeatedly noted that while many patients benefit from lithium monotherapy, a substantive number of young patients do not fully achieve remission when prescribed lithium alone. In addition, rapid discontinuation and noncompliance are associated with a high relapse rate (Madaan and Chang, 2007). Several clinical factors that have been reported as possibly predictive of a poor response to lithium treatment in PBD include prepubertal onset and the presence of comorbid ADHD, substance abuse, conduct disorder, and personality disorder (Kowatch and DelBello, 2005). Furthermore, mixed mania episodes and rapid cycling, which are commonly seen in adolescents, may have a poorer response to lithium treatment (Kowatch and DelBello, 2005).

One study, funded by the National Institute of Mental Health, sought to compare the efficacy of lithium, divalproex sodium, and placebo in the acute treatment of symptomatic children and adolescents with bipolar I disorder, mixed or manic episodes. One hundred fifty-three outpatient subjects between the ages of 7 and 17 years were randomized in a double-blind protocol to lithium, divalproex, and placebo. At the end of eight weeks, divalproex demonstrated efficacy on the primary outcome measures, whereas lithium did not. Although there was a definitive trend toward efficacy for lithium, lithium did not separate from placebo in this study (Kowatch *et al.*, 2007).

Another study investigated the effectiveness and tolerability of lithium for the acute treatment of depression in adolescents with bipolar I disorder. Twenty-seven adolescents ages 12–18 were included in this open-label trial. All subjects were diagnosed with a current episode of depression associated with bipolar I disorder. At the end of the six week trial, lithium was found to have statistically significant improvements in response and remission rates based on the trial's outcome measures. In addition, lithium was relatively well tolerated. This study indicates that lithium may be beneficial in the treatment of acute episodes of depression in PBD but that controlled studies are needed (Patel *et al.*, 2006).

In summary, despite the lack of definitive efficacy and tolerability studies, lithium appears to be a reasonably safe and generally effective treatment of acute mixed and manic states in pediatric patients. Further studies in the treatment of depressive states are needed. Furthermore, definitive studies pertaining to the use of lithium in pediatric bipolar disorder (The Collaborative Lithium Trials – CoLT) are currently underway under the auspices of National Institute of Child Health and Human Development supported studies (Findling, 2009; Findling *et al.*, 2008a). The multidisciplinary CoLT trials should provide more definitive information that will help establish evidence-based dosing strategies for lithium in PBD as well as help determine the pharmacokinetics and biodisposition, acute and long term efficacy, and tolerability of lithium in the treatment of youth suffering from bipolarity.

17.3 ANTICONVULSANTS

Several medications originally marketed as anticonvulsants have been shown to be beneficial in treating bipolar disorder in adults. As a result, it was believed that these medications may have mood-stabilizing properties in pediatric bipolar disorder as well. Please refer to Table 17.2 for a summary of selected studies of anticonvulsants in the treatment of pediatric bipolar disorder. What follows is a summary of what is known about this class of medication in PBD.

17.3.1 CARBAMAZEPINE

While there have been studies demonstrating the efficacy of carbamazepine in the treatment of adults with mania, there are limited data regarding the safety and efficacy of this drug in the treatment of PBD. In an open-label study in which patients were randomly assigned to receive lithium, divalproex, or carbamazepine, clinically meaningful benefit was reported for all three study groups. In this study, carbamazepine was reasonably well tolerated with no serious adverse outcomes reported (Kowatch *et al.*, 2000). Some case reports have suggested that carbamazepine might be effective in adolescents with mania who have been nonresponsive to lithium.

Conversely, on a cautionary note, there have been case reports that suggest that carbamazepine may actually worsen mania. In addition, because of this drug's stimulation of the hepatic P450 isoenzyme system, there may be clinically significant drug-drug interactions that may make its clinical use difficult. Despite these preliminary observations, there are no randomized placebo-controlled studies on the use of carbamazepine in the treatment of bipolar disorder in children and adolescents, and the definitive safety, tolerability, and efficacy, both as monotherapy and as an agent used in combination with other compounds, remains to be seen (Danielyan and Kowatch, 2005).

17.3.2 SODIUM DIVALPROEX

Sodium divalproex has demonstrated efficacy in the treatment of adults with acute mania. However, much of the data on the use of divalproex in the pediatric population are from case reports. One randomized, double blind, industry-sponsored study investigating the use of divalproex extended-release in 150 children and adolescents with bipolar disorder found no statistically significant improvement in acute manic symptoms when compared

Table 17.2 Findings from selected studies of anticonvulsants in the treatment of pediatric bipolar disorder.

Medication	Author (yr)	Type of study	Sample size (number receiving study drug)	Age range (yr)	Patient diagnosis	Dosing	Study duration (wk)	Side effects	Outcome
Carbamazepine	Kowatch et al. (2000)	OL	42 (13)	8–18	Bipolar I or II, mixed or manic episode	15 mg/kg/day, with goal serum levels of 7–11 µg/l	6	Nausea, sedation, rash, dizziness	Carbamazepine, lithium, and divalproex sodium all showed a large effect size
Divalproex sodium	Kowatch et al. (2007)	RCT	153 (56)	7–17	Bipolar I, mixed or manic stated	Initial = 15 mg/kg, Week 1 = 20 mg/kg (target levels: 85–110 µg/ml)	8	—	Divalproex demonstrated efficacy when compared to placebo
Divalproex Sodium	Findling et al. (2003)	OL	90 (90)	5–17	Bipolar I or II disorder	20 mg/kg with goal serum levels of 50–100 µg/ml	Up to 20 wk, mean time 11.3 wk	GI upset, enuresis, tremor, increased thirst	Combination divalproex and lithium showed statistically significant improvement
Divalproex extended-release	Wagner et al. (2009)	RCT	150 (74)	10–17	Bipolar I, mixed or manic episode	Initiated at 15 mg/kg/day and titrated to serum levels of 80–125 µg/ml or max 35 mg/kg/d	4	Headache, GI upset, somnolence, rash	Divalproex ER did not separate from placebo

Drug	Study	Design	N (completed)	Age	Diagnosis	Dosing	Ref	Side effects	Results
Topiramate	DelBello et al. (2005)	RCT	56 (29)	6–17	Bipolar I, mixed or manic episode	Starting dose of 50 mg/day to target dose of 400 mg/d over five days	4	GI side effects, paresthesia, somnolence	Results are inconclusive because of premature termination of study resulting in limited sample size, however, preliminary data indicate that topirimate may have been more effective than placebo had the study continued
Oxcarbazepine	Wagner et al. (2006)	RCT	116 (59)	7–18	Bipolar I, mixed or manic episode	Titrated by 300 mg/day every two days to max of 900–2400 mg/day	7	Dizziness, nausea, somnolence, diplopia	Oxcarbazepine was not significantly superior to placebo
Lamotrigine	Chang, Saxena, and Howe (2006)	OL	20 (20)	12–17	Bipolar I, II, or NOS, depressive episode	Initiated at 12.5 or 25 mg/d with target dose of 50–200 mg/d	8	Headache, fatigue, nausea, sweating, difficulty sleeping	Appeared to be some improvement in depression
Lamotrigine	Pavuluri et al. (2009)	OL	46 (46)	8–18	Bipolar I, mixed or manic or Bipolar II, hypomanic episode	Initiated at 12.5 mg/d with gradual eight week titration	14	Sedation, stomachache, increased urination, increased appetite	Appeared effective in maintaining symptom control of manic and depressive symptoms

GI, gastrointestinal; Li, lithium; OL, open label; RCT, randomized control trial, ER, extended-release.

with placebo (Wagner *et al.*, 2009). However, a randomized, NIMH-supported double blind trial investigating 153 youth found that divalproex was superior to placebo for treating children and adolescents with bipolar disorder during a mixed or manic episode (Kowatch *et al.*, 2007). A possible explanation for the discrepant results of these two studies may be due to issues related to between-site variability. The NIMH-supported study was conducted at substantively fewer sites than the industry-supported trial. Furthermore, there have been combination pharmacotherapy studies that suggest that divalproex may be beneficial when co-administered with lithium, quetiapine, or risperidone (Findling and Kuich, 2008).

Common side effects of divalproex in children are weight gain, nausea, sedation, and tremor. In addition, particular concern has been raised regarding the relationship between divalproex and the development of polycystic ovarian syndrome (PCOS) in girls. Therefore, it is recommended that clinicians should monitor female patients treated with divalproex for any signs of PCOS including weight gain, menstrual abnormalities, hirsutism, or acne (Kowatch and DelBello, 2006).

17.3.3   TOPIRAMATE

Preliminary data has indicated that topirimate may be effective for pediatric bipolar disorder. These data come primarily from a pilot controlled trial of topiramate for mania in pediatric bipolar disorder that was discontinued prematurely when adult mania trials with topiramate failed to show efficacy. However, when these preliminary data were analyzed from the pediatric study, it was found that topiramate might have proven beneficial should the study have continued (DelBello *et al.*, 2005). Key side effects of topiramate include anorexia, weight loss, and sedation. It should be mentioned that although there are no methodologically rigorous data on this topic, some clinicians appear to utilize topiramate's weight loss properties and prescribe this drug as an adjunctive treatment for youth with bipolar disorder who have gained weight as a result of treatment with other psychotropic agents (Kowatch and DelBello, 2006).

17.3.4   OXCARBAZEPINE

One randomized, double-blind placebo controlled study investigated the use of oxcarbazapine versus placebo in 116 youth with bipolar disorder. The authors found that treatment with oxcarbazepine was no different than the response seen with placebo. As a result, these findings do not support the use of oxcarbazepine as monotherapy in the treatment of the manic phase of PBD (Wagner *et al.*, 2006).

17.3.5   GABAPENTIN

Gabapentin has not been found to be effective for the treatment of bipolar disorder in adults, and there is currently no evidence to support its use in the treatment of pediatric bipolar disorder (Smarty and Findling, 2007). Furthermore, gabapentin has been reported to cause behavioral disinhibition in younger children (Kowatch, 2009).

17.3.6 LAMOTRIGINE

Lamotrigine has been shown to be efficacious for the maintenance treatment of bipolar disorder in adults and data supports its use in the long-term treatment of bipolar depression in adults. There have been open studies indicating that lamotrigine may be beneficial for adolescents with bipolar depression. However, randomized, controlled trials are still needed. The risk of potentially lethal cutaneous reactions, such as Stevens-Johnson syndrome and toxic epidermal necrolysis, is greater in youth younger than 16 years old than in adults. However, dosing guidelines using a more conservative dose titration may lower the risk of such serious rashes (Kowatch and DelBello, 2006).

17.4 ANTIPSYCHOTICS

Atypical antipsychotics have been shown to be efficacious in treating bipolar disorder in adults. Several recent placebo-controlled trials provide evidence that atypical antipsychotics may be beneficial for the acute treatment of manic and/or mixed states in youths suffering from bipolar disorder as well. However, as with adults, the possible metabolic complications of these drugs are important considerations, particularly over the long-term. Unfortunately, there is limited information about the long-term effects of these agents in the pediatric population. In addition, there are no methodologically-stringent studies that have specifically compared the safety and efficacy of one atypical to another. Moreover, there are almost no data about the use of typical antipsychotics in this patient population. Further methodologically-stringent, placebo-controlled studies investigating the use of antipsychotics and their acute and long-term efficacy and safety in the treatment of children and adolescents suffering from bipolarity are needed. Please refer to Table 17.3 for a summary of selected studies of atypical antipsychotics in the treatment of pediatric bipolar disorder.

17.4.1 RISPERIDONE

Risperidone, either as monotherapy or in combination with a mood stabilizer, has been reported to be effective in the treatment of juvenile bipolarity in case reports and open label studies. In addition, in 2007 risperidone was given the first FDA indication for an atypical antipsychotic for the treatment of acute mania or mixed episodes associated with bipolar I disorder in children and adolescents ages 10–17 years of age. One randomized, placebo-controlled study of youth with bipolar disorder found that risperidone was efficacious and relatively well tolerated at doses as low as 0.5–2.5 mg per day in the acute treatment of manic or mixed episodes in children and adolescents ages 10–17 (Haas et al., 2009).

Table 17.3 Findings from selected studies of atypical antipsychotics in the treatment of pediatric bipolar disorder.

Medication	Author (year)	Type of study	Sample size (number receiving study drug)	Age range (yr)	Patient diagnosis	Dosing	Study duration (wk)	Side effects	Outcome
Aripiprazole	Chang et al. (2007)	RCT	296 (197)	10–17	Bipolar I, mixed or manic episode	10 or 30 mg reached after a 5 or 13 d titration	4	Somnolence, extrapyramidal side effects, fatigue	Aripiprazole was significantly superior to placebo
Aripiprazole	Wagner et al. (2007)	RCT	296 (197)	10–17	Bipolar I, mixed or manic episode	10 or 30 mg reached after a 5 or 13 d titration	30	Somnolence, extrapyramidal side effects, fatigue	Over 30 weeks, aripiprazole sustained superiority to placebo
Aripiprazole	Correll et al. (2007)	RCT	296 (197)	10–17	Bipolar I, mixed or manic episode	10 or 30 mg reached after a 5 or 13 d titration	30	Somnolence, extrapyramidal side effects, fatigue	Over 30 weeks, most adverse events were mild to moderate; EPS and somnolence appear dose-related
Aripiprazole	Biederman et al. (2007)	OL	19 (19)	6–17	Bipolar I, II, or NOS, manic, or mixed episode	9.4 ± 4.2 mg/d	8	Sedation, GI problems	Aripiprazole was beneficial
Ziprasidone	DelBello et al. (2008)	RCT	238 (150)	10–17	Bipolar I, mixed or manic episode	80–160 mg/d	4	Sedation, somnolence, nausea, dizziness	Ziprasidone found to be effective and generally well tolerated

Drug	Study	Design	N (completers)	Age	Diagnosis	Dose	Duration (weeks)	Side effects	Conclusion
Ziprasidone	Findling et al. (2008b)	OL	162 (162)	10–17	Bipolar I, mixed or manic episode	40–160 mg/d	26	Sedation, headache, somnolence, insomnia, GI side effects	Ziprasidone was associated with benefit and generally well tolerated
Quetiapine	DelBello et al. (2007)	RCT	277 (188)	10–17	Bipolar I, manic episode	400 or 600 mg/d	3	Somnolence, sedation, dizziness, headache	Quetiapine was superior to placebo
Quetiapine	DelBello et al. (2008)	OL	380 (205 with bipolar, 175 with schizophrenia)	10–18	Bipolar I disorder or schizophrenia	400–800 mg/d	26	Somnolence, headache, sedation, weight gain, GI side effects	Quetiapine was generally well tolerated
Quetiapine	DelBello et al. (2006)	RCT	50 (25)	12–18	Bipolar I, mixed or manic episode	400–600 mg/d	4	Sedation, dizziness, GI upset, dry mouth	Quetiapine as effective as divalproex with quicker reduction in manic symptoms
Quetiapine	DelBello et al. (2009)	RCT	32 (17)	12–18	Bipolar I, depressive episode	300–600 mg/d	8	GI upset, sedation, dizziness	Quetiapine was not found to be more effective than placebo for depressed episodes
Risperidone	Haas et al. (2009)	RCT	169 (111)	10–17	Bipolar I, mixed or manic episode	0.5–2.5 mg/day or 3–6 mg/d	3	Somnolence, headache, fatigue	Risperidone was efficacious and generally well tolerated at low doses

(Continued Overleaf)

Table 17.3 (Continued)

Medication	Author (year)	Type of study	Sample size (number receiving study drug)	Age range (yr)	Patient diagnosis	Dosing	Study duration (wk)	Side effects	Outcome
Olanzapine	Tohen et al. (2007)	RCT	161 (107)	13–17	Bipolar I, mixed or manic episode	2.5–20 mg/d	3	Weight gain, increases in levels of hepatic enzymes, prolactin, fasting glucose, fasting total cholesterol, and uric acid	Olanzapine was effective but was associated with significant weight gain and metabolic changes
Olanzapine	Kryzhanovskaya et al. (2009)	Pooled analysis of 4 clinical trials (both RCT and OL)	Placebo controlled: 268 (179); overall adolescent exposure database: 454 (454)	13–17	Bipolar I or schizophrenia	Mean daily dose of the four trials was 10.6 mg/d	(Study 1—6, 26; study 2—3, 26; study 3—4.5; study 4—24)	Increased weight, somnolence, increased appetite, sedation, dry mouth, headache; changes in fasting glucose, total cholesterol, triglycerides, and alanine aminotransferase	Types of adverse events in adolescents appeared similar to adults; however, the magnitude and incidence of weight and prolactin changes were greater in adolescents than adults

OL, open label; RCT, randomized control trial; GI, gastrointestinal; EPS, extrapyramidal symptoms.

17.4.2   OLANZAPINE

Several open-label studies have reported efficacy for the use of olanzapine in pediatric bipolar disorder. In 2007, one double-blind, randomized placebo-controlled trial in adolescents 13–17 years of age with a manic or mixed episode found that olanzapine, at doses between 2.5 and 20 mg per day, was superior to placebo in treatment of these adolescent patients. However, the study also found that those youths treated with olanzapine had significantly greater weight gain and increases in the levels of hepatic enzymes, prolactin, fasting glucose, fasting total cholesterol, and uric acid when compared to those treated with placebo. The mean baseline-to-endpoint increases in weight were 3.66 kg in the olanzapine group versus 0.30 kg in the placebo group over the three week study period. The research team calculated a risk-benefit ratio around weight gain and treatment response and found that although the probability of responding favorably to olanzapine is good, the probability of gaining weight is even greater (Tohen *et al.*, 2007). Another study sought to describe the safety of olanzapine treatment in adolescents diagnosed with bipolar I disorder or schizophrenia and to compare the data to that of adults treated with olanzapine. This study analyzed data from four clinical trials of adolescents 13–17 years of age treated with olanzapine for up to 32 weeks. The adolescent data were then compared with data pooled from up to 84 clinical trials of adults treated with olanzapine. The analysis revealed that the types of adverse events in olanzapine-treated adolescents appeared similar to those of adults. The most common adverse events included increased weight, somnolence, and increased appetite. However, the magnitude and incidence of weight and prolactin changes were greater in adolescents than adults. In up to 32 weeks of treatment, when compared with adults, adolescents treated with olanzapine gained statistically more weight (7.4 kg vs 3.2 kg, $p < 0.001$), and significantly more adolescents gained $\geq 7\%$ of their baseline weight (65.1% vs 35.6%, $p < 0.001$) (Kryzhanovskaya *et al.*, 2009). Ultimately, the benefits of olanzapine for the treatment of pediatric bipolar disorder should be considered within the context of its safety profile.

17.4.3   QUETIAPINE

Quetiapine was one of the first atypical antipsychotics to be studied in a double-blind, placebo-controlled trial for the treatment of mania in adolescents. This study found that combination therapy with quetiapine and divaloproex was more effective than divalproex and placebo in the acute treatment of adolescents suffering from manic or mixed episodes (DelBello *et al.*, 2006). In addition, a randomized, placebo-controlled study of 277 participants, ages 10–17, concluded that quetiapine, at doses of 400 and 600 mg per day, was significantly more effective than placebo in treating acute manic symptoms in children and adolescents with bipolar disorder (DelBello *et al.*, 2007). More recently, a pilot study comparing the effects of quetiapine and placebo for the treatment of depressive episodes in adolescents with bipolar I disorder was conducted. This study included 32 adolescents ages 12–18 treated with doses of 300–600 mg per day over an eight week period.

Ultimately, the results suggested that quetiapine monotherapy was no more effective than placebo for depressive episodes in this patient population (DelBello *et al.*, 2009).

The safety and tolerability of quetiapine was investigated in a 26-week, open label study of 380 youth ages 10–18 with a diagnosis of bipolar I disorder or schizophrenia. Quetiapine was flexibly dosed at 400–800 mg/day with the option to decrease to 200 mg/day based on tolerability. Sixty-two percent of patients completed the study. Ultimately, quetiapine was found to be generally safe and well tolerated, with the most common adverse events including somnolence, headache, sedation, weight gain, and vomiting (DelBello *et al.*, 2008a).

17.4.4   ZIPRASIDONE

Ziprasidone has been shown to be effective in treating mania in adults. In addition, ziprasidone is typically associated with less weight gain than risperidone and olanzapine. One randomized, double blind, placebo-controlled study of 238 youth ages 10–17 years old with bipolar disorder found that ziprasidone at doses of 80–160 mg per day was effective and generally well tolerated for the treatment of mania in children and adolescents (DelBello *et al.*, 2008b).

A 26-week, open-label extension study investigating the long-term safety and tolerability of ziprasidone was conducted in 162 patients ages 10–17 years diagnosed with bipolar I disorder. Patients were treated with flexible dosing of ziprasidone from 40 to 160 mg/day. The study found that ziprasidone was generally safe and well tolerated in this population with the most common adverse events including sedation, headache, somnolence, insomnia, upper abdominal pain, and nausea (Findling *et al.*, 2008b).

17.4.5   ARIPIPRAZOLE

Aripiprazole is indicated by the FDA for the acute and maintenance treatment of manic and mixed episodes associated with bipolar I disorder in pediatric patients ages 10–17 years. One randomized, double blind, placebo-controlled study of 296 youth ages 10–17 with bipolar I disorder has shown that aripiprazole, at doses of 10 and 30 mg, is superior to placebo in the acute treatment of manic and mixed episodes (Chang, Nyilas, and Aurang, 2007). Patients completing this four-week, double-blind trial were continued in randomly assigned treatments for an additional 26 weeks. At the completion of the study, aripiprazole was found to remain significantly superior to placebo in the long-term treatment of pediatric bipolar patients (Wagner *et al.*, 2007). Data from this 4-week acute-phase and 26-week continuation phase were analyzed to assess the long-term safety and efficacy of aripiprazole in this patient population. Over the 30 weeks, most of the adverse events were mild to moderate. The three most common adverse events included somnolence, extrapyramidal disorder, and fatigue. In addition, extrapyramidal symptoms and fatigue appeared to be dose-related (Correll *et al.*, 2007).

17.4.6   CLOZAPINE

There is some evidence from open trials and case reports that clozapine may be beneficial in the treatment of pediatric bipolar patients that have not shown adequate response to other agents (Masi, Mucci, and Millepiedi, 2002). However, clozapine's side effect profile, which may include sedation, weight gain, increased salivation, seizures, myocarditis as well as potentially lethal agranulocytosis limit the usage of this medication. For these reasons, clozapine is generally recommended only for children and adolescents who have not responded to multiple treatment courses with other medications.

17.5   CONCLUSION

Historically, pharmacological treatment of pediatric bipolar disorder in clinical practice was based on data collected from the treatment of adults with this disorder. However, more recently, clinical trials have been conducted in PBD and new data are now available, particularly concerning the efficacy of the atypical antipsychotics in treating children and adolescents. However, some medications that have been shown to be useful in treating adult patients remain unstudied in children. In addition, long-term safety and efficacy data are lacking for many drugs. Thus, unknown risks to this vulnerable population may exist. Furthermore, ongoing research in the depressed phase of PBD, the treatment of psychiatric comorbidities, and the treatment of symptomatic genetically at-risk youth require further attention. Ultimately, with continued research and forthcoming data from ongoing trials, clinical decisions based on essential acute and long-term efficacy, and safety data will become increasingly feasible.

DISCLOSURES

Dr. Findling receives or has received research support, acted as a consultant and/or served on a speaker's bureau for Abbott, Addrenex, AstraZeneca, Biovail, Bristol-Myers Squibb, Forest, GlaxoSmithKline, Johnson & Johnson, KemPharm Lilly, Lundbeck, Neuropharm, Novartis, Organon, Otsuka, Pfizer, Sanofi-Aventis, Sepracore, Shire, Solvay, Supernus Pharmaceuticals, Validus, and Wyeth.

References

Biederman, J., Mick, E., Spencer, T. *et al.* (2007) An open-label trial of aripiprazole monotherapy in children and adolescents with bipolar disorder. *CNS Spectr.*, **12** (9), 683–689.

Campbell, M., Silva, R.R., Kafantaris, V. *et al.* (1991) Predictors of side effects associated with lithium administration in children. *Psychopharmacol. Bull.*, **27** (3), 373–380.

Chang, K.D., Nyilas, M., Aurang, C. *et al.* (2007) Efficacy of aripiprazole in children (10–17 years old) with mania. Poster presented at the Annual Meeting of the American Academy of Child and Adolescent Psychiatry, October 23–28, 2007, Boston, MA.

Chang, K., Saxena, K., and Howe, M. (2006) An open-label study of lamotrigine adjunct or monotherapy for the treatment of adolescents with bipolar depression. *J. Am. Acad. Child Adolesc. Psychiatry*, **45** (3), 298–304.

Correll, C.U., Nyilas, M., Aurang, C. *et al.* (2007) Safety and tolerability of aripiprazole in children (10–17) with mania. Poster presented at the Annual Meeting of the American Academy of Child and Adolescent Psychiatry, October 23–28, 2007, Boston, MA.

Danielyan, A. and Kowatch, R.A. (2005) Management options for bipolar disorder in children and adolescents. *Paediatr. Drugs*, **7** (5), 277–294.

DelBello, M.P., Chang, K., Welge, J.A. *et al.* (2009) A double-blind, placebo-controlled pilot study of quetiapine for depressed adolescents with bipolar disorder. *Bipolar Disord.*, **11**, 483–493.

DelBello, M.P., Findling, R.L., Earley, W.R. *et al.* (2007) Efficacy of quetiapine in children and adolescents with bipolar mania: a 3-week, double-blind, randomized, placebo-controlled trial. Poster presented at the Annual Meeting of the American Academy of Child and Adolescent Psychiatry, October 24–29, 2007, Boston, MA.

DelBello, M.P., Findling, R.L., Earley, W.R. *et al.* (2008a) Safety and tolerability of quetiapine in children and adolescents with bipolar I disorder and adolescents with schizophrenia: a 26-week, open-label study. Poster presented at the Annual Meeting of the American Academy of Child and Adolescent Psychiatry, October 28–November 2, 2008, Chicago, IL.

DelBello, M.P., Findling, R.L., Wang, P.P. *et al.* (2008b) Efficacy and safety of ziprasidone in pediatric bipolar disorder. Poster presented at the Annual Meeting of American Psychiatric Association, May 3–8, 2008, Washington, DC.

DelBello, M.P., Findling, R.L., Kushner, S. *et al.* (2005) A pilot controlled trial of topiramate for mania in children and adolescents with bipolar disorder. *J. Am. Acad. Child. Adolesc. Psychiatry*, **44** (6), 539–547.

DelBello, M.P., Kowatch, R.A., Adler, C.M. *et al.* (2006) A double-blind randomized pilot study comparing quetiapine and divalproex for adolescent mania. *J. Am. Acad. Child Adolesc. Psychiatry*, **45** (3), 305–313.

Findling, R.L. (2009) Treatment of childhood-onset bipolar disorder, in *Bipolar Depression: Molecular Neurobiology, Clinical Diagnosis and Pharmacotherapy* (eds C.A. Zarate and H.K. Manji), Birkhauser, Verlag, Switzerland, pp. 241–252.

Findling, R.L., Frazier, J.A., Karantaris, V. *et al.* (2008a) The collaborative lithium trials (CoLT): specific aims, methods, and implementation. *Child Adolesc. Psychiatry Ment. Health*, **2** (1), 21.

Findling, R.L., DelBello, M.P., Wang, P.P. *et al.* (2008b) Long-term safety and tolerability of ziprasidone in children and adolescents with bipolar disorder. Poster presented at the Annual Meeting of American Psychiatric Association, May 3–8, 2008, Washington, DC.

Findling, R.L. and Kuich, K. (2008) Bipolar disorders, in *Clinical Manual of Child and Adolescent Psychopharmacology* (ed. R.L. Findling), Guilford Press, New York, pp. 229–263.

Findling, R.L. and Pavuluri, M.N. (2008) Lithium, in *Treatment of Bipolar Disorder in Children and Adolescents* (eds B. Geller and M. DelBello) The Guilford Press, New York, pp. 43–68.

Findling, R.L., McNamara, N.K., Gracious, B.L. *et al.* (2003) Combination lithium and divalproex sodium in pediatric bipolarity. *J. Am. Acad. Child Adolesc. Psychiatry*, **42** (8), 895–901.

Haas, M., DelBello, M.P., Pandina, G. *et al.* (2009) Risperidone for the treatment of acute mania in children and adolescents with bipolar disorder: a randomized, double-blind, placebo-controlled study. *Bipolar Disord.*, **11**, 687–700.

Hagino, O.R., Weller, E.B., and Weller, R.A. (1995) Untoward effects of lithium treatment in children aged four through six years. *J. Am. Acad. Child Adolesc. Psychiatry*, **34** (12), 1584–1590.

Kafantaris, V., Coletti, D., Dicer, R. *et al.* (2003) Lithium treatment of acute mania in adolescents: a large open trial. *J. Am. Acad. Child Adolesc. Psychiatry*, **42** (9), 1038–1045.

Kowatch, R.A. (2009) Pharmacotherapy 1: mood Stabilizers, in *Clinical Manual for Management of Bipolar Disorder in Children and Adolescents* (eds R.A. Kowatch and M.A. Fristad), American Psychiatric Publishing, Inc., Arlington, VA, pp. 133–156.

Kowatch, R.A. and DelBello, M.P. (2005) Pharmacotherapy of children and adolescents with bipolar disorder. *Psychiatr. Clin. N. Am.*, **28** (2), 385–397.

Kowatch, R.A. and DelBello, M.P. (2006) Pediatric bipolar disorder: emerging diagnostic and treatment approaches. *Child Adolesc. Psychiatr. Clin. N. Am.*, **15** (1), 73–108.

Kowatch, R.A., Findling, R.L., Scheffer, R.E. *et al.* (2007) Pediatric bipolar collaborative mood stabilizer trial. Poster presented at the Annual Meeting of the American Academy of Child and Adolescent Psychiatry, October 23–28, 2007, Boston, MA.

Kowatch, R.A., Suppes, T., Carmody, T.J. *et al.* (2000) Effect size of lithium, divalproex sodium, and carbamazepine in children and adolescents with bipolar disorder. *J. Am. Acad. Child Adolesc. Psychiatry*, **39** (6), 713–720.

Kryzhanovskaya, L.A., Robertson-Plouch, C.K., Xu W. *et al.* (2009) The safety of olanzapine in adolescents with schizophrenia or bipolar I disorder: a pooled analysis of 4 clinical trials. *J. Clin. Psychiatry*, **70** (2), 247–258.

Madaan, V. and Chang, K.D. (2007) Pharmacotherapeutic strategies for pediatric bipolar disorder. *Exp. Opin. Pharmacother.*, **8** (12), 1801–1819.

Masi, G., Mucci, M., and Millepiedi, S. (2002) Clozapine in adolescent inpatient mania. *J. Child Adolesc. Psychopharmacol.*, **12** (2), 93–99.

McClellan, J., Kowatch, R., and Findling, R.L. (2007) Practice parameter for the assessment and treatment of children and adolescents with bipolar disorder. *J. Am. Acad. Child Adolesc. Psychiatry*, **46** (1), 107–125.

Patel, N.C., DelBello, M.P., Bryan, H.S. *et al.* (2006) Open-Label Lithium for the treatment of adolescents with bipolar depression. *J. Am. Acad. Child Adolesc. Psychiatry*, **45** (3), 289–297.

Pavuluri, M.N., Henry, D.B., Moss, M. *et al.* (2009) Effectiveness of lamotrigine in maintaining symptom control in pediatric bipolar disorder. *J. Child Adolesc. Psychopharmacol.*, **19** (1), 75–82.

Smarty, S. and Findling, R.L. (2007) Psychopharmacology of pediatric bipolar disorder: a review. *Psychopharmacology*, **191** (1), 39–54.

Tohen, M., Kryzhanovskaya, L., Carlson, G. *et al.* (2007) Olanzapine versus placebo in the treatment of adolescents with bipolar mania. *Am. J. Psychiatry*, **164**, 1547–1556.

Wagner, K.D., Kowatch, R.A., Emslie, G.J. *et al.* (2006) A double-blind, randomized, placebo-controlled trial of oxcarbazepine in the treatment of bipolar disorder in children and adolescents. *Am. J. Psychiatry*, **163** (7), 1179–1186.

Wagner, K.D., Nyilas, M., Johnson, B. *et al.* (2007) Long-term efficacy of aripiprazole in children (10–17 years old) with mania. Poster presented at the Annual Meeting of the American Academy of Child and Adolescent Psychiatry, October 23–28, 2007, Boston, MA.

Wagner, K.D., Redden, L., Kowatch, R.A. *et al.* (2009) A double-blind, randomized, placebo-controlled trial of divalproex extended-release in the treatment of bipolar disorder in children and adolescents. *J. Am. Acad. Child Adolesc. Psychiatry*, **48** (5), 519–532.

Wiznitzer, M. and Findling, R.L. (2003) Why do psychiatric drug research in children? *Lancet*, **361**, 1147–1148.

18

Treatment of Bipolar Disorder in Old Age

**Kenneth I. Shulman[1], Nathan Herrmann[1]
and Martha Sajatovic[2]**

[1]Department of Psychiatry, Faculty of Medicine, Sunnybrook Health Sciences Centre,
University of Toronto, Ontario, Canada
[2]Department of Psychiatry, Case Western Reserve University School of Medicine and
University Hospitals Case Medical Centre, Ohio, USA

18.1 TREATMENT OF BIPOLAR DISORDER IN OLD AGE

Although the focus of this chapter is on pharmacotherapy, the clinical issues unique to old age will be reviewed first. To treat effectively, clinicians require a clear understanding of classification, nosology, and subtypes of bipolarity in late life in order to make informed clinical decisions about drug therapy. In this chapter, we will highlight those aspects of the clinical understanding of bipolarity that are unique to older bipolar patients. This includes its relatively late age of onset, long-term clinical course, and the high prevalence of comorbidity including cognitive impairment, other psychiatric disorders, and neurobiological features. Before addressing the management of issues specific to older adults, we will summarize the determinants of bipolarity in old age and review its implications for assessment and clinical diagnosis.

18.1.1 CLASSIFICATION ISSUES AND SUBTYPES

Relevant to this discussion is the concept of secondary mania (Krauthammer and Klerman, 1978) that implies that cerebral organic (neurologic) factors are responsible for the manic syndrome. In a parallel literature, the neurologists use the term "disinhibition syndrome" that describes a condition that is essentially identical to the concept of secondary mania with a similar clinical spectrum. Clearly, diagnostic subtypes may have a strong influence on treatment approach.

Bipolar Psychopharmacotherapy: Caring for the patient, Second Edition. Edited by Hagop S. Akiskal and Mauricio Tohen.
© 2011 John Wiley & Sons, Ltd. Published 2011 by John Wiley & Sons, Ltd.

18.1.2   AGE OF ONSET

By and large, bipolar disorder in old age is associated with a late age of onset. In a retrospective study in which the mean age of index elderly bipolar patients was 70, their mean age of first psychiatric hospitalization was age 55 (Shulman *et al.*, 1992). Wylie *et al.* (1999) used a cut-off of 49 years to define a late onset group of elderly bipolar patients who demonstrated an increase in cerebrovascular risk factors.

While the community prevalence of bipolar disorder decreases from a high of 1.4% in young adults (Weissman, Bruce, and Leak, 1991) to a negligible prevalence of <0.1%, the opposite trend applies to the incidence of hospital admissions for bipolar disorder. Almost 20% of first admissions of patients with bipolar disorders in Finland occurred after the age of 60 (Rasanen, Tiihonen, and Hakko, 1998). These elderly bipolars are very different from the very early age of onset found in most community surveys such as the Epidemiologic Catchment Area (ECA) study (Weissman, Bruce, and Leak, 1991) and the U.S National Comorbidity (Kessler *et al.*, 1997) who reported a mean age of onset of bipolar disorder at 21 years. However a relatively small number of elderly bipolar inpatients are known to experience their first manic episode before the age of 40 (Shulman *et al.*, 1992; Snowdon, 1991) and we have not yet answered the question "where have all the young bipolars gone?" Whether this is related to a relatively higher mortality rate and suicide in bipolar patients has not yet been determined.

Age of onset is also a variable that may help to identify sub-types of mania and thereby reduce the genetic heterogeneity that is inherent in the bipolar spectrum (Leboyer *et al.*, 2005). Age of onset is also significantly influenced by the age cut-off, that is, used for the identification of an "elderly proband" and most studies use age 60 or 65 as such a cut-off. While 50 is the most common cut-off for "early versus late onset" bipolar disorder. Moorhead and Young (2003) used the psychiatric case registry in the United Kingdom to determine age of onset in bipolar I patients. They noted that those subjects without a family history were more likely to have a later age of onset with a modal onset of 49 years. In this latter sub-group, they concluded that nongenetic factors were more relevant and agreed that age 50 would indeed be a useful cut-off for late onset.

This late onset disorder is understandably associated with a high level of neuro-logic comorbidity characterized by a heterogeneous group of right hemisphere lesions (Starkstein *et al.*, 1990; Strakowski *et al.*, 1994; Steffens and Krishnan, 1998). Even when compared to age and sex-matched unipolar depressives, elderly bipolars had a significantly higher rate of coarse neurologic disorders (36% versus 8%) (Shulman *et al.*, 1992). A subgroup whose first affective episode was mania in old age were even more likely to present with coarse neurological abnormalities (71%) than elderly patients with multiple previous episodes of bipolar disease (28%). Braun *et al.* (2008) collected a series of single case reports of unilateral lesions involving at least one manic symptom. They assembled a sub-group of 59 clearly defined manic patients, the majority of whom had right hemisphere lesions. However, elation alone without a manic symptom complex was not significantly predicted by lesion side. Rather, the association of right hemisphere lesions with mania is primarily related to disinhibition rather than a shift of mood as a result of the release of left hemisphere influence. Cerebrovascular disease featured as the predominant type of disorder in groups of elderly manic patients as well as those considered to be suffering from secondary mania (Tohen, Shulman, and Satlin, 1994). Lin, Tsai, and Lee (2007) used two study cohorts identified in the Taiwan National Health Insurance Research Database. Patients hospitalized with bipolar disorder compared to those undergoing appendectomy had twice the likelihood of developing stroke. The presence of cerebrovascular disease associated with mania has led to the proposal of a bipolar vascular sub-type (Steffens and Krishnan, 1998). Similar to the vascular depression hypothesis of Alexopoulos, Meyers, and Young (1993), vascular mania is defined in the context of a finding of cerebrovascular disease based on clinical or neuroimaging findings with further evidence of cognitive impairment. The cohort of elderly manic patients with cerebrovascular disease may fit in the proposed vascular subtype although the hypothesis still needs better data for corroboration. Using a cut-off of 49 years, Wylie *et al.* (1999) found that the late onset group had more cerebrovascular risk factors which are elaborated on below. Hays *et al.* (1998) also found an increase in vascular comorbidity in their sample of elderly bipolar patients whose mean age was 74 years. Silent cerebral infarctions were found to occur most commonly in late onset mania when compared to age and sex-matched group of depressive patients (Fujikawa, Yamawaki, and Touhouda, 1995). The proportion of manic patients over the age of 60 found to have silent cerebral infarctions was greater than 20% with a relatively modest family history in first degree relatives.

18.1.3   COGNITIVE DYSFUNCTION

A recent systematic literature review of older bipolar patients, supplemented by a cross-sectional sample of 70 such patients concluded that there was an overall pattern of significant cognitive impairment that did not correlate with the level of mania and were considered persistent deficits in euthymic older patients (Young *et al.*, 2006). Similar conclusions were drawn by two other groups including Tsai *et al.* (2007) and Gildengers *et al.* (2004). Schouws *et al.* (2009) conducted an assessment of cognitive functioning in 119 older patients including those with a late onset disorder which they defined as over 40 years. They noted a greater level of cognitive impairment in the late onset compared to the early onset group.

It is now quite clear that euthymic bipolar patients demonstrate significant and persistent cognitive dysfunction not dissimilar to younger euthymic bipolar patients (Schouws *et al.*, 2007). Radanovic *et al.* (2008) demonstrated language impairment in euthymic elderly bipolar patients compared to controls while Gunning-Dixon *et al.* (2008) noted impairment of executive functioning in a group of nondemented bipolar subjects compared to depressive subjects and controls.

18.1.4   NEUROIMAGING RESEARCH

Neuroimaging research has demonstrated increased hyperintensities on MRI scans in older bipolar subjects (Steffens and Krishnan, 1998). These hyperintensities are associated with risk factors such as hypertension, atherosclerotic heart disease, and diabetes mellitus and strengthens the relationship of mania to cerebrovascular pathology. Other studies have shown an increased prevalence of silent cerebral infarctions on neuroimaging in late onset mania when compared to depression and earlier ages of onset for mood disorder (Kobayashi, Okada, and Yamashita, 1991; Fujikawa, Yamawaki, and Touhouda, 1995). The proportion of elderly manic patients whose onset was over the age of 60 with silent cerebral infarctions was more than 65% in these samples. Neuroimaging and other studies provide additional support for the proposal that there is indeed a vascular subtype of mania which may affect treatment choice and outcome. The examination of cortical atrophy has not been as frequent as that of hyperintensities and silent cerebral infarcts but Beyer *et al.* (2004) found a decreased right caudate volume in older bipolar patients compared with controls related to the duration of illness. This was most pronounced in a late onset sub-group and points to the role of the caudate in the emotional brain circuitry involving the prefrontal cortex, the amygdala, thalamus, and other basal ganglia structures. Another interesting associated finding from Beyer, Kuchibhatla, and Payne (2004) was an increase in left hippocampal volume in elderly bipolar patients. They hypothesized that lithium treatment may have been responsible for this and point to the possible neuroplasticity and cellular resilience in this region of the brain possibly induced by lithium (Manji and Duman, 2001a).

18.1.5 CLINICAL COURSE, PRESENTATION, AND HEALTH SERVICE UTILIZATION

Clinical course and outcome in elderly bipolars, even when compared to age and sex-matched unipolars, shows a very high rate of comorbidity and mortality. In one study, half of the elderly manic patients had died at a mean six year follow-up compared to only 20% of age and sex-matched elderly depressives. For the one-half of elderly bipolar patients whose first episode is depression, a long latency averaging 15 years, precedes the onset of the first manic episode (Shulman *et al.*, 1992). Almost one-quarter of this subgroup experienced a latency of more than 25 years between first depression and first manic episode. This apparent conversion to bipolarity, after numerous episodes and many years of a unipolar course, suggests that comorbid neurologic disorders do indeed play a significant role. A very small subgroup of bipolar elderly patients meets criteria for a course of unipolar mania (Shulman and Tohen, 1994). These unipolar manic patients were among the very few elderly patients whose illness began early in life, suggesting that they may have a different etiology and pathogenesis compared to other subtypes of bipolarity.

The presentation of bipolar disorder remains fairly constant across the lifespan including the general range of symptoms (Sajatovic *et al.*, 2004; Broadhead and Jacoby, 1990). Subsequent studies including those by Bartels *et al.* (2000) report that elderly bipolar patients had greater severity of symptoms and impairment of community living skills compared to age-matched older adults with unipolar depression. Moreover, they used almost four times the total amount of mental health services, including hospitalization (Sajatovic *et al.*, 2004; Bartels *et al.*, 2000). Generally, bipolar patients are found to have greater medical comorbidity, more cognitive impairment, and a less robust response to treatment (Sajatovic *et al.*, 2004; Bartels *et al.*, 2000). Depp *et al.* (2005) noted that elderly bipolar patients were less likely to use hospital facilities compared to younger bipolar patients, but were more likely to use case management services. Kessing (2006) used a nation-wide psychiatric registry in Denmark to study different diagnostic subtypes of bipolar disorder in patients with late onset (over 50) and early onset. He found that those bipolar patients whose first psychiatric hospitalization occurred after the age of 50 tended to present with less psychotic manic episodes and more severe depressions including psychosis compared to younger onset patients.

Beyer *et al.* (2008) examined stressful life events in older bipolar patients. They showed that the number of serious stressful life events in the 12 months prior to a manic episode was no different in older or younger bipolar patients. In general, negative life events were more prevalent in both older and younger bipolar patients compared to a control group. Depp *et al.* (2006a) noted that psychotic depressive symptoms as well as cognitive impairment in elderly adults with bipolar disorder contributed to the finding of a lower health related quality of life and functioning in this sample.

Older adults with new or persistent bipolar disorder are profoundly affected by their illness, resulting in a significant impact on their quality of life. These disorders represent a significant challenge to geriatric and psychiatric services because of the high levels of comorbidity and mortality.

18.1.6 DETERMINANTS OF BIPOLARITY IN OLD AGE AND CLINICAL IMPLICATIONS

Three factors appear most relevant to the manifestation of manic syndromes and bipolarity in old age.

1. Genetic loading is not as prominent as in early onset disorders yet elderly manic bipolar patients still have a very significant familial prevalence of mood disorder (50–85%) in first degree relatives (Shulman and Herrmann, 2002). An "affective predisposition" is common and this may include psychological rather than genetic vulnerability.
2. The long latency seen between first onset depression and later manifestation of mania in old age may reflect degenerative changes associated with normal aging in affectively vulnerable individuals.
3. Heterogeneous brain lesions (especially cerebrovascular) associated with mania in late life affecting the right orbital frontal cortex may be specific factors in the manifestation of mania late in life.

Affective vulnerability emerges as a significant factor in late life bipolar disorder. However, clinical experience suggests that this is not based solely on genetics (Shulman *et al.*, 1992; Fujikawa, Yamawaki, and Touhouda, 1995). Psychological events in early life such as early loss and trauma in childhood may very well be significant risk factors for affective vulnerability later in life. Beyer *et al.* (2008) have demonstrated that stressful life events do play a role in late life but are not more prevalent than in younger bipolar patients. It appears that the perfect storm of genetics, psychological stressors, and vulnerability as well as the localization of brain lesions to the right hemisphere involving the right orbital frontal circuit may be critical for mania to become manifest in old age. This may have heuristic value in shedding light on the nature and pathogenesis of mania in a much larger mixed-age population. How this translates to differences in management and pharmacological treatment is addressed in the next section on treatment.

18.2 MANAGEMENT OF BIPOLAR DISORDER IN THE ELDERLY

There are numerous reviews and treatment recommendations that have been published describing the management of bipolar disorder in the elderly (Shulman and Herrmann, 1999; Young et al., 2004a; Sajatovic, Madhusoodanan, and Coconcea, 2005; Aziz, Lorberg, and Tampi, 2006a). It is important to recognize however that because there has never been a single double-blind randomized placebo-controlled trial of any type of treatment conducted in an exclusively elderly patient population, none of these clinical practice guidelines are based on high quality evidence. Rather, they rely on anecdotal and nonrandomized trials or simply apply recommendations from young and mixed-age populations to the elderly. This methodology is highly problematic for a number of reasons. As noted previously, the etiology of bipolar disorder in late life might differ from this condition whose onset is most common in young adulthood, and therefore similar therapies might yield vastly different responses. Multiple psychiatric and medical comorbidity will also require consideration, and alterations to typical therapies that would be used in other patient populations are necessary. Similarly, age-related changes in drug metabolism and reduced tolerance to medication side-effects will require modification in terms of choice of drug, dosage of drug used, and treatment monitoring. Finally, as has become clear in the randomized placebo controlled trials of atypical antipsychotics in elderly dementia patient populations, older adults may have specific adverse events that differ from younger patient populations and therefore may result in a completely different risk/benefit ratio.

In an attempt to deal with the lack of randomized placebo-controlled data, some investigators have attempted to pool studies of mixed-age populations and do sub-analyses with the elderly subjects. Unfortunately, because many trials only enroll subjects up to the age of 65, few of these post-hoc analyses are available, and those that have been published are sub-optimal given the actual numbers included as well as the age of the "elderly" patients they include. For example, in a recent post-hoc analysis of two randomized placebo-controlled trials of an atypical antipsychotic for the treatment of mania, only 59 out of 604 patients were over the age of 55 and the average age of the treatment groups in this analysis was only 61 and 63, hardly what most geriatric psychiatrists would consider to be an elderly patient population (Sajatovic, Calabrese, and Mullen, 2008).

This lack of high quality evidence from randomized trials will also continue to plague the profession for at least the near future. For example, a review of the American Clinical

Trial Registry (clinicaltrials.gov) revealed only four trials recruiting elderly patients with bipolar disorder (Health NIo, 2009). None of the four trials are placebo-controlled and the only randomized trial, comparing lithium to valproate, has already been recruiting for over four years.

As noted previously, despite the absence of specific trials in the elderly, attempts have been made to apply adult treatment guidelines to geriatric patient populations. In an open-labelled trial of 31 elderly bipolar patients (Gildengers, Mulsant, and Begley, 2005), standardized treatment based on the Systematic Treatment Enhanced Program for Bipolar Disorder (STEP-BD) were successfully applied (Sachs *et al.*, 2003). Unfortunately, while patients demonstrated significant clinical improvement, only 10% of study participants experienced sustained recovery. It is, therefore, obvious that larger trials are essential in order to document efficacy and safety of treatment in the bipolar elderly patient population.

18.2.1   TREATMENT OF ACUTE MANIA IN THE ELDERLY

Clinical practice guidelines for the treatment of acute mania recommend lithium, valproic acid (or the combination) or an atypical antipsychotic as first-line therapy (American Psychiatric Association, 2002a; Yatham *et al.*, 2006). Carbamazepine, oxcarbazepine, and electroconvulsive therapy (ECT) are generally included under second-line therapies, while clozapine would be considered third-line treatment. Similar recommendations have been suggested for elderly patient populations as well (Shulman and Herrmann, 1999; Young *et al.*, 2004a; Aziz, Lorberg, and Tampi, 2006a). In the past two decades, there has been a significant shift in treatment utilization of these therapies in the elderly which likely parallels changes in the treatment of bipolar disorder in general. For example, even though lithium remains a commonly used mood stabilizer in late life (Head and Dening, 1998) and was the most commonly prescribed treatment used in the standardized treatment trial mentioned previously (Gildengers, Mulsant, and Begley, 2005), valproic acid now appears to be more commonly prescribed in the elderly. In a study conducted between 1993 and 2000, the new use of lithium carbonate fell consistently, while the use of valproic acid increased eventually surpassing the use of lithium (Shulman *et al.*, 2003). The use of atypical antipsychotics has also increased dramatically in the elderly. For example, in a recently published cohort study of a large outpatient population of elderly bipolar patients, while 54% were taking a classic mood stabilizer (lithium or valproic acid), up to 46% were taking an atypical antipsychotic. This study also highlighted the growing trend toward using polypharmacy for bipolar patients. Even though geriatric psychiatrists have traditionally eschewed polypharmacy, almost half of the elderly bipolar patients in this large cohort were taking three or more psychotropic drugs (Kupfer *et al.*, 2009).

While there is no data on the use of psychotherapy, ECT, transcranial magnetic stimulation or benzodiazepines for elderly manic patients, these interventions have still been recommended in treatment practice guidelines (Sajatovic, 2002).

18.2.1.1 Lithium Carbonate

Evidence of lithium's effectiveness and safety in the elderly comes from a surprisingly small number of open-label naturalistic and retrospective studies (Gildengers, Mulsant, and Begley, 2005; Van der Velde, 1970; Himmelhoch *et al.*, 1980; Schaffer and Garvey, 1984; Chen *et al.*, 1999). Age-related changes in creatinine clearance and glomerular filtration rate have significant effects on lithium pharmacokinetics, with at least one study documenting that the rate of lithium excretion in the elderly was half that of younger patients (Hardy, Shulman, and Mackenzie, 1987). There are also reports of increased sensitivity to lithium adverse events and toxicity which can occur even at lithium serum levels considered within the therapeutic range as reported by most laboratories (Roose *et al.*, 1979; Murray *et al.*, 1983; Sproule, Hardy, and Shulman, 2000). A recent study confirmed the need to keep serum lithium levels low in the elderly (Forester *et al.*, 2009). This magnetic resonance spectroscopy study demonstrated that there was no correlation between lithium serum lithium levels and brain lithium levels, and that higher brain levels of lithium were associated with frontal lobe cognitive dysfunction and higher depression rating scale scores. Studies such as this have also contributed to the controversy regarding lithium dosages and serum levels recommended for the elderly. While some authors have recommended levels as low as 0.5 mmol/l (Shulman, Mackenzie and Hardy, 1987), others have argued that higher levels are needed to obtain better clinical outcomes (Chen *et al.*, 1999, Young, 1996). In general, the published studies of lithium in the elderly utilized dosages that were 25–50% lower with serum levels typically below 0.7 mmol/l (Aziz, Lorberg, and Tampi, 2006a).

Treatment with lithium in the elderly requires consideration of age-specific adverse events and potential drug interactions with the numerous medications used to treat concomitant medical conditions. As well as lithium-induced tremor, Parkinsonian symptoms, and other extrapyramidal effects, lithium has been associated with cognitive impairment and even delirium in the elderly. In an administrative health database study, the rate of hospitalization for lithium-induced delirium was 2.5 per 100 person years, though this was not significantly different from the rate of delirium associated with valproate use (Shulman *et al.*, 2005a). Lithium-induced hypothyroidism might be more common in the elderly than in younger populations. In a community study of elderly lithium users, one-third had elevated levels of thyroid stimulating hormone or were being treated with thyroid replacement (Head and Dening, 1998). In an administrative health database study of 1705 new elderly lithium users, 6% were being treated for hypothyroidism which the authors estimated to be about twice the expected prevalence from a mixed-age population (Shulman *et al.*, 2005b).

Drug-drug interactions associated with reduced lithium clearance and potential for lithium toxicity include reactions with angiotensin-converting enzyme inhibitors, non-steroidal anti-inflammatory drugs, and diuretics (Shulman and Herrmann, 1999). Besides thiazide diuretics, furosemide also appears to be associated with lithium toxicity. For example, in a nested case controlled study of elderly lithium users were 4% were hospitalized for lithium toxicity, new use of a loop diuretic such as furosemide increased the risk of hospitalization by five- to sevenfold (Juurlink *et al.*, 2004).

18.2.1.2 Valproic Acid

Open-label and retrospective studies suggest that valproic acid is effective and well tolerated in the treatment of acute mania in the elderly (Gildengers, Mulsant, and Begley, 2005; Chen *et al.*, 1999; McFarland, Miller, and Straumfjord, 1990; Risinger, Risby, and Risch, 1994; Kando *et al.*, 1996; Noaghiul, Narayan, and Nelson 1998; Mordecai, Sheikh, and Glick, 1999; Niedermier and Nasrallah 1998; Puryear, Kunik, and Workman, 1995). Dosages used in these studies have ranged between 250 and 2250 mg per day with serum levels between 25 and 120 µg/ml. Dose dependent changes in valproic acid metabolism, including prolonged elimination half-life which may increase the risk of toxicity have been described (Felix *et al.*, 2003; Bryson *et al.*, 1983). Besides the frequent and well documented adverse events of excessive sedation and gastrointestinal intolerance, under-recognized, and important side-effects in the elderly include thrombocytopenia (Trannel, Ahmed, and Goebert, 2001) and hyperammonemia leading to delirium (Beyenburg *et al.*, 2007). In an administrative health database study, there were no differences found between the rates of hospitalization for delirium when comparing valproate to lithium (Shulman *et al.*, 2005a).

18.2.1.3 Other Anticonvulsants

There are only a small number of open-label and naturalistic studies reported on the use of carbamazepine in the elderly (Kellner and Neher, 1991; Schneier and Kahn, 1990). There are also concerns about the tolerability of carbamazepine in the elderly, its potential for neurotoxicity and significant potential for drug interactions (Young, 1996; Janicak, 1993). While there is one small series of gabapentin used in elderly manics (Sethi, Mehta, and Devanand, 2003), there is no data on other anticonvulsants including oxcarbazepine, topiramate, or zonisamide.

18.2.1.4 Atypical Antipsychotics

Studies in adult populations have suggested that the atypical antipsychotics appear to have mood stabilizing properties leading to their recommendation as first-line agents for the treatment of acute mania (Yatham *et al.*, 2006). In contrast to the numerous randomized placebo-controlled trials of atypical antipsychotics that have published with elderly dementia patients, there are no randomized placebo-controlled trials of atypical antipsychotics for elderly bipolar patients. Small case series and case reports have suggested that olanzapine (Madhusoodanan *et al.*, 1999), risperidone (Madhusoodanan *et al.*, 1995), and clozapine (Shulman, Singh, and Shulman, 1997; Frye, Altshuler, and Bitran, 1996) can be effective for elderly bipolar patients. With respect to clozapine, elderly patients may be at greater risk of developing leukopenia and agranulocytosis compared to younger patient populations (Gareri *et al.*, 2008). Finally, in a post-hoc analysis from two randomized placebo-controlled trials of quetiapine for mania, significant benefit in reducing mania rating scale scores in an elderly sub-population was noted as early as day 4 and by the end of the studies (Sajatovic, Calabrese, and Mullen, 2008). These studies used daily doses of approximately 550 mg per day and a significant number of patients discontinued prematurely because of adverse events.

While clearly recognized in younger schizophrenic patients, it is still unclear how significant metabolic adverse effects are in the elderly (Herrmann and Lanctot, 2006). For example, neither the randomized placebo-controlled trials in elderly dementia patients nor the population-based studies that have been performed, consistently demonstrate increases in weight, glucose intolerance, and hyperlipidemia with drugs including clozapine, olanzapine, quetiapine, and risperidone (Herrmann and Lanctot, 2006). Most recently, data from the CATIE-AD study with elderly dementia patients did suggest significant weight gain in elderly females treated with atypical antipsychotics (Zheng *et al.*, 2009) and in a population-based study of elderly patients with pre-existing diabetes new atypical antipsychotic use was associated with a dramatically increased risk of hyperglycemia-related events (Lipscombe, Levesque, and Gruneir, 2009).

Similarly, based on both randomized placebo-controlled trials in elderly dementia patients as well as administrative health database studies, both typical and atypical antipsychotics appear to increase the risk of cerebrovascular adverse events as well as mortality (Herrmann and Lanctot, 2006; Herrmann and Lanctot, 2005). It is unclear, however, whether elderly bipolar patients have similar risks for cerebrovascular adverse events and mortality as patients with dementia.

18.3 TREATMENT OF BIPOLAR DEPRESSION IN OLDER ADULTS

Depressive symptoms occur three times more frequently than manic symptoms among individuals with bipolar illness, and are a severe and pervasive problem across the life span (Judd *et al.*, 2002; Kupka *et al.*, 2007). Furthermore, disability associated with bipolar depression is disproportionately greater compared with bipolar mania (Post *et al.*, 2003; Judd *et al.*, 2005) and depressed mood among individuals with bipolar disorder is known to contribute to completed suicide (Vieta *et al.*, 1997).

Among middle-aged and older adults with bipolar disorder, depressive symptom significantly reduce quality of life (Depp *et al.*, 2006b). In depressed bipolar elders, treatments directed at mood dysregulation can reduce disability (Klausner *et al.*, 1998), and may avoid "behavioral disuse atrophy" (Alexopoulos *et al.*, 1995; Lehman *et al.*, 2002).

In spite of the fact that most randomized controlled trials (RCTs) in bipolar disorder have been mania treatment trials (Smith *et al.*, 2007), it appears that the most salient issue for those with bipolar disorder appears to be treatments for bipolar depression. A study that surveyed 469 individuals with bipolar disorder found that patients identified reduction of depression as a top priority (Johnson *et al.*, 2007).

Unfortunately, there remains a scarcity of evidence-based treatments for bipolar depression, and information on this topic has accumulated only recently (Fontoulakis *et al.*, 2008). Pharmacotherapies for bipolar depression in mixed-age populations include lithium, the anticonvulsants valproate, lamotrigine, and carbamazepine as well as the atypical antipsychotics and combination therapy with antidepressant medications adjunct to mood stabilizers (Fontoulakis *et al.*, 2008; Gijsman *et al.*, 2004). Fontoulakis *et al.* (2008) reported that research-based evidence supported by at least one placebo-controlled trial of "sufficient" magnitude is only available for selected atypical antipsychotic compounds including olanzapine and quetiapine monotherapies and olanzapine in combination with fluoxetine. The International Consensus Group (ICG) identified only three compounds (lithium, lamotrigine, quetiapine) which appear to have first-level evidence for the treatment of acute and long term bipolar depression as monotherapies (Kaspar *et al.*, 2008). A recently published study of add-on lamotrigine with lithium in bipolar depression demonstrated significant improvement and very good tolerability in mixed age (mean 45.2 years) patients (Van der Loos *et al.*, 2009).

Finally, the use of antidepressants in bipolar depression is controversial due to the possible likelihood of precipitating manic switching and rapid cycling. For this reason, the ICG does not recommend the use of antidepressants generally for individuals with bipolar depression (Kaspar *et al.*, 2008). Treatment guidelines by the American Psychiatry Association (APA) (American Psychiatric Association, 2002b), recommend that antidepressants be used cautiously and parsimoniously in those with bipolar depression, with use discontinued once the depressive episode has resolved.

Uncontrolled and secondary analyses in late-life bipolar depression suggest a possible role for the traditional mood stabilizing medications lithium and for lamotrigine (Young *et al.*, 2004b; Aziz, Lorberg, and Tampi, 2006b). Sajatovic and colleagues have recently conducted a 12-week, open label trial of lamotrigine for older adults (age 60 and older) with type I or type II bipolar depression conducted at five academic medical centers in the U.S. (Sajatovic *et al.*, 2009). In addition to age and diagnostic criteria confirmed via the SCID-I/P (First *et al.*, 1996), all individuals had a 24-item Hamilton Depression Scale (HAM-D 24) (Hamilton, 1960) total score of 18 or higher. Primary study outcome was changed from baseline to endpoint on the Montgomery Asberg Depression Rating Scale (MADRS) (Montgomery and Asberg, 1979). In a preliminary data analysis report (Sajatovic *et al.*, 2009), 56 nondemented bipolar depressed elders (mean age 66.9, range 6–90 years) received lamotrigine therapy (mean dose 138.5 mg/day, range 12.5–400 mg/day) adjunct to bipolar maintenance treatments which included lithium, valproate, and antipsychotic compounds. There was significant improvement from baseline to endpoint on the MADRS with a baseline mean of 25.8, SD = 8.36, range 9–48 to endpoint mean of 7.8, SD = 6.31, range 0–21 (p < 0.0001). Functional status was improved on most domains in these bipolar elders including self-care, life activities, ability to understand and communicate, participation in society, and getting along with people as measured by the World Health Organization-Disability Assessment Schedule II (WHO-DAS II). Lamotrigine was fairly well tolerated in this population with no significant change in group means from baseline in body weight, serum glucose, total cholesterol, and triglycerides.

18.3.1   ATYPICAL ANTIPSYCHOTICS

Atypical antipsychotic compounds, which are commonly utilized in mixed-age bipolar populations, may also be of benefit in late-life bipolar depression. A secondary analysis focusing on an older adult sub-sample evaluated combined results from two eight-week, double-blind, randomized, placebo-controlled studies of quetiapine in fixed doses (300 or 600 mg/day) in the treatment of depressive episodes associated with bipolar I or II disorder (Sajatovic and Paulsson, 2007; Calabrese *et al.*, 2005; Thase *et al.*, 2006). Primary efficacy endpoint was MADRS total score change from baseline to endpoint. The older group comprised 72 individuals (mean age $\pm$ SD 58.4 $\pm$ 2.6 years; n = 23, 23, and 26 for quetiapine 300 mg/day, quetiapine 600 mg/day, and placebo, respectively) and the younger group comprised 906 individuals aged 18 to <55 years (mean 35.7 $\pm$ 9.9 years; n = 304, 298, and 304, respectively). Illness characteristics, including DSM-IV diagnoses and baseline depression scores, were similar between older and younger groups. In older adults, least square mean $\pm$ SE MADRS score decreased 13.4 $\pm$ 2.4 with quetiapine 300 mg/day and 14.2 $\pm$ 2.5 with quetiapine 600 mg/day versus 8.0 $\pm$ 2.3 with placebo (p = 0.097 and 0.057, respectively, versus placebo). In younger adults, mean MADRS score decreased 16.8 $\pm$ 0.7 and 16.5 $\pm$ 0.7 versus 11.2 $\pm$ 0.7, respectively (p < 0.001, both doses versus placebo). Quetiapine (both doses) significantly decreased HAM-D and CGI-S scores and increased CGI-I scores relative to placebo in older and younger adults. The most frequent adverse effects in both age groups were dry mouth, somnolence, sedation, and dizziness. Treatment-related study participation withdrawal rates were similar in older and younger adults.

The atypical antipsychotic aripiprazole was evaluated in a small sample (N = 20) of older adults with type I bipolar disorder (Sajatovic *et al.*, 2008). Bipolar elders who were sub-optimally responsive to their bipolar pharmacologic treatments received 12 weeks of adjunct open-label aripiprazole (Sajatovic *et al.*, 2008). Aripiprazole was initiated at 5 mg daily and increased as tolerated. Primary study outcomes were changed from baseline in the MADRS and Young Mania Rating Scale (YMRS). Mean age of the sample was 59.6 years, range 50–83 years. The majority of individuals had bipolar depression. Individuals had significant reductions in HAM-D and YMRS scores and significant improvements level of functioning as measured by the Global Assessment Scale (GAS). Mean daily dose of aripiprazole was 10.26 mg/day SD $\pm$ 4.9, range 5–20 mg/day. Overall, aripiprazole was efficacious and relatively well tolerated. Of particular note were the improvements in bipolar depression in this older population receiving aripiprazole therapy. While the limited data with atypicals is somewhat promising in bipolar elderly, this must be tempered by concerns regarding antipsychotic drugs in the population discussed above.

18.3.2 ANTIDEPRESSANTS

While concern regarding negative effects of antidepressant therapy in mixed-age bipolar populations has been noted by groups of bipolar experts (Fontoulakis *et al.*, 2008; American Psychiatric Association, 2002c), there is preliminary data in geriatric bipolar depression which suggests that antidepressants can have beneficial effects on some health outcomes. One study found decreased rates of hospitalization for manic/mixed episodes during a 5135 person-years follow-up study of antidepressant use among bipolar elders (Schaffer *et al.*, 2006). Another report found that bipolar elders with a recent history of suicide attempts were less likely to have received treatment with mood stabilizers and antidepressants compared to bipolar elders with no recent history of suicide attempts (Aizenberg, Olmer, and Barak, 2006). In addition to pharmacotherapies, ECT is known to an efficacious and well-tolerated treatment that should be considered for more severely ill bipolar depressed elderly (Van der Wurff _et al._, 2003).

18.3.3 MAINTENANCE TREATMENT OF BIPOLAR DISORDER IN OLDER ADULTS

Minimal data is available on maintenance or longer-term treatments for geriatric bipolar disorder. A recent retrospective analysis of elders with unipolar depression and with bipolar disorder demonstrated that lithium maintenance significantly reduced the probability of relapse and recurrence, suicidal behavior, and severity of mood disturbance (Lepkifker _et al._, 2006).

A secondary analysis of pooled data from two placebo-controlled, double-blind bipolar maintenance treatment studies focused on older adults (age 55 and older) and compared patients randomized to treatment with lamotrigine, lithium, or placebo for up to 18 months (Sajatovic _et al._, 2005). Primary outcome was time-to-intervention for any mood episode while secondary outcomes included time-to-intervention for depression and mania/hypomania/mixed mood. There were 98 older adults, mean age 61 years (±SD 6.0, range 55–82 years) included in the total group of 638 patients. Among older adults, lamotrigine, but not lithium, significantly delayed time-to-intervention for any mood episode compared with placebo. Lamotrigine also significantly delayed time-to-intervention for a depressive episode compared with lithium and placebo. Lithium did significantly better than lamotrigine for time-to-intervention for mania. Lamotrigine and lithium were associated with side effects that were generally mild to moderate. Rates of skin rash were 3% for lamotrigine and 5% for lithium while daily drug doses were 240 and 750 mg/day respectively.

An accumulating body of data suggests that lithium may provide neuroprotective/neurotrophic effects as a result of maintenance treatment (Kessing _et al._, 2008; Forester _et al._, 2008; Nunes, Forlenza, and Gattaz, 2007). Lithium is known to inhibit glycogen synthase kinase-3, which is a key enzyme in the metabolism of amyloid precursor protein and in the phosphorylation of tau protein involved in the pathogenesis of Alzheimer's disease (Manji and Duman, 2001b; Caccamo _et al._, 2007). A case-control, Brazilian study found that maintenance lithium treatment reduced the prevalence of Alzheimer's disease in bipolar elders to levels similar to that found in the general population (Nunes, Forlenza, and Gattaz, 2007), while a Danish healthy registry study suggested that maintenance lithium treatment is associated with a reduced rate of dementia (Kessing _et al._, 2008).

Al Jurdi and colleagues (2008) compared prescription patterns and recovery status among older and younger adults from the NIMH-funded STEP-BD. "Recovery" was defined as eight consecutive weeks without significant symptoms. Treatment regimes and doses were compared between younger participants (N = 3364), 20–59 years old, and older participants 60 and above (N = 246). Of the 3615 STEP-BD patients, 67.6% (N = 2442) achieved a recovered status – 78.5% (N = 193) of older patients vs. 66.8% of the younger patients. Recovered patients received an average of 2.05 medications with no age group difference. There were 37.8% of younger patients who received lithium vs. 29.5% of older patients. Lithium, valproate, and risperidone daily dosages were all lower in older patients. Significant reduction in lithium dosing was observed among individuals aged 50 and older although 42.1% of recovered bipolar elders achieved recovery with lithium alone compared with only 21.3% of the younger individuals. The STEP-BD older-adult sub-set analysis suggests that more than one bipolar medication treatment is needed for recovery.

It has been suggested that older adults with bipolar disorder appear to benefit from psychotherapy that facilitates coping with both mental illness and aging-related issues (McBride and Bauer, 2007). Kilbourne and colleagues (2008) have described a manual-based medical care model (BCM) that appears feasible for implementation in bipolar elderly. The BCM includes sessions on bipolar symptom patient self-management, use of nurse-run coordination/management, and dissemination of guidelines to care providers on cardiovascular disease risk in bipolar elders (Kilbourne *et al.*, 2008). Integrated therapies that address both bipolar and medical conditions are particularly attractive for geriatric bipolar populations.

18.3.4   ADHERENCE TO TREATMENT

In mixed-age samples, nearly one in two individuals with bipolar disorder is nonadherent with treatment (Lingam and Scott, 2002; Perlick, 2004). Nonadherence may be predicted to some extent by age, marital status, gender, educational level, and psychiatric comorbidity, in particular substance abuse (Lingam and Scott, 2002; Berk, Berk, and Castle, 2004; Aagaard, Vestergaard, and Maarbjerg, 1988). A large VA case registry study (N = 73 964) evaluated antipsychotic medication adherence in bipolar patients using pharmacy refill patterns (Sajatovic *et al.*, 2007). Among bipolar elders, 61.0% (N = 3350) were fully adherent, while 19% (N = 1043) were partially adherent and 20% (N = 1098) were nonadherent. Among younger adults, 49.5% (N = 10 644) were fully adherent, while 21.8% (N = 4680) were partially adherent, and 28.7% (N = 6170) were nonadherent. As in younger bipolar populations, among bipolar elderly, comorbid substance abuse, and homelessness predict nonadherence.

18.4   THE FUTURE

The future directions in the pharmacological management of bipolar disorder in old age need to build on the existing knowledge base and clinical experience in spite of the limited systematic data that is currently available. The following issues will likely help advance our understanding in managing bipolar disorder later in life:

1.   The elucidation of the pathogenesis of bipolarity in old age should lead to heuristically valuable subtypes that can be targeted for specific treatments and outcome studies. Shulman and Herrmann (2008) have proposed four subtypes for consideration. These include:

(a) Primary bipolar disorder. These are individuals with early onset of mood disorder continuing into old age. These patients are largely treated as outpatients and generally do not require hospitalization.
(b) Latent bipolar disorder which includes those individuals with an onset of depression in mid-life and a "conversion" to mania late in life often after a long latency and multiple depressive episodes. This conversion may be due to "cerebral organic" factors that may be due to normal degenerative changes with aging.
(c) Secondary mania (disinhibition syndromes). This group of generally late onset manic syndromes occurs with a decreased history of familial predisposition or prior history of mood disorder. They tend to be associated with clear-cut neurologic disorders or other systemic medical disorders.
(d) A less common group of unipolar manics who have their onset early in life and continue to persist into old age with manic-only episodes.

Each of these subtypes may require a different pharmacological approach on the assumption that they each have a different underlying pathogenesis.

2. It may be useful to determine whether there is a differential response of bipolarity in older adults to mood stabilizers or antipsychotics dependent on the subtype. In particular, we need to determine whether manic syndromes that are associated with neurologic comorbidity require long-term stabilization or whether these conditions can be treated with short-term atypical antipsychotic agents. We need better information to determine whether the new "mood stabilizers" are as effective as lithium in older adults.
3. Only the completion of a multi-center RCT in elderly bipolars patients will provide sufficient efficacy data for the most commonly used pharmacological agents.
4. Until the completion of such an RCT, pharmaco-epidemiologic data, and Consensus Conferences can help to guide treatment decisions. It seems likely that combination therapies will be more common, especially for refractory and rapid-cycling cases (Mondimore, Fuller, and De Paulo, 2003).

References

Aagaard, J., Vestergaard, P., and Maarbjerg, K. (1988) Adherence to lithium prophylaxis: II. Multivariate analysis of clinical, social, and psychosocial predictors of nonadherence. *Pharmacopsychiatry*, **21**, 166–170.

Aizenberg, D., Olmer, A., and Barak, Y. (2006) Suicide attempts amongst elderly bipolar patients. *J. Affect. Disord.*, **91**, 91–94.

Alexopoulos, G.S., Meyers, B.S., Young, R.C. *et al.* (1993) The course of geriatric depression with "reversible dementia": a controlled study. *Am. J. Psychiatry*, **150** (11), 1693–1699.

Alexopoulos, G.S., Vrontou, C., Kakuma, T. *et al.* (1995) *Disability in Geriatric Depression*, American Psychological Association.

Al Jurdi, R.K., Marangell, L.B., Petersen, N.J. *et al.* (2008) Prescription patterns of psychotropic medications in elderly compared with younger participants who achieved a "recovered" status in the systematic treatment enhancement program for bipolar disorder. *Am. J. Geriatr. Psychiatry*, **16**, 922–933.

American Psychiatric Association (2002a) *Practice Guidelines for the Treatment of Patients with Bipolar Disorder*, American Psychiatric Press, Washington, DC.

American Psychiatric Association (2002b) Practice guideline for the treatment of patients with bipolar disorder (Revision). *Am. J. Psychiatry* **159** (Suppl. 4), 1–50.

American Psychiatric Association (2002c) *Practice Guidelines for The Treatment of Patients With Bipolar Disorder*, American Psychiatric Press, Washington, DC.

Aziz, R., Lorberg, B., and Tampi, R.R. (2006a) Treatments for late-life bipolar disorder. *Am. J. Geriatr. Pharmacother.*, **4** (4), 347–364.

Aziz, R., Lorberg, B., and Tampi, R.R. (2006b) Treatments for late-life bipolar disorder. *Am. J. Geriatr. Pharmacothe.*, **4**, 347–364.

Bartels, S.J., Forester, B., Miles, K.M. *et al.* (2000) Mental health service use by elderly patients with bipolar disorder and unipolar major depression. *Am. J. Geriatr. Psychiatry*, **8** (2), 160–166.

Berk, M., Berk, L., and Castle, D. (2004) A collaborative approach to the treatment alliance in BPD. *Bipolar Disord.*, **6**, 504–518.

Beyenburg, S., Back, C., Diederich, N. *et al.* (2007) Is valproate encephalopathy under-recognised in older people? A case series. *Age Ageing*, **36** (3), 344–346.

Beyer, J.L., Kuchibhatla, M., Cassidy, F. *et al.* (2008) Stressful life events in older bipolar patients. *Int. J. Geriatr. Psychiatry*, **23** (12), 1271–1275.

Beyer, J.L., Kuchibhatla, M., and Payne, M.E. (2004) Hippocampal volume measurement in older adults with bipolar disorder. *Am. J. Geriatr. Psychiatry*, **12** (6), 613–620.

Beyer, J.L., Kuchibhatla, M., Payne, M. *et al.* (2004) Caudate volume measurement in older adults with bipolar disorder. *Int. J. Geriatr. Psychiatry*, **19** (2), 109–114.

Braun, C.M., Daigneault, R., Gaudelet, S. *et al.* (2008) Diagnostic and statistical manual of mental disorders, fourth edition symptoms of mania: which one(s) result(s) more often from right than left hemisphere lesions? *Compr. Psychiatry*, **49** (5), 441–459.

Broadhead, J. and Jacoby, R. (1990) Mania in old age: a first prospective study. *Int. J. Geriatr. Psychiatry*, **5**, 215.

Bryson, S.M., Verma, N., Scott, P.J. *et al.* (1983) Pharmacokinetics of valproic acid in young and elderly subjects. *Br. J. Clin. Pharmacol.*, **16** (1), 104–105.

Caccamo, A., Oddo, S., Tran, L.X. *et al.* (2007) Lithium reduces tau phosphorylation but not a beta or working memory deficits in a transgenic model with both plaques and tangles. *Am. J. Pathol.*, **170**, 1669–1675.

Calabrese, J., Keck, P.E., Macfadden, W. Jr. *et al.* (2005) A randomized, double-blind, placebo-controlled trial of quetiapine in the treatment of bipolar I or II depression. *Am. J. Psychiatry*, **162**, 1351–1360.

Chen, S.T., Altshuler, L.L., Melnyk, K.A. *et al.* (1999) Efficacy of lithium vs. valproate in the treatment of mania in the elderly: a retrospective study. *J. Clin. Psychiatry*, **60** (3), 181–186.

Depp, C.A., Davis, C.E., Mittal, D. *et al.* (2006a) Health-related quality of life and functioning of middle-aged and elderly adults with bipolar disorder. *J. Clin. Psychiatry*, **67** (2), 215–221.

Depp, C.A., Davis, C.E., Mittal, D. *et al.* (2006b) Health-related quality of life and functioning of middle-aged and elderly adults with bipolar disorder. *J. Clin. Psychiatry*, **67**, 215–221.

Depp, C.A., Lindamer, L.A., Folsom, D.P. *et al.* (2005) Differences in clinical features and mental health service use in bipolar disorder across the lifespan. *Am. J. Geriatr. Psychiatry*, **13** (4), 290–298.

Felix, S., Sproule, B.A., Hardy, B.G. *et al.* (2003) Dose-related pharmacokinetics and pharmacodynamics of valproate in the elderly. *J. Clin. Psychopharmacol.*, **23** (5), 471–478.

First, M.B., Spitzer, R.L., Gibbon, M. *et al.* (1996) *Structured Clinical Interview for DSM-IV Axis I Disorders- Patient Edition (SCID-I/P, Version 2.0)*, Biometrics Research Department, New York State Psychiatric Institute, New York.

Fontoulakis, K.N., Vieta, E., Bouras, C. *et al.* (2008) A systematic review of existing data on long-term lithium therapy: neuroprotective or neurotoxic? *Int. J. Neuropsychopharmacol.*, **11**, 269–287.

Forester, P.B., Fin, C.T., Berlow, Y.A. *et al.* (2008) Grain lithium, N-acetyl aspartate and myo-inositol levels in older adults with bipolar disorder treated with lithium: a lithium-7 and proton magnetic resonance spectroscopy study. *Bipolar Disord.*, **10**, 691–700.

Forester, B.P., Streeter, C.C., Berlow, Y.A. *et al.* (2009) Brain lithium levels and effects on cognition and mood in geriatric bipolar disorder: a lithium-7 magnetic resonance spectroscopy study. *Am. J. Geriatr. Psychiatry*, **17** (1), 13–23.

Frye, M.A., Altshuler, L.L., and Bitran, J.A. (1996) Clozapine in rapid cycling bipolar disorder. *J. Clin. Psychopharmacol.*, **16** (1), 87–90.

Fujikawa, T., Yamawaki, S., and Touhouda, Y. (1995) Silent cerebral infarctions in patients with late-onset mania. *Stroke*, **126** (6), 946–949.

Gareri, P., De Fazio, P., Russo, E. *et al.* (2008) The safety of clozapine in the elderly. *Exp. Opin. Drug Saf.*, **7** (5), 525–538.

Gijsman, H.J., Geddes, J.R., Rendell, J.M. *et al.* (2004) Antidepressants for bipolar depression: a systematic review of randomized, controlled trials. *Am. J. Psychiatry*, **161**, 1537–1547.

Gildengers, A.G., Butters, M.A., Seligman, K. *et al.* (2004) Cognitive functioning in late-life bipolar disorder. *Am. J. Psychiatry*, **161** (4), 736–738.

Gildengers, A.G., Mulsant, B.H., and Begley, A.E. (2005) A pilot study of standardized treatment in geriatric bipolar disorder. *Am. J. Geriatr. Psychiatry*, **13** (4), 319–323.

Gunning-Dixon, F.M., Murphy, C.F., Alexopoulos, G.S. *et al.* (2008) Executive dysfunction in elderly bipolar manic patients. *Am. J. Geriatr. Psychiatry*, **16** (6), 506–512.

Hamilton, M. (1960) A rating scale for depression. *J. Neurol. Neurosurg. Psychiatry*, **23** (1), 56–62.

Hardy, B.G., Shulman, K.I., and Mackenzie, S.E. (1987) Pharmacokinetics of lithium in the elderly. *J. Clin. Psychopharmacol.*, **7** (3), 153–158.

Hays, J.C., Krishnan, K.R., George, L.K. *et al.* (1998) Age of first onset of bipolar disorder: demographic, family history, and psychosocial correlates. *Depress. Anxiety*, **7** (2), 76–82.

Head, L. and Dening, T. (1998) Lithium in the over-65s: who is taking it and who is monitoring it? A survey of older adults on lithium in the Cambridge Mental Health Services catchment area. *Int. J. Geriatr. Psychiatry*, **13** (3), 164–171.

Health NIo (2009) www.clinicaltrials.gov.

Herrmann, N. and Lanctot, K.L. (2005) Do atypical antipsychotics cause stroke? *CNS Drugs*, **19** (2), 91–103.

Herrmann, N. and Lanctot, K.L. (2006) Atypical antipsychotics for neuropsychiatric symptoms of dementia: malignant or maligned? *Drug Saf.*, **29** (10), 833–843.

Himmelhoch, J.M., Neil, J.F., May, S.J. *et al.* (1980) Age, dementia, dyskinesias, and lithium response. *Am. J. Psychiatry*, **137** (8), 941–945.

Janicak, P.G. (1993) The relevance of clinical pharmacokinetics and therapeutic drug monitoring: anticonvulsant mood stabilizers and antipsychotics. *J. Clin. Psychiatry*, **54**, 35–41; discussion 55–56.

Johnson, F.R., Ozdemir, S., Manjunath, R. *et al.* (2007) Factors that affect adherence to bipolar disorder treatments: a stated-preference approach. *Med. Care*, **45**, 545–552.

Judd, L.L., Akiskal, H.S., Schettler, P.J. *et al.* (2002) The long-term natural history of the weekly symptomatic status of bipolar I disorder. *Arch. Gen. Psychiatry*, **59**, 530–537.

Judd, L.L., Akiskal, H.S., Schettler, P.J. *et al.* (2005) Psychosocial disability in the course of bipolar I and II disorders: a prospective, comparative, longitudinal study. *Arch. Gen. Psychiatry*, **62**, 1322–1330.

Juurlink, D.N., Mamdani, M.M., Kopp, A. *et al.* (2004) Drug-induced lithium toxicity in the elderly: a population-based study. *J. Am. Geriatr. Soc.*, **52** (5), 794–798.

Kando, J.C., Tohen, M., Castillo, J. *et al.* (1996) The use of valproate in an elderly population with affective symptoms. *J. Clin. Psychiatry*, **57** (6), 238–240.

Kaspar, S., Calabrese, J., Johnson, G. *et al.* (2008) International Consensus Group on the evidence-based pharmacologic treatment of bipolar I and II depression. *J. Clin. Psychiatry*, **69**, 1632–1646.

Kellner, M.B. and Neher, F. (1991) A first episode of mania after age 80. *Can. J. Psychiatry*, **36** (8), 607–608.

Kessing, L.V. (2006) Diagnostic subtypes of bipolar disorder in older versus younger adults. *Bipolar Disord.*, **8** (1), 56–64.

Kessing, L.V., Søndergaard, L., Forman, J.L. *et al.* (2008) Lithium treatment and risk of dementia. *Arch. Gen. Psychiatry*, **65**, 1331–1335.

Kessler, R.C., Rubinow, D.R., Holmes, C. *et al.* (1997) The epidemiology of DSM-III-R bipolar I disorder in a general population survey. *Psychol. Med.*, **27** (5), 1079–1089.

Kilbourne, A.M., Post, E.P., Nossek, A. *et al.* (2008) Improving medical and psychiatric outcomes among individuals with bipolar disorder: a randomized controlled trial. *Psychiatr. Serv.*, **59**, 760–768.

Klausner, E.J., Clarkin, J.F., Lieberman, S. *et al.* (1998) Late-life depression and functional disability: the role of goal-focused group psychotherapy. *Int. J. Geriatr. Psychiatry*, **13**, 707–716.

Kobayashi, S., Okada, K., and Yamashita, K. (1991) Incidence of silent lacunar lesion in normal adults and its relation to cerebral blood flow and risk factors. *Stroke*, **22** (11), 1379–1383.

Krauthammer, C. and Klerman, G.L. (1978) Secondary mania: manic syndromes associated with antecedent physical illness or drugs. *Arch. Gen. Psychiatry*, **35** (11), 1333–1339.

Kupfer, D.J., Axelson, D.A., Birmaher, B. *et al.* (2009) Bipolar disorder center for Pennsylvanians: implementing an effectiveness trial to improve treatment for at-risk patients. *Psychiatr. Serv.*, **60** (7), 888–897.

Kupka, R.W., Altshuler, L.L., Nolen, W.A. *et al.* (2007) Three times more days depressed than manic or hypomanic in both bipolar I and bipolar II disorder. *Bipolar Disord.*, **9**, 531–535.

Leboyer, M., Henry, C., Paillere-Martinot, M.L. *et al.* (2005) Age at onset in bipolar affective disorders: a review. *Bipolar Disord.*, **7** (2), 111–118.

Lehman A.F., Alexopoulos G.S., Goldman H., *et al.* (2002) in *Mental Disorders and Disability. Time to Re-Evaluate The Relationship: Research Agenda for DSM-V* (eds D.J. Kupfer, M.B. First, and D.A. Regier), American Psychiatric Press, Washington, DC.

Lepkifker, E., Iancu, I., Horesh, N. *et al.* (2006) Lithium therapy for unipolar and bipolar depression among the middle-aged and older adult patient subpopulation. *Depress. Anxiety*, **24**, 571–576.

Lin, H.-C., Tsai, S.-Y., and Lee, H.-C. (2007) Increased risk of developing stroke among patients with bipolar disorder after an acute mood episode: a six-year follow-up study. *J. Affect. Disord.*, **100**, 49–54.

Lingam, R. and Scott, J. (2002) Treatment non-adherence in affective disorders. *Acta Psychiatr. Scand.*, **105**, 164–172.

Lipscombe, L.L., Levesque, L., and Gruneir, A. (2009) Antipsychotic drugs and hyperglycemia in older patients with diabetes. *Arch. Intern. Med.*, **169** (14), 1282–1289.

Madhusoodanan, S., Brenner, R., Araujo, L. *et al.* (1995) Efficacy of risperidone treatment for psychoses associated with schizophrenia, schizoaffective disorder, bipolar disorder, or senile dementia in 11 geriatric patients: a case series. *J. Clin. Psychiatry*, **56** (11), 514–518.

Madhusoodanan, S., Suresh, P., Brenner, R. *et al.* (1999) Experience with the atypical antipsychotics--risperidone and olanzapine in the elderly. *Ann. Clin. Psychiatry*, **11** (3), 113–118.

Manji, H.K. and Duman, R.S. (2001a) Impairments of neuroplasticity and cellular resilience in severe mood disorders: implications for the development of novel therapeutics. *Psychopharmacol. Bull.*, **35** (2), 5–49.

Manji, H.K. and Duman, R.S. (2001b) Impairments of neuroplasticity and cellular resilience in severe mood disorders: implications for the development of novel therapeutics. *Psychopharmacol. Bull.*, **35**, 5–49.

McBride, L. and Bauer, M.S. (2007) Psychosocial Interventions for Older Adults with Bipolar Disorder, in *Bipolar Disorders in Later Life* (eds M. Sajatovic and F. Blow), Johns Hopkins Press, Baltimore, MD.

McFarland, B.H., Miller, M.R., and Straumfjord, A.A. (1990) Valproate use in the older manic patient. *J. Clin. Psychiatry*, **51** (11), 479–481.

Mondimore, F.M., Fuller, G.A., and De Paulo, J.R. Jr. (2003) Drug combinations for mania. *J. Clin. Psychiatry*, **54**, 25–31.

Montgomery, S.A. and Asberg, M. (1979) A new depression scale designed to be sensitive to change. *Br. J. Psychiatry*, **134**, 382–389.

Moorhead, S.R. and Young, A.H. (2003) Evidence for a late onset bipolar-I disorder sub-group from 50 years. *J. Affect. Disord.*, **73** (3), 271–277.

Mordecai, D.J., Sheikh, J.I., and Glick, I.D. (1999) Divalproex for the treatment of geriatric bipolar disorder. *Int. J. Geriatr. Psychiatry*, **14** (6), 494–496.

Murray, N., Hopwood, S., Balfour, D.J. *et al.* (1983) The influence of age on lithium efficacy and side-effects in out-patients. *Psychol. Med.*, **13** (1), 53–60.

Niedermier, J.A. and Nasrallah, H.A. (1998) Clinical correlates of response to valproate in geriatric inpatients. *Ann. Clin. Psychiatry*, **10** (4), 165–168.

Noaghiul, S., Narayan, M., and Nelson, J.C. (1998) Divalproex treatment of mania in elderly patients. *Am. J. Geriatr. Psychiatry*, **6** (3), 257–262.

Nunes, P.V., Forlenza, O.V., and Gattaz, W.F. (2007) Lithium and risk for Alzheimer's disease in elderly patients with bipolar disorder. *Br. J. Psychiatry*, **190**, 359–360.

Perlick, D.A. (2004) Medication non-adherence in BPD: a patient – centered review of research findings. *Clin. Approaches Bipolar Disord.*, **3**, 56–54.

Post, R.M., Denicoff, K.D., Leverich, G.S. *et al.* (2003) Morbidity in 258 bipolar outpatients followed for 1 year with daily prospective ratings on the NIMH life chart method. *J. Clin. Psychiatry*, **64**, 680–690.

Puryear, L.J., Kunik, M.E., and Workman, R. Jr. (1995) Tolerability of divalproex sodium in elderly psychiatric patients with mixed diagnoses. *J. Geriatr. Psychiatry Neurol.*, **8** (4), 234–237.

Radanovic, M., Nunes, P.V., Gattaz, W.F. *et al.* (2008) Language impairment in euthymic, elderly patients with bipolar disorder but no dementia. *Int. Psychogeriatr.*, **20** (4), 687–696.

Rasanen, P., Tiihonen, J., and Hakko, H. (1998) The incidence and onset-age of hospitalized bipolar affective disorder in Finland. *J. Affect. Disord.*, **48** (1), 63–68.

Risinger, R.C., Risby, E.D., and Risch, S.C. (1994) Safety and efficacy of divalproex sodium in elderly bipolar patients. *J. Clin. Psychiatry*, **55** (5), 215.

Roose, S.P., Bone, S., Haidorfer, C. *et al.* (1979) Lithium treatment in older patients. *Am. J. Psychiatry*, **136** (6), 843–844.

Sachs, G.S., Thase, M.E., Otto, M.W. *et al.* (2003) Rationale, design, and methods of the systematic treatment enhancement program for bipolar disorder (STEP-BD). *Biol. Psychiatry*, **53** (11), 1028–1042.

Sajatovic, M. (2002) Treatment of bipolar disorder in older adults. *Int. J. Geriatr. Psychiatry*, **17** (9), 865–873.

Sajatovic, M., Blow, F.C., Kales, H.C. *et al.* (2007) Age comparison of treatment adherence with antipsychotic medications among individuals with bipolar disorder. *Int. J. Geriatr. Psychiatry*, **22**, 992–998.

Sajatovic, M., Blow, F.C., Ignacio, R.V. *et al.* (2004) Age-related modifiers of clinical presentation and health service use among veterans with bipolar disorder. *Psychiatr. Serv.*, **55** (9), 1014–1021.

Sajatovic, M., Calabrese, J.R., and Mullen, J. (2008) Quetiapine for the treatment of bipolar mania in older adults. *Bipolar Disord.*, **10** (6), 662–671.

Sajatovic, M., Coconcea, N., Ignacio, R.V. *et al.* (2008) Aripiprazole therapy in 20 older adults with bipolar disorder: A 12-week, open label trial. *J. Clin. Psychiatry*, **69**, 41–46.

Sajatovic, M., Gildengers, A., Al Jurdi, R. *et al.* (2009) *Multi-Site, Open-Label, Prospective Trial of Lamotrigine for Geriatric Bipolar Depression*, American College of Neuropsychopharmacology (ACNP), Hollywood, FL, December 7.

Sajatovic, M., Gyulai, L., Calabrese, J.R. *et al.* (2005) Maintenance treatment outcomes in older patients with bipolar I disorder. *Am. J. Geriatr. Psychiatry*, **13**, 305–311.

Sajatovic, M., Madhusoodanan, S., and Coconcea, N. (2005) Managing bipolar disorder in the elderly: defining the role of the newer agents. *Drugs Aging*, **22** (1), 39–54.

Sajatovic, M. and Paulsson, B. (2007) Quetiapine for the treatment of depressive episodes in adults aged 55 to 65 years with bipolar disorder. New research poster presented at the American Association of Petroleum Geologists (AAPG) Annual Meeting, New Orleans, Louisiana, March.

Schaffer, C.B. and Garvey, M.J. (1984) Use of lithium in acutely manic elderly patients. *Clin. Gerontology*, **3**, 58–60.

Schneier, H.A. and Kahn, D. (1990) Selective response to carbamazepine in a case of organic mood disorder. *J. Clin. Psychiatry*, **51** (11), 485.

Schaffer, A., Mamdani, M., Levitt, A. *et al.* (2006) Effect of antidepressant use on admissions to hospital among elderly bipolar patients. *Int. J. Geriatr. Psychiatry*, **13**, 275–280.

Schouws, S.N., Comijs, H.C., Stek, M.L. *et al.* (2009) Cognitive impairment in early and late bipolar disorder. *Am. J. Geriatr. Psychiatry*, **17** (6), 508–515.

Schouws, S.N., Zoeteman, J.B., Comijs, H.C. *et al.* (2007) Cognitive functioning in elderly patients with early onset bipolar disorder. *Int. J. Geriatr. Psychiatry*, **22** (9), 856–861.

Sethi, M.A., Mehta, R., and Devanand, D.P. (2003) Gabapentin in geriatric mania. *J. Geriatr. Psychiatry Neurol.*, **16** (2), 117–120.

Shulman, K.I. and Herrmann, N. (1999) The nature and management of mania in old age. *Psychiatr. Clin. N. Am.*, **22** (3), 649–665.

Shulman, K.I. and Herrmann, N. (2002) Bipolar disorder in old age, in *Bipolar Disorders: 100 Years after Manic-Depressive Insanity* (eds A. Marneros and J. Angst), Kluwer Academic Publishers, Great Britain, pp. 153–174.

Shulman, K.I. and Herrmann, N. (2008) Manic syndromes in old age, in *Oxford Textbook of Old Age Psychiatry* (eds R. Jacoby, C Oppehnheimer, and T. Denin), Oxford University Press, pp. 563–572.

Shulman, K.I. and Tohen, M. (1994) Unipolar mania reconsidered: evidence from an elderly cohort. *Br. J. Psychiatry*, **164** (4), 547–549.

Shulman, K.I., Mackenzie, S., and Hardy, B. (1987) The clinical use of lithium carbonate in old age: a review. *Prog. Neuropsychopharmacol. Biol. Psychiatry*, **11** (2–3), 159–164.

Shulman, K.I., Rochon, P., Sykora, K. *et al.* (2003) Changing prescription patterns for lithium and valproic acid in old age: shifting practice without evidence. *Br. Med. J.*, **326** (7396), 960–961.

Shulman, R.W., Singh, A., and Shulman, K.I. (1997) Treatment of elderly institutionalized bipolar patients with clozapine. *Psychopharmacol. Bull.*, **33** (1), 113–118.

Shulman, K.I., Sykora, K., Gill, S. *et al.* (2005a) Incidence of delirium in older adults newly prescribed lithium or valproate: a population-based cohort study. *J. Clin. Psychiatry*, **66** (4), 424–427.

Shulman, K.I., Sykora, K., Gill, S.S. *et al.* (2005b) New thyroxine treatment in older adults beginning lithium therapy: implications for clinical practice. *Am. J. Geriatr. Psychiatry*, **13** (4), 299–304.

Shulman, K.I., Tohen, M., Satlin, A. *et al.* (1992) Mania compared with unipolar depression in old age. *Am. J. Psychiatry*, **149** (3), 341–345.

Smith L.A., Cornelius V., Warnock A. *et al.* (2007) Pharmacological interventions for acute bipolar mania: a systematic review of randomized placebo-controlled trials. *Bipolar Disord.* **9**, 551–560.

Snowdon, J. (1991) A retrospective case-note study of bipolar disorder in old age. *Br. J. Psychiatry*, **158**, 485–490.

Sproule, B.A., Hardy, B.G., and Shulman, K.I. (2000) Differential pharmacokinetics of lithium in elderly patients. *Drugs Aging*, **16** (3), 165–177.

Starkstein, S.E., Mayberg, H.S., Berthier, M.L. *et al.* (1990) Mania after brain injury: neuroradiological and metabolic findings. *Ann. Neurol.*, **27** (6), 652–659.

Steffens, D.C. and Krishnan, K.R. (1998) Structural neuroimaging and mood disorders: recent findings, implications for classification, and future directions. *Biol. Psychiatry*, **43** (10), 705–712.

Strakowski, S.M., MeElroy, S.L., Keck, P.W. Jr. *et al.* (1994) The co-occurrence of mania with medical and other psychiatric disorders. *Int. J. Psychiatry Med.*, **24** (4), 305–328.

Thase, M.E., Macfadden, W., Weisler, R.H. *et al.* (2006) Efficacy of quetiapine monotherapy in bipolar I and II depression: a double-blind, placebo-controlled study (the BOLDER II study). *J. Clin. Psychopharmacol.*, **26**, 600–609.

Tohen, M., Shulman, K.I., and Satlin, A. (1994) First-episode mania in late life. *Am. J. Psychiatry*, **151** (1), 130–132.

Trannel, T.J., Ahmed, I., and Goebert, D. (2001) Occurrence of thrombocytopenia in psychiatric patients taking valproate. *Am. J. Psychiatry*, **158** (1), 128–130.

Tsai, S.Y., Lee, H.C., Chen, C.C. *et al.* (2007) Cognitive impairment in later life in patients with early-onset bipolar disorder. *Bipolar Disord.*, **9** (8), 868–875.

Van der Loos, M.L., Mulder, P.G., Hartong, E.G. *et al.* (2009) Efficacy and safety of lamotrigine as add-on treatment to lithium in bipolar depression: a multi-center, double-blind, placebo-controlled trial. *J. Clin. Psychiatry*, **70** (2), 223–231.

Van der Velde, C.D. (1970) Effectiveness of lithium carbonate in the treatment of manic-depressive illness. *Am. J. Psychiatry*, **127** (3), 345–351.

Van der Wurff, F.B., Stek, M.L., Hoogendijk, W.J.G. *et al.* (2003) The efficacy and safety of ECT in depressed older adults, a literature review. *Int. J. Geriatr. Psychiatry*, **18**, 894–904.

Vieta, E., Benabarre, A., Colom, F. *et al.* (1997) Suicidal behavior in bipolar I and bipolar II disorder. *J. Nerv. Ment. Dis.*, **185**, 407–409.

Weissman, M.M., Bruce, M.L., and Leak, P.J. (1991) Affective disorders, in *Psychiatric Disorders in America: The Epidemiologic Catchment Area Study* (eds L.N. Robins and D.A. Regier), Free Press, New York, pp. 53–80.

Wylie, M.E., Mulsant, B.H., Pollock, B.G. *et al.* (1999) Age at onset in geriatric bipolar disorder. Effects on clinical presentation and treatment outcomes in an inpatient sample. *Am. J. Geriatr. Psychiatry*, **7** (1), 77–83.

Yatham, L.N., Kennedy, S.H., O'Donovan, C. *et al.* (2006) Canadian network for mood and anxiety treatments (CANMAT) guidelines for the management of patients with bipolar disorder: update 2007. *Bipolar Disord.* **8** (6), 721–739.

Young, R.C. (1996) Treatment of geriatric mania, in *Mood Disorders Across The Life Span* (eds K.I. Shulman, M. Tohen, and S.P. Kutcher), Wiley-Liss, New York, pp. 411–425.

Young, R.C., Gyulai, L., Mulsant, B.H. *et al.* (2004a) Pharmacotherapy of bipolar disorder in old age: review and recommendations. *Am. J. Geriatr. Psychiatry*, **12** (4), 342–357.

Young, R.C., Gyulai, L., Mulsant, B.H. *et al.* (2004b) Pharmacotherapy of bipolar disorder in old age: review and recommendations. *Am. J. Geriatr. Psychiatry*, **12**, 342–357.

Young, R.C., Murphy, C.F., Heo, M. *et al.* (2006) Cognitive impairment in bipolar disorder in old age: literature review and findings in manic patients. *J. Affect. Disord.*, **92** (1), 125–131.

Zheng, L., Mack, W.J., Dagerman, K.S. *et al.* (2009) Metabolic changes associated with second-generation antipsychotic use in Alzheimer's disease patients: the CATIE-AD study. *Am. J. Psychiatry*, **166** (5), 583–590.

19

Diagnosis and Treatment of Mixed States

Alan C. Swann

Department of Psychiatry and Behavioral Sciences, The University
of Texas Health Science Center at Houston, TX, USA

19.1 WHAT IS A MIXED STATE?

19.1.1 THE CONCEPT OF MIXED STATE – HISTORY AND DEVELOPMENT

Mixed states are an unusual challenge in bipolar disorder. They are considered to be difficult to treat and to represent a more complicated course of illness. Perhaps the greatest challenge presented by mixed states, however, is that they force us to redefine what is meant by an episode in bipolar disorder, and to consider bipolar disorder in a manner different from its usual formulation as an illness with discrete symptomatic affective states.

The concept of mixed states is old, predating that of bipolar disorder itself. Combinations of depressive and manic behavior were described by Areteaus of Cappadocia and in the Bible (Angst and Marneros, 2001; Jackson, 1986). Case reports in the medical literature predate the formulation of recurrent affective disorders by Kraepelin (1921), much less that of bipolar disorder by Leonhardt (Angst and Marneros, 2001; Jackson, 1986).

Kraepelin realized that symptomatic states of bipolar disorder did not consist simply of affective symptom complexes, but as combinations of more fundamental behavioral disturbances, which he considered to be increased or decreased mood, thought, and activity (Kraepelin, 1921). He observed that, in his patients, these basic behavioral disturbances formed a variety of combinations, which included pure depressive (mood, action, and thought all inhibited) and manic (mood, action, and thought all disinhibited) states, but also states where aspects of depression and mania were mixed. He also observed that mixed states were, in some way, more severe, both in symptomatic state and course of illness, than nonmixed depressive or manic states (Kraepelin, 1921). As information on neurobiology has grown, the idea that more basic elements of behavior underlie affective disorders has developed to include elements with more identifiable neurobehavioral bases (Carroll, 1983; van Praag et al., 1990).

Bipolar Psychopharmacotherapy: Caring for the patient, Second Edition. Edited by Hagop S. Akiskal and Mauricio Tohen.
© 2011 John Wiley & Sons, Ltd. Published 2011 by John Wiley & Sons, Ltd.

Unfortunately, this formulation of mixed states was lost in the descriptive psychiatry of the late twentieth century, where mixed states were defined, in DSM-III and DSM-IV, as a variant of mania that included, essentially, a major depressive episode as well (American Psychiatric Association, 1995). This model did not allow for mixed states with hypomania, in bipolar II disorder, or with predominately depressive affect (Akiskal and Benazzi, 2005a). Largely as a result, data on treatment of mixed states is almost entirely derived from studies of manic episodes that happened to also include subjects who were experiencing full syndromal depression.

More recent data suggests a broader range of mixed states, that is, closer to the Kraepelinian model of permutations of basic behavioral disturbances (McElroy *et al.*, 1992; Akiskal and Benazzi, 2004). Salient features include the following:

1. Manic episodes with subsyndromal depressive symptoms resemble DSM-IV mixed states in their response to treatment and course of illness (Swann *et al.*, 1997).
2. Predominately depressive mixed states are at least as prevalent as predominately manic mixed states (Benazzi, 2008).
3. Predominately depressive and predominately manic mixed states are similar in their more severe course of illness (Swann *et al.*, 2001; Maj *et al.*, 2006) and in the treacherous manner in which they combine hopelessness with behavioral activation (Akiskal and Benazzi, 2005b). The resulting increase in risk for suicide was first described over 70 years ago (Jameison, 1936) and has been documented repeatedly (Dilsaver *et al.*, 1995; Strakowski *et al.*, 1996; Berk and Dodd, 2005; Goldberg *et al.*, 1998, 2009; Balazs *et al.*, 2006).
4. There may be a continuum across predominately depressive and manic mixed states, with the degree to which mixed symptoms are present being proportional to severity of the underlying course of illness (Swann *et al.*, 2007, 2009), as originally proposed by Kraepelin (1921). Accordingly, catecholaminergic activity in mixed states is substantially higher than that in nonmixed manic episodes, even though manic symptoms are not (Swann *et al.*, 1994).

Summary: the Models and Concepts of Mixed States

Mixed states combine depressive and manic features in the same episode and are a severe presentation of bipolar disorder. They were described long before the concept of bipolar disorder was developed. Current nosology calls for full superimposed syndromal depression and mania, but the historical evolution of the concept, and the clinical characteristics of the patients, are more consistent with a model where activation and depression are combined dimensionally.

19.1.2 QUESTIONS ABOUT MIXED STATES AND TARGETS FOR TREATMENT

In order to understand mixed states and their treatment, it may be necessary to depart from our accepted model where bipolar disorder is defined as depressive or manic episodes for one in which episodes are defined by their dominant polarity and the extent to which depressive and manic symptoms are mixed. Basic questions include

1. Should there be integrated treatment, or separate treatments aimed at depression and mania? The answer to this question depends on whether one assumes the presence of a mechanism that drives the mixed episodes, or assumes that the episode consists of more independent components.
2. Should predominately depressive or manic mixed states be addressed as distinctive episode types, or as a continuum? Or, expressed otherwise, is there essentially one mixed state, or are there many?

In this review, we will attempt to address these questions in a practical manner.

19.1.3   DIAGNOSIS AND CLINICAL CHARACTERISTICS OF MIXED STATES

Mixed states have to be identified before they can be properly treated. Mixed states can be predominately manic or predominately depressive. Each presents its own diagnostic challenges.

19.1.3.1   Predominately Manic

This includes the mixed state, that is, defined in DSM III/IV. Its diagnosis requires a full manic episode with, essentially, a superimposed depressive episode lasting at least a week (American Psychiatric Association, 1995). Comparisons of the nature of manic symptoms in mixed compared to nonmixed manic episodes vary; generally there is less euphoria in mixed states, but grandiosity, irritability, and increased goal-directed activity are prominent (Swann *et al.*, 1986; Henry *et al.*, 2003). Depression-related symptoms include anhedonia, hopelessness, and suicidal ideation (Swann *et al.*, 1986; Henry *et al.*, 2003). Anxiety is especially prominent, to the extent that Kraepelin referred to these episodes interchangeably as anxious or depressive mania (Kraepelin, 1921).

Multivariate analyses and investigations of treatment response have shown that the DSM-IV criterion is unnecessarily narrow (Swann *et al.*, 2001; Bertschy *et al.*, 2007; Gonzalez-Pinto *et al.*, 2003). Treatment response, clinical characteristics, and course of illness are already quite different if two or more depressive symptoms are present (Swann *et al.*, 1997; Akiskal *et al.*, 1998). Several authors have suggested that a continuum or spectrum of mixed characteristics across manic episodes was a more accurate description than a dichotomy requiring full superimposed manic and depressive episodes (Swann *et al.*, 1997; Henry *et al.*, 2003; Akiskal *et al.*, 1998).

19.1.3.2   Predominately Depressive

Predominately depressive mixed states, where a depressive episode is combined with hypomania or subsyndromal hypomanic symptoms, may be more common than predominately manic mixed episodes – yet are not recognized in DSM-IV (American Psychiatric Association, 1995). Flight of ideas/racing thoughts, agitation/hyperactivity, and irritability were the most consistent hypomanic symptoms identifying mixed depressive states (Akiskal and Benazzi, 2004; Goldberg *et al.*, 2009; Benazzi, 2003; Benazzi and Akiskal, 2006). As with mixed states based on mania, the course of illness was more severe than with nonmixed depression, including early onset, frequent episodes, suicidal behavior, and comorbidities (Akiskal and Benazzi, 2004; Goldberg *et al.*, 2009; Swann *et al.*, 2007). Clinical features including more severe course of illness emerge with modest, subsyndromal levels of hypomanic symptoms, in a manner that also resembles predominately manic mixed states (Swann *et al.*, 2007).

19.1.3.3   Mixed States and Agitated Depression: Boundaries of Bipolar Disorder

Mixed states are a subset of agitated depressive episodes, but not all agitated depressive episodes are mixed states of bipolar disorder. Agitation can be an expression of excited hyperactivity, as occurs in mania or mixed states, or painful inner tension, as occurs in depressive or mixed states (Akiskal and Benazzi, 2005b; Swann *et al.*, 1993). Noradrenergic function is higher in mixed states than in agitated depression without hypomanic symptoms (Swann *et al.*, 1994). Agitated depressive episodes that include noneuphoric hypomanic symptoms are different from those that do not, in a manner consistent with the presence of bipolar disorder: early onset, risky behaviors, addictive disorders, and family history of bipolar disorder are all increased in agitated depressed patients who have noneuphoric hypomanic symptoms compared to those who do not (Maj *et al.*, 2006; Zimmermann *et al.*, 2009; Akiskal *et al.*, 2005). It has been suggested that these episodes should be considered excited, rather than agitated, depressions (Akiskal *et al.*, 2005). The excitement can be expressed cognitively or motorically (Akiskal and Benazzi, 2004).

Some patients with agitated depression and noneuphoric hypomanic symptoms may have bipolar disorder with a predominately depressive presentation, but have not had their first hypomanic or manic episode yet (O'Donovan *et al.*, 2007). For such patients, the initial hypomanic or manic episode, and the accurate diagnosis of bipolar disorder, may be delayed by 10 years or more (Rosa *et al.*, 2008). Others, however, may have a presentation of bipolar disorder where hypomanic (or manic) episodes occur only during depressive episodes (Benazzi and Akiskal, 2008).

Summary: Mixed Presentations in Bipolar Disorder

Mixed states, whether predominately depressive or manic, are similar with respect to course of illness and clinical characteristics. "Mixed" characteristics emerge with modest (two or three symptoms) levels of depression during manic episodes or of mania during depressive episodes. These findings suggest that there may be a continuum of mixed states, with the degree to which symptoms are mixed being more salient than whether symptoms are mostly depressive or manic.

19.1.4   MIXED STATES ARISE FROM AN UNSTABLE COURSE OF ILLNESS IN BIPOLAR DISORDER

The course of bipolar disorder is heterogeneous in two ways. Both are related to the concept of mixed states:

19.1.4.1   Predominately Depressive versus Manic Course

Bipolar disorder can have a life course with predominately depressive or predominately manic episodes (Quitkin, Rabkin, and Prien, 1986). Bipolar I disorder can be associated with either predominately depressive or manic episodes, while the course of bipolar II disorder tends to be predominately depressive (Colom *et al.*, 2006). The first episode usually predicts the course pattern (Chaudhury *et al.*, 2007). While the course of illness appears more severe when the first episode is depressive, this may be a result of initial misdiagnosis and treatment with antidepressive agents without concurrent mood-stabilizing treatments (Rosa *et al.*, 2008).

Mixed states may occur in either depression- or mania-prone bipolar disorder, but may be more common in the depression-prone form (Perugi *et al.*, 2000). In a minority of cases, the first episode is mixed (Perugi *et al.*, 2000; Cassidy and Carroll, 2001). Usually, the first episode is not mixed (depressive more often than manic), and mixed episodes develop later (Cassidy and Carroll, 2001; Kessing, 2008). Once a mixed episode has occurred, the likelihood of further episodes being mixed is increased (Kessing, 2008); within the same patient, depressive or manic mixed episodes tend to recur true to type (Cassidy, Ahearn, and Carroll, 2001; Mitropoulou *et al.*, 2003).

19.1.4.2   Predominately Episodic-Stable versus Inherently Unstable Course

Second, the course of bipolar disorder is heterogeneous in terms of susceptibility to frequent episodes or complications. There are two basic course patterns:

1. **Episodic-stable pattern**: Episodes may be severe, but they are relatively infrequent, recovery from an episode is relatively complete, and comorbid disturbances tend to be episode-bound. This course of illness is familial and is associated with robust response to lithium treatment (Duffy *et al.*, 2002).
2. **Inherently unstable pattern**: Episodes may not be as severe as in the episodic-stable pattern (although they may be) but they are more frequent, with earlier onset, and with less opportunity for recovery between episodes. Episodes of illness can be mixed or polyphasic (changing in dominant polarity within the same symptomatic period (Turvey *et al.*, 1999). Comorbid disturbances, like substance use or anxiety disorders, are more frequent and are not necessarily episode-bound (Turvey *et al.*, 1999; Dilsaver *et al.*, 1997). This course pattern is also familial and is associated with relative lithium-resistance (Duffy *et al.*, 2002).

Susceptibility to mixed states in general is strongly related to an unstable course of illness. Individuals with mixed states have more previous episodes of illness, with greater frequency and earlier onset, than those without mixed states (Swann *et al.*, 2001; Goldberg *et al.*, 2009; Swann *et al.*, 2007; Cassidy and Carroll, 2001), regardless of whether the mixed state is predominately manic (Swann *et al.*, 2001) or depressive (Swann *et al.*, 2007). Mixed states are also associated with greater inter-episode affective lability (Benazzi, 2006). Most of the time, the first episode was not mixed, but once subjects have experienced a mixed episode, further mixed episodes become more likely (Cassidy and Carroll, 2001; Kessing, 2008; Cassidy, Ahearn, and Carroll, 2001; Sato *et al.*, 2004).

Also consistent with the inherently unstable illness course pattern, individuals who experience mixed states are more likely to have comorbid conditions (perhaps best regarded as complications of bipolar disorder) than those without mixed states (Goldberg *et al.*, 2009; Himmelhoch and Garfinkel, 1986; Goldberg and McElroy, 2007). These include substance-use disorders (perhaps especially alcohol) and anxiety disorders (Goldberg *et al.*, 2009; Dilsaver *et al.*, 1997). Presence of these disturbances complicates treatment and further worsens the course of illness.

Summary: Mixed States and Course of Illness

In terms of illness course pattern, mixed states appear to be associated with an inherently unstable course of illness. Whether the mixed state is predominately depressive or manic may depend on whether the individual has a predominately depressive or manic course pattern.

19.1.5   INDIVIDUALS EXPERIENCING MIXED EPISODES ARE UNUSUALLY SUSCEPTIBLE TO BEHAVIORAL ACTIVATION AND AFFECTIVE INSTABILITY

19.1.5.1   Mixed States and Mood Instability

Rather than sporadic events, mixed states are part of a lifetime pattern of susceptibility to mood instability. Susceptibility to mood instability is a hallmark of mixed states. Models for mixed states have tended to emphasize them as a stable entity, with simultaneous depressive and manic symptoms, or as rapidly alternating symptoms, or both (Maggini *et al.*, 2000). Frequently, mixed states appear polyphasic (Turvey *et al.*, 1999), with syndromal shifts during the symptomatic period (Goldberg *et al.*, 2000). Kraepelin (1921) proposed that the pathophysiology of mixed states involves a more severe underlying illness, with greater hyperarousal, than is present in nonmixed states. This is consistent with the disproportionate increase in noradrenergic activity (both central and peripheral) in mixed states (Swann *et al.*, 1994), the strong relationships between mixed states and anxiety (Swann *et al.*, 1993; Dilsaver *et al.*, 1997; Barbee, 1998) or emotional excitability

(Henry et al., 2007a, 2007b), and the relationship between mixed states and interepisode affective lability (Benazzi, 2006).

19.1.5.2 Susceptibility to Behavioral Activation in Mixed States

This susceptibility to affective instability can predispose to treatment-induced behavioral activation. Behavioral activation by antidepressive agents is associated with illness-course characteristics resembling those of mixed states, including presence of a substance-use disorder (Goldberg and Whiteside, 2002) and unstable illness course (O'Donovan et al., 2007), and can precipitate mixed states in susceptible individuals (Dilsaver and Swann, 1995). Morning light therapy also induced mixed states in similar patients (Sit et al., 2007). This susceptibility to behavioral activation may be related to treatment-emergent suicidal behavior in mixed depressive patients (Berk and Dodd, 2005).

19.1.5.3 Anxiety in Mixed States

Kraepelin described "frantic anxiety" in mixed states as a manifestation of the severe over-arousal experienced by these patients (Kraepelin, 1921). Anxiety, and comorbid anxiety disorders, are prominent in mixed states, regardless of the predominate polarity (Swann et al., 1993; Dilsaver et al., 1997): anxiety correlates with depression in manic episodes, and with mania in depressive episodes (Swann et al., 2009). Patients with bipolar disorder and severe anxiety have increased overall severity, including poor lithium response, addictive disorders, suicide attempts, early onset, and increased family history of bipolar disorder (Keller, 2006).

19.1.5.4 Mixed States and Suicidal Behavior

The combination of depression and excitation is conducive to suicidal behavior. Patients who are susceptible to mixed states appear susceptible to behavioral activation even during nonmixed depressive episodes, where environmental or pharmacological stimulation can lead to excitation superimposed on depression (Berk and Dodd, 2005; Akiskal et al., 2005; O'Donovan et al., 2007). Two routes whereby mixed states or their emergence can increase risk for suicidal behavior are:

- In manic patients, depressive symptoms, especially hopelessness, can lead to emergence of suicidality (Dilsaver et al., 1995; Goldberg et al., 1998). Accordingly, Strakowski et al. reported a correlation between suicidality and depressive symptoms in manic patients (Strakowski et al., 1996).
- In depressed patients, activated symptoms, such as racing thoughts, hyperactivity, and mood lability, are associated with increased suicidality (Akiskal and Benazzi, 2005b), as part of the natural history of their illness (Bronisch et al., 2005; Swann et al., 2005), or from treatment with antidepressive or other potentially activating agents (Colom et al., 2006). This phenomenon is especially treacherous in depressed patients who have not yet been diagnosed as bipolar (Akiskal et al., 2005; O'Donovan et al., 2007).

Summary: Mixed States, Over-Arousal, and Affective Instability

Consistent with the underlying course of illness, mixed episodes of bipolar disorder are marked by hyperarousal and by combinations of depression (most notably hopelessness and anhedonia), activation (most notably motor hyperactivity and racing thoughts), and behavioral arousal (most notably emotional lability and anxiety). Individuals with mixed states are susceptible to excessive activation, whether pharmacological or environmental. This combination of depression and stimulation increases risk for suicidal behavior, whether spontaneous or treatment-emergent.

19.2 GENERAL CONSIDERATIONS FOR TREATMENT STRATEGIES IN MIXED STATES

19.2.1 TARGETS OF TREATMENTS

Because clinical trials and diagnostic criteria have focused on depressive and manic syndromes, we will initially classify treatment studies in terms of effects on depressive or manic states. Treatment can address the depressive and manic components of a mixed episode. Treatments aimed at mania, however, can predispose to depression (Vieta, 2005); as discussed above, treatments aimed solely at depression can produce problematic behavioral activation (Colom *et al.*, 2006). Alternatively, treatments can address the underlying affective instability that presumably gives rise to the combination of depression and activation.

Therefore, our overall aim will be to understand integrated treatment of mixed states. Treatments optimal for mixed states may be different from those that are effective for manic or depressive syndromes in other contexts.

19.2.2 GENERAL MEDICAL CONSIDERATIONS

Perhaps even more than with other episodes of bipolar disorder, mixed states require general medical alertness. Patients with mixed states are more likely to have other illnesses that can complicate the episode:

- Substance-use disorders, with potential for intoxication, withdrawal, drug toxicity, and pharmacokinetic interactions with treatments.
- Other medical disorders, including either diagnosed or undiagnosed neurological, endocrine, or cardiovascular illnesses.
- Trauma
- Pharmacokinetic considerations: individuals with mixed episodes are likely to be taking more psychotropic agents than are other patients with bipolar disorder, in addition to treatments for other medical problems.

19.2.3 ENVIRONMENTAL AND NON-PHARMACOLOGICAL CONSIDERATIONS

Successful treatment of mixed states requires the precautions that are necessary for both manic and depressive episodes, regardless of dominant polarity. These include

- Environmental and interpersonal consistency and protection against overstimulation
- Vigilant attention toward risk for suicide, aggression, or escalation, being mindful of the potential for affective and behavioral lability,
- Ascertainment of environmental, legal, family, financial, and medical factors that might be contributing to or complicating the episode.

19.3 TREATING MANIA IN MIXED STATES

19.3.1 PREDOMINATELY MANIC

19.3.1.1 What Treatments Work According to Randomized Controlled Trials?

Most controlled studies of treatment in mixed states has focused on mixed states as a subset of manic episodes, and have therefore focused mainly on how effectively treatments reduce manic symptoms (Kruger, Trevor, and Braunig, 2005). Divalproex (Swann et al., 1997; Bowden et al., 1994), carbamazepine (Weisler, Kalali, and Ketter, 2004), olanzapine (Baldessarini et al., 2003), ziprasidone (Keck et al., 2003), aripiprazole (Suppes et al., 2008), and asenapine (McIntyre et al., 2009) all reduced mania rating scale scores similarly in mixed and nonmixed manic episodes. Antimanic effects of lithium were significantly less in mixed than in nonmixed episodes (Swann et al., 1997; Freeman et al., 1992). The initial trials with quetiapine excluded patients in mixed episodes, but did include subjects with significant subclinical depressive symptoms (Weisler et al., 2008).

19.3.1.2 Lithium in Mixed Manic States

In uncontrolled studies, Himmelhoch reported that lithium treatment was less effective in outpatients with mixed, compared to nonmixed, episodes (Himmelhoch et al., 1976). The NIMH Collaborative Study on the Psychobiology of Depression (Biological Studies) also found lithium to be relatively ineffective in mixed states (Swann et al., 1986). In a controlled study comparing lithium, divalproex, and placebo, response to divalproex and lithium was similar overall but lithium was not effective in mixed episodes or in manic episodes with subsyndromal depression (Swann et al., 1997). Similarly, in a double-blind comparison of lithium and valproate, response to valproate was better than response to lithium in subjects with depressive symptoms (Freeman et al., 1992). Response to lithium was also reduced in patients who had experienced mixed episodes in the past (Backlund et al., 2009), consistent with the fact that these patients were more likely to have experienced the inherently unstable course pattern, which appears relatively resistant to lithium monotherapy (Duffy et al., 2002).

The relative ineffectiveness of lithium (at least as monotherapy) in mixed episodes may be related to greater severity of illness in mixed states (Himmelhoch and Garfinkel,

1986). Substance-use disorders (Goldberg *et al.*, 1999) and histories of early onset and/or frequent episodes (Goldberg *et al.*, 2009; Backlund *et al.*, 2009; Swann *et al.*, 1999), both increased in mixed states, are related to reduced response to lithium (Duffy *et al.*, 2002). However, in each case, these factors are negatively related to lithium response regardless of episode subtype (Goldberg *et al.*, 1999; Swann *et al.*, 1999), so differential effects of lithium in mixed states are not solely related to comorbidities or recurrence of illness.

Mixed states are more likely than other affective episodes to require multiple treatments (Dilsaver *et al.*, 1993; McIntyre, 2008). Lithium may be less effective as monotherapy than some other treatments are, but in patients not responding to a single agent, lithium can be an extremely useful augmenting agent in a combined treatment strategy. This is especially the case considering the high lifetime risk of suicidal behavior in patients with mixed episodes (Goldberg *et al.*, 1998, 2009; Swann *et al.*, 2007). Even when it is not effective in reducing depressive or manic symptoms, lithium appears to reduce the lethality of suicide attempts (McIntyre *et al.*, 2008), possibly as a result of its anti-aggressive effects (Sheard *et al.*, 1976).

19.3.1.3 Problems with RCTs in Mixed Mania

Few randomized clinical trials have focused on mixed manic episodes. Generally studies included both mixed and nonmixed episodes and analyzed effects on mixed states as a subgroup, comparing them to nonmixed manic subjects. Statistical power for detecting differences between mixed and nonmixed subjects was potentially inadequate, since the studies were generally powered for differences between active drug and placebo for the overall group.

In general, mixed states were categorically defined according to DSM-IV. A study that investigated alternative definitions of mixed states found lithium response to be sensitive to the number of depressive symptoms, being reduced with subsyndromal symptoms (Swann *et al.*, 1997).

Patients experiencing mixed states are more likely to have other complications of illness, like substance-use or medical disorders, or to be more severely ill (Goldberg *et al.*, 2009; Cassidy and Carroll, 2001). Therefore, they may be less likely to be included in placebo-controlled studies than other patients with bipolar disorder, and those who are included are likely to be less severely ill than patients with mixed episodes in general (Licht, 1998).

19.3.2 PREDOMINATELY DEPRESSIVE: MIXED HYPOMANIA OR MIXED DEPRESSION

Recent studies describing patients with combined hypomanic and depressive syndromes, or mixed hypomania, have found them to resemble patients with mixed mania in terms of course of illness (Swann *et al.*, 2001, 2009; Goldberg *et al.*, 2009; Azorin *et al.*, 2009). These patients can have either bipolar I or bipolar II disorder (Akiskal and Benazzi, 2005a; Maj *et al.*, 2003). As is the case with hypomania in general, there is little information about pharmacological effects on hypomanic symptoms in these patients. It is generally assumed that these symptoms will respond to effective antimanic treatments.

19.4 TREATING DEPRESSION IN MIXED STATES

19.4.1 PREDOMINATELY MANIC

19.4.1.1 Independent Treatment of Depression and Mania

Effective treatment of mixed states may result in improvement of both depressive and manic symptoms. Alternatively, depressive and manic symptoms may have a more parallel and independent response to treatment.

Some early data suggested at least partial dissociation of depressive and manic symptom response. In the NIMH Collaborative Study noted above, lithium appeared to improve depressive symptoms even when mania did not improve, though the number of subjects was too small for definitive conclusions (Swann *et al.*, 1986). More recently, Brown *et al.* investigated effects of an added antidepressive agent (bupropion) in subjects whose mania had responded to multiple treatments (usually at least two of an anticonvulsant, and antipsychotic agent, and lithium) but who had persistent depressive symptoms two weeks after resolution of mania. These depressive symptoms improved after addition of bupropion (Brown *et al.*, 1994). These results support the use of antidepressive agents, but only after antimanic treatment has reduced behavioral activation.

19.4.1.2 Combined Treatment of Depression and Mania

In apparent contrast to these earlier studies, most randomized controlled trials of second generation antipsychotic agents and anticonvulsants have shown depressive symptoms to improve with the same treatments that were effective in reducing mania rating scores (Kruger, Trevor, and Braunig, 2005; McIntyre, 2008). This would support the idea that treatment of the underlying affective episode can resolve both depressive and manic symptoms in mixed states. Two factors to be taken into account are that (i) the general severity of illness is likely to have been lower in these randomized clinical trial participants than in the general population of manic patients (Licht, 1998) and (ii) in the randomized clinical trials, changes in depressive symptoms were not always reported separately in mixed and nonmixed subjects, although, when they were, subjects in mixed states did generally have significant reductions in depressive symptoms (Kruger, Trevor, and Braunig, 2005).

Treatment of Predominately Manic Mixed States

Most, but not all, treatments that are effective for mania also reduce depressive symptoms in manic episodes, including valproate, second generation antipsychotic agents, and carbamazepine. Monotherapy with lithium is an exception, but lithium is a valuable second treatment. Mixed episodes are more likely than nonmixed episodes to require multiple treatments for an optimal response.

19.4.2 PREDOMINATELY DEPRESSIVE

19.4.2.1 Mood-Stabilizing Treatments

Consistent with the case for bipolar depression in general, there is little information on treatment response of depression in predominately depressive mixed states. Randomized controlled trials suggest that quetiapine may be effective (Calabrese *et al.*, 2005). Other nonantidepressant treatments with suggested effectiveness in bipolar depressive episodes, including lithium (Swann *et al.*, 1986), valproate (Ghaemi *et al.*, 2007), or lamotrigine (Geddes, Calabrese, and Goodwin, 2009), have potential promise.

In the case of lamotrigine, five randomized controlled trials in bipolar depressive episodes were negative for the primary end point (Calabrese *et al.*, 2008) (one was positive for a secondary end point (Calabrese *et al.*, 1999)), but meta-analysis showed an overall positive effect, especially for patients with relatively severe depression (MADRS > 24) (Geddes, Calabrese, and Goodwin, 2009).

19.4.2.2 Antidepressive Agents

It is tempting to use antidepressive agents in treating these patients, and the incidence of antidepressive treatments is high (Azorin *et al.*, 2009; Ghaemi, 2008). However, there is little evidence for effectiveness of antidepressive agents even in bipolar disorder as a whole (Ghaemi, 2008), much less in patients experiencing mixed states, who appear to be unusually sensitive to mood destabilization and behavioral activation. The STEP-BD, in 380 patients given antidepressants in depressive mixed states, reported increased manic symptoms with limited or no benefit for depression (Goldberg *et al.*, 2007).

Treatment of Predominately Depressive Mixed States

In these episodes, it is necessary to recognize the importance of the underlying mood instability. Antimanic agents that are also effective against mixed states are primary treatments, especially those like quetiapine and valproate that also have evidence suggesting effectiveness against bipolar depression. Favored second treatments are lithium or other potentially mood-stabilizing treatments, including lamotrigine. Because these patients are susceptible to pharmacological mood destabilization, it is prudent to defer unimodal antidepressive treatments until after mood stabilizing treatments have been instituted and determined not to elicit an adequate response.

19.5 NONPHARMACOLOGICAL TREATMENTS

Nonpharmacological treatments, including electroconvulsive treatment (ECT) and transcranial magnetic stimulation, can be aimed at either depressive or manic syndromes. Vagal nerve stimulation is a potential treatment for depressive episodes. ECT is the only nonpharmacological treatment with substantial supporting data for mixed states. It has the advantages of potential effectiveness for either depression or mania, many years of experience, and recent technical advances. Most evidence is from case series. A meta-analysis supported its effectiveness in full bipolar mixed states (Valenti *et al.*, 2008), as have other studies where it was effective in patients who had not responded to vigorous conventional treatment (Gruber *et al.*, 2000). In a randomized study, ECT was superior to lithium in acute mania; the difference emerged from the superior effectiveness of ECT in subjects with mixed features (Small *et al.*, 1988).

19.6 AN INTEGRATED MODEL FOR TREATING MIXED STATES

19.6.1 PROVISIONAL, OPERATIONALIZED DEFINITION OF MIXED STATE

For the purpose of recommending practical treatment, we will define mixed states in a manner that reflects the combination of activation and depression, the similarity in course of illness between predominately depressive and manic mixed states, and the apparently continuous nature of mixed symptoms, ranging from mania with modest depressive symptoms or depression with modest manic symptoms to full manic and depressive syndromes (Swann *et al.*, 2009). Our definition is based on evidence that differences in course of illness and treatment response emerge in manic episodes with two or more depressive symptoms, and in depressive episodes with two or more manic symptoms (Swann *et al.*, 1997; Maj *et al.*, 2006; Swann *et al.*, 2009; Akiskal *et al.*, 1998; Benazzi and Akiskal, 2001).

Provisional Definition of a Mixed State

- Mania, hypomania, or depression is present, and
- There are two or more symptoms of the opposite polarity. This excludes symptoms that overlap between depressive and manic states, including insomnia, and agitation as defined broadly (McElroy *et al.*, 1992). Decreased need for sleep and increased goal-directed activity, however, are considered mixed symptoms in depressive episodes.

19.6.2 INTEGRATED PHARMACOLOGICAL TREATMENT STRATEGY

These general guidelines depend on the individual's previous history of psychopharmacological response and toleration. Because of the complexity of mixed states, treatment will need to be individualized (Dilsaver and Benazzi, 2008):

1. **Initial treatment**: If the patient is not receiving treatment, institute treatment with one or two of the following medicines, which have been reported to be effective, in placebo-controlled studies, for mania and for mixed mania, and not to worsen depression or cause mood destabilization:

   (a) Valproate (Swann *et al.*, 1997; Bowden *et al.*, 1994)
   (b) A second-generation antipsychotic agent: Olanzapine (Baldessarini *et al.*, 2003), risperidone (Khanna *et al.*, 2005), quetiapine (initial mania studies excluded mixed states but did include subsyndromal depression (Weisler *et al.*, 2008), and efficacy against depression in bipolar I and II disorders has been demonstrated (Calabrese *et al.*, 2005)), ziprasidone (Keck *et al.*, 2003; Vieta *et al.*, 2008) (initially IM or with at least 500 kcal of food (Citrome, 2009)), aripiprazole (Suppes *et al.*, 2008), or asenapine (McIntyre *et al.*, 2009)
   (c) Lithium (not as monotherapy (Swann *et al.*, 1997))
   (d) Lamotrigine (efficacy against mania has never been demonstrated and evidence against depression is limited, so only in depressive mixed state, and not as monotherapy)
   (e) Carbamazepine (Weisler, Kalali, and Ketter, 2004) or oxcarbazepine, allowing for potential pharmacokinetic interactions in patients receiving multiple treatments.

2. **Second treatment**: If the patient is already receiving one of the treatments above (McIntyre, 2008),

   (a) Maximize the dose, and
   (b) Add another treatment from (1), but not a second antipsychotic agent

3. **Additional treatment**: If the patient is already receiving, or has not responded to two treatments from (1)

   (a) Add a third treatment from the list in part 1, or
   (b) Add clozapine if predominately manic (Suppes *et al.*, 1992), or
   (c) Institute bilateral ECT (Valenti *et al.*, 2008)

4. **Residual depression**: If the patient has experienced improvement in manic symptoms using the above strategy, but is still depressed after two weeks:

   (a) Add lithium or lamotrigine if they are not already being given, or, if the patient is not receiving an antipsychotic agent, consider quetiapine (Calabrese *et al.*, 2005); or
   (b) Add a nontricyclic antidepressive agent with a relatively low incidence of mood destabilization, such as bupropion (Brown *et al.*, 1994); or
   (c) If depression or history of treatment-emergent mood instability is severe, consider ECT (Valenti *et al.*, 2008).

5. Long-term treatment:

   (a) As for other episodes of bipolar disorder, treatments considered essential for resolution of the episode should be adjusted for tolerability and continued.

    (b) Due to the relative lack of long term prophylactic efficacy of antidepressive agents (Ghaemi, 2008), their gradual taper and discontinuation should be considered, generally after the patient has had time to recuperate from the episode and to recover pre-episode functionality, unless the specific patient's past history shows consistent relapse into depression after antidepressant discontinuation.

    (c) In patients who had poor responses to pharmacological treatments and responded to ECT, maintenance ECT should be considered.

    (d) Because of these patients' susceptibility to a severe and unstable course of illness, additional measures to preserve affective and behavioral stability are vital, including symptom monitoring, management of substance-use disorders and other complications of bipolar disorder, and protection of social and sleep-activity rhythms.

19.7 CONCLUSIONS

Mixed states are a serious manifestation of bipolar disorder, where symptoms are not limited to depressive or manic syndromes, and substantial affective and behavioral instability occurs in the specific episode and in the course of illness. They are characterized by a course with early onset and frequent recurrences, poor response to conventional treatments, substance use disorders, and susceptibility to suicidal behavior. Their treatment requires identification of the mixed state, and vigorous treatment of the underlying severe bipolar disorder that generates the episode.

References

Akiskal, H.S. and Benazzi, F. (2004) Validating Kraepelin's two types of depressive mixed states: "depression with flight of ideas" and "excited depression". *World J. Biol. Psychiatry*, **5** (2), 107–113.

Akiskal, H.S. and Benazzi, F. (2005a) Toward a clinical delineation of dysphoric hypomania – operational and conceptual dilemmas. *Bipolar Disord.*, **7** (5), 456–464.

Akiskal, H.S. and Benazzi, F. (2005b) Psychopathologic correlates of suicidal ideation in major depressive outpatients: is it all due to unrecognized (bipolar) depressive mixed states? *Psychopathology*, **38** (5), 273–280.

Akiskal, H.S., Benazzi, F., Perugi, G. *et al.* (2005) Agitated "unipolar" depression re-conceptualized as a depressive mixed state: implications for the antidepressant-suicide controversy. *J. Affect. Disord.*, **85** (3), 245–258.

Akiskal, H.S., Hantouche, E.G., Bourgeois, M.L. *et al.* (1998) Gender, temperament, and the clinical picture in dysphoric mixed mania: findings from a French national study (EPIMAN). *J. Affect. Disord.*, **50** (2–3), 175–186.

American Psychiatric Association (1995) *Diagnostic and Statistical Manual of Mental Disorders*, 4th edn, APA, Washington, DC.

Angst, J. and Marneros, A. (2001) Bipolarity from ancient to modern times: conception, birth and rebirth. *J. Affect. Disord.*, **67** (1–3), 3–19.

Azorin, J.M., Aubrun, E., Bertsch, J. *et al.* (2009) Mixed states vs. pure mania in the French sample of the EMBLEM study: results at baseline and 24 months – European mania in bipolar longitudinal evaluation of medication. *BMC Psychiatry*, **9**, 33.

Backlund, L., Ehnvall, A., Hetta, J. *et al.* (2009) Identifying predictors for good lithium response – a retrospective analysis of 100 patients with bipolar disorder using a life-charting method. *Eur. Psychiatry*, **24** (3), 171–177.

Balazs, J., Benazzi, F., Rihmer, Z. *et al.* (2006) The close link between suicide attempts and mixed (bipolar) depression: implications for suicide prevention. *J. Affect. Disord.*, **91** (2–3), 133–138.

Baldessarini, R.J., Hennen, J., Wilson, M. *et al.* (2003) Olanzapine versus placebo in acute mania: treatment responses in subgroups. *J. Clin. Psychopharmacol.*, **23** (4), 370–376.

Barbee, J.G. (1998) Mixed symptoms and syndromes of anxiety and depression: diagnostic, prognostic, and etiologic issues. *Ann. Clin. Psychiatry*, **10** (1), 15–29.

Benazzi, F. (2003) Bipolar II depressive mixed state: finding a useful definition. *Compr. Psychiatry*, **44** (1), 21–27.

Benazzi, F. (2006) Impact of temperamental mood lability on depressive mixed state. *Psychopathology*, **39** (1), 19–24.

Benazzi, F. (2008) Reviewing the diagnostic validity and utility of mixed depression (depressive mixed states). *Eur. Psychiatry*, **23** (1), 40–48.

Benazzi, F. and Akiskal, H.S. (2001) Delineating bipolar II mixed states in the Ravenna-San Diego collaborative study: the relative prevalence and diagnostic significance of hypomanic features during major depressive episodes. *J. Affect. Disord.*, **67** (1–3), 115–122.

Benazzi, F. and Akiskal, H.S. (2006) Psychometric delineation of the most discriminant symptoms of depressive mixed states. *Psychiatry Res.*, **141** (1), 81–88.

Benazzi, F. and Akiskal, H.S. (2008) How best to identify a bipolar-related subtype among major depressive patients without spontaneous hypomania: superiority of age at onset criterion over recurrence and polarity? *J. Affect. Disord.*, **107** (1–3), 77–88.

Berk, M. and Dodd, S. (2005) Are treatment emergent suicidality and decreased response to antidepressants in younger patients due to bipolar disorder being misdiagnosed as unipolar depression? *Med. Hypotheses*, **65** (1), 39–43.

Bertschy, G., Gervasoni, N., Favre, S. *et al.* (2007) Phenomenology of mixed states: a principal component analysis study. *Bipolar Disord.*, **9** (8), 907–912.

Bowden, C.L., Brugger, A.M., Swann, A.C. *et al.*, The Depakote Mania Study Group (1994) Efficacy of divalproex vs lithium and placebo in the treatment of mania. *J. Am. Med. Assoc.*, **271** (12), 918–924.

Bronisch, T., Schwender, L., Hofler, M. *et al.* (2005) Mania, hypomania, and suicidality: findings from a prospective community study. *Arch. Suicide Res.*, **9** (3), 267–278.

Brown, E.S., Dilsaver, S.C., Shoaib, A.M. *et al.* (1994) Depressive mania: response of residual depression to bupropion. *Biol. Psychiatry*, **35** (7), 493–494.

Calabrese, J.R., Bowden, C.L., Sachs, G.S. *et al.* (1999) A double-blind placebo-controlled study of lamotrigine monotherapy in outpatients with bipolar I depression. Lamictal 602 study group. *J. Clin. Psychiatry*, **60** (2), 79–88.

Calabrese, J.R., Huffman, R.F., White, R.L. *et al.* (2008) Lamotrigine in the acute treatment of bipolar depression: results of five double-blind, placebo-controlled clinical trials. *Bipolar Disord.*, **10** (2), 323–333.

Calabrese, J.R., Keck, P.E. Jr., Macfadden, W. *et al.* (2005) A randomized, double-blind, placebo-controlled trial of quetiapine in the treatment of bipolar I or II depression. *Am. J. Psychiatry*, **162** (7), 1351–1360.

Carroll, B.J. (1983) Neurobiologic dimensions in depression and mania, in *The Origins of Depression* (ed. J Angst), Springer, Berlin, pp. 163–186.

Cassidy, F., Ahearn, E., and Carroll, B.J. (2001) A prospective study of inter-episode consistency of manic and mixed subtypes of bipolar disorder. *J. Affect. Disord.*, **67** (1–3), 181–185.

Cassidy, F. and Carroll, B.J. (2001) The clinical epidemiology of pure and mixed manic episodes. *Bipolar Disord.*, **3** (1), 35–40.

Chaudhury, S.R., Grunebaum, M.F., Galfalvy, H.C. *et al.* (2007) Does first episode polarity predict risk for suicide attempt in bipolar disorder? *J. Affect. Disord.*, **104** (1–3), 245–250.

Citrome, L. (2009) Using oral ziprasidone effectively: the food effect and dose-response. *Adv. Ther.*, **26** (8), 739–748.

Colom, F., Vieta, E., Daban, C. *et al.* (2006) Clinical and therapeutic implications of predominant polarity in bipolar disorder. *J. Affect. Disord.*, **93**, 13–17.

Dilsaver, S.C. and Benazzi, F. (2008) Treating depressive mixed states in bipolar disorders. *J. Clin. Psychiatry*, **69** (8), e23.

Dilsaver, S.C., Chen, Y.R., Swann, A.C. *et al.* (1995) Suicidality in patients with pure and depressive mania. *Am. J. Psychiatry*, **151**, 1312–1315.

Dilsaver, S.C., Chen, Y.R., Swann, A.C. *et al.* (1997) Suicidality, panic disorder, and psychosis in bipolar depression, depressive-mania, and pure mania. *Psychiatry Res.*, **73**, 47–56.

Dilsaver, S.C. and Swann, A.C. (1995) Mixed mania: apparent induction by a tricyclic antidepressant in five consecutively treated patients with bipolar depression. *Biol. Psychiatry*, **37**, 60–62.

Dilsaver, S.C., Swann, A.C., Shoaib, A.M. *et al.* (1993) Mixed mania associated with non-response to antimanic agents. *Am. J. Psychiatry*, **150**, 1548–1551.

Duffy, A., Alda, M., Kutcher, S. *et al.* (2002) A prospective study of the offspring of bipolar parents responsive and nonresponsive to lithium treatment. *J. Clin. Psychiatry*, **63** (12), 1171–1178.

Freeman, T.W., Clothier, J.L., Pazzaglia, P. *et al.* (1992) A double-blind comparison of valproate and lithium in the treatment of acute mania. *Am. J. Psychiatry*, **149**, 108–111.

Geddes, J.R., Calabrese, J.R., and Goodwin, G.M. (2009) Lamotrigine for treatment of bipolar depression: independent meta-analysis and meta-regression of individual patient data from five randomised trials. *Br. J. Psychiatry*, **194** (1), 4–9.

Ghaemi, S.N. (2008) Why antidepressants are not antidepressants: STEP-BD, STAR*D, and the return of neurotic depression. *Bipolar Disord.*, **10** (8), 957–968.

Ghaemi, S.N., Gilmer, W.S., Goldberg, J.F. *et al.* (2007) Divalproex in the treatment of acute bipolar depression: a preliminary double-blind, randomized, placebo-controlled pilot study. *J. Clin. Psychiatry*, **68** (12), 1840–1844.

Goldberg, J.F., Garno, J.L., Leon, A.C. *et al.* (1998) Association of recurrent suicidal ideation with nonremission from acute mixed mania. *Am. J. Psychiatry*, **155** (12), 1753–1755.

Goldberg, J.F., Garno, J.L., Leon, A.C. *et al.* (1999) A history of substance abuse complicates remission from acute mania in bipolar disorder. *J. Clin. Psychiatry*, **60** (11), 733–740.

Goldberg, J.F., Garno, J.L., Portera, L. *et al.* (2000) Qualitative differences in manic symptoms during mixed versus pure mania. *Compr. Psychiatry*, **41** (4), 237–241.

Goldberg, J.F. and McElroy, S.L. (2007) Bipolar mixed episodes: characteristics and comorbidities. *J. Clin. Psychiatry*, **68** (10), e25.

Goldberg, J.F., Perlis, R.H., Bowden, C.L. *et al.* (2009) Manic symptoms during depressive episodes in 1,380 patients with bipolar disorder: findings from the STEP-BD. *Am. J. Psychiatry*, **166** (2), 173–181.

Goldberg, J.F., Perlis, R.H., Ghaemi, S.N. *et al.* (2007) Adjunctive antidepressant use and symptomatic recovery among bipolar depressed patients with concomitant manic symptoms: findings from the STEP-BD. *Am. J. Psychiatry*, **164** (9), 1348–1355.

Goldberg, J.F. and Whiteside, J.E. (2002) The association between substance abuse and antidepressant-induced mania in bipolar disorder: a preliminary study. *J. Clin. Psychiatry*, **63** (9), 791–795.

Gonzalez-Pinto, A., Ballesteros, J., Aldama, A. *et al.* (2003) Principal components of mania. *J. Affect. Disord.*, **76** (1–3), 95–102.

Gruber, N.P., Dilsaver, S.C., Shoaib, A.M. *et al.* (2000) ECT in mixed affective states: a case series [In Process Citation]. *J. ECT*, **16** (2), 183–188.

Henry, C., M'Bailara, K., Desage, A. *et al.* (2007a) Towards a reconceptualization of mixed states, based on an emotional-reactivity dimensional model. *J. Affect. Disord.*, **101** (1–3), 35–41.

Henry, C., M'Bailara, K., Poinsot, R. *et al.* (2007b) Evidence for two types of bipolar depression using a dimensional approach. *Psychother. Psychosom.*, **76** (6), 325–331.

Henry, C., Swendsen, J., Van Den Bulke, D. *et al.* (2003) Emotional hyper-reactivity as a fundamental mood characteristic of manic and mixed states. *Eur. Psychiatry*, **18** (3), 124–128.

Himmelhoch, J.M. and Garfinkel, M.E. (1986) Sources of lithium resistance in mixed mania. *Psychopharmacol. Bull.*, **22**, 613–620.

Himmelhoch, J.M., Mulla, D., Neil, J.F. *et al.* (1976) Incidence and severity of mixed affective states in a bipolar population. *Arch. Gen. Psychiatry*, **33**, 1062.

Jackson, S. (1986) *The Various Relationships of Mania and Melancholia. Melancholia and Depression: From Hippocratic Times to Modern Times*, Yale University Press, New Haven, pp. 249–273.

Jameison, G.R. (1936) Suicide and mental disease: a clinical analysis of one hundred cases. *Arch. Neurol. Psychiatry*, **36**, 1–12.

Keck, P.E., Jr., Versiani, M., Potkin, S. *et al.* (2003) Ziprasidone in the treatment of acute bipolar mania: a three-week, placebo-controlled, double-blind, randomized trial. *Am. J. Psychiatry*, **160** (4), 741–748.

Keller, M.B. (2006) Prevalence and impact of comorbid anxiety and bipolar disorder. *J. Clin. Psychiatry*, **67** (Suppl. 1), 5–7.

Kessing, L.V. (2008) The prevalence of mixed episodes during the course of illness in bipolar disorder. *Acta Psychiatr. Scand.*, **117** (3), 216–224.

Khanna, S., Vieta, E., Lyons, B. *et al.* (2005) Risperidone in the treatment of acute mania: double-blind, placebo-controlled study. *Br. J. Psychiatry*, **187**, 229–234.

Kraepelin, E. (1921) *Manic-Depressive Illness and Paranoia*, E & S Livingstone, Edinburgh, Scotland.

Kruger, S., Trevor, Y.L., and Braunig, P. (2005) Pharmacotherapy of bipolar mixed states. *Bipolar Disord.*, **7** (3), 205–215.

Licht, R.W. (1998) Drug treatment of mania: a critical review. *Acta Psychiatr. Scand.*, **97** (6), 387–397. [Review] [89 refs].

Maggini, C., Salvatore, P., Gerhard, A. *et al.* (2000) Psychopathology of stable and unstable mixed states: a historical view. *Compr. Psychiatry*, **41** (2), 77–82.

Maj, M., Pirozzi, R., Magliano, L. *et al.* (2003) Agitated depression in bipolar I disorder: prevalence, phenomenology, and outcome. *Am. J. Psychiatry*, **160** (12), 2134–2140.

Maj, M., Pirozzi, R., Magliano, L. *et al.* (2006) Agitated "unipolar" major depression: prevalence, phenomenology, and outcome. *J. Clin. Psychiatry*, **67** (5), 712–719.

McElroy, S.L., Keck, P.E. Jr., Pope, H.G. Jr. *et al.* (1992) Clinical and research implications of the diagnosis of dysphoric or mixed mania or hypomania. *Am. J. Psychiatry*, **149**, 1633–1644.

McIntyre, R.S. (2008) Acute treatment of patients with bipolar mixed episodes. *J. Clin. Psychiatry*, **69** (4), e10.

McIntyre, R.S., Cohen, M., Zhao, J. *et al.* (2009) A 3-week, randomized, placebo-controlled trial of asenapine in the treatment of acute mania in bipolar mania and mixed states. *Bipolar Disord.*, **11** (7), 673–686.

McIntyre, R.S., Muzina, D.J., Kemp, D.E. *et al.* (2008) Bipolar disorder and suicide: research synthesis and clinical translation. *Curr. Psychiatry Rep.*, **10** (1), 66–72.

Mitropoulou, V., Trestman, R.L., New, A.S. *et al.* (2003) Neurobiologic function and temperament in subjects with personality disorders. *CNS Spectr.*, **8** (10), 725–730.

O'Donovan, C., Garnham, J.S., Hajek, T. *et al.* (2007) Antidepressant monotherapy in pre-bipolar depression; predictive value and inherent risk. *J. Affect. Disord.*, **107**, 93–298.

Perugi, G., Micheli, C., Akiskal, H.S. *et al.* (2000) Polarity of the first episode, clinical characteristics, and course of manic depressive illness: a systematic retrospective investigation of 320 bipolar I patients. *Compr. Psychiatry*, **41** (1), 13–18.

van Praag, H.M., Asnis, G.M., Kahn, R.S. *et al.* (1990) Monoamines and abnormal behavior: a multi-aminergic perspective. *Br. J. Psychiatry*, **157**, 723–734.

Quitkin, F.M., Rabkin, J.G., and Prien, R.F. (1986) Bipolar disorder: are there manic-prone and depressive-prone forms? *J. Clin. Psychopharmacol.*, **6** (3), 167–172.

Rosa, A.R., Andreazza, A.C., Kunz, M. *et al.* (2008) Predominant polarity in bipolar disorder: diagnostic implications. *J. Affect. Disord.*, **107** (1–3), 45–51.

Sato, T., Bottlender, R., Sievers, M. *et al.* (2004) Evaluating the inter-episode stability of depressive mixed states. *J. Affect. Disord.*, **81** (2), 103–113.

Sheard, M.H., Marini, J.L., Bridges, C.I. *et al.* (1976) The effect of lithium on impulsive aggressive behavior in man. *Am. J. Psychiatry*, **133** (12), 1409–1413.

Sit, D., Wisner, K.L., Hanusa, B.H. *et al.* (2007) Light therapy for bipolar disorder: a case series in women. *Bipolar Disord.*, **9** (8), 918–927.

Small, J.G., Klapper, M.H., Kellams, J.J. *et al.* (1988) Electroconvulsive treatment compared with lithium in the management of manic states. *Arch. Gen. Psychiatry*, **45**, 727–732.

Strakowski, S.M., McElroy, S.L., Keck, P.E. Jr. *et al.* (1996) Suicidality among patients with mixed and manic bipolar disorder. *Am. J. Psychiatry*, **153** (5), 674–676.

Suppes, T., Eudicone, J., McQuade, R. *et al.* (2008) Efficacy and safety of aripiprazole in subpopulations with acute manic or mixed episodes of bipolar I disorder. *J. Affect. Disord.*, **107** (1–3), 145–154.

Suppes, T., McElroy, S.L., Gilbert, J. *et al.* (1992) Clozapine in the treatment of dysphoric mania. *Biol. Psychiatry*, **32** (3), 270–280.

Swann, A.C., Bowden, C.L., Calabrese, J.R. *et al.* (1999) Differential effect of number of previous episodes of affective disorder on response to lithium or divalproex in acute mania. *Am. J. Psychiatry*, **156**, 1264–1266.

Swann, A.C., Bowden, C.L., Morris, D. *et al.* (1997) Depression during mania: treatment response to lithium or divalproex. *Arch. Gen. Psychiatry*, **54**, 37–42.

Swann, A.C., Dougherty, D.M., Pazzaglia, P.J. *et al.* (2005) Increased impulsivity associated with severity of suicide attempt history in patients with bipolar disorder. *Am. J. Psychiatry*, **162** (9), 1680–1687.

Swann, A.C., Gerard, M.F., Steinberg, J.L. *et al.* (2007) Manic symptoms and impulsivity during bipolar depressive episodes. *Bipolar Disord.*, **9** (3), 206–212.

Swann, A.C., Janicak, P.G., Calabrese, J.R. *et al.* (2001) Structure of mania: depressive, irritable, and psychotic clusters with distinct courses of illness in randomized clinical trial participants. *J. Affect. Disord.*, **67**, 123–132.

Swann, A.C., Secunda, S.K., Katz, M.M. *et al.* (1986) Lithium treatment of mania: clinical characteristics, specificity of symptom change, and outcome. *Psychiatry Res.*, **18**, 127–141.

Swann, A.C., Secunda, S.K., Katz, M.M. *et al.* (1993) Specificity of mixed affective states: Clinical comparison of mixed mania and agitated depression. *J. Affect. Disord.*, **28**, 81–89.

Swann, A.C., Steinberg, J.L., Lijffijt, M. *et al.* (2009) Continuum of depressive and manic mixed states in patients with bipolar disorder: quantitative measurement and clinical features. *World Psychiatry*, **8** (3), 166–172.

Swann, A.C., Stokes, P.E., Secunda, S. *et al.* (1994) Depressive mania vs agitated depression: bio-genic amine and hypothalamic-pituitary-adrenocortical function. *Biol. Psychiatry*, **35**, 803–813.

Turvey, C.L., Coryell, W.H., Solomon, D.A. *et al.* (1999) Long-term prognosis of bipolar I disorder. *Acta Psychiatr. Scand.*, **99** (2), 110–119.

Valenti, M., Benabarre, A., Garcia-Amador, M. *et al.* (2008) Electroconvulsive therapy in the treatment of mixed states in bipolar disorder. *Eur. Psychiatry*, **23** (1), 53–56.

Vieta, E. (2005) The treatment of mixed states and the risk of switching to depression. *Eur. Psychiatry*, **20** (2), 96–100.

Vieta, E., Ramey, T., Keller, D. *et al.* (2008) Ziprasidone in the treatment of acute mania: a 12-week, placebo-controlled, haloperidol-referenced study. *J. Psychopharmacol.*, **24**, 547–558.

Weisler, R.H., Calabrese, J.R., Thase, M.E. *et al.* (2008) Efficacy of quetiapine monotherapy for the treatment of depressive episodes in bipolar I disorder: a post hoc analysis of combined results from 2 double-blind, randomized, placebo-controlled studies. *J. Clin. Psychiatry*, **69** (5), 769–782.

Weisler, R.H., Kalali, A.H., and Ketter, T.A. (2004) A multicenter, randomized, double-blind, placebo-controlled trial of extended-release carbamazepine capsules as monotherapy for bipolar disorder patients with manic or mixed episodes. *J. Clin. Psychiatry*, **65** (4), 478–484.

Zimmermann, P., Bruckl, T., Nocon, A. *et al.* (2009) Heterogeneity of DSM-IV major depres-sive disorder as a consequence of subthreshold bipolarity. *Arch. Gen. Psychiatry*, **66** (12), 1341–1352.

Rapid Cycling of Bipolar Patients

**Athanasios Koukopoulos[1], G. Serra[2], F. Zazzara[1],
A. E. Koukopoulos[2] and G. Sani[2]**

[1]Centro Lucio Bini Roma, Rome, Italy
[2]Azienda Ospedaliera Sant'Andrea, Università La Sapienza Roma, Rome, Italy

> We have never observed a complete recovery, not even a lasting improvement.
>
> *La folie circulaire*. J.P. Falret, 1854

20.1 INTRODUCTION

In Dunner and Fieve (1974) defined as Rapid cyclers (RCs) those patients who had a course of four or more affective episodes in the previous 12 months and this course specifier was adopted by the DSM-IV (American Psychiatric Association, 1994). They were identified because of their failure to respond to lithium treatment. Lithium prophylaxis had failed in 82% of these patients.

According to the DSM-IV criteria, the four episodes in the previous 12 months should meet the criteria for a major depressive, manic, mixed, or hypomanic episode. Today, most clinicians waive the duration criterion of episodes and intervals because in many cases the episodes become progressively shorter and we see ultra-rapid (within the course of weeks or days) and ultradian cyclers (mood shifts within 24 hours). Some patients indeed show an alternation of phase within a few hours.

RC were well described in the pioneering work of J. P. Falret *Folie Circulaire* (1854) and J. Baillarger *Folie à double forme* (1854).

It is significant that the alternating course of mania and depression, called by German psychiatrists *Circuläres Irresein*, constituted for Kraepelin the core of his entire conception of manic-depressive illness. Likewise, the authors of this chapter consider the rapid-cycling course the most essential and complete expression of the bipolar spectrum because of its clear bipolarity and the autonomous evolution of its course.

20.2 EPIDEMIOLOGICAL DATA

The general impression of clinicians today is that the course of recurrences of manic-depressive illness has substantially changed in the last 40 years. The recurrences of many

Bipolar Psychopharmacotherapy: Caring for the patient, Second Edition. Edited by Hagop S. Akiskal and Mauricio Tohen.
© 2011 John Wiley & Sons, Ltd. Published 2011 by John Wiley & Sons, Ltd.

patients have become more frequent. One sees more manias and hypomanias and therefore more bipolar cases than before, more RCs, and more chronic depressions (Koukopoulos *et al.*, 1983; Ghaemi, 2008). This phenomenon is today called mood destabilization.

It is difficult to verify and quantify all these changes, because comparisons in psychiatry, especially among statistical data gathered over long time intervals, are very hard to make. Nevertheless, reading the older literature, one has a clear impression that the course of the disease was different then.

In his monograph on *la folie a double forme*, Ritti (1883) presented only 17 cases with a rapid course; he collected them from various French and German authors. Kraepelin (1913) illustrated one case with a rapid cycling course in his graphs of type of course. This was case C, and he commented, "I had to seek for a long time in my cases until I finally found at least one course of the type that case C represents." J. Lange (1928) speaks of only one patient with two cycles per year Brodwall (1941) found only two circular cases among 110 patients. Lundquist (1945) referred to only "a few cases" with circular courses among 319 manic depressive patients Stenstedt (1952) found only one case of circular psychosis among 216 manic-depressive patients. Many authors do not mention rapid courses at all. Today, on the contrary, rapid courses have become a frequent and serious therapeutic problem.

In a meta-analysis of eight studies including 2054 bipolar patients, Kupka *et al.* (2003) found a percentage of 16.3% of RCs women and bipolar II patients were slightly but significantly more prevalent.

Maj *et al.* (1994) found a prevalence of 19.5% of RC among 67 BPI patients.

Among the first 500 BP patients of the STEP-BD study 20% were RC while in 2008 among 1742 BD patients the percentage at entry was 32% (Schneck *et al.*, 2008).

Among women, rapid cycling is more frequent than among men and the age of onset of the bipolar disorder is earlier than among nonrapid cycling patients (Yildiz and Sachs, 2004).

Particularly frequent is rapid cycling among prepubertal and early adolescent bipolar patients. Geller *et al.* (1998) found a proportion of 83.3% rapid, ultra-rapid, or ultradian cyclers among such young patients.

Significant differences in the prevalence of RC patients among bipolar patients in different countries were found by the EMBLEM study (Cruz *et al.*, 2007): Norway 28.6%, Switzerland 24%, Germany 22.3%, Italy 21.3%, UK/Ireland 20.9%, Denmark 18.7%, Belgium 17.6%, France 17.5%, the Netherlands 13.8%, Greece 12.7%, Finland 12.5%, Spain 10.3%, and Portugal 5.6%.

20.3   SPONTANEOUS AND INDUCED RAPID CYCLING

The investigation of the course of manic-depressive illness is a difficult task in itself, and the investigation of possible factors that influence this course is extremely difficult. Yet the above-mentioned changes and the general increase of bipolar cases today make this investigation necessary. Of all the possible factors that unfavorably influence the course of the disease what most urgently need to be studied are the treatments themselves – first, because they certainly influence the disease, and second, because treatments are given by the doctor and therefore can be easily modified. This is certainly not the case of other factors like menopause, older age, life situations, and so forth.

During the first years of the use of antidepressant drugs some papers appeared that indicated a clear increase of recurrences in comparison to the previous course treated with electroconvulsive therapy (ECT) or otherwise. We draw attention to the work of Freyhan (1960), Lauber (1964), Arnold and Kryspin-Exner (1965), Hoheisel (1966), and Till and Vuckovic (1970).

Today many clinicians recognize that in many cases the RC course is iatrogenically induced by antidepressive treatments or other stimulant drugs. In a study of 1983, our group (Kukopulos *et al.*, 1983) found that, among 118 RCs, 32 of them had a rapid-cycling course from the beginning of the disorder while 82 of them (73%) had a different course at the beginning and became RCs following treatment with antidepressants. Among these 82 patients, the link with antidepressants was more evident in 52 because earlier they had had other treatment like ECT, anxiolytics and psychotherapy without becoming RCs.

Tondo *et al.* (1981) found that of 67 patients who became RCs, 40 patients underwent the change after intense or protracted use of antidepressant drugs.

In a study performed by Wehr *et al.* (1988), 73% of his 53 patients began to cycle rapidly when they were treated with tricyclic antidepressants.

In a study performed by our group in 2003 (Koukopoulos *et al.*, 2003) on 109 patients, we found that in 13 patients (12%), RC emerged spontaneously and in 96 patients (88%), it was associated with antidepressant and other treatments. In 19 women (28% of all women) RC course started in perimenopausal age (45–54 years).

The common feature of the transformation of previous courses into rapid cyclic ones was the appearance for the first time in the course of the disease of a hypomanic episode after the depression, or the accentuation of a hypomania that had been of milder intensity in previous recurrences. It was after one or more such depression-hypomania cycles (more rarely, depression-mania) that the following depression occurred without interval and that continuous circularity was established. The transformation in RC course under the action of antidepressants in some cases is accomplished after a few recurrences. In other cases it takes years, through a progressive shortening of the episodes and free intervals. As Goodwin and Jamison say (1990): "We consider a phenomenon, that is, the virtual opposite of the prophylaxis: the apparent capacity of antidepressant drugs, in some patients, to accelerate the underlying cyclic process of the illness." In order to explain the successive recurrences without a triggering cause, R. Post *et al.* (1997) advances the hypothesis of sensitization and kindling: once the animal has experienced the repeated pharmacological or electrical stimulation, the neuronal pathways involved become more and more susceptible to have a reactivation without a new stimulation.

On the other hand, Coryell, Endicott, and Keller (1992) did not find any correlation between the use of antidepressants, both tricyclic and serotonergic, and the onset of rapid cyclicity. Bauer *et al.* (1994), however, found that, of the 60 rapid-cycling patients who were followed for at least 12 months, the RC course persisted through the follow-up period in 39 patients (63%) while only 8 patients (13.3%) had no relapses. Baldessarini *et al.* (2000) found that 22.2% of their RC patients showed no improvement and only 29.4% had no recurrences of mania or depression during treatment.

In the STEP-BD, antidepressant use during follow-up was associated with more frequent mood episodes (Schneck *et al.*, 2008).

The clinical practice, however, shows everyday the association of the acceleration of the cyclic course of illness with the use of antidepressants. Ghaemi remarks: "In my own clinical experience, most of the cases of refractory bipolar disorder, usually of the rapid cycling variety, are due to the mood-destabilizing effects of antidepressants." Ghaemi (2008)

20.4 TEMPERAMENT AND RAPID CYCLING

In order to explain the acceleration of the course of the illness under the action of antidepressants, we should take into account the fact that most of the RCs have a premorbid temperament of the cyclothymic or hyperthymic type. They are very energetic, very emotional and reactive (Kukopoulos *et al.*, 1983). One could posit the hypothesis that they are equally reactive to chemical stimulations. Because of this temperament they are diagnosed often as borderline personality disorders and in the past as hysterics. In patients with cyclothymic temperament the rapid-cycling course could be viewed as the accentuation of longstanding subclinical mood oscillations. In patients with iatrogenic RC course we have found a cyclothymic temperament in 44% of the cases and a hyperthymic temperament in another 44% of the cases (Kukopoulos *et al.*, 1983).

20.5 COURSE

In the study of 2003, we examined the evolution of the course of 109 RC patients (68 women and 41 men) followed for a minimum of 2 years and up to 36 years, beginning with the index episode when the RC course was diagnosed. The follow-up period varied from 2 to 5 years for 25 patients, 6 to 10 years for 24 patients, 11 to 15 years for 24 patients, 16 to 20 years for 19 patients, 21 to 25 years for 13 patients, and 30 to 36 years for 4 patients.

The mean duration of RC course during the follow-up period was 7.86 years (range 1–32) and its total duration (including RC course prior to the follow-up period) was 11 years (range 1–40). The total duration of the affective disorder, from the first episode to the end of the follow-up, was 21.78 years (range 1–70). At the end of the follow-up, 36 patients (33%) had complete remission for at least the past year, 44 (40%) stayed RCs with severe episodes (6 of this group committed suicide), while 15 (14%) were rapid cycling but with attenuated episodes. The other 14 patients (13%) became long cyclers, 8 with severe episodes and 6 with milder ones. The two main distinguishing features between those who remitted from and those who persisted in the RC course were first, the initial cycle pattern: patients with Depression-Hypomania (mania)-free interval cycles (53 patients) had a worse outcome: 26.4% remitted and 52.8% persisted in the RC course through to the end of the follow-up period. The Mania/Hypomania-Depression-free interval cycles (22 patients) had a significantly better outcome, with 50% remitted and 27.2% persisting RC. Second, the occurrence of the switch process from depression to hypomania/mania and the occurrence of agitated depressions made the prognosis worse. Of 25 that had at least one switch and one agitated depression 68% remained RC through the follow-up time.

Wehr *et al.* (1988), in their study of the outcome of 51 RC patients after five years of follow-up found that RC course persisted in 41% of the patients while complete remission was 31%. The percentage of patients who had further recurrences but with long cycles was 16%. In our study of 2003, 40% persisted in their RC course, 33% recovered, and 13% changed to long cycles.

Coryell, Endicott, and Keller (1992) in their five-year follow-up study of 45 rapid-cycling bipolar patients, found that only one of the 39 patients who completed five years of follow-up met criteria for rapid-cycling over the entire five years. They remarked, "rapid-cycling is in the large majority of cases, a transient, nonfamilial manifestation of bipolar affective disorder." They also noted that the use of TCAs and MAOIs did not seem to anticipate rapid-cycling and that the prognosis of patients with rapid cycling is more benign than generally assumed. Maj *et al.* (1994) in a two to five-year follow-up of 37 rapid-cycling patients found that only 7 of them (18.9%) had >4 affective episodes per year throughout the follow-up period, whatever its duration. They also found that rapid-cycling patients with a pole-switching pattern during the year preceding intake were significantly more likely than other rapid-cycling patients to have >4 affective episodes during each of the first four years of follow-up.

In the STEP-BD, at entry, 32% of the patients met the DSM-IV criteria for rapid cycling in the pre-study year. At the end of 12 months, only 5% of the patients could be classified as RCs, 34% had no further mood episodes, 34% experienced one episode, and 27% had two or three episodes (Schneck *et al.*, 2008).

In our work of 2003 we found that the patients more likely to remain RCs for many years are those with a DM1 or DmI cycle patterns, those with a switch process and/or agitated depression in their course and those who have not recovered after the first year of an adequate treatment.

The main feature of the course of RCs is the absence of a real free interval between the episodes. Often the change from one episode to another of opposite polarity occurs as a switch in a very short time. In our 2003 work, 59 (54%) of the total 109 RC patients had switches from depression to mania or hypomania before or during the RC course.

When a free interval exists it is always very short and it is probably only the transition from one episode to another.

Baillarger states: "When the attacks are brief, the change from one phase to the other occurs rapidly and, usually, during sleep. This change, on the contrary, occurs slowly and gradually when the episodes are long."

This absence of real free interval must be the main cause of the refractoriness of RCs to prophylactic treatments.

20.6   CLINICAL PICTURE OF RAPID CYCLING

In an early study (1980) of our group of 87 patients (20% of 207 BPI and 227 BPII) had a continuous circular course with short episodes (four or more per year). In this group the number of women was more than twice that of men (61 women and 26 men). Only 16 patients had one or more severe manias, while 71 had only hypomanic episodes. The depression was usually severe, with both inhibitory and anxiety symptoms. The depression was moderate and of the inhibitory type in only 11 cases, all of which had severe manias. The duration of the episodes was usually of two to three months, and depressions were slightly longer than hypomanias. This type of duration of the episodes follows often a seasonal pattern with hypomania in the spring and in autumn and depression in the summer and in the winter. This seasonal pattern is often changed by the treatments. As the years pass by the episodes however become shorter and shorter and ultradian switches appear.

The transition from depression to hypomania was very often rapid, like a switch, while the transition from mania or hypomania to depression was very often gradual. More than half of RC patients showed one or more switches from depression to mania/hypomania (Koukopoulos et al., 2003). Maj et al. (1994) found that 67% of RC patients had had at least a switch during the previous year.

20.7 NEUROBIOLOGY OF RAPID CYCLING BIPOLAR DISORDER: THE ROLE OF DOPAMINE D2 RECEPTORS, SENSITIZATION

A large body of preclinical and clinical evidence suggests a key role of dopamine (DA) in the pathogenesis of bipolar mood disorders. Mania should be associated with an increased DA activity, while a decreased DA neurotransmission might underlie depressive syndromes (Serra et al., 1992; Berk et al., 2007).

In 1979 we first suggested that antidepressants increase DA transmission and that this effect may play an important role both in the therapeutic action and in the switches from depression to mania induced by these drugs (Serra et al., 1979; Gershon, Vishne, and Grunhaus, 2007).

The increased DA transmission induced by antidepressants is due to the development of a DA D2 receptors sensitization in the mesolimbic DA system (Serra et al., 1990; Collu et al., 1997).

Thus, it may be suggested that the sensitization of DA D2 receptors induced by antide-pressants, may be responsible for the switches from depression to mania/hypomania, which, in turn, accelerates the course and finally establishes a rapid cycling course (Serra and D'Aquila, 2008).

Currently mood stabilizers fail to antagonize antidepressant-induced DA D2 receptor sensitization, an observation predictive of their failure to prevent antidepressant-induced mania/hypomania and, in turn, of their ineffectiveness in rapid cycling bipolar disorder.

On the contrary, blockade of NMDA receptors antagonizes antidepressant-induced DA D2 receptors sensitization (D'Aquila et al., 1992).

In keeping with our experimental observations we have hypothesized that Memantine, an uncompetitive NMDA receptor blocker, may have an antimanic and mood stabilizing effect, and should be particularly effective in Rapid Cycling Bipolar Patients.

20.8   TREATMENT

The treatment of RCs is difficult and requires prolonged effort. It is necessary to know the life of the patients, their premorbid temperament and personality, the history of the illness, and its course, the treatments used in the past, and the events and treatments associated with the onset of rapid cycling.

Patients with rapid cycling course are usually of cyclothymic or hyperthymic temperament, therefore particularly excitable and emotional persons. It is important to advise them to avoid coffee, tea, alcohol, and all psychostimulant substances, intense physical exercise and also to avoid, as much as possible, stressful situations and events. Sleep is particularly important and they should go to sleep early and try to sleep for as long as possible.

An evaluation of the thyroid function, and if necessary a TRH test, is useful in order to detect subclinical deficiency and to compensate it by the administration of thyroxine. Bauer and Whybrow (1991) advise adding high doses of levothyroxine to lithium and anticonvulsant treatment, even for patients with normal thyroid function. Subsequent studies have raised doubts about the link between subclinical hypothyroidism and rapid cycling (Post et al., 1997).

The resistance of RCs to all mood-stabilizing treatments is well established. Baldessarini et al. (2002) in a review of 905 RC vs 951 nonRC in 2002, found that nonimprovement was 2.9-fold greater in RC patients treated with carbamazepine, lamotrigine, lithium, topiramate, or valproate. None of these treatments showed a clear advantage over the others. The authors, however, agree with Muzina (2009) about the fundamental importance of lithium in the treatment of RCs. Other mood stabilizers or anti-psychotics should be added to lithium.

We apply the following strategy. Given that most cases of rapid cycling are induced by antidepressants, it is of primary importance to suspend the antidepressants and to continue the treatment with mood stabilizing agents. In most cases without antidepressants the depressive phase will last longer but the following mania/hypomania will be less intense. The anti-manic action of mood stabilizers will be more effective in the absence of antidepressants. Gradually, both the excitatory and the depressive phase will lessen and stabilization will eventually be achieved, over a variable period of time. This therapeutic strategy is based on the idea that the suppression of the excitatory phase prevents or attenuates the following depression (Koukopoulos and Ghaemi, 2009). Indeed, all mood stabilizers like lithium, anticonvulsants, calcium antagonists, and old or new neuroleptics are essentially anti-excitatory agents.

Calabrese et al. (1992) report data showing that the combination of lithium and divalproex sodium administered continuously over six months appears to result in marked acute and continuation antimanic efficacy in 85% of patients and marked antidepressive efficacy in 60%.

In the presence of suicide risk, ECT could be used to end the depressive phase and immediately afterwards mood stabilizing treatment should be administered. A study from Sainte-Anne hospital in Paris shows that maintenance ECT is effective against the RC course, with full or partial remission for 100% of RC patients (Vanelle et al., 1994).

Minnai *et al.* (2009) report that of 14 RC patients treated with maintenance ECT 8 (58%) did not relapse during the two year follow-up period. Similar good results are reported by (G. Fazzàri, personal communication).

The possible antimanic action of Memantine, the only safe NMDA receptor antagonist available for clinical use, prompted us to use it as an antimanic and mood stabilizing agent. We administered Memantine 10–30 mg/die to 15 bipolar patients: 12 BP I (8 women and 4 men) and 3 BP II (2 women and 1 man). Seven of these 15 patients were RCs and 6 were continuous circular with long cycles. Twelve exhibited frequent psychotic symptoms. Mean age 41. These patients had been ill for an average of 21 (4–38) years and, they were all resistant to very intense standard treatments, including lithium, anti-epileptics, typical, and atypical antipsychotics. The Memantine treatment was added to the ongoing ineffective treatment which was left unmodified. Four patients improved within seven days After 24 weeks of Memantine treatment 73% of patients were very much or much improved (Koukopoulos *et al.*, 2009).

20.9 DISCUSSION

Rapid-cycling course certainly existed before the use of antidepressant drugs but it was rare. Many classical authors including Kraepelin hardly mentioned it. The high frequency we observe today is undoubtedly linked to antidepressants. Stimulant recreational drugs like cocaine contribute in some cases. In our samples of bipolar patients examined over the last 40 years, RC course was associated and indeed started with the use of antidepressants in the large majority of cases. This clinical fact supports the hypothesis that excitatory processes are of primary importance in the genesis of bipolar disorder (Koukopoulos and Ghaemi, 2009). Indeed, the most useful mood stabilizers are lithium and anti-epileptic drugs. The good results obtained with Memantine in our short naturalistic study should be explained by its antimanic action due to the blocking effect on the NMDA receptor.

Particularly harmful seems to be the prolongation of antidepressant treatment beyond the end of the depression. The large majority of our patients became rapid-cyclers in association with antidepressants or other stimulating treatments. Many of them initially had a unipolar depressive course. After a period of many years these unipolars first evolved into bipolar and later into rapid-cycling patients. The lag of several years between the first episode and start of rapid cyclicity may not be due only to age-related factors. Some cases require repeated AD treatments before they become RCs. The prevalent premorbid temperament of these "unipolar" depressives was hyperthymic or cyclothymic. These unipolar depressives are probably latent bipolars and have been called unipolar II by Kupfer *et al.* (1975) and pseudo-unipolar by Akiskal (1983).

It is obvious that not all depressions treated with antidepressant drugs undergo an acceleration of their course. Our material shows that those patients who tend to develop a hypomania after depression are the most likely to undergo an acceleration under the action of antidepressants. Patients with a cyclothymic or hyperthymic temperament clearly have this tendency (Kukopulos, 1983). We think that these highly energetic persons have periods of latent hypomania, which is intensified by antidepressants. The same is true for mild hypomanias of the cyclothymic temperament. Akiskal *et al.* (1977) found that 11 of 25 cyclothmyic patients who were treated with tricyclics experienced hypomania. We believe that this intensification of hypomanic processes will, in turn, accentuate the depressive oscillation that follows, which otherwise would have passed unperceived or would not have taken place at all. We derive this hypothesis from the clinical fact that most manias are followed by a depression. At this point the question should arise as to why an intensified hypomania precipitates the following depression in advance. As little is known about the underlying chemical processes, this question cannot be answered. It is conceivable, however, that the energetic processes that sustain a mild hypomania or the free interval of a very active person are depleted more rapidly when they are intensified, and the free interval ends more quickly. The role of temperament appears to be of decisive importance. Kilzieh and Akiskal (1999) state that "it would be logical to assume that RC represents a natural accentuation of the cyclothymic's tendency toward cycling on a lower plane of severity." Brieger and Marneros (1997) state that "Cyclothymic disorder operationalized as a subaffective dimension or temperament appears to be a likely precursor or ingredient of the construct of bipolar II disorder." Kraepelin (1913), reporting that the cyclothymic disposition among almost a thousand cases observed in Munich was 3–4%, adds "but without doubt in reality it is much more frequent, as is the invariable introduction to the slightest forms of manic-depressive insanity which run their course outside of institutions." In our study (Kukopulos *et al.*, 1983), dealing with the premorbid temperament of RCs, we found that 44% had a cyclothymic temperament and another 44% had a hyperthymic temperament.

The data on the duration and stability of the RC course are contrasting.

We think these contradictory data regarding the stability of the RC course are due to the powerful effect of treatments on the duration of episodes and probably the intervals too. Many bipolar cases may become "transient rapid-cyclers" (Kukopulos *et al.*, 1975). These periods of transient rapid-cyclicity are mere iatrogenic artifacts of the course of bipolar disorder which do not involve endogenous rhythms. We would like to suggest that only patients who have had four or more episodes for two or more years should be considered RCs, at least for research purposes. This would permit a more accurate investigation of the biological and clinical features that contribute to the creation of long-lasting rapid cycling. It is, in fact, the stable rapid-cyclers who constitute a major therapeutic problem and have a poorer outcome than the other cases and, hence, are more likely to be represented in a mood clinic which is known for its expertise in taking care of such patients. Dunner, Stallone, and Fieve (1976) in their study included patients who had two years of RC course. A two-year duration criterion would correspond to the criterion of other such chronic affective disorders as Dysthymia and Cyclothymia.

The DSM system considers rapid cyclicity as a course specifier. For its continuous and completely autonomous cycling in clear bipolar alternation, rapid cyclicity could be viewed as the core form of the entire Bipolar Spectrum.

The most important feature of RCs is their refractoriness to treatment. Actually they were identified by this feature. We think that the cause of this refractoriness is the absence or the shortness of the intervals between the episodes. Probably the short intervals seen in RCs are transitions between the episodes and not real free intervals. It is well known that the best responders to prophylactic treatment have long intervals especially if they precede a manic/hypomanic episode (Kukopulos *et al.*, 1980; Grof *et al.*, 1987; Haag *et al.*, 1987; Maj, Piroizi, and Starace, 1989; Faedda *et al.*, 1991). The hypothesis could be proposed that the gradually emerging manic process during the interval is easily suppressed by the continuous prophylactic treatment. It is conceivable that rapidly emerging manic processes are more resistant to treatment.

References

Akiskal, H.S. (1983) The bipolar spectrum: new concepts in classification and diagnosis, in *Psychiatry Update: The American Psychiatry Association Annual Review* (ed. L. Grinspoon), American Psychiatry Press, Washington. DC., pp. 271–292.

Akiskal, H.S., Djenderedjian, A.H., Rosenthal, R.H. *et al.* (1977) Cyclothimic disorder: validating criteria for inclusion in the bipolar affective group. *Am. J. Psychiatry*, **134**, 1227–1233.

American Psychiatric Association (1994) *DSM-IV*, American Psychiatric Association, Washington, DC.

Arnold, O.H. and Kryspin-Exner, K. (1965) Zur Frage der Beeinflussung des Venlaufes des manish- depressiven Krankheitsgeschehens durch Antidepressiva. *Wien. Med. Wochenschr.*, **45/46**, 929–934.

Baillarger, J. Note sur un genre de folie. *Bulletin de l'Acad. Imperiale de Med. Tome XIX*, 1853–1854.

Baldessarini, R.J., Tondo, L., Floris, G., and Hennen, J. (2000) Effects of rapid cycling on response to Lithium maintenance treatment in 360 bipolar I and 11 disorder patients. *J. Affect. Disord.*, **61**, 13–22.

Baldessarini, R.J., Tondo, L., Hennen, J., and Viguera, A.C. (2002) Is lithium still worth using? An update of selected recent research. *Harv. Rev. Psychiatry*, **10** (2), 59–75 (Review).

Bauer, M.S., Calabrese, J., Dunner, D.L. *et al.* (1994) Multisite data reanalysis of the validity of rapid cycling as a course modifier for bipolar disorder in DSM-IV. *Am. J. Psychiatry*, **151**, 506–515.

Bauer, M.S. and Whybrow, P.C. (1991) Rapid cycling bipolar disorder: clinical features, treatment and etiology, *Refractory Depression*, Advances in Neuropsychiatry and Psychopharmacology, Vol. **2**, Raven Press Ltd, Amsterdam, JD.

Berk, M., Dodd, S., Kauer-Sant'anna, M. *et al.* (2007) Dopamine dysregulation syndrome: implications for a dopamine hypothesis of bipolar disorder. *Acta Psychiatr. Scand. Suppl.*, **434**, 41–49.

Brieger, P. and Marneros, A. (1997) Dysthymia and cyclothymia: historical origins and contemporary development. i. *Affect. Disord.*, **45**, 117–126.

Brodwall, O. (1941) The course of the manic-depressive psychosis. *Acta Psychiatr. Neurol.*, **22**, 195–210.

Calabrese, J.R., Markovitz, P.J., Kimmel, S.E., and Wagner, S.C. (1992) Spectrum of efficacy of vaiproate in 78 rapid-cycling bipolar patients. *J. Clin. Psychopharmacol.*, **12** (Suppl. I), 53S–56S.

Collu, M., Poggiu, A.S., Devoto, P. and Serra, G. (1997) Behavioural sensitization of D2 mesolimbic dopamine receptors in chronic fluoxetine treated rats. *Eur. J. Pharm.*, **322**, 123–127.

Coryell, W., Endicott, I., and Keller, M. (1992) Rapidly cycling affective disorder. *Arch. Gen. Psychiatry*, **49**, 126–131.

Cruz, N., Vieta, E., Comes, M. *et al.* (2007) Rapid-cycling bipolar I disorder: course and treatment outcomes of a large sample across Europe (EMBLEM). *J. Psychiatr. Res.*, **42**, 1068–1075.

D'Aquila, P.S., Sias, A., Gessa, G.L., and Serra, G. (1992) The NMDA receptor antagonist MK-801 prevents imipramine-induced supersensitivity to quinpirole. *Eur. J. Pharmacol.*, **224**, 199–202.

Dunner, D.L. and Fieve, R.R. (1974) Clinical factors in lithium carbonate prophylaxis failure. *Arch. Gen. Psychiatry*, **30**, 229–233.

Dunner, D.L., Stallone, F., and Fieve, R.R. (1976) Lithium carbonate and affective disorders. *Arch. Gen. Psychiatry*, **33**, 117–120.

Faedda, G.L., Baldessarini, T.J., Tohen, M. *et al.* (1991) Episode sequence in bipolar disorder and response to lithium treatment. *Am. J. Psychiatry*, **148**, 1237–1239.

Falret, J.P. (1854) *Lecons Cliniques de Medicine Mentale*, Premiere Partie, Paris.

Freyhan, F.A. (1960) Zur modernen psychiatrischen Behandlung der Depressionen. *Nervenarzt*, **31**, 112–118.

Geller, B., Williams, M., Zimerman, B. *et al.* (1998) Prepubertal and early adolescent bipolarity. *J. Affect Disord.*, **51** (2), 81–91.

Gershon, A.A., Vishne, T., and Grunhaus, L. (2007) Dopamine D2-like receptors and the antidepressant response. *Biol. Psychiatry*, **61** (2), 145–153.

Ghaemi, S.N. (2008) Treatment of rapid-cycling bipolar disorder: are antidepressants mood destabilizers? *Am. J. Psychiatry*, **165**, 3.

Goodwin, F.K. and Jamison K.R. (1990) *Manic-Depressive Illness*, Oxford University Press.

Grof, E., Haag, M., Grof, P., and Haag, H. (1987) Lithium response and the sequence of episode polarities: preliminary report on a Hamilton sample. *Prog. Neuropsychopharmacol. Biol. Psychiatry*, **11**, 199–203.

Haag, H., Heidorn, A., Haag, M., and Greili, W. (1987) Sequence of affective polarity and Lithium response: preliminary report on a Munich sample. *Prog. Neuropsychopharmacol. Biol. Psychiatry*, **11**, 205–208.

Hoheisel, H.P. (1966) Zur Frage der Verkiirzung von Intervallzeiten psychopharmakologisch behandelter phasischer Psychosen. *Nervenarzt*, **37**, 259–263.

Kilzieh, N. and Akiskal, H. (1999) Rapid-cycling bipolar disorder: overview. *Psychiatr. Clin. North Am.*, **22**, 585–607.

Koukopoulos, A. and Ghaemi, S.N. (2009) The Primacy of Mania. A reconsideration of mood disorders. *Eur Psychiatry*, **24** (2), 125–134.

Koukopoulos, A., Reginaldi, D., Serra, G. *et al.* (2010) Antimanic and mood stabilizing effect of memantine as augmenting agent in bipolar resistant patients. *Bipolar Disord.*, **12**, 348–349.

Koukopoulos, A., Sani, G., Koukopoulos, A.E. *et al.* (2003) Duration and stability of the rapid-cycling course: a long-term personal follow-up of 109 patients. *J Affect Disord.*, **73**, 75–85.

Kraepelin, E. (1913) *Psychiatry*, 8th edn, Barth, Leipzig.

Kukopulos, A. (variant of Koukopoulos), Caliari, B., Tundo, A. *et al.* (1983) Rapid cyclers.temperament and antidepressants. *Compr. Psychiatry*, **24**, 249–258.

Kukopulos, A. (variant of Koukopoulos), Reginaldi, D., Girardi, P., and Tondo, L. (1975) Course of manic-depressive recurrences under lithium. *Compr. Psychiatry*, **16**, 517–524.

Kukopulos, A. (variant of Koukopoulos), Reginaldi, D., Laddomada, P. *et al.* (1980) Course of the manic-depressive cycle and changes caused by treatments. *Pharmakopsychiatry*, **13**, 156–167.

Kupfer, D.J., Packar, D., Himmelhoch, J.M., and Detre, T.P. (1975) Are there two types of unipolar depression? *Arch. Gen. Psychiatry*, **32**, 866–871.

Kupka, R.W., Luckenbaugh, D.A., Post, R.M. *et al.* (2003) Rapid and non-rapid cycling bipolar disorder: a meta-analysis of clinical studies. *J. Clin. Psychiatry*, **64** (12), 1483–1494.

Lange, J. (1928) The endogenen und reaktiven Gemutskrankhejten und die manisch- depressive Konstitution, in *Handbuch der Geisteskrankeiten*, Spezieller Teil II, Band **6** (ed. O. Bumke), Springer, Berlin, p. 181.

Lauber, H. (1964) Studie zur Frage der Krankheitsdauer unter Behandlung mit Psychopharmaka. *Nervenarzt*, **35**, 488–491.

Lundquist, G. (1945) Prognosis and course in manic-depressive psychoses. *Acta Psych Neurl.*, (Suppl. 35), 1–96.

Maj, N.I., Piroizi, R., and Starace, F. (1989) Previous pattern of course of the illness as a predictor of response to lithium prophylaxis in bipolar patients. *J. Affect. Disord.*, **7**, 237–241.

Maj, M., Magliano, L., Pirozzi, R. *et al.* (1994) Validity of rapid cycling as a course specifier for bipolar disorder. *Am. J. Psychiatry*, **151**, 1015–1019.

Minnai, G.P., Salis, P.G., Oppo, R. *et al.* Effectiveness of maintenance electroconvulsive therapy (m-ECT) in rapid cycling bipolar disorder. (2009) *J. ECT*, in press.

Muzina, D.J. (2009) Pharmacologic treatment of rapid cycling and mixed states in bipolar disorder: an argument for the use of lithium. *Bipolar Disord.*, **11** (Suppl. 2), 84–91 (Review).

Post, R.M., Kramlinger, K.G., Joffe, R.T. *et al.* (1997) Rapid cycling affective disorder: lack of relation to hypothyroidism. *Psychiatry Res.*, **72** (1), 1–7.

Ritti, A. (1883) *Traité Clinique de la Folieà Double Forme*, Octave Doin, Paris.

Schneck, C.D., Miklowitz, D.J., Miyahara, S. *et al.* (2008) The prospective course of rapid-cycling bipolar disorder: findings from the STEP-BD. *Am. J. Psychiatry*, **165** (3), 370–377.

Serra, G., Argiolas, A., Klimek, V. *et al.* (1979) Chronic treatment with antidepressants prevents the inhibitory effect of small doses of apomorphine on dopamine synthesis and motor activity. *Life Sci.*, **25**, 415–424.

Serra, G., Collu, M., D'Aquila, P.S. *et al.* (1990) Possible role of dopamine D1 receptor in the behavioural supersensitivity to dopamine agonists induced by chronic treatment with antidepressant. *Brain Res.*, **527**, 234–243.

Serra, G., Collu, M., D'Aquila, P.S., and Gessa, G.L. (1992) Role of mesolimbic dopamine system in the mechaniasm of action of antidepressants. *Pharmacol. Toxicol.*, **71** (Suppl. I), 72–85.

Serra, G. and D'Aquila, P.S. (2008) Do antidepressants induce mania and rapid cycling by increasing dopaminergic transmission? TDM 2008 International Meeting – Bologna ottobre 2008, pp. 554–552.

Stenstedt, A. (1952) A study in manic depressive psychosis. *Acta Psychiatr. Scand.*, **79**, 1–111.

Till, E. and Vuckovic, S. (1970) Ueber den Einfluss der thymoleptischen Behandlung auf den Verlauf endogener Depressionen. *Im Pharmacopsychiatry*, **4**, 210–219.

Tondo, L., Laddomada, P., Serra, G. *et al.* (1981) Rapid Cyclers and Antidepressants. *Int. Pharmacopsychiatry*, **16**, 119–223.

Vanelle, J.M., Loo, H., Galinowski, A. *et al.* (1994) Maintenance ECT in intractable manicdepressive disorders. *Convuls. Ther.*, **10** (3), 195–205.

Wehr, T.A., Sack, D.A., Rosenthal, N.E., and Cowdry, R.W. (1988) Rapid cycling affective disorder: contributing factors and treatment responses in 51 patients. *Am. J. Psychiatry*, **145**, 179–184.

Yildiz, A. and Sachs, G.S. (2004) Characteristics of rapid cycling bipolar I patients in a bipolar speciality clinic. *J Affect. Disord.*, **79** (1–3), 247–251.

21

Novel Therapeutic Approaches for Treating Bipolar Disorder

Rodrigo Machado-Vieira, Ioline Henter, Jacqueline Baumann, David Latov, Cristina Wheeler-Castillo and Carlos A. Zarate

Experimental Therapeutics and Pathophysiology Branch, Intramural Research Program, National Institute of Mental Health, National Institutes of Health, Bethesda, MD, USA

21.1 INTRODUCTION

Bipolar disorder (BPD) is a serious, chronic, and heterogeneous disorder characterized by high rates of persistent subsyndromal symptoms as well as frequent episode relapses and recurrences that often result in psychosocial dysfunction and disability. Recent estimates suggest that BPD affects 1–2% of the general population (Goodwin and Jamison, 2007). Currently available treatments are associated with both lack of efficacy and tolerability, making them far from ideal for many patients with BPD (Judd *et al.*, 2002). It is also surprising to note that, to date, no agent has been developed exclusively to treat BPD; indeed, with the exception of lithium, all medications currently used to treat the disorder were initially developed for another indication (for example, antipsychotics, anticonvulsants). Thus, there is an urgent need to identify novel therapeutic targets for BPD.

Here, we review several potential new drugs and targets worthy of further consideration in the development of novel therapies for BPD. These include: (i) the dynorphin opioid neuropeptide system, (ii) the purinergic system, (iii) the melatonergic system, (iv) the glutamatergic system, (v) the tachykinin neuropeptides system, (vi) the glucocorticoid system, (vii) the arachidonic acid (AA) cascade, (viii) the endocannabinoid system, (ix) oxidative stress and bioenergetics, and (x) intracellular signaling cascades. The compounds reviewed below have shown either antimanic or antidepressant effects in individuals with BPD or in preclinical models of mania and depression. However, it is important to note at the outset that the extrapolation of animal studies to humans requires cautious interpretation.

Bipolar Psychopharmacotherapy: Caring for the patient, Second Edition. Edited by Hagop S. Akiskal and Mauricio Tohen.
© 2011 John Wiley & Sons, Ltd. Published 2011 by John Wiley & Sons, Ltd.

21.2 THE DYNORPHIN OPIOID NEUROPEPTIDE SYSTEM

The dynorphin opioid neuropeptide family modulates diverse behavioral aspects including mood, cognition, and motor function. Similar to other neuropeptides, dynorphins are produced from a biologically inactive precursor protein. The three opioid receptors (delta, mu, and kappa) are coupled to different intracellular effector systems and are widely distributed in the ventral tegmental area, nucleus accumbens, and prefrontal cortex; these areas have been critically linked to mood regulation, drive, and motivation (Berrocoso, Sanchez-Blazquez, and Garzon, 2009).

Opioid peptides and their receptors are potential candidates for the development of novel treatments for mood disorders. These endogenous peptides are coexpressed in brain areas critically implicated in the action of various antidepressants (Schwarzer, 2009). Also, stress has been found to elevate dynorphin levels in limbic brain areas, and these elevations were reversed by treatment with antidepressants (Chartoff *et al.*, 2009; Shirayama *et al.*, 2004). Related to the neurobiology of BPD, a significant decrease (37–38%) in pro-dynorphin messenger RNA (mRNA) expression levels in the amygdalo-hippocampal area and in the parvicellular division of the accessory basal area was noted in patients with BPD (Hurd, 2002). In addition, some clinical reports described the efficacy of opioid agonists such as oxymorphone and buprenorphine in the treatment of refractory major depressive disorder (MDD) (Bodkin *et al.*, 1995; Stoll and Rueter, 1999). Patients with comorbid depression and anxiety have also been found to have decreased serum β-endorphin levels (Darko *et al.*, 1992). Furthermore, standard monoaminergic antidepressants have been shown to activate the opioid system, while the opioid antagonist naloxone blocked this effect. For instance, naloxone blocked the antidepressant-like effects of clomipramine, desipramine, and venlafaxine in the forced swim test, a well-known rodent model of depression (Berrocoso, Rojas-Corrales, and Mico, 2004; Devoize *et al.*, 1984).

Mu receptors are densely distributed in several brain regions implicated in stress response and emotional stimuli. Mu opioid receptor agonists have been shown to have antidepressant-like effects in animal models (Besson *et al.*, 1996; Rojas-Corrales *et al.*, 2002; Tejedor-Real *et al.*, 1995), and these effects are reversed by the nonselective opioid antagonist naloxone (Besson *et al.*, 1996). The synthetic opioid tramadol, an atypical agent that binds weakly to Mu receptors, also has monoaminergic properties. Although it is an analgesic, studies conducted with tramadol suggest it has antidepressant-like effects in various animal models (Rojas-Corrales *et al.*, 2004; Rojas-Corrales, Gibert-Rahola, and Mico, 1998; Yalcin *et al.*, 2007). In clinical studies of individuals with treatment-resistant MDD, tramadol showed rapid antidepressant efficacy either as monotherapy or as an add-on; it was also associated with antisuicidal properties (Shapira, Verduin, and DeGraw, 2001; Spencer, 2000).

Delta receptors have a high affinity for the endogenous opioid peptide proenkephalin. For instance, proenkephalin-knockout (KO) mice are at increased risk for anxiety- and depressive-like behaviors (Ragnauth *et al.*, 2001). Supporting the role of opioid delta receptors as potential therapeutics for the treatment of mood disorders, preclinical studies suggest that several of these receptor agonists have antidepressant-like properties (Jutkiewicz, 2006). For instance, the delta agonist SNC80 induced significant antidepressant-like effects in the olfactory bulbectomized model of depression (Saitoh *et al.*, 2008), which also involves mediation by the monoaminergic system. In addition, acute treatment with a delta opioid agonist simultaneously increased expression of brain derived neurotrophic factor (BDNF) and produced antidepressant-like effects (Torregrossa *et al.*, 2006). However, clinical evidence is still lacking.

With regard to kappa opiate receptors, studies have shown that activation of this system induces depressive symptoms in both humans and animals (Barber and Gottschlich, 1997; Carlezon *et al.*, 2006). Thus, it is possible that kappa opiate agonists may bring about antimanic effects; however, activation of opioid receptors may also induce psychotomimetic effects (Rimoy *et al.*, 1994; Walsh *et al.*, 2001). In animal models, the highly selective kappa opioid receptor agonist Salvinorin-A *(Salvia divinorum)* was associated with depressive-like behaviors (Carlezon *et al.*, 2006), while the kappa opioid antagonist MCL-144B had antidepressant-like effects (Mague *et al.*, 2003; Reindl *et al.*, 2008). This suggests that blocking these receptors may be relevant to the treatment of mood disorders.

In one uncontrolled study, 10 individuals with BPD who were experiencing a manic episode received two doses of the partial kappa agonist pentazocine (Talwin, 50-mg, 2 hours apart) added to their existing medications for BPD. Within an hour of each dose, manic symptoms were significantly reduced (>44% after the first dose and 41% after the second dose) (Cohen and Murphy, 2008). No significant or severe adverse events were described. Presently, no selective kappa agonist has been clinically evaluated as monotherapy for the treatment of BPD; however, activation of this system has induced depressive symptoms in healthy volunteers. Future controlled proof-of-concept studies are needed to clarify the relevance of kappa opioid receptors in the pathophysiology and therapeutics of BPD.

21.3   THE PURINERGIC SYSTEM

Recent genetic and clinical studies have supported the role of this system in the pathophysiology and therapeutics of BPD (Barden *et al.*, 2006; Lucae *et al.*, 2006; Machado-Vieira *et al.*, 2008). The purinergic system is mostly mediated by adenosine triphosphate (ATP) and adenosine, and plays an important role in modulating several neurotransmitters involved in the pathophysiology of mood disorders, including dopamine, serotonin, and gamma aminobutyric acid (GABA) (Burnstock, 2007). This system directly regulates cognition, sleep, motor activity, appetite, memory, and social interaction (Machado-Vieira *et al.*, 2002). Four subtypes of P1 receptors have been cloned: A_1, A_{2A}, A_{2B}, and A_3. The neuromodulator adenosine is widely distributed in the brain and acts mostly through the A_1 and A_{2A} receptors. Adenosine has been shown to have antidepressant and anticonvulsant-like effects in preclinical paradigms (Burnstock, 2007; Kaster *et al.*, 2004). On the other hand, adenosine antagonists such as caffeine increase irritability, anxiety, and insomnia in BPD, all of which trigger manic episodes (Ogawa and Ueki, 2003). In contrast, adenosine agonists appear to have sedative, anticonvulsant, anti-aggressive, and antipsychotic-like properties in animal models (Lara *et al.*, 2006).

Recently, a single nucleotide polymorphism in the purinergic P2RX7 gene was described as a possible susceptibility gene for BPD (Barden *et al.*, 2006). Interestingly,

P2X7 receptor KO mice show an antidepressant-like profile in the tail suspension and forced swim tests – two well-known animal models of depression – compared to mice treated with imipramine; no such effects were noted in preclinical models of anxiety (Basso *et al.*, 2009). Blockade of the adenosine A_{2A} receptor also induced antidepressant-like effects (El Yacoubi *et al.*, 2001) in animal models. A_1 receptor agonists have been shown to limit the activating effects of caffeine, while A_1 receptor antagonists induced stimulating behavioral effects similar to those of caffeine (Antoniou *et al.*, 2005). In animal models of mania, the ATP P2 receptor antagonist pyridoxalphosphate-6-azophenyl-2'4'-disulfonic acid (PPADS) blocked amphetamine-induced motor hyperactivity (Kittner, Krugel, and Illes, 2001).

With regard to clinical studies, studies conducted over 40 years ago noted that remission in mania was associated with increased excretion of uric acid (Anumonye *et al.*, 1968). Subsequently, it was proposed that purinergic system dysfunction was directly involved in the neurobiology of mania (Machado-Vieira *et al.*, 2002). In support of this theory, the purinergic modulator allopurinol, which has been used for many years to treat gout, was found to have antimanic efficacy, particularly in patients with hyperuricemia (Machado-Vieira *et al.*, 2001). Two double-blind, placebo-controlled studies lend further support to these findings. In the first study, Akhondzadeh *et al.* (2006) studied the antimanic efficacy of allopurinol (300 mg/day) compared to placebo, administered adjunctively to lithium plus haloperidol for eight weeks. Posthoc comparisons showed a significant improvement in manic symptoms as early as Day 7, as assessed by Young Mania Rating Scale (YMRS) scores; this difference between groups was also statistically significant at endpoint (eight weeks) (Akhondzadeh *et al.*, 2006). More recently, a four-week, double-blind, placebo-controlled study involving 180 subjects with acute bipolar mania compared the efficacy and safety of allopurinol (600 mg/day), dipyridamole (an adenosine reuptake inhibitor) (200 mg/day), and placebo added to lithium (Machado-Vieira *et al.*, 2008). Antipsychotics were not used in the study. Allopurinol was found to be significantly superior to dipyridamole and placebo in decreasing manic symptoms; few side effects were observed. Antimanic effects induced by allopurinol were significantly associated with uric acid levels, reinforcing the role of purinergic dysfunction in mania. Further large controlled studies assessing allopurinol as a maintenance treatment for BPD, and evaluating selective purinergic modulators, may help to determine specific, relevant targets within this system.

21.4 THE MELATONERGIC SYSTEM

Melatonin receptors (MT1 and MT2) are highly expressed in the brain and produce their biological effects mostly through G protein-coupled receptors. The role of this system in the pathophysiology of BPD has focused on dysfunction of the circadian system and sleep-wake rhythms. Supersensitivity to melatonin suppression by light was shown in patients with BPD, as well as in the nonaffected offspring of probands with BPD and monozygotic twins discordant for BPD; however, these findings were not confirmed by a similar study evaluating euthymic individuals with BPD (Hallam, Olver, and Norman, 2005; Lewy *et al.*, 1981, 1985; Nurnberger *et al.*, 2000).

In genetic studies, a significant association between the δ 502–505 polymorphism in GPR50 (H9, melatonin-related receptor) and increased risk for BPD was observed in one study but was not subsequently replicated (Alaerts *et al.*, 2006; Thomson *et al.*, 2005). Agomelatine, a potent, nonselective agonist of melatonin MT1 and MT2 receptors was shown to resynchronize disrupted circadian rhythms and has circadian phase-advancement properties (Armstrong *et al.*, 1993; Nagayama, 1996; Redman and Francis, 1998). In animal models, agomelatine had significant antidepressant-like effects in the forced swim, chronic mild stress, and learned helplessness tests (Bertaina-Anglade *et al.*, 2006; Millan *et al.*, 2005; Papp *et al.*, 2003). Agomelatine is also known to increase synaptic levels of both norepinephrine and dopamine and to increase cell proliferation and neurogenesis in the ventral dentate gyrus (Banasr *et al.*, 2006; Van Oekelen, Luyten, and Leysen, 2003).

No controlled clinical studies have evaluated the use of melatonin in subjects with BPD, and existing case reports have described conflicting results (Van Oekelen, Luyten, and Leysen, 2003; Bersani and Garavini, 2000). However, a recent open-label trial evaluating 21 patients with bipolar depression receiving agomelatine (25 mg/day) adjunctive to either lithium or valpromide for six weeks found that 81% of patients had significantly improved by study endpoint; 47% of these showed response during the first week of treatment (Calabrese, Guelfi, and Perdrizet-Chevallier, 2007). Agomelatine has also been used in the treatment of MDD. Three large, controlled, multicenter clinical trials have found it to be well-tolerated, and consistently more effective than placebo (Kennedy and Emsley, 2006; Loo, Hale, and D'Haenen, 2002; Montgomery and Kasper, 2007). Despite a growing body of evidence suggesting a role for the melatonergic system in mood disorders, additional placebo-controlled studies specifically addressing its potential therapeutic role in BPD are needed.

21.5 THE GLUTAMATERGIC SYSTEM

Glutamate regulates diverse physiological functions, including learning, synaptic plasticity, and memory (Bannerman *et al.*, 1995; Collingridge, 1994; Collingridge and Bliss, 1995; Watkins and Collingridge, 1994). Altered glutamatergic regulation appears to be directly involved in the altered neuroplasticity and cellular resilience associated with BPD (Zarate, Singh, and Manji, 2006a).

In recent years, several glutamatergic modulators have been tested in proof-of-concept studies in mood disorders; these agents mostly target N-methyl-D-aspartate (NMDA), alpha-amino-3-hydroxyl-5-methyl-4-isoxazole-propionate (AMPA), and metabotropic receptors in pre- and post-synaptic neurons as well as glia (Machado-Vieira, Manji, and Zarate, 2009).

21.5.1 IONOTROPIC GLUTAMATE RECEPTORS

NMDA receptor antagonists have antidepressant-like effects in diverse animal models of depression (reviewed in Zarate *et al.* (2002, 2003)). For instance, animal models assessing the effectiveness of the NMDA antagonists dizocilpine (MK-801) and CGP 37849 found that these agents had significant antidepressant-like effects as monotherapy or in combination with standard antidepressants (Meloni _et al._, 1993; Padovan and Guimaraes, 2004; Papp and Moryl, 1993; Skolnick _et al._, 1992; Trullas and Skolnick, 1990).

AMPA receptor potentiators have also been tested as potential therapeutics for mood disorders. These agents decrease receptor desensitization and/or deactivation rates (Bleakman and Lodge, 1998). Interestingly, AMPA receptor trafficking (including receptor insertion, internalization, and delivery to synaptic sites), which is believed to be involved in the antidepressant effects of AMPA receptor potentiators, plays a critical role in regulating activity-dependent regulation of synaptic strength, as well as various forms of neural and behavioral plasticity (Sanacora _et al._, 2008). AMPA potentiators have significant antidepressant-like effects in preclinical paradigms of depression (reviewed in Black (2005); Du _et al._ (2007), and Miu _et al._ (2001)). For instance, the AMPA potentiator ampalex exerted antidepressant-like effects during the first days of treatment (Knapp _et al._, 2002). In addition, the AMPA receptor antagonist Talampanel (GYKI 53773; formerly LY 300164) has completed Phase II clinical trials, where it demonstrated preliminary efficacy (Traynor _et al._, 2006). The competitive AMPA receptor antagonist NS1209 has been tested for the treatment of refractory status epilepticus (Rogawski, 2006), and may be a potential therapeutic for the treatment of BPD; the agent showed good central nervous system bioavailability and was well-tolerated in Phase I/II clinical trials. NS1209 also induced more rapid and consistent anticonvulsant effects than diazepam in animal models (Pitkanen _et al._, 2007).

21.5.2   METABOTROPIC GLUTAMATE RECEPTORS (mGluRs)

The metabotropic glutamate receptors (mGluRs) family comprises eight receptor subtypes (mGluR1 to GluR8) classified into three groups based on their sequence homology, agonist selectivity, and second messenger system-coupled receptors. Group I mGluRs (mGluR1 and mGluR5) are coupled to the phospholipase C signal transduction pathway. Group II (mGluR2 and mGluR3) and III (mGluR4 and mGluR6 to mGluR8) receptors are both coupled to the adenylyl cyclase signal transduction pathway in an inhibitory manner.

Diverse Group I mGluR1 and mGluR5 antagonists induce antidepressant-like effects in animal models (Machado-Vieira, Manji, and Zarate, 2009). In preclinical studies, the potent and selective mGluR5 antagonist fenobam was found to have anxiolytic effects, but studies were discontinued because of its psychostimulant effects (Palucha and Pilc, 2007). Also, the mGluR5-positive allosteric modulator _3-cyano-N-(1,3-diphenyl-1Hpyrazol- 5-yl)benzamide_ reversed amphetamine-induced locomotor activity in rodents, thus suggesting that it is potentially useful in treating mania (Kinney _et al._, 2005).

The Group II mGluR2 and mGluR2/3 receptors limit excessive glutamate release into the synapse; diverse group II mGluRs modulators (for example, LY341495) have been found to induce dose-dependent antidepressant-like effects in preclinical paradigms (reviewed in Zarate _et al._ (2002)). Furthermore, Group III mGluR agonists showed antidepressant-like effects in the forced swim and behavioral despair tests (Palucha and Pilc, 2007; Gasparini _et al._, 1999). In addition, mGluR7 KO mice displayed an antidepressant phenotype in the forced swim and tail suspension tests (Cryan _et al._, 2003).

Another recent study noted that Group III GluR6 KO mice showed increased motor activity when exposed to amphetamine, with elevated risk-taking and aggressive behavior; these manifestations were abolished after chronic treatment with lithium (Shaltiel *et al.*, 2008). To date, no Group III mGluR agonists have been tested clinically in BPD, but based on the evidence from animal studies, this class of compounds has potential clinical utility in treating both depressive and manic episodes.

21.5.3 GLUTAMATERGIC MODULATORS

21.5.3.1 Riluzole, Ketamine, and Cytidine

In addition to preclinical animal models, several clinical trials have been conducted using glutamatergic modulators in the treatment of mood disorders. Riluzole is approved by the U.S. Food and Drug Administration (FDA) for the treatment of amyotrophic lateral sclerosis (ALS), and has well-defined neuroprotective properties. This blood-brain-penetrant glutamatergic agent upregulates AMPA trafficking by membrane insertion of GluR1 and GluR2 subunits, and also inhibits glutamate release. It has also been found to enhance glutamate reuptake and to activate the synthesis of neurotrophins (Frizzo *et al.*, 2004; Mizuta *et al.*, 2001). In animal models of mood disorders, pretreatment with 10 mg/kg riluzole (but not 3 mg/kg) moderately reduced amphetamine-induced hyperlocomotion (Lourenco Da Silva *et al.*, 2003). Also, a variety of changes induced by chronic unpredictable stress (an animal model of depression) were reversed and/or blocked by riluzole, including anhedonia/helplessness, decreased glial metabolism, and decreased glial fibrillary acidic protein (GFAP) mRNA expression (Banasr *et al.*, 2010).

In humans, riluzole showed significant antidepressant effects and was well-tolerated in two open-label studies evaluating its use in treatment-resistant unipolar and bipolar depression (Zarate *et al.*, 2004, 2005), respectively. In the first study, 13 patients with MDD completed the trial and all showed significant improvement by week 6 (Zarate *et al.*, 2004), with similar antianxiety effects (29% decrease in total Hamilton Anxiety Rating Scale (HAM-A) scores). In the second trial, significant antidepressant effects were noted in 14 patients with bipolar depression who received riluzole (100–200 mg per day) adjunctively to lithium for six weeks (Zarate *et al.*, 2005). Another recent study found that riluzole (50 mg/twice daily) produced antidepressant effects after one week of treatment in a group of treatment-resistant patients with MDD who were also receiving antidepressants; a significant decrease (36%) in Hamilton Depression Rating Scale (HAM-D) scores was noted among completers (Sanacora *et al.*, 2007). Double-blind, placebo-controlled trials are necessary to confirm these data.

Ketamine is a high affinity NMDA receptor antagonist that induces significant presynaptic release of glutamate by enhancing the firing of glutamatergic neurons after disinhibiting GABAergic inputs (Moghaddam *et al.*, 1997). Diverse preclinical studies have demonstrated that ketamine has anxiolytic and antidepressant effects (Aguado *et al.*, 1994; Garcia *et al.*, 2008; Maeng *et al.*, 2008; Mickley *et al.*, 1998; Silvestre *et al.*, 1997). Recently, animal studies have further shown that blocking AMPA activation abolishes ketamine's antidepressant effects, thus suggesting that its antidepressant properties occur by enhancing AMPA throughput (Maeng *et al.*, 2008).

In clinical studies, ketamine has been associated with significant antidepressant effects for the treatment of MDD. An initial study described improvement 72 hours after ketamine infusion in treatment-resistant patients with MDD (Berman *et al.*, 2000). Subsequently, a double-blind placebo-controlled, crossover study evaluating ketamine in treatment-resistant MDD found a rapid (within 2 hours) and relatively sustained (lasting one to two weeks) antidepressant effect after ketamine infusion (single-dose, 0.5 mg/kg for 40 minutes) (Zarate, Singh, and Manji, 2006b). In that study, more than 70% of patients met criteria for response (50% improvement) 24 hours post-infusion, and 35% showed a sustained response after one week. Significant improvement in HAM-D scores was associated with ketamine over placebo from 110 minutes through seven days.

To date, ketamine and riluzole have served as the prototypes for developing the next generation of glutamatergic modulators with antidepressant and mood stabilizing effects. More recently, cytidine has been tested in bipolar depression. Cytidine is a pyrimidine component of RNA and glutamatergic modulator that regulates dysfunctional neuronal-glial glutamate cycling and affects cerebral phospholipid metabolism, catecholamine synthesis, and mitochondrial function. A double-blind, placebo-controlled, add-on study evaluated the effects of cytidine in 35 patients with bipolar depression (Yoon *et al.*, 2009). Patients received valproate plus either cytidine or placebo for 12 weeks. Those patients who received cytidine showed earlier improvement of depressive symptoms (at one week); this improvement was directly correlated with decreased midfrontal glutamate/glutamine levels ($p = 0.001$). This study suggests that cytidine supplementation may have therapeutic effects in treating bipolar depression, and that these effects are potentially mediated by decreased cerebral glutamate/glutamine levels. Trials testing additional subtype-selective NMDA antagonists as well as other glutamatergic modulators are underway to help establish which of these agents have antidepressant effects.

21.6 THE TACHYKININ NEUROPEPTIDES SYSTEM

Over the past decade, diverse studies have noted the potential therapeutic role of tachykinin in mood disorders. Tachykinin neuropeptides include substance P, neurokinin A, neurokinin B, and their receptors (NK1, NK2, NK3) (Ebner, Sartori, and Singewald, 2009). These peptides act as neuromodulators and neurotransmitters, directly interacting with the monoaminergic system in several brain areas implicated in emotion processing and mood regulation. The activity of these neuropeptides is directly regulated by G-protein coupled receptors, leading to increased intracellular calcium via phospholipase C, inositol trisphosphate, and diacylglycerol signaling cascades (Khawaja and Rogers, 1996). Altered tachykinin transmission has been demonstrated in mood disorders; for instance, increased substance P has been found in the CSF and serum of individuals with MDD (Ebner, Sartori, and Singewald, 2009). Thus, diverse tachykinin receptor modulators have been tested as potential antidepressant or antipsychotic agents.

In Phase II and III clinical trials, diverse neurokinin receptor antagonists were associated with heterogeneous results. For instance, two double-blind, randomized, placebo-controlled Phase II clinical trials evaluated three different NK1 receptor antagonists: MK869, L759274, and CP122721. These agents significantly reduced depressive symptoms compared with placebo; in addition, both MK869 and CP122721 caused fewer side effects than the active comparators (paroxetine and fluoxetine) (Kramer *et al.*, 1998, 2004). However, the demonstrated efficacy of MK869 was not replicated in a subsequent multi-site, placebo-controlled, Phase III trial (Keller *et al.*, 2006). Similarly, three other studies evaluating NK1 and NK3 receptor antagonists failed to show antidepressant efficacy compared to active agents or placebo (Kramer *et al.*, 2002; Rupniak and Kramer, 1999). The NK3 receptor antagonist SR142801 (osanetant) was also not superior to either placebo or paroxetine in a six-week Phase II trial (Holmes *et al.*, 2003). In contrast, a Phase III trial evaluating the NK2 receptor antagonist SR48968 (saredudant) in adult and elderly patients with MDD found it to be effective in treating depressive symptoms, as well as well-tolerated and safe (Ebner, Sartori, and Singewald, 2009).

In addition to the clinical data noted above, preclinical studies have noted that tachykinin antagonists induce antidepressant-like effects in diverse animal models, with special relevance for the NK2 receptor system (Dableh *et al.*, 2005; Louis *et al.*, 2008; Micale *et al.*, 2008; Steinberg *et al.*, 2001). Interestingly, some of the tachykinin neuropeptides are believed to potentiate the therapeutic effects of selective serotonin reuptake inhibitors (SSRIs) based on the behavioral effects of serotonin reuptake inhibition by neurokinin receptor antagonism. Ongoing studies may continue to shed light on the potential role of these agents as therapeutics for mood disorders.

21.7 THE GLUCOCORTICOID SYSTEM

The hypothalamic pituitary adrenal (HPA) axis is a major "stress pathway" involved in the pathophysiology of severe mood disorders. It starts in the hypothalamic lateral ventricular nucleus, which stimulates the production of adrenocorticotropin-releasing hormone (ACTH) in the pituitary via corticotropin-releasing factor (CRF). ACTH subsequently induces the production of glucocorticoids such as cortisol. Hyperactivity of this system has been shown to induce injury and cell atrophy in hippocampal neurons (which express high levels of glucocorticoid receptors (GRs)) (Brown *et al.*, 2003; Duman and Monteggia, 2006). Glucocorticoids limit the expression of BDNF in the hippocampus, which may possibly explain the deleterious effects induced by chronic corticosteroids in cellular resilience. Thus, antiglucocorticoid therapy – including glucocorticoid synthesis inhibitors (aminoglutethimide, ketoconazole, metyrapone), GR antagonists (for example, mifepristone) (Belanoff *et al.*, 2002), and dehydroepiandrosterone (DHEA) (reviewed by Quiroz *et al.* (2004)) – is a valuable proof-of-concept tool for the treatment of mood disorders.

The non-selective GR antagonist mifepristone (RU-486) was reported to have antidepressant and antipsychotic effects in psychotic depression (Belanoff *et al.*, 2002). In a six-week trial in individuals with bipolar depression, mifepristone (600 mg/day) improved depressive symptoms and cognitive functioning compared to placebo (Young *et al.*, 2004). In contrast, a recent letter to the editor reported that this compound lacked antidepressant efficacy in two large Phase III studies of individuals with psychotic depression (Carroll and Rubin, 2008). Future studies are needed to clarify whether mifepristone elicits a different response in MDD with psychotic features versus bipolar depression. However, it is important to note that short-term benefits may be expected only during acute depressive episodes, as long-term treatment could be associated with significant side effects (for example, adrenal insufficiency, hepatic injury, antiprogesterone effects (Grunberg *et al.*, 2006; Rothschild, 2003)).

Glucocorticoid synthesis inhibitors such as ketoconazole and metyrapone appear to have an antidepressant profile in clinical and preclinical studies (Quiroz *et al.*, 2004). In a double-blind, randomized, controlled trial in MDD, metyrapone showed superior efficacy to placebo as an add-on therapy, accelerating the onset of antidepressant action (Jahn *et al.*, 2004). Similarly, ketoconazole (up to 800 mg/day) was given as an add-on treatment in six treatment-resistant BPD patients experiencing a depressive episode (Brown, Bobadilla, and Rush, 2001). Three patients receiving a dose of at least 400 mg/day had reduced depressive symptoms and no induction of manic symptoms; ketoconazole also reduced cortisol levels. Overall, five trials evaluating antiglucocorticoids in nonpsychotic depression (MDD or BPD) found a significant difference in favor of treatment (reviewed in Gallagher *et al.* (2008)).

Preclinical studies suggested that altered CRF1 receptor activity critically regulates depressive-like behaviors; thus, diverse nonpeptide CRF1 receptor antagonists have also recently been tested as potential antidepressant agents (reviewed in Valdez (2009)). Antalarmin (10 mg/kg) (a novel pyrrolopyrimidine compound that significantly reduces CRF-stimulated ACTH release) and fluoxetine (10 mg/kg) significantly improved measures of physical state, weight gain, and emotional response in mice undergoing chronic restraint stress (Ducottet, Griebel, and Belzung, 2003). Similarly, the CRF inhibitor CP-154 526 induced antidepressant-like properties in the learned helplessness model in rodents. Also, a 2-aminothiazole derivative (SSR125543A) that displays a high affinity for human CRF R1 receptors improved depressive-like symptoms and reduced aggressive behavior in three different animal models (Alonso *et al.*, 2004; Farrokhi *et al.*, 2004; Griebel *et al.*, 2002). In humans, an open label study using the CRF1 antagonist R-121919 found that it decreased anxiety and depressive symptoms in patients with MDD (Zobel *et al.*, 2000). Taken together, these findings support the notion that GRs, which are potentially associated with regulatory effects targeting plasticity pathways, may be relevant to therapeutic response in mood disorders.

21.8 THE ARACHIDONIC ACID (AA) CASCADE

The AA signaling pathway has recently been implicated in the pathophysiology and therapeutics of mood disorders. The AA pathway exerts critical modulatory effects as an intermediary of second messenger pathways in the brain, thus resulting in the release of AA and cyclooxygenase (COX)-mediated eicosanoid metabolites such as prostaglandins and thromboxanes. In rats, chronic administration of the mood stabilizers lithium, carbamazepine, valproate, or lamotrigine limits AA turnover in brain phospholipids, as well as the production of prostaglandin E(2), and/or the expression of AA cascade enzymes, including cytosolic phospholipase A(2), COX-2, and/or acyl-CoA synthetase (Rapoport *et al.*, 2009). More specifically, valproate decreases AA turnover, protein levels of COX-1 and COX-2, and frontal cortex COX-2 mRNA levels (Rao *et al.*, 2007). COX-2 also protects against neurotoxicity promoted by excessive concentrations of glutamate. Strong evidence also suggests that cytokine dysregulation plays a role in the pathophysiology of depression (Khairova *et al.*, 2009).

In two rodent models of mania (amphetamine-stimulated locomotor activity and blocked cocaine sensitization), the nonselective COX inhibitors indomethacin and piroxicam prevented the induction of manic-like effects (Ross *et al.*, 2002). In clinical studies of individuals with MDD, the COX-2 inhibitor celecoxib (400 mg/day) showed significant antidepressant effects compared to placebo as an add-on to reboxetine (Müller *et al.*, 2006). In a recent six-week, double-blind, placebo-controlled study of individuals with BPD experiencing a depressive or mixed episode, celecoxib (400 mg/day) showed superior antidepressant effects only during the first week of treatment as an add-on to mood stabilizers (Nery *et al.*, 2008). It is important to note that the degree of celecoxib's ability to penetrate the blood brain barrier is not well-established, and that the increased risk of adverse cardiovascular outcomes may limit the long-term use of selective COX-2 inhibitors (Velentgas *et al.*, 2006).

Also, minocycline, a second-generation tetracycline, has shown promising results in preclinical animal models of depression and as an antidepressant augmentation strategy in patients with MDD (Pae *et al.*, 2008). This agent also produces anti-inflammatory and neuroprotective effects; the latter are believed to occur through inhibition of 5-lipoxygenase, which mediates the generation of leukotrienes from AA (Song *et al.*, 2004). Overall, the brain AA cascade may represent a common target of mood stabilizers in mania, which may be associated with excess AA signaling via D(2)-like and NMDA receptors (Rapoport *et al.*, 2009); future studies using agents that directly target this system may clarify its utility in treating mood disorders.

21.9 THE ENDOCANNABINOID SYSTEM

Recent preclinical evidence suggests that cannabinoid agonists and endocannabinoid enhancers, such as fatty acid amide hydrolase (FAAH) inhibitors, have potential antidepressant effects. Nevertheless, little is known about the putative mechanisms involved in these antidepressant-like and anxiolytic-like effects (Manzanares *et al.*, 2004). Endocannabinoids are lipid retrograde messengers that regulate electrochemical transmission of diverse neurotransmitters, including GABA, glutamate, D-aspartate, acetylcholine, dopamine, norepinephrine (or noradrenaline), and 5-hydroxytryptamine (or serotonin). Cannabinoid agonists and endocannabinoid enhancers elevate serotonin and noradrenergic neuronal firing activity, increase serotonin release in the hippocampus, and promote neurogenesis (Bambico *et al.*, 2009). Diverse clinical and preclinical studies have compared the efficacy of endocannabinoid enhancers to standard antidepressants. In preclinical studies, these agents decrease immobility (an antidepressant-like effect) and aggressive behavior, and increase social interaction. These effects take place preferentially by augmenting serotonergic and noradrenergic transmission (Bambico *et al.*, 2009). Studies using cannabinoid receptor 1 (CB1) and FAAH KO mice have obtained similar results (Bambico *et al.*, 2009).

A recent FDA report showed that 26% of people taking 20 mg of the CB1 antagonist rimonabant during an obesity study experienced adverse psychiatric effects (mainly depression or anxiety) (Mitchell and Morris, 2007). These subjects also reported increased suicidal ideation or risk of suicide attempts. Ultimately, factors limiting the use of such agents as therapeutics include the possible peripheral consequences of endocannabinoid potentiation, the risk of abuse, and the relationship between endocannabinoids and other lipids.

21.10 OXIDATIVE STRESS AND BIOENERGETICS

21.10.1 CREATINE

Creatine, which has recently been implicated in BPD, plays a critical role in brain energy homeostasis. Brain creatine kinase is altered in the hippocampus in animal models of mania as well as in subjects with BPD experiencing a manic episode (Segal *et al.*, 2007; Streck *et al.*, 2008). Also, decreased creatine kinase mRNA expression was found in the hippocampus and dorsolateral prefrontal cortex in BPD (MacDonald *et al.*, 2006). Thus, it is possible that creatine supplementation may modify brain high-energy phosphate metabolism and be a useful therapeutic approach in individuals with BPD. A recent open-label study of 10 treatment-resistant depressed patients (including subjects with BPD) found that 3–5 mg/day of creatine monohydrate as an adjunctive treatment significantly improved depressive symptoms (Roitman *et al.*, 2007). However, two subjects with bipolar depression did experience transient hypomanic/manic symptoms. It was also recently shown that the acute use of ketamine and imipramine elevated cerebellar and prefrontal cortex creatine kinase activity in rats (Assis *et al.*, 2009). Overall, further studies are needed to clarify the role of creatine in the pathophysiology and therapeutics of BPD (Quiroz *et al.*, 2008).

21.10.2 N-ACETYL CYSTEINE (NAC)

Increasing evidence suggests that altered oxidative stress parameters play a direct role in the pathophysiology of BPD (Andreazza *et al.*, 2008; Machado-Vieira *et al.*, 2007). Glutathione is the most abundant antioxidant substrate in all tissues, and its altered levels have been described in individuals with BPD (Andreazza *et al.*, 2007; Kuloglu *et al.*, 2002). N-Acetylcysteine (NAC), a precursor of glutathione, increases glutathione levels. In a recent, randomized, double-blind, multicenter, placebo-controlled study, 75 patients with BPD received NAC (1 g twice daily) as an add-on to their usual treatment for 24 months, followed by a four-week washout phase. NAC showed superior antidepressant effects compared to placebo, with moderate to high effect sizes on measures of depression as assessed by the Montgomery-Asberg Depression Rating Scale (MADRS), the Bipolar Depression Rating Scale (BDRS), and quality of life and functionality scores (Berk *et al.*, 2008). Patients were not necessarily selected for experiencing a major depressive episode and there was a considerable lag in the benefits obtained. The authors hypothesized that NAC's efficacy might be due to its ability to reverse increased oxidative stress during mood episodes.

21.11 THE INTRACELLULAR SIGNALING PATHWAYS

21.11.1 GLYCOGEN SYNTHASE KINASE-3 (GSK-3)

Glycogen Synthase Kinase (GSK-3) is a highly active and multifunctional serine/threonine kinase that regulates diverse signaling pathways (for example, the phosphoinositide 3-kinase pathway, the Wnt pathway, protein kinase A (PKA), and protein kinase C (PKC)). In general, increased activity of GSK-3 is proapoptotic, whereas inhibiting GSK-3 attenuates or prevents apoptosis. GSK-3 is a key modulator of glycogen synthesis, gene transcription, synaptic plasticity, apoptosis (cell death), cellular structure and resilience, and the circadian cycle (Jope, 2003), all of which have been directly implicated in the pathophysiology of severe recurrent mood disorders. Also, GSK-3 directly regulates behavior through its effects at β-catenin, glutamate receptors, circadian rhythms, and serotonergic transmission (reviewed in Beaulieu *et al.* (2008)).

Lithium and other mood stabilizers have been shown to directly target GSK-3 activity (Beaulieu *et al.*, 2008). Lithium also induces neurotrophic and neuroprotective effects in rodents, in part due to GSK-3 inhibition (reviewed in Gould and Manji (2005)). Mice overexpressing a constitutively active form of brain GSK-3β have increased locomotor activity and decreased habituation in the open field test. In addition, in preclinical studies the GSK-3 inhibitor AR-A014418 had both antidepressant-like effects in the forced swim test and antimanic-like effects in the D-amphetamine hyperlocomotion model (Gould *et al.*, 2004; Gould *et al.*, 2006). However, the use of GSK-3 inhibitors would be limited, due to GSK-3's involvement with diverse pathways and multiple substrates that may induce side effects and/or toxicity (Rayasam *et al.*, 2009). Presently, no blood brain barrier-penetrant GSK-selective inhibitor has been clinically tested. Proof-of-principle studies with selective and safe GSK-3 inhibitors are needed to assess the therapeutic relevance and safety of this target in BPD.

21.11.2 THE PKC SIGNALING CASCADE

PKC plays a key role in regulating neuronal excitability, neurotransmitter release, and long-term alterations in gene expression and plasticity. PKC isoforms differ in their structure, subcellular localization, tissue specificity, mode of activation, and substrate specificity. Diverse studies support the involvement of PKC and its substrates in the pathophysiology and therapeutics of BPD (Chen *et al.*, 1994; Friedman *et al.*, 1993; Hahn and Friedman, 1999; Manji *et al.*, 1993; Manji and Lenox, 1999; Young *et al.*, 1999).

In addition to studies showing that PKC is directly regulated by lithium and valproate (Chen *et al.*, 1994; Manji and Lenox, 1999), a recent clinical trial provided further evidence for the involvement of this system in bipolar mania. Although well known for its anti-estrogenic properties, tamoxifen is also a potent PKC inhibitor at high concentrations, with demonstrated ability to decrease amphetamine-induced hyperactivity in a large open field (Einat *et al.*, 2007). In a single-blind study, tamoxifen had significant antimanic effects in five of seven subjects with BPD (Bebchuk *et al.*, 2000). In another four-week, three-arm, double-blind, placebo-controlled, add-on study involving

13 women, tamoxifen (n = 5) was compared to medroxyprogesterone acetate (n = 4) and placebo (n = 4). Subjects in the tamoxifen group had a significantly greater decrease in manic and positive psychotic symptoms than the placebo group. All patients received concomitant treatment consisting of either lithium (0.8–1.0 mmol/l) and/or valproate (Kulkarni et al., 2006). These initial findings were confirmed by two recent three-week, double-blind, placebo-controlled, monotherapy studies (Yildiz et al., 2008; Zarate et al., 2007). The main difference between the studies was that Zarate and colleagues tested higher doses (up to 140 mg/day) and ratings were obtained daily during the first week, thus permitting the assessment of early antimanic effects. In contrast, Yildiz and colleagues used doses of up to 80 mg/day and obtained weekly ratings, but because of the large sample size, they were able to assess the effects of tamoxifen on other specific domains (for example, psychosis and depression) and to perform multivariate regression models of response. Taken together, the results of these studies suggest that tamoxifen's antimanic effects were not related to its sedative effects, and no increased risk of depression was observed. However, it is possible that some of tamoxifen's antimanic effects may be due to its anti-estrogen effects (see (Goldstein, 1986)). Additional controlled studies with selective PKC inhibitors in acute bipolar mania are necessary to cement the role of PKC in the therapeutics of BPD.

21.12 FINAL REMARKS

Recently, animal studies assessed diverse targets/compounds that are now at the proof-of-concept stage. Ultimately, these may result in putative novel treatments for BPD. These include (i) the dynorphin opioid neuropeptide system, (ii) the purinergic system, (iii) the melatonergic system, (iv) the glutamatergic system, (v) the tachykinin neuropeptides system, (vi) the glucocorticoid system, (vii) the AA cascade, (viii) the endocannabinoid system, (ix) oxidative stress and bioenergetics, and (x) intracellular signaling cascades. It is important to note that none of these new treatments are FDA-approved for the treatment of BPD. Also, important methodological differences exist regarding how specific compounds are evaluated. For instance, most of the evidence presented in this chapter comes from case reports, case series, or proof-of-concept studies, some with small sample sizes. Nevertheless, these findings may guide important future research directions in drug development for BPD.

References

Aguado, L., San Antonio, A., Perez, L. et al. (1994) Effects of the NMDA receptor antagonist ketamine on flavor memory: conditioned aversion, latent inhibition, and habituation of neophobia. Behav. Neural Biol., 61, 271–281.

Akhondzadeh, S., Milajerdi, M.R., Amini, H. et al. (2006) Allopurinol as an adjunct to lithium and haloperidol for treatment of patients with acute mania: a double-blind, randomized, placebo-controlled trial. Bipolar Disord., 8, 485–489.

Alaerts, M., Venken, T., Lenaerts, A.S. et al. (2006) Lack of association of an insertion/deletion polymorphism in the G protein-coupled receptor 50 with bipolar disorder in a Northern Swedish population. Psychiatr. Genet., 16, 235–236.

Alonso, R., Griebel, G., Pavone, G. *et al.* (2004) Blockade of CRF(1) or V(1b) receptors reverses stress-induced suppression of neurogenesis in a mouse model of depression. *Mol. Psychiatry*, **9**, 278–286, 24.

Andreazza, A.C., Cassini, C., Rosa, A.R. *et al.* (2007) Serum S100B and antioxidant enzymes in bipolar patients. *J. Psychiatr. Res.*, **41**, 523–529.

Andreazza, A.C., Kauer-Sant'anna, M., Frey, B.N. *et al.* (2008) Oxidative stress markers in bipolar disorder: a meta-analysis. *J. Affect. Disord.*, **111**, 135–144.

Antoniou, K., Papadopoulou-Daifoti, Z., Hyphantis, T. *et al.* (2005) A detailed behavioral analysis of the acute motor effects of caffeine in the rat: involvement of adenosine A1 and A2A receptors. *Psychopharmacology (Berl.)*, **183**, 154–162.

Anumonye, A., Reading, H.W., Knight, F. *et al.* (1968) Uric-acid metabolism in manic-depressive illness and during lithium therapy. *Lancet*, **1**, 1290–1293.

Armstrong, S.M., McNulty, O.M., Guardiola-Lemaitre, B. *et al.* (1993) Successful use of S20098 and melatonin in an animal model of delayed sleep-phase syndrome (DSPS). *Pharmacol. Biochem. Behav.*, **46**, 45–49.

Assis, L.C., Rezin, G.T., Comim, C.M. *et al.* (2009) Effect of acute administration of ketamine and imipramine on creatine kinase activity in the brain of rats. *Rev. Bras. Psiquiatr.*, **31**, 247–252.

Bambico, F.R., Duranti, A., Tontini, A. *et al.* (2009) Endocannabinoids in the treatment of mood disorders: evidence from animal models. *Curr. Pharm. Des.*, **15**, 1623–1646.

Banasr, M., Chowdhury, G.M., Terwilliger, R. *et al.* (2010) Glial pathology in an animal model of depression: reversal of stress-induced cellular, metabolic and behavioral deficits by the glutamate-modulating drug riluzole. *Mol. Psychiatry*, **15** (5), 501–511.

Banasr, M., Soumier, A., Hery, M. *et al.* (2006) Agomelatine, a new antidepressant, induces regional changes in hippocampal neurogenesis. *Biol. Psychiatry*, **59**, 1087–1096.

Bannerman, D.M., Good, M.A., Butcher, S.P. *et al.* (1995) Distinct components of spatial learning revealed by prior training and NMDA receptor blockade. *Nature*, **378**, 182–186.

Barber, A. and Gottschlich, R. (1997) Novel developments with selective, non-peptidic kappa-opioid receptor agonists. *Expert. Opin. Investig. Drugs*, **6**, 1351–1368.

Barden, N., Harvey, M., Gagne, B. *et al.* (2006) Analysis of single nucleotide polymorphisms in genes in the chromosome 12Q24.31 region points to P2RX7 as a susceptibility gene to bipolar affective disorder. *Am. J. Med. Genet. B Neuropsychiatr. Genet.*, **141B**, 374–382.

Basso, A.M., Bratcher, N.A., Harris, R.R. *et al.* (2009) Behavioral profile of P2X7 receptor knock-out mice in animal models of depression and anxiety: relevance for neuropsychiatric disorders. *Behav. Brain Res.*, **198**, 83–90.

Beaulieu, J.M., Zhang, X., Rodriguiz, R.M. *et al.* (2008) Role of GSK3 beta in behavioral abnormalities induced by serotonin deficiency. *Proc. Natl. Acad. Sci. U.S.A.*, **105**, 1333–1338.

Bebchuk, J.M., Arfken, C.L., Dolan-Manji, S. *et al.* (2000) A preliminary investigation of a protein kinase C inhibitor in the treatment of acute mania. *Arch. Gen. Psychiatry*, **57**, 95–97.

Belanoff, J.K., Rothschild, A.J., Cassidy, F. *et al.* (2002) An open label trial of C-1073 (mifepristone) for psychotic major depression. *Biol. Psychiatry*, **52**, 386–392.

Berk, M., Copolov, D.L., Dean, O. *et al.* (2008) N-acetyl cysteine for depressive symptoms in bipolar disorder--a double-blind randomized placebo-controlled trial. *Biol. Psychiatry*, **64**, 468–475.

Berman, R.M., Cappiello, A., Anand, A. *et al.* (2000) Antidepressant effects of ketamine in depressed patients. *Biol. Psychiatry*, **47**, 351–354.

Berrocoso, E., Rojas-Corrales, M.O., and Mico, J.A. (2004) Non-selective opioid receptor antagonism of the antidepressant-like effect of venlafaxine in the forced swimming test in mice. *Neurosci. Lett.*, **363**, 25–28.

Berrocoso, E., Sanchez-Blazquez, P., Garzon, J. *et al.* (2009) Opiates as antidepressants. *Curr. Pharm. Des.*, **15**, 1612–1622.

Bersani, G. and Garavini, A. (2000) Melatonin add-on in manic patients with treatment resistant insomnia. *Prog. Neuropsychopharmacol. Biol. Psychiatry*, **24**, 185–191.

Bertaina-Anglade, V., la Rochelle, C.D., Boyer, P.A. *et al.* (2006) Antidepressant-like effects of agomelatine (S 20098) in the learned helplessness model. *Behav. Pharmacol.*, **17**, 703–713.

Besson, A., Privat, A.M., Eschalier, A. *et al.* (1996) Effects of morphine, naloxone and their interaction in the learned-helplessness paradigm in rats. *Psychopharmacology (Berl.)*, **123**, 71–78.

Black, M.D. (2005) Therapeutic potential of positive AMPA modulators and their relationship to AMPA receptor subunits. A review of preclinical data. *Psychopharmacology (Berl.)*, **179**, 154–163.

Bleakman, D. and Lodge, D. (1998) Neuropharmacology of AMPA and kainate receptors. *Neuropharmacology*, **37**, 1187–1204.

Bodkin, J.A., Zornberg, G.L., Lukas, S.E. *et al.* (1995) Buprenorphine treatment of refractory depression. *J. Clin. Psychopharmacol.*, **15**, 49–57.

Brown, E.S., Bobadilla, L., and Rush, A.J. (2001) Ketoconazole in bipolar patients with depressive symptoms: a case series and literature review. *Bipolar Disord.*, **3**, 23–29.

Brown, E.S., Frol, A., Bobadilla, L. *et al.* (2003) Effect of lamotrigine on mood and cognition in patients receiving chronic exogenous corticosteroids. *Psychosomatics*, **44**, 204–208.

Burnstock, G. (2007) Physiology and pathophysiology of purinergic neurotransmission. *Physiol. Rev.*, **87**, 659–797.

Calabrese, J.R., Guelfi, J.D., and Perdrizet-Chevallier, C. (2007) Agomelatine adjunctive therapy for acute bipolar depression: preliminary open data. *Bipolar Disord.*, **9**, 628–635.

Carlezon, W.A., Jr., Beguin, C., DiNieri, J.A. *et al.* (2006) Depressive-like effects of the kappa-opioid receptor agonist salvinorin A on behavior and neurochemistry in rats. *J. Pharmacol. Exp. Ther.*, **316**, 440–447.

Carroll, B.J. and Rubin, R.T. (2008) Mifepristone in psychotic depression? *Biol. Psychiatry*, **63**, e1; author reply e3.

Chartoff, E.H., Papadopoulou, M., MacDonald, M.L. *et al.* (2009) Desipramine reduces stress-activated dynorphin expression and CREB phosphorylation in NAc tissue. *Mol. Pharmacol.*, **75**, 704–712.

Chen, G., Manji, H.K., Hawver, D.B. *et al.* (1994) Chronic sodium valproate selectively decreases protein kinase C alpha and epsilon in vitro. *J. Neurochem.*, **63**, 2361–2364.

Cohen, B.M. and Murphy, B. (2008) The effects of pentazocine, a kappa agonist, in patients with mania. *Int. J. Neuropsychopharmacol.*, **11**, 243–247.

Collingridge, G.L. (1994) Long-term potentiation. A question of reliability. *Nature*, **371**, 652–653.

Collingridge, G.L. and Bliss, T.V. (1995) Memories of NMDA receptors and LTP. *Trends Neurosci.*, **18**, 54–56.

Cryan, J.F., Kelly, P.H., Neijt, H.C. *et al.* (2003) Antidepressant and anxiolytic-like effects in mice lacking the group III metabotropic glutamate receptor mGluR7. *Eur. J. Neurosci.*, **17**, 2409–2417.

Dableh, L.J., Yashpal, K., Rochford, J. *et al.* (2005) Antidepressant-like effects of neurokinin receptor antagonists in the forced swim test in the rat. *Eur. J. Pharmacol.*, **507**, 99–105.

Darko, D.F., Risch, S.C., Gillin, J.C. *et al.* (1992) Association of beta-endorphin with specific clinical symptoms of depression. *Am. J. Psychiatry*, **149**, 1162–1167.

Devoize, J.L., Rigal, F., Eschalier, A. *et al.* (1984) Influence of naloxone on antidepressant drug effects in the forced swimming test in mice. *Psychopharmacology (Berl.)*, **84**, 71–75.

Du, J., Suzuki, K., Wei, Y. *et al.* (2007) The anticonvulsants lamotrigine, riluzole, and valproate differentially regulate AMPA receptor membrane localization: relationship to clinical effects in mood disorders. *Neuropsychopharmacology*, **32**, 793–802.

Ducottet, C., Griebel, G., and Belzung, C. (2003) Effects of the selective nonpeptide corticotropin-releasing factor receptor 1 antagonist antalarmin in the chronic mild stress model of depression in mice. *Prog. Neuropsychopharmacol. Biol. Psychiatry*, **27**, 625–631.

Duman, R.S. and Monteggia, L.M. (2006) A neurotrophic model for stress-related mood disorders. *Biol. Psychiatry*, **59**, 1116–1127.

Ebner, K., Sartori, S.B., and Singewald, N. (2009) Tachykinin receptors as therapeutic targets in stress-related disorders. *Curr. Pharm. Des.*, **15**, 1647–1674.

Einat, H., Yuan, P., Szabo, S.T. *et al.* (2007) Protein kinase C inhibition by tamoxifen antagonizes manic-like behavior in rats: implications for the development of novel therapeutics for bipolar disorder. *Neuropsychobiology*, **55**, 123–131.

El Yacoubi, M., Ledent, C., Parmentier, M. *et al.* (2001) Adenosine A2A receptor antagonists are potential antidepressants: evidence based on pharmacology and A2A receptor knockout mice. *Br. J. Pharmacol.*, **134**, 68–77.

Farrokhi, C., Blanchard, D.C., Griebel, G. *et al.* (2004) Effects of the CRF1 antagonist SSR125543A on aggressive behaviors in hamsters. *Pharmacol. Biochem. Behav.*, **77**, 465–469.

Friedman, E., Hoau Yan, W., Levinson, D. *et al.* (1993) Altered platelet protein kinase C activity in bipolar affective disorder, manic episode. *Biol. Psychiatry*, **33**, 520–525.

Frizzo, M.E., Dall'Onder, L.P., Dalcin, K.B. *et al.* (2004) Riluzole enhances glutamate uptake in rat astrocyte cultures. *Cell. Mol. Neurobiol.*, **24**, 123–128.

Gallagher, P., Malik, N., Newham, J. *et al.* (2008) Antiglucocorticoid treatments for mood disorders. *Cochrane Database Syst. Rev.* (DOI number: 10.1002/14651858.CD005168.pub2).

Garcia, L.S., Comim, C.M., Valvassori, S.S. *et al.* (2008) Acute administration of ketamine induces antidepressant-like effects in the forced swimming test and increases BDNF levels in the rat hippocampus. *Prog. Neuropsychopharmacol. Biol. Psychiatry*, **32**, 140–144.

Gasparini, F., Bruno, V., Battaglia, G. *et al.* (1999) (R,S)-4-phosphonophenylglycine, a potent and selective group III metabotropic glutamate receptor agonist, is anticonvulsive and neuroprotective in vivo. *J. Pharmacol. Exp. Ther.*, **289**, 1678–1687.

Goldstein, J.A. (1986) Danazol and the rapid-cycling patient. *J. Clin. Psychiatry*, **47**, 153–154.

Goodwin, F.K. and Jamison, K.R. (2007) *Manic-Depressive Illness:Bipolar Disorders and Recurrent Depression*, 2nd edn, Oxford University Press, Oxford.

Gould, T.D., Einat, H., Bhat, R. *et al.* (2004) AR-A014418, a selective GSK-3 inhibitor, produces antidepressant-like effects in the forced swim test. *Int. J. Neuropsychopharmacol.*, **7**, 387–390.

Gould, T.D. and Manji, H.K. (2005) Glycogen synthase kinase-3: a putative molecular target for lithium mimetic drugs. *Neuropsychopharmacology*, **30**, 1223–1237.

Gould, T.D., Picchini, A.M., Einat, H. *et al.* (2006) Targeting glycogen synthase kinase-3 in the CNS: implications for the development of new treatments for mood disorders. *Curr. Drug Targets*, **7**, 1399–1409.

Griebel, G., Simiand, J., Steinberg, R. *et al.* (2002) 4-(2-Chloro-4-methoxy-5-methylphenyl)-N-[(1S)-2-cyclopropyl-1-(3-fluoro-4- methylphenyl)ethyl]5-methyl-N-(2-propynyl)-1, 3-thiazol-2-amine hydrochloride (SSR125543A), a potent and selective corticotrophin-releasing factor(1) receptor antagonist. II. Characterization in rodent models of stress-related disorders. *J. Pharmacol. Exp. Ther.*, **301**, 333–345.

Grunberg, S.M., Weiss, M.H., Russell, C.A. *et al.* (2006) Long-term administration of mifepristone (RU486): clinical tolerance during extended treatment of meningioma. *Cancer Invest.*, **24**, 727–733.

Hahn, C.G. and Friedman, E. (1999) Abnormalities in protein kinase C signaling and the pathophysiology of bipolar disorder. *Bipolar Disord.*, **1**, 81–86.

Hallam, K.T., Olver, J.S., and Norman, T.R. (2005) Melatonin sensitivity to light in monozygotic twins discordant for bipolar I disorder. *Aust. N. Z. J. Psychiatry*, **39**, 947.

Holmes, A., Heilig, M., Rupniak, N.M. *et al.* (2003) Neuropeptide systems as novel therapeutic targets for depression and anxiety disorders. *Trends Pharmacol. Sci.*, **24**, 580–588.

Hurd, Y.L. (2002) Subjects with major depression or bipolar disorder show reduction of prodynorphin mRNA expression in discrete nuclei of the amygdaloid complex. *Mol. Psychiatry*, **7**, 75–81.

Jahn, H., Schick, M., Kiefer, F. *et al.* (2004) Metyrapone as additive treatment in major depression: a double-blind and placebo-controlled trial. *Arch. Gen. Psychiatry*, **61**, 1235–1244.

Jope, R.S. (2003) Lithium and GSK-3: one inhibitor, two inhibitory actions, multiple outcomes. *Trends Pharmacol. Sci.*, **24**, 441–443.

Judd, L.L., Akiskal, H.S., Schettler, P.J. *et al.* (2002) The long-term natural history of the weekly symptomatic status of bipolar I disorder. *Arch. Gen. Psychiatry*, **59**, 530–537.

Jutkiewicz, E.M. (2006) The antidepressant-like effects of delta-opioid receptor agonists. *Mol. Interv.*, **6**, 162–169.

Kaster, M.P., Rosa, A.O., Rosso, M.M. *et al.* (2004) Adenosine administration produces an antidepressant-like effect in mice: evidence for the involvement of A1 and A2A receptors. *Neurosci. Lett.*, **355**, 21–24.

Keller, M., Montgomery, S., Ball, W. *et al.* (2006) Lack of efficacy of the substance p (neurokinin1 receptor) antagonist aprepitant in the treatment of major depressive disorder. *Biol. Psychiatry*, **59**, 216–223.

Kennedy, S.H. and Emsley, R. (2006) Placebo-controlled trial of agomelatine in the treatment of major depressive disorder. *Eur. Neuropsychopharmacol.*, **16**, 93–100.

Khairova, R.A., Machado-Vieira, R., Du, J. *et al.* (2009) A potential role for pro-inflammatory cytokines in regulating synaptic plasticity in major depressive disorder. *Int. J. Neuropsychopharmacol.*, **12**, 561–578.

Khawaja, A.M. and Rogers, D.F. (1996) Tachykinins: receptor to effector. *Int. J. Biochem. Cell. Biol.*, **28**, 721–738.

Kinney, G.G., O'Brien, J.A., Lemaire, W. *et al.* (2005) A novel selective positive allosteric modulator of metabotropic glutamate receptor subtype 5 has in vivo activity and antipsychotic-like effects in rat behavioral models. *J. Pharmacol. Exp. Ther.*, **313**, 199–206.

Kittner, H., Krugel, U., and Illes, P. (2001) The purinergic P2 receptor antagonist pyridoxalphosphate-6-azophenyl-2'4'-disulphonic acid prevents both the acute locomotor effects of amphetamine and the behavioural sensitization caused by repeated amphetamine injections in rats. *Neuroscience*, **102**, 241–243.

Knapp, R.J., Goldenberg, R., Shuck, C. *et al.* (2002) Antidepressant activity of memory-enhancing drugs in the reduction of submissive behavior model. *Eur. J. Pharmacol.*, **440**, 27–35.

Kramer, L., Bauer, E., Funk, G. *et al.* (2002) Subclinical impairment of brain function in chronic hepatitis C infection. *J. Hepatol.*, **37**, 349–354.

Kramer, M.S., Cutler, N., Feighner, J. *et al.* (1998) Distinct mechanism for antidepressant activity by blockade of central substance P receptors. *Science*, **281**, 1640–1645.

Kramer, M.S., Winokur, A., Kelsey, J. *et al.* (2004) Demonstration of the efficacy and safety of a novel substance P (NK1) receptor antagonist in major depression. *Neuropsychopharmacology*, **29**, 385–392.

Kulkarni, J., Garland, K.A., Scaffidi, A. *et al.* (2006) A pilot study of hormone modulation as a new treatment for mania in women with bipolar affective disorder. *Psychoneuroendocrinology*, **31**, 543–547.

Kuloglu, M., Ustundag, B., Atmaca, M. *et al.* (2002) Lipid peroxidation and antioxidant enzyme levels in patients with schizophrenia and bipolar disorder. *Cell. Biochem. Funct.*, **20**, 171–175.

Lara, D.R., Dall'Igna, O.P., Ghisolfi, E.S. *et al.* (2006) Involvement of adenosine in the neuro-biology of schizophrenia and its therapeutic implications. *Prog. Neuropsychopharmacol. Biol. Psychiatry*, **30**, 617–629.

Lewy, A.J., Nurnberger, J.I., Jr., Wehr, T.A. *et al.* (1985) Supersensitivity to light: possible trait marker for manic-depressive illness. *Am. J. Psychiatry*, **142**, 725–727.

Lewy, A.J., Wehr, T.A., Goodwin, F.K. *et al.* (1981) Manic-depressive patients may be supersen-sitive to light. *Lancet*, **1**, 383–384.

Loo, H., Hale, A., and D'Haenen, H. (2002) Determination of the dose of agomelatine, a melatonin-ergic agonist and selective 5-HT(2C) antagonist, in the treatment of major depressive disorder: a placebo-controlled dose range study. *Int. Clin. Psychopharmacol.*, **17**, 239–247.

Louis, C., Stemmelin, J., Boulay, D. *et al.* (2008) Additional evidence for anxiolytic- and antidepressant-like activities of saredutant (SR48968), an antagonist at the neurokinin-2 receptor in various rodent-models. *Pharmacol. Biochem. Behav.*, **89**, 36–45.

Lourenco Da Silva, A., Hoffmann, A., Dietrich, M.O. *et al.* (2003) Effect of riluzole on MK-801 and amphetamine-induced hyperlocomotion. *Neuropsychobiology*, **48**, 27–30.

Lucae, S., Salyakina, D., Barden, N. *et al.* (2006) P2RX7, a gene coding for a purinergic ligand-gated ion channel, is associated with major depressive disorder. *Hum. Mol. Genet.*, **15**, 2438–2445.

MacDonald, M.L., Naydenov, A., Chu, M. *et al.* (2006) Decrease in creatine kinase messenger RNA expression in the hippocampus and dorsolateral prefrontal cortex in bipolar disorder. *Bipolar Disord.*, **8**, 255–264.

Machado-Vieira, R., Andreazza, A.C., Viale, C.I. *et al.* (2007) Oxidative stress parameters in unmedicated and treated bipolar subjects during initial manic episode: a possible role for lithium antioxidant effects. *Neurosci. Lett.*, **421**, 33–36.

Machado-Vieira, R., Lara, D.R., Souza, D.O. *et al.* (2001) Therapeutic efficacy of allopurinol in mania associated with hyperuricemia. *J. Clin. Psychopharmacol.*, **21**, 621–622.

Machado-Vieira, R., Lara, D.R., Souza, D.O. *et al.* (2002) Purinergic dysfunction in mania: an integrative model. *Med. Hypotheses*, **58**, 297–304.

Machado-Vieira, R., Manji, H.K., and Zarate, C.A. (2009) The role of the tripartite glutamatergic synapse in the pathophysiology and therapeutics of mood disorders. *Neuroscientist.*, **15** (5), 525–539.

Machado-Vieira, R., Soares, J.C., Lara, D.R. *et al.* (2008) A double-blind, randomized, placebo-controlled 4-week study on the efficacy and safety of the purinergic agents allopurinol and dipyridamole adjunctive to lithium in acute bipolar mania. *J. Clin. Psychiatry*, **69**, 1237–1245.

Maeng, S., Zarate, C.A., Jr., Du, J. *et al.* (2008) Cellular mechanisms underlying the antidepressant effects of ketamine: role of alpha-amino-3-hydroxy-5-methylisoxazole-4-propionic acid recep-tors. *Biol. Psychiatry*, **63**, 349–352.

Mague, S.D., Pliakas, A.M., Todtenkopf, M.S. *et al.* (2003) Antidepressant-like effects of kappa-opioid receptor antagonists in the forced swim test in rats. *J. Pharmacol. Exp. Ther.*, **305**, 323–330.

Manji, H.K., Etcheberrigaray, R., Chen, G. *et al.* (1993) Lithium decreases membrane-associated protein kinase C in hippocampus: selectivity for the alpha isozyme. *J. Neurochem.*, **61**, 2303–2310.

Manji, H.K. and Lenox, R.H. (1999) Ziskind-Somerfeld Research Award. Protein kinase C signaling in the brain: molecular transduction of mood stabilization in the treatment of manic-depressive illness. *Biol. Psychiatry*, **46**, 1328–1351.

Manzanares, J., Uriguen, L., Rubio, G. *et al.* (2004) Role of endocannabinoid system in mental diseases. *Neurotox. Res.*, **6**, 213–224.

Meloni, D., Gambarana, C., De Montis, M.G. *et al.* (1993) Dizocilpine antagonizes the effect of chronic imipramine on learned helplessness in rats. *Pharmacol. Biochem. Behav.*, **46**, 423–426.

Micale, V., Tamburella, A., Leggio, G.M. *et al.* (2008) Behavioral effects of saredutant, a tachykinin NK2 receptor antagonist, in experimental models of mood disorders under basal and stress-related conditions. *Pharmacol. Biochem. Behav.*, **90**, 463–469.

Mickley, G.A., Schaldach, M.A., Snyder, K.J. *et al.* (1998) Ketamine blocks a conditioned taste aversion (CTA) in neonatal rats. *Physiol. Behav.*, **64**, 381–390.

Millan, M.J., Brocco, M., Gobert, A. *et al.* (2005) Anxiolytic properties of agomelatine, an antidepressant with melatoninergic and serotonergic properties: role of 5-HT2C receptor blockade. *Psychopharmacology (Berl.)*, **177**, 448–458.

Mitchell, P.B. and Morris, M.J. (2007) Depression and anxiety with rimonabant. *Lancet*, **370**, 1671–1672.

Miu, P., Jarvie, K.R., Radhakrishnan, V. *et al.* (2001) Novel AMPA receptor potentiators LY392098 and LY404187: effects on recombinant human AMPA receptors in vitro. *Neuropharmacology*, **40**, 976–983.

Mizuta, I., Ohta, M., Ohta, K. *et al.* (2001) Riluzole stimulates nerve growth factor, brain-derived neurotrophic factor and glial cell line-derived neurotrophic factor synthesis in cultured mouse astrocytes. *Neurosci. Lett.*, **310**, 117–120.

Moghaddam, B., Adams, B., Verma, A. *et al.* (1997) Activation of glutamatergic neurotransmission by ketamine: a novel step in the pathway from NMDA receptor blockade to dopaminergic and cognitive disruptions associated with the prefrontal cortex. *J. Neurosci.*, **17**, 2921–2927.

Montgomery, S.A. and Kasper, S. (2007) Severe depression and antidepressants: focus on a pooled analysis of placebo-controlled studies on agomelatine. *Int. Clin. Psychopharmacol.*, **22**, 283–291.

Müller, N., Schwarz, M.J., Dehning, S. *et al.* (2006) The cyclooxygenase-2 inhibitor celecoxib has therapeutic effects in major depression: results of a double-blind, randomized, placebo controlled, add-on pilot study to reboxetine. *Mol. Psychiatry*, **11**, 680–684.

Nagayama, H. (1996) Chronic administration of imipramine and lithium changes the phase-angle relationship between the activity and core body temperature circadian rhythms in rats. *Chronobiol. Int.*, **13**, 251–259.

Nery, F.G., Monkul, E.S., Hatch, J.P. *et al.* (2008) Celecoxib as an adjunct in the treatment of depressive or mixed episodes of bipolar disorder: a double-blind, randomized, placebo-controlled study. *Hum. Psychopharmacol.*, **23**, 87–94.

Nurnberger, J.I., Jr., Adkins, S., Lahiri, D.K. *et al.* (2000) Melatonin suppression by light in euthymic bipolar and unipolar patients. *Arch. Gen. Psychiatry*, **57**, 572–579.

Ogawa, N. and Ueki, H. (2003) Secondary mania caused by caffeine. *Gen. Hosp. Psychiatry*, **25**, 138–139.

Padovan, C.M. and Guimaraes, F.S. (2004) Antidepressant-like effects of NMDA-receptor antagonist injected into the dorsal hippocampus of rats. *Pharmacol. Biochem. Behav.*, **77**, 15–19.

Pae, C.U., Marks, D.M., Han, C. *et al.* (2008) Does minocycline have antidepressant effect? *Biomed. Pharmacother.*, **62**, 308–311.

Palucha, A. and Pilc, A. (2007) Metabotropic glutamate receptor ligands as possible anxiolytic and antidepressant drugs. *Pharmacol. Ther.*, **115**, 116–147.

Papp, M., Gruca, P., Boyer, P.A. *et al.* (2003) Effect of agomelatine in the chronic mild stress model of depression in the rat. *Neuropsychopharmacology*, **28**, 694–703.

Papp, M. and Moryl, E. (1993) New evidence for the antidepressant activity of MK-801, a noncompetitive antagonist of NMDA receptors. *Pol. J. Pharmacol.*, **45**, 549–553.

Pitkanen, A., Mathiesen, C., Ronn, L.C. *et al.* (2007) Effect of novel AMPA antagonist, NS1209, on status epilepticus. An experimental study in rat. *Epilepsy Res.*, **74**, 45–54.

Quiroz, J.A., Gray, N.A., Kato, T. *et al.* (2008) Mitochondrially mediated plasticity in the patho-physiology and treatment of bipolar disorder. *Neuropsychopharmacology*, **33**, 2551–2565.

Quiroz, J.A., Singh, J., Gould, T.D. *et al.* (2004) Emerging experimental therapeutics for bipolar disorder: clues from the molecular pathophysiology. *Mol. Psychiatry*, **9**, 756–776.

Ragnauth, A., Schuller, A., Morgan, M. *et al.* (2001) Female preproenkephalin-knockout mice display altered emotional responses. *Proc. Natl. Acad. Sci. U.S.A.*, **98**, 1958–1963.

Rao, J.S., Bazinet, R.P., Rapoport, S.I. *et al.* (2007) Chronic treatment of rats with sodium valproate downregulates frontal cortex NF-kappaB DNA binding activity and COX-2 mRNA. *Bipolar Disord.*, **9**, 513–520.

Rapoport, S.I., Basselin, M., Kim, H.W. *et al.* (2009) Bipolar disorder and mechanisms of action of mood stabilizers. *Brain Res. Rev.*, **61** (2), 185–209.

Rayasam, G.V., Tulasi, V.K., Sodhi, R. *et al.* (2009) Glycogen synthase kinase 3: more than a namesake. *Br. J. Pharmacol.*, **156**, 885–898.

Redman, J.R. and Francis, A.J. (1998) Entrainment of rat circadian rhythms by the melatonin agonist S-20098 requires intact suprachiasmatic nuclei but not the pineal. *J. Biol. Rhythms*, **13**, 39–51.

Reindl, J.D., Rowan, K., Carey, A.N. *et al.* (2008) Antidepressant-like effects of the novel kappa opioid antagonist MCL-144B in the forced-swim test. *Pharmacology*, **81**, 229–235.

Rimoy, G.H., Wright, D.M., Bhaskar, N.K. *et al.* (1994) The cardiovascular and central nervous system effects in the human of U-62066E. A selective opioid receptor agonist. *Eur. J. Clin. Pharmacol.*, **46**, 203–207.

Rogawski, M.A. (2006) Diverse mechanisms of antiepileptic drugs in the development pipeline. *Epilepsy Res.*, **69**, 273–294.

Roitman, S., Green, T., Osher, Y. *et al.* (2007) Creatine monohydrate in resistant depression: a preliminary study. *Bipolar Disord.*, **9**, 754–758.

Rojas-Corrales, M.O., Berrocoso, E., Gibert-Rahola, J. *et al.* (2002) Antidepressant-like effects of tramadol and other central analgesics with activity on monoamines reuptake, in helpless rats. *Life Sci.*, **72**, 143–152.

Rojas-Corrales, M.O., Berrocoso, E., Gibert-Rahola, J. *et al.* (2004) Antidepressant-like effect of tramadol and its enantiomers in reserpinized mice: comparative study with desipramine, fluvox-amine, venlafaxine and opiates. *J. Psychopharmacol.*, **18**, 404–411.

Rojas-Corrales, M.O., Gibert-Rahola, J., and Mico, J.A. (1998) Tramadol induces antidepressant-type effects in mice. *Life Sci.*, **63**, PL175–PL180.

Ross, B.M., Brooks, R.J., Lee, M. *et al.* (2002) Cyclooxygenase inhibitor modulation of dopamine-related behaviours. *Eur. J. Pharmacol.*, **450**, 141–151.

Rothschild, A.J. (2003) Challenges in the treatment of depression with psychotic features. *Biol. Psychiatry*, **53**, 680–690.

Rupniak, N.M. and Kramer, M.S. (1999) Discovery of the antidepressant and anti-emetic efficacy of substance P receptor (NK1) antagonists. *Trends Pharmacol. Sci.*, **20**, 485–490.

Saitoh, A., Yamada, M., Yamada, M. *et al.* (2008) Antidepressant-like effects of the delta-opioid receptor agonist SNC80 ([(+)-4-[(alphaR)-alpha-[(2S,5R)-2,5-dimethyl-4-(2-propenyl)-1-piperazinyl]-(3-methoxyphenyl)methyl]-N,N-diethylbenzamide) in an olfactory bulbectomized rat model. *Brain Res.*, **1208**, 160–169.

Sanacora, G., Kendell, S.F., Levin, Y. *et al.* (2007) Preliminary evidence of riluzole efficacy in antidepressant-treated patients with residual depressive symptoms. *Biol. Psychiatry*, **61**, 822–825.

Sanacora, G., Zarate, C.A., Krystal, J.H. *et al.* (2008) Targeting the glutamatergic system to develop novel, improved therapeutics for mood disorders. *Nat. Rev. Drug. Discov.*, **7**, 426–437.

Schwarzer, C. (2009) 30 years of dynorphins--new insights on their functions in neuropsychiatric diseases. *Pharmacol. Ther.*, **123**, 353–370.

Segal, M., Avital, A., Drobot, M. *et al.* (2007) Serum creatine kinase level in unmedicated nonpsychotic, psychotic, bipolar and schizoaffective depressed patients. *Eur. Neuropsychopharmacol.*, **17**, 194–198.

Shaltiel, G., Maeng, S., Malkesman, O. *et al.* (2008) Evidence for the involvement of the kainate receptor subunit GluR6 (GRIK2) in mediating behavioral displays related to behavioral symptoms of mania. *Mol. Psychiatry*, **13**, 858–872.

Shapira, N.A., Verduin, M.L., and DeGraw, J.D. (2001) Treatment of refractory major depression with tramadol monotherapy. *J. Clin. Psychiatry*, **62**, 205–206.

Shirayama, Y., Ishida, H., Iwata, M. *et al.* (2004) Stress increases dynorphin immunoreactivity in limbic brain regions and dynorphin antagonism produces antidepressant-like effects. *J. Neurochem.*, **90**, 1258–1268.

Silvestre, J.S., Nadal, R., Pallares, M. *et al.* (1997) Acute effects of ketamine in the holeboard, the elevated-plus maze, and the social interaction test in Wistar rats. *Depress. Anxiety*, **5**, 29–33.

Skolnick, P., Miller, R., Young, A. *et al.* (1992) Chronic treatment with 1-aminocyclopropanecarboxylic acid desensitizes behavioral responses to compounds acting at the N-methyl-D-aspartate receptor complex. *Psychopharmacology (Berl.)*, **107**, 489–496.

Song, Y., Wei, E.Q., Zhang, W.P. *et al.* (2004) Minocycline protects PC12 cells from ischemic-like injury and inhibits 5-lipoxygenase activation. *Neuroreport*, **15**, 2181–2184.

Spencer, C. (2000) The efficacy of intramuscular tramadol as a rapid-onset antidepressant. *Aust. N. Z. J. Psychiatry*, **34**, 1032–1033.

Steinberg, R., Alonso, R., Griebel, G. *et al.* (2001) Selective blockade of neurokinin-2 receptors produces antidepressant-like effects associated with reduced corticotropin-releasing factor function. *J. Pharmacol. Exp. Ther.*, **299**, 449–458.

Stoll, A.L. and Rueter, S. (1999) Treatment augmentation with opiates in severe and refractory major depression. *Am. J. Psychiatry*, **156**, 2017.

Streck, E.L., Amboni, G., Scaini, G. *et al.* (2008) Brain creatine kinase activity in an animal model of mania. *Life Sci.*, **82**, 424–429.

Tejedor-Real, P., Mico, J.A., Maldonado, R. *et al.* (1995) Implication of endogenous opioid system in the learned helplessness model of depression. *Pharmacol. Biochem. Behav.*, **52**, 145–152.

Thomson, P.A., Wray, N.R., Thomson, A.M. *et al.* (2005) Sex-specific association between bipolar affective disorder in women and GPR50, an X-linked orphan G protein-coupled receptor. *Mol. Psychiatry*, **10**, 470–478.

Torregrossa, M.M., Jutkiewicz, E.M., Mosberg, H.I. *et al.* (2006) Peptidic delta opioid receptor agonists produce antidepressant-like effects in the forced swim test and regulate BDNF mRNA expression in rats. *Brain Res.*, **1069**, 172–181.

Traynor, B.J., Bruiin, L., Conwit, R. *et al.* (2006) Neuroprotective agents for clinical trials in ALS: a systematic assessment. *Neurology*, **67**, 20–27.

Trullas, R. and Skolnick, P. (1990) Functional antagonists at the NMDA receptor complex exhibit antidepressant actions. *Eur. J. Pharmacol.*, **185**, 1–10.

Valdez, G.R. (2009) CRF receptors as a potential target in the development of novel pharmacotherapies for depression. *Curr. Pharm. Des.*, **15**, 1587–1594.

Van Oekelen, D., Luyten, W.H., and Leysen, J.E. (2003) 5-HT2A and 5-HT2C receptors and their atypical regulation properties. *Life Sci.*, **72**, 2429–2449.

Velentgas, P., West, W., Cannuscio, C.C. *et al.* (2006) Cardiovascular risk of selective cyclooxygenase-2 inhibitors and other non-aspirin non-steroidal anti-inflammatory medications. *Pharmacoepidemiol. Drug Saf.*, **15**, 641–652.

Walsh, S.L., Strain, E.C., Abreu, M.E. *et al.* (2001) Enadoline, a selective kappa opioid agonist: comparison with butorphanol and hydromorphone in humans. *Psychopharmacology (Berl.)*, **157**, 151–162.

Watkins, J. and Collingridge, G. (1994) Phenylglycine derivatives as antagonists of metabotropic glutamate receptors. *Trends Pharmacol. Sci.*, **15**, 333–342.

Yalcin, I., Aksu, F., Bodard, S. *et al.* (2007) Antidepressant-like effect of tramadol in the unpredictable chronic mild stress procedure: possible involvement of the noradrenergic system. *Behav. Pharmacol.*, **18**, 623–631.

Yildiz, A., Guleryuz, S., Ankerst, D.P. *et al.* (2008) Protein kinase C inhibition in the treatment of mania: a double-blind, placebo-controlled trial of tamoxifen. *Arch. Gen. Psychiatry*, **65**, 255–263.

Yoon, S.J., Lyoo, I.K., Haws, C. *et al.* (2009) Decreased glutamate/glutamine levels may mediate cytidine's efficacy in treating bipolar depression: a longitudinal proton magnetic resonance spectroscopy study. *Neuropsychopharmacology*, **34**, 1810–1818.

Young, A.H., Gallagher, P., Watson, S. *et al.* (2004) Improvements in neurocognitive function and mood following adjunctive treatment with mifepristone (RU-486) in bipolar disorder. *Neuropsychopharmacology*, **29**, 1538–1545.

Young, L.T., Wang, J.F., Woods, C.M. *et al.* (1999) Platelet protein kinase C alpha levels in drug-free and lithium-treated subjects with bipolar disorder. *Neuropsychobiology*, **40**, 63–66.

Zarate, C.A., Du, J., Quiroz, J. Jr. *et al.* (2003) Regulation of cellular plasticity cascades in the pathophysiology and treatment of mood disorders: role of the glutamatergic system. *Ann. N. Y. Acad. Sci.*, **1003**, 273–291.

Zarate, C.A., Payne, J.L., Quiroz, J. Jr. *et al.* (2004) An open-label trial of riluzole in patients with treatment-resistant major depression. *Am. J. Psychiatry*, **161**, 171–174.

Zarate, C.A., Quiroz, J., Payne, J. *et al.* (2002) Modulators of the glutamatergic system: implications for the development of improved therapeutics in mood disorders. *Psychopharmacol. Bull.*, **36**, 35–83.

Zarate, C.A., Jr., Quiroz, J.A., Singh, J.B. *et al.* (2005) An open-label trial of the glutamate-modulating agent riluzole in combination with lithium for the treatment of bipolar depression. *Biol. Psychiatry*, **57**, 430–432.

Zarate, C.A.J., Singh, J., and Manji, H.K. (2006a) Cellular plasticity cascades: targets for the development of novel therapeutics for bipolar disorder. *Biol. Psychiatry*, **59**, 1006–1020.

Zarate, C.A. Jr., Singh, J.B., Carlson, P.J. *et al.* (2006b) A randomized trial of an N-methyl-D-aspartate antagonist in treatment-resistant major depression. *Arch. Gen. Psychiatry*, **63**, 856–864.

Zarate, C.A. Jr., Singh, J.B., Carlson, P.J. *et al.* (2007) Efficacy of a protein kinase C inhibitor (tamoxifen) in the treatment of acute mania: a pilot study. *Bipolar Disord.*, **9**, 561–570.

Zobel, A.W., Nickel, T., Kunzel, H.E. *et al.* (2000) Effects of the high-affinity corticotropin-releasing hormone receptor 1 antagonist R121919 in major depression: the first 20 patients treated. *J. Psychiatr. Res.*, **34**, 171–181.

The Pivotal Role of Psycho-Education in the Long-Term Treatment of Bipolar Disorder

Francesc Colom and Andrea Murru

Barcelona Bipolar Disorders Program, IBIBAPS, Institute of Neurosciences, Hospital Clinic, Barcelona, Spain

22.1 INTRODUCTION

The relationship between the doctor and his patient is becoming – and should become – more horizontal and interactive. Trust is replacing authority. Partnership takes the place of paternalism. Prevention replaces intervention. Agreement replaces orders. And finally, education replaces hierarchy.

This is true for each and every branch of medicine. In fact, a good number of severe medical illnesses may improve their outcome by including in their regular treatment some aspects concerning healthy habits, behavioral changes that may benefit the course of the illness, symptoms management, and adherence issues. This new model of "horizontal medicine" based on education has shown its efficacy in several medical conditions including cardiovascular disease (Linden, 2000), diabetes (Olmsted *et al.*, 2002), and asthma (Durna and Ozcan, 2003).

The need for horizontal and educational models is even clearer when it comes to psychiatric disorder due to its very own nature where behavior and decisions-taking are often altered. And, amongst all psychiatric disorders, bipolar disorders are by far the ones that may benefit the most from education.

The ancestors of psycho-education were the so called "lithium clinics," which appeared both in Europe and the US in the 1970s. Those resources were typically composed by a team consisting of a psychiatrist and support staff (nurses and sometimes psychologists) and provided a wise combination of pharmacological care and patient education. Patients' education was supplemented by support groups to facilitate destigmatization, peer-based learning, and mutual support. Unfortunately, despite its quick worldwide implementation, the efficacy of this interesting approach has not been properly tested.

Other interesting studies come from the Netherlands, a country with a long tradition both of psycho-education and self-help/advocacy groups; the studies by Eduard van Gent

Bipolar Psychopharmacotherapy: Caring for the patient, Second Edition. Edited by Hagop S. Akiskal and Mauricio Tohen.
© 2011 John Wiley & Sons, Ltd. Published 2011 by John Wiley & Sons, Ltd.

(2000) showed, initially, a remarkable effect on stigma and self-esteem and, later on, in a three-year follow-up, a significant decrease of adherence problems and hospitalizations amongst psycho-educated patients.

However, the last decade must be considered as the golden period for bipolar psycho-education. Despite the pioneering psycho-education studies were published by Peet and Harvey back in the early 1990s (Harvey and Peet, 1991; Peet and Harvey, 1991), those studies were not enough to reach conclusions regarding psycho-education's prophylactic efficacy, as they did not provide any clinical outcome measures.

Nowadays, a psychological intervention, at least for some months, is almost a must in the maintenance treatment, as the benefits in terms of less relapses and hospitalizations are very clear and the cost very low (Scott et al., 2009).

Psycho-education – as every efficacious psychological intervention – is essentially based on common sense and should be considered as a clinically oriented technique. Psycho-education goes far beyond a mere delivery of information. Psycho-education is aimed at providing the bipolar patients with a theoretical and practical approach towards understanding and coping with the consequences of illness – in the context of a medical model-, and allows them to actively collaborate with the physician in some aspects of the treatment. Briefly, the main goals of psycho-education are the enhancement of adherence, the improvement of illness management skills such as early recognition of episode recurrence and development of strategies for effective coping with symptoms, and the improvement of social and occupational function and quality of life (Table 22.1).

Psycho-education, has shown the efficacy of group psycho-education in preventing all sorts of bipolar episodes and increasing time to relapse at two-year follow-up (Colom et al., 2003). One hundred and twenty bipolar patients – type I or II – who had been euthymic for at least six months (YMRS < 6, HDRS, 8) were included in the study. Patients were randomly assigned to receiving 21 sessions of group psycho-education or 21 sessions of nonspecific group meetings during a period of six months as an add-on to the naturalistic pharmacological treatment. At the two-year follow-up, 55 subjects (92%) in the control group fulfilled criteria for recurrence versus 40 patients (67%) in the psycho-education group ($p < 0.001$), whilst the total number of recurrences and the number of depressive episodes was significantly lower for psycho-educated patients. As for time to recurrence, the survival analysis showed an advantage of psycho-education for time to any recurrence (log rank $= 13.453$, df $= 1$, $p < 0.0002$), time to depressive recurrence (log rank $= 15.473$, df $= 1$, $p < 0.0001$), time to mixed recurrence (log rank $= 7.95$, df $= 1$, $p < 0.05$) and time to manic or hypomanic recurrence (log rank $= 7.79$, df $= 1$, $p < 0.006$). Another interesting outcome had to do with hospitalizations; although no difference was found regarding the number of patients who required hospitalization, there was a significant difference concerning the number of hospitalizations per patient at the two-year follow-up (0.304 for the psycho-educated patients vs. 0.780, U $= -2.14$, $p < 0.05$). Thus, psycho-education appeared to be avoiding the constant re-hospitalization of the most severe subset of patients, a phenomenon which is usually known as "revolving door."

Group psycho-education has shown its efficacy even in those complex patients fulfilling criteria for a comorbid personality disorder (Colom et al., 2004). This might be particularly interesting if we consider on the one hand the poor outcome of comorbid

Table 22.1 Sessions of the Barcelona Psycho-education Program (Colom and Vieta, 2006).

Session 1 is just an **introductory session**, to allow people introduce themselves and have a first
contact with the therapist and the other participants. The goals for the sessions aimed
specifically at improving illness awareness are as follows:

Session 2. What is bipolar disorder?

To introduce patients to the concept of bipolar disorder and to dispel the numerous myths about
it, stressing the biological nature of the disorder and attempting to overcome its social stigma.

Session 3. Etiological and triggering factors

To explain the biological nature of the disorder and learn to distinguish between the "causal"
concept of the disorder – underscored as biological – and the "triggering" concept – which can
be either biological or environmental.

Session 4. Symptoms (i): mania and hypomania

To have patients get familiar with what a manic or hypomanic episode is. The purpose of session
4 is not yet to teach patients how to detect a manic or hypomanic episode in time, but rather
try to show them what a hypomanic or manic episode is and, particularly, why hypomania is a
syndrome and not a gift.

Session 5. Symptoms (ii): depression and mixed episodes

To convey to our patients the idea that depression is a medical illness, moving away from
pejorative and blameful social considerations or popular meanings associated with the concept.
A further aim is to help to differentiate normal emotions from pathological ones.

Session 6: Course and outcome

To focus on the chronic and recurring character of the bipolar disorder, further emphasizing the
difference between causal and triggering factors, reminding the patient of the cyclic character
of the disorder based on the life chart technique, which the patient must master by the end of
the session.

Session 7. Treatment (I): mood stabilizers

To inform the patients of the various types of mood stabilizers, their differences and specific
indications, their advantages and side effects. Although it may be arguable, due to the recent
data on mood-stabilizing properties of some second-generation antipsychotics, drugs included
under this umbrella are lithium, valproate, carbamazepine, and lamotrigine.

Session 8. Treatment (II): antimanic drugs

To share updated information on the pharmacological treatment of the manic and hypomanic
phases in order to improve patient adherence in these phases, since it is usually deficient.
Again, although lithium and some anticonvulsants have antimanic properties, this session is
devoted exclusively to antipsychotics. The term antimanic is preferred over antipsychotic in
the context of bipolar disorder.

Session 9. Treatment (III): antidepressants

To inform about the pharmacological treatment of depressive episodes, which of course may
include other options. The session includes specific information about the relatively limited
evidence base for the use of antidepressants in bipolar depression and the potential risk of
switch, but also the need to take them if prescribed, particularly in combination with
mood-stabilizers and/or antimanic drugs.

(Continued Overleaf)

Table 22.1 (Continued)

Session 10. Plasma levels of mood stabilizers

To help the patient understand the need for periodic blood tests in order to determine serum levels. Many patients do not do these serum determinations regularly, either because they forget, because they do not understand their importance or because they are afraid of needles.

Session 11. Pregnancy and genetic advice

This session is especially addressed to women, since its objective is to tackle the problematic relationship between psychotropic drugs and pregnancy, but men should attend too. The core message of the session is that in all events, the patient must always consult her psychiatrist before deciding to become pregnant, in order to be able to have rigorous control along with her gynecologist. Disorder inheritance issues are also discussed.

Session 12. Psychopharmacology vs. alternative therapies

To explain to our patients difference between scientifically tested and non-tested therapies.

Session 13. Risks associated with interruption of the treatment

To fix the contents of all the above mentioned sessions and make the patients understand the risk of relapse associated with treatment withdrawal.

Session 14. Alcohol, coffee, and street drugs

To stress the problems associated with the intake of several substances. A major importance is paid to substances such as coffee and alcohol whose danger is estimated as "low" by the general population.

Session 15. Early detection of mania and hypomanic episodes

To train patients detect their (hypo)manic relapses in time, and make their own lists of operational early signs so that these are available for identification of future episodes.

Session 16. Early detection of depressive and mixed episodes

To train patients to detect their depressive episodes as soon as possible; this is not as easy as it sounds because many of them have difficulty in detecting the first signs, especially in the case of inhibited or anergic depressions with a low cognitive load and limited mental suffering.

Session 17. What to do when a new phase is detected?

To build up, together with each patient, a structured action plan for oncoming episodes.

Session 18. Regularity of habits

To enter into greater depth on the need for regular habits. Sleep-hygiene habits are reviewed.

Session 19. Stress control techniques

To emphasize the importance of stress as a trigger for relapses and to let the patients know of the existence of various psychological techniques that can help them to better cope with stress and anxiety.

Session 20. Problem-solving strategies

Decision-making is usually difficult for bipolar patients. Some user-friendly problem-solving strategies, stressing its use in bipolar disorder, are introduced.

Session 21. Summary and farewell

The experience of sharing a program for 20 weeks usually creates strong bonds between patients and to the therapist, so a proper closure has a strong emotional value.

bipolar patients and on the other hand the complexity of its treatment. Integrated care, including psycho-educative contents, has also been proven effective for bipolar patients with substance dependence.

The usefulness of care packages containing psycho-education as a core element has also been shown. To these regards, two studies should be stressed:

1. The Life-Goals Program, developed by Bauer and colleagues (2003) is a team-based intervention originally designed to test the "real world" efficacy – or effectiveness – of a specific program of care for bipolar disorders. Thus, this intervention is quite different from the randomized clinical trials by (i) including severely ill patients with comorbidities, (ii) minimizing the provider-based variability typical of medical-surgical and mental health care, and (iii) minimizing the system-related barriers characteristic of chronic care to allow patients a proactive illness management. The Life-Goals Program consists consisted of patient psycho-education to improve self-management skills, simplified clinical practice guidelines, and use of a nurse care coordinator working in collaboration with a supervising psychiatrist to enhance continuity of care and information flow. This program, when compared to usual care in a three-year study has shown a significant reduction in time spent acutely ill – including reduction in weeks of manic episodes, and a nonsignificant reduction in weeks of depression-, reducing weeks in episode by 14%, weeks manic by 23%, and weeks depressed by 11%. Mean intervention three-year costs were $61 398 compared with $64 379 in costs for usual care. The authors did not report any significant effect of the treatment regarding hospitalizations.

2. The Systematic Care Program designed by Simon et al. (2002) is another multicomponent intervention designed to be provided by psychiatric nurses in collaboration with the psychiatrist. This program last for two years and includes five distinct components, namely: "Assessment and Care Planning" (which includes medication, early warning signs, and identification of a care partner – family member or significant other), "Structured Monthly Telephone Calls" (the nurse called each patient monthly to complete structured clinician ratings of symptoms, current medication use and medication adverse effects), "Feedback to the Mental Health Treatment Team," "Structured Group Psycho-educational Program" (consisting on 48 sessions) and "As-Needed Support, Education, and Care Coordination." In a randomized trial of 24-month follow-up period (Simon et al., 2006), the mean mania severity ratings were lower in the intervention group. Unfortunately, there was no significant difference in the depression ratings between the two treatment groups. Regarding the costs of the intervention, it should be underlined that patients in the intervention group had more medication management visits and consumed more atypical antipsychotic medications than the usual care group, but neither of these differences was statistically significant at the 5% level. The direct costs of the intervention program were approximately $500 during the first year and $300 during the second year. The total costs in the intervention group were $1251 (95% confidence interval, $55–2446) higher than those in the usual care group.

22.2   ON THE NEED FOR PSYCHO-EDUCATION

Psycho-education fits nicely on the medical model of the illness, overcoming old-fashioned and stigmatizing views of the condition. This is why psycho-education has been happily accepted by professionals all over the world because, in a certain way, they felt they had been implementing psycho-education for many years – sometimes using other similar names. This phenomena, which does not apply to other academia-based psychological therapies, is explained by the fact that, psycho-education, more than a technique is an attitude when treating the patient. Since bipolar disorder is a chronic condition, bipolar patients not having learnt to live with it will be at risk of feeling unable of leading their own life and may, hence, have a mostly painful life experience of "learned helplessness" ("no matter what I do, I will relapse"), which might seriously limit their well-being, performance, and quality of life. Psycho-education does not cure bipolar disorder, but it cures incomprehension, alleviates stigma, deals effectively with guilt, and prevents learned helplessness. Psycho-education replaces guilt by responsibility, helplessness by proactive care, and denial by awareness. Patients included in a psycho-education group are able to sense from our explanations about their disorder that psychiatry has already described and understood situations that they may be living through with shame, isolation, or convinced that they are unique and nontransferable. The psycho-educated patient "knows that we know" and that results in an improvement in the therapeutic relationship. Of course, psycho-education should include an acceptance by both parts – therapist and patient – of a certain paradigm that encourages the patient to have a proactive attitude in dealing with his bipolar disorder, but only through acknowledging the need for proper training which must be on the basis of such proactive attitude. Hence, it is not necessarily true that the "patient is an expert in his own condition": although the patient lives with the condition, proper tools should be delivered by health professionals to upgrade him to expertise on it, and psycho-education is a way of providing them.

22.3   THE FIVE INGREDIENTS OF PSYCHO-EDUCATION

The following (Figure 22.1) are the main components integrating the Barcelona Psycho-education Program, which consists of 21 sessions (Colom and Vieta, 2006). They were chosen on the basis of clinical experience and the needs referred both by patients and clinicians in the everyday coping with bipolar disorder. They are present in most therapeutic packages for bipolar disorder existing all over the world, and they proved to be efficacious altogether to prevent recurrences.

22.3.1   ILLNESS AWARENESS

More than a half of bipolar patients have difficulties to obtain good insight and denial is not at all uncommon, representing one of the main problems in order to start a treatment. Despite the association between lack of insight and neuropsychological impairment has been solidly reported, social stigma and myths surrounding bipolar disorders and psychiatric conditions in general gives diagnosis a high likelihood to be rejected by patients themselves.

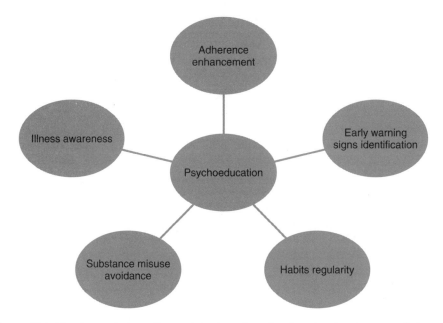

Figure 22.1 The five main ingredients of the Barcelona Psycho-education Program (Colom and Vieta, 2006).

On the other hand, clinicians' attitude and language does not always help illness acceptance. This is why several sessions are devoted to illness acceptance before moving to other essential issues such as symptom-management or medication adherence. Thus, it is not casual that "Illness awareness" is the first component to be approached, as it will introduce concepts that will later be absolutely necessary during the group program.

Patients generally feel comfortable within the medical model of the illness, as it is perceived as very practical, treatment-oriented, and exonerating. As the general population is generally unaware of the origin and nature of psychiatric disorders, the first sessions are usually quite "open," allowing to learn which illness model is managed by the patients and which prejudices they may have, since they are often useful to cope with guilt and frustration. Certain patients react to the medical model with a certain degree of initial resistance. If this is the case, it is quite useful to allow group members to discuss freely, as in most cases the rest of group members will be more consistent in managing other patients' reluctance to the medical model than even the therapist, who might be seen as defending his own *beliefs* or *opinions*.

The topic of illness awareness is central and will regularly appear in all the sessions of the program.

22.3.2 ADHERENCE ENHANCEMENT

Improving treatment adherence must be one of the main objectives of any psychological intervention in bipolar disorders, since the problem of poor adherence explains a high rate of relapses and the poor outcome of many patients (Colom *et al.*, 2000). Some crucial issues to consider regarding treatment non-adherence include:

1. Practically all bipolar patients seriously think at one time in their life of abandoning treatment.
2. Almost a half the patients stop taking medication without indication from their psychiatrists, even during euthymia.
3. The reasons for nonadherence are quite unspecific and patient-dependent, although substance and personality comorbidities play a major role.
4. Medication withdrawal is the most common cause of relapse amongst bipolar patients. The risk of hospitalization is four times higher among the patients who do not duly comply with their maintenance treatment. Mortality, especially by suicide, is also higher in nonadherent patients.
5. Nonadherence is usually underestimated by clinicians.
6. Lack of adherence is often explained by irrational fears, prejudice, and misinformation.

Poor adherence can be defined as the inability of the patient to follow some or all of the instructions given by his psychiatrist and psychologist, including drug prescription and the facilitation of health-promoting behavior or habits. In the sessions devoted to improve treatment adherence, it may be useful to cover all the different presentations of nonadherence, and also the following 10 points:

1. Inform the patient on the existing different types of psychotropic medications for bipolar disorder.
2. Review brand names of psychotropic medications. Explain the difference between brand name and generic name.
3. Stress the idea that pharmacological treatment is highly individualized.
4. Learn on the purpose of each medication and how a drug may have more than one purpose.
5. Learn on common side effects of medications.
6. Discuss strategies to deal with side effects.
7. Learn the importance of serum levels determination, especially in the case of lithium, but also valproate and carbamazepine.
8. Learn to identify the signs of severe toxicity with lithium and other drugs.
9. Inform on drug-drug and drug-food interactions.
10. Inform on appropriate administration.

It is positive to open a debate on several fears and prejudices regarding medication for psychiatric diseases. Amongst them, the most common has to do with the risk of becoming dependant to psychopharmacological agents; the therapy should clearly state that psychotropic drugs are not addictive – except for benzodiazepines, if not properly used – that they do not "brainwash" or cause "idiocy" – as both fears are frequently expressed by patients-, that most medications are not either sedatives just aimed at keeping people quiet, or stimulants which replace the will of those who take them.

Despite some sessions on adherence may look much more informative than behavioral, the practice points at the contrary, as the number of debates, exercises, and patient-to-patient interactions. For instance, we encourage a debate on how to cope with relevant side effects (tremor, weight gain, or diarrhea) or another one on how to remind to take the medication on a daily basis.

Another issue that usually comes up during these sessions is the social stigma associated with psychotropic drugs, because in many cases the social group or even the patient's family do not understand the need to take medication and, hence, may send messages such as "you are going to become stupid from so much medication," "if you try harder you wouldn't need so many pills," or "this medication is drugging you, you look like a zombie," which obviously have a very negative impact on adherence. In general, it may be good to advise all patients to speak about their need for treatment with special emphasis on the more biological aspects of the disorder.

During these sessions, it may be also helpful to discuss on the inefficacy of alternative therapies for bipolar disorder, given that bipolar patients are especially prone to seek for this sort of "help." According to a recently published US-based study (Kilbourne et al., 2007), more than a half of the patients are using alternative remedies such as prayer/spiritual healing (54%), meditation or herbs (50%), being patients on anticonvulsants or atypical antipsychotics more likely to use them. It will be worth explaining the scientific method to our patients, so they will be able to learn the distinction between a fact and an opinion. Later on, we could explain to our patients what a randomized clinical trial is. This will be of great help when explaining what is meant by "non-tested" treatments, and will be valid not only to talk about drugs but also – and maybe even more – to emphasize the difference between tested and nontested psychotherapies.

Specific attention should also be paid to teratogenic effects of medication: the main message here should be to get the patient to learn how not only medications may be harmful for the fetus, but also how mania or depression can cause damage by altering some healthy habits which are badly needed during pregnancy, and which are the risks of postpartum episodes. If the patient learns that there is a delicate balance between benefits and risks of medication during pregnancy that needs to be personalized, then he or she can be in a better position to decide when this situation comes up in the future.

The efficacy of psycho-education on improving adherence has been proven. The patients who were on lithium and were receiving psycho-education, for instance, had more stable lithium serum levels than those who did not receive psycho-education (Colom et al., 2005).

22.4 SUBSTANCE MISUSE AVOIDANCE

The largest study on co-occurrence of bipolar disorders and substance use disorders was conducted as part of the National Epidemiologic Survey on Alcohol and Related Conditions (NESARC) which assessed more than 40 000 people in the US (Grant et al., 2005). According to this study, there was a lifetime prevalence for co-occurring alcohol use disorders reaching almost 60% of bipolar I patients, and a 38% lifetime prevalence of any drug use disorder, a finding that is supported in general by all the existing literature. According to the Epidemiological Catchment Area data, nearly half of bipolar II patients would have a comorbid substance use disorder (Regier et al., 1990). Thus, the risk for a bipolar patient to suffer a substance related problem is six fold higher than that of the general population. Alcohol seems to be the most frequently used drug amongst bipolar patients, as opposed to schizophrenic patients, who would be more prone to the use of stimulants. Substance use is associated with a poorer outcome: Increased episodes of depression, increased adherence problems, and delayed symptomatic recovery. Data coming from the Systematic Treatment Enhancement Program for Bipolar Disorder (STEP-BD) suggest that substance related disorders are strongly associated with an increased number of hospitalizations (Simon *et al.*, 2004). Suicidal attempts are also more frequent amongst patients with such comorbidity (Baldassano, 2006).

On the other hand, many patients do not meet the criteria for substance abuse or dependence even though they consume alcohol or other substances with a certain assiduity, and the mere consumption of alcohol, cannabis, and other toxics, even without reaching abuse quantities, can act as a trigger for new episodes.

Although patients with severe comorbid substance abuse or dependence may need a specific program that tackles dual pathology, it is very useful to target the regular use of substances with psychotropic effects. In other words, the idea is to prevent substance consumption in order to control a potential triggering factor. To achieve this objective, it may be useful not only to focus on alcohol and street drugs but also on apparently harmless substances such as caffeine, as many patients may drink coffee or other stimulant drinks in order to compensate their subdepressive clinical condition or to get "higher," which obviously implies a risk, especially because of its impact on the quality of sleep. The importance of avoiding substance use to improve prognosis will be present throughout the program despite there is only one session specifically devoted to the topic (Session 14). Hence, this issue will come up again and again in many other sessions (such causes and triggers, course and outcome, alternative treatments, early intervention, symptoms management, lifestyle regularity, and so on). During all these sessions the following contents can be addressed:

- **Alcohol** may trigger depression, increase anxiety, worsen sleep, reduce impulse control, cause cognitive impairment, increase aggressiveness, and the appearance of psychotic symptoms and mania.
- **Marijuana** may cause an amotivational syndrome characterized by great apathy; it may also trigger depression and mania, interfere with sleep, increase anxiety, and psychotic symptoms.
- **Cocaine** and **hallucinogens** all by themselves can trigger any type of episode, and also rapid cycling, anxiety, aggressiveness, psychotic symptoms, poor sleep, and cognitive impairment.
- The danger of **coffee** is mainly its ability to alter sleep structure and increase anxiety.
- As for cigarettes **smoking**, it is important to advise on how to stop smoking, but also on *when* to stop smoking, by means of five important points:

  1. It is generally not a good idea to try to quit smoking during an episode.
  2. The best time to quit smoking is during periods of long-duration euthymia (six months euthymia or more).
  3. Do not try to stop suddenly.

4. The use of substitutes is recommended (nicotine chewing gum or patch) to avoid the withdrawal syndrome, which may give rise to anxiety and irritability.
5. The use of anti-craving drugs such as bupropion is absolutely contraindicated in bipolar patients who are not depressed, as they are antidepressants and might eventually destabilize the disorder.

Amongst the psychological interventions who have targeted specifically the comorbidity of substance and bipolar disorders, it is worth mentioning the Integrated Group Therapy (IGT), a highly – structured group treatment consisting of 20 weekly group sessions (Weiss *et al.*, 2007). The core principle guiding the treatment is that the same kinds of thoughts and behaviors that facilitate recovery from substance-related disorders will also be helpful in order to reach affective stability. Unfortunately, the evidence does not seem to support this last point, as IGT has shown its usefulness in decreasing the days of substance use and other measures regarding the severity of the substance disorder, but not the outcome of bipolar disorder.

22.5 EARLY WARNING SIGNS – DETECTION

The detection of early warning signs is one of the key elements of a psycho-education program and, probably, the one which requires more skills from the therapist. Although the Barcelona program devotes a session to early detection of elation and another one to early detection of depression, the former keeps on appearing during several oncoming sessions as to stress its importance mainly because:

- The speed with which elation early warning symptoms become a full-blown episode is far greater than in the case of depression. While in depression several weeks usually elapse between the first warning signs and the actual episode, in the case of hypomania and mania this can happen in a matter of days or hours.
- There are almost-immediate-acting drugs to slow down the start of a manic episode, while this is not mostly true for depression.
- Many patients have greater difficulty in identifying a hypomanic episode, due to its subtle appearance and the pleasure that often implies, whilst in the case of depression, psychic pain (sadness, anxiety, and fatigue) would work as a relapse alarm. However, this is not true for all bipolar patients, many of whom have depression "without sadness," featured mainly by fatigue, inhibition, and apathy, sometimes with little suffering or desperation.
- Many patients tend to "give themselves permission" to live through their first hypomanic symptoms without taking any action to abort the episode, and this happens because very often the patient has a near-addictive relationship with mania. This is why any action identifying the early signs of hypomania as something pathological and a cause for concern by the patient is especially important.

One useful comparison to help the patients understand the need for early detection and treatment of (hypo)mania is the *avalanche*: a manic episode works like a snow avalanche. At the beginning, it's just a little snowball sliding smoothly down the slope, apparently harmless, which could be easily stopped with your hand, but, as it rolls down the side of the mountain, it starts to gain on volume, weight, and speed, coming to a point where the disaster can not be avoided.

Another key element of these sessions is the early intervention plan. Although it should be tailored to each single case, a list of general tips could be provided. It is very important to train patients to give priority to some interventions (such as increase sleeping or avoid stimulants) that could be crucial for each episode, avoiding general advices as "try to calm down."

The issue of "rescue medication" (encouraging patient's self-administration of small doses of antipsychotics (antimanics) as an emergency resource once early warning signs of hypomania are detected) will appear during these sessions, and will be quite controversial. In any event, the antipsychotic is something that must be prescribed by the psychiatrist at an individual appointment with the patient, and not in the context of a psycho-education group, as to a large degree it depends on the patient's mental level, his ability to identify episodes correctly, and know what type they are, his response to antipsychotics, whether there is a history of substance abuse, and the relationship with the psychiatrist. So this is not advice to be generalized to all cases, but some patients may do well with some self-prescription in the case of *hypomania*. On the contrary, it is not advisable at the current stage of knowledge to let the patient change the drug prescription if a *depressive* episode is suspected. Many patients have a degree of addiction to their elation stages and may abuse antidepressants if the psychiatrist opens the door to this possibility, small though it may be. Other patients habitually hover around the border of subsyndromal depression; they might misinterpret this fluctuation and start using antidepressants.

In order to build up an emergency plan, it is very useful for the patient to have contact telephone numbers handy for their psychiatrist, psychologist, nurse, and other related health caregivers. It may be good to give to the patients some sort of "fire extinguisher card" bearing the clinics telephone number, the name and telephone number of their psychiatrist or other psychiatrists who could take care of him or her, the psychologist, the team nurse, and an emergency telephone number.

Identifying early signs consists on three steps; of these, the first and second are generally worked during the group program, while the third step usually requires individual intervention, although this is not essential in all cases.

22.6   LIFESTYLE REGULARITY (AND MISCELLANEA)

Regular habits and stress management are extremely important in bipolar disorder and constitute the foundational ingredient of Interpersonal Social Rhythm Therapy (IPSRT) (Frank *et al.*, 1997). Moreover, improving habits regularity by means of IPSRT is efficacious to prevent newer relapses in bipolar patients. Psycho-education just tries to encourage patients towards healthy habits, and a tailored intervention such as IPSRT will be needed to improve this aspect in more depth. There are two major concerns regarding lifestyle that should be covered during a psycho-education group.

1. **Sleeping habits/circadian rhythm.** Sleeping and social-rhythm disruptions have mood-destabilizing effects. Sleep duration is a key factor in predicting manic and

depressive symptoms. There is robust evidence that sleep deprivation can induce manic symptoms among nondepressed bipolar individuals. Increasing the duration of night sleep may have some effect on treating manic symptoms, whilst total sleep deprivation has been reported to be associated with remission in unipolar depression, but its use in bipolar disorder is much more controversial. The general advice in psycho-education is to sleep between seven and nine hours, avoid daytime sleep, and use sleep both as an indicator of relapse and as a helper to deal with oncoming episodes (by reducing or augmenting the number of sleeping hours within a reasonable frame).

On the other hand, many bipolar patients tend to organize their time rather erratically. Regular schedules and better structuring of activities should be one of the key points in any individual intervention with a bipolar patient. In the group, what can be done is to get across the importance of these aspects, presenting them as information, as there is not enough time to work on techniques such as recording activities, which are usually useful for bipolar patients. It is important for the patient to keep the proper balance between the schedule that maintains his euthymia and schedules that favor social adjustment and quality of life. To this regard, it is crucial to attend to the individual needs of each patient, something that goes far beyond what will be offered in a psycho-education group.

2. **Physical exercise.** Chronic medical conditions such as dyslipidemia, hypertension, diabetes, and obesity occur more often among bipolar patients than in the general population. This may be due to poor general medical care seeking, medication side-effects, and negligence of proactive health behaviors; many bipolar patients have extremely unbalanced nutrition habits and have – especially if depressed – sedentary habits. Thus, doing physical exercise is highly recommended for bipolar patients, not only to improve general health but also to improve mood. To date, there is evidence of the usefulness of physical exercise as an add-on to medication and psychological interventions in many psychiatric conditions, including anxiety and depression and to prevent depressive relapses in unipolar recurrent patients. Speculations on the "antidepressant" action of physical activity include various elements such as enhancement of monoamines transmission, endorphins release, distraction from negative stimuli, promotion of self-efficacy, and social interaction. Physical activity may also favorably influence brain plasticity, possibly mediated through neurotrophic factors, enhance executive cognitive functions and temper the activities of stress neural circuitries. A recent retrospective trial, including nearly 70 bipolar patients, showed some benefit of physical exercise regarding some measures of depressive symptoms, anxiety, and stress (Ng et al., 2007). However, the use of physical activity in bipolar disorder should be selective, following basically three axioms:

(a) Physical exercise should not be done 3–4 hours before going to bed, as its stimulant properties may worsen the quality of sleep.
(b) Physical exercise should be stopped if a manic, hypomanic, or mixed relapse is suspected. Similarly, should be increased if a depressive relapse is suspected.
(c) Physical exercise often implies some risk of dehydration. This should be kept in mind especially with those patients on lithium, due to intoxication risk.

22.7   PSYCHO-EDUCATION WITH THE FAMILY

There is evidence that stressful events inside family environment are often related to exacerbations of bipolar disorder; expressed emotion has been described as an important predictor of symptoms severity (Miklowitz *et al.*, 1988). Bipolar disorder may represent a significant psychological burden for family members and other caregivers. Thus, bipolar disorder affects family relationships and family relationships affect bipolar disorder.

Keeping these facts in mind – and reminding the positive evidence in schizophrenia-, it sounded quite logical to essay family psychosocial interventions for bipolar disorder since the pre-pharmacological treatment era (Reinares *et al.*, 2002).

It is well-known that under the name of family therapy one can find very different kinds of interventions with diverse concepts in foundation, going from poorly evidence-based systemic or dynamic interventions to family psycho-education, which is strongly supported by data.

Family-focused therapy was adapted for bipolar patients from a previous psychosocial intervention model created for schizophrenic patients, and consists roughly of three components: psycho-education about bipolar disorder, communication enhancement training, and problem-solving skills training. It is administered in 21 one-hour session. It has shown its efficacy, mainly in the prevention of depressive relapses.

Another interesting model is the "Multifamily Psycho-educational Group Therapy," a short (six sessions), semi-structured intervention with small groups of patients and their relatives (Fristad *et al.*, 2009). The intervention focused mainly on information and coping strategies. The psychotherapists encouraged patients and family members to share their perspectives on family interactions. Unfortunately, there is no outcome published yet on the efficacy of this approach.

Psycho-educational family intervention consists of 12 90-minute group sessions for patients' caregivers, and follows – roughly – the model presented so far, stressing also on coping strategies. At the one-year follow-up, it has shown efficacy in the prevention of manic phases, but not depressive (Reinares *et al.*, 2008).

A major limitation of family based therapies is quite obvious: about 40–60% of bipolar patients, depending on the cultural context, are not residing with their family. Hence, the number of patients that may benefit from this approach is limited.

22.8   LONG-TERM FOLLOW-UP

Psychological interventions in bipolar disorder claim to be a maintenance tool. But, by definition, any maintenance tool must show its efficacy in the long term. Unfortunately, most of the studies mentioned during this chapter examined the efficacy of several psychological interventions at a maximum of two-year follow-up, but little is known about the longer-term maintenance efficacy of such treatments. According to this, the long term efficacy of many interventions can no longer be sustained. This fact is strongly at odds with the widespread belief, shared by many clinicians, that psychotherapy has a long-term mechanism – even a "curative" action, according to some obsolete paradigms – whilst drugs are useful "just" to manage symptoms.

However, group psycho-education has long-term (five years) data, supporting its efficacy. At the five-year follow-up, psycho-educated patients showed a longer time to recurrence (log rank = 9.953, $P < 00202$) and less recurrences than non-psycho-educated patients (3.86 vs. 8.37, $t = 4.33$, p < 0.001). On the other hand, psycho-educated patients spent much less time acutely ill than nonpsycho-educated patients (Colom et al., 2009). This is mainly due to the dramatic differences accounting for time spent on depression (364 days vs. 399, $t = 5.387$, p < 0.0001). Interestingly enough, the number of days depressed has reported to be a strong predictor of recurrences according to the STEP-BD data (Perlis et al., 2006).

At the five-year follow-up (Colom et al., 2009) the number of hospitalizations per patient, is also clearly better for psycho-educated patients with 0.24 (SD = 0.52) admissions vs. 0.59 (SD = 0.96) in the control group ($t = 2.284$, $P = .025$). The mean number of days of hospitalization per hospitalized patient was also lower for psychoeducated patients; 68.26 days (SD = 65.13) in the control group vs 31.66 (SD = 16.40) in the treatment group ($t = 2.57$, $P = 0.016$).

Thus, group psycho-education is the first intervention showing efficacy at the longer term, whilst other psychological therapies may lose effect with the passing of time. This is interesting, especially if we note that psycho-educated patients did not participate in any kind of booster sessions, which means that a time-limited single intervention is able to cause a major improvement on the outcome of bipolar disorders at the longer term (five years). Group psycho-education may enhance behavioral and attitudinal changes that seem to be maintained along the years.

As in every proper training, the passing of time plays, in fact, in favor of the intervention: prevention of mania seems to be more powerful at the longer-term (Cohen's d effect size 0.4 at two years vs. 0.57 at five years), probably due to the fact that changes concerning habits regularity and, specially, early detection, may be more noticeable at the longer-term. This is also valid for any recurrence (Cohen's d effect size for prevention of all sorts of episodes 0.79 vs. 0.87).

22.9 THE FUTURE

Psycho-education is part of the standard maintenance treatment of bipolar disorder, according to the most outstanding guidelines. However, it is yet to be implemented regularly in clinical settings and this would be a major advance in the routine care of bipolar patients.

As for research, there are a number of interesting issues that should be clarified on the oncoming few years, namely:

- To investigate which psycho-education "ingredient" explains most of the efficacy of the intervention.
- To assess its effectiveness in clinical and demographic special populations (bipolar II, schizoaffective, elderly, children, and so on.).
- To introduce modules focused on physical health and on neurocognitive remediation to make it even more comprehensive.
- To research the neurobiological basis of response to psycho-education.

Many of these challenges will find an answer in the oncoming years. Similarly, we hope that more and more of our patients will find, by means of psycho-education, stability, and well-being.

22.10   FUNDING SOURCES AND ACKNOWLEDGMENTS

Francesc Colom would like to thank the support and funding of the Spanish Ministry of Health, Instituto de Salud Carlos III, CIBER-SAM. Dr. Colom is also funded by the Spanish Ministry of Science and Innovation, Instituto Carlos III,, through a "Miguel Servet" postdoctoral contract (CP08/00140) and a FIS (PS09/01044).

References

Baldassano, C.F. (2006) Illness course, comorbidity, gender, and suicidality in patients with bipolar disorder. *J. Clin. Psychiatry*, **67** (Suppl. 11), 8–11.

Bauer, M.S., Callaway, B.J., and McBride, L. (2003) *Structured Group Psychotherapy for Bipolar Disorder: The Life Goals Program*, 2nd edn, Springer Publishing Company.

Colom, F. and Vieta, E. (2006) *Psychoeducation Manual for Bipolar Disorder*, Cambridge University Press, Cambridge.

Colom, F., Vieta, E., Martínez-Arán, A. *et al.* (2000) Clinical factors associated to treatment non-compliance in euthymic bipolar patients. *J. Clin. Psychiatry*, **61**, 549–554.

Colom, F., Vieta, E., Martínez-Arán, A. *et al.* (2003) A randomized trial on the efficacy of group psychoeducation in the prophylaxis of recurrences in bipolar patients whose disease is in remission. *Arch. Gen. Psychiatry*, **60**, 402–407.

Colom, F., Vieta, E., Sánchez-Moreno, J. *et al.* (2004) Psychoeducation in bipolar patients with comorbid personality disorders. *Bipolar Disord.*, **6** (4), 294–298.

Colom, F., Vieta, E., Sánchez-Moreno, J. *et al.* (2005) Stabilizing the stabilizer: group psychoeducation enhances the stability of serum lithium levels. *Bipolar Disord.*, **7** (Suppl. 5), 32–36.

Colom, F., Vieta, E., Sánchez-Moreno, J. *et al.* (2009) Group psychoeducation for stabilised bipolar disorders: 5-year outcome of a randomized clinical trial. *Br. J. Psychiatry*, **194** (3), 260–265.

Durna, Z. and Ozcan, S. (2003) Evaluation of self-management education for asthmatic patients. *J. Asthma.*, **40**, 631–643.

Frank, E., Hlastala, S., Ritenour, A. *et al.* (1997) Inducing lifestyle regularity in recovering bipolar disorder patients: results from the maintenance therapies in bipolar disorder protocol. *Biol. Psychiatry*, **41** (12), 1165–1173.

Fristad, M.A., Verducci, J.S., Walters, K., and Young, M.E. (2009) Impact of multifamily psychoeducational psychotherapy in treating children aged 8 to 12 years with mood disorders. *Arch. Gen. Psychiatry*, **66** (9), 1013–1021.

Grant, B.F., Hasin, D.S., Stinson, F.S. *et al.* (2005) Co-occurrence of 12-month mood and anxiety disorders and personality disorders in the US: results from the national epidemiologic survey on alcohol and related conditions. *J. Psychiatr. Res.*, **39** (1), 1–9.

Harvey, N.S. and Peet, M. (1991) Lithium maintenance: effects of personality and attitude on health information acquisition and compliance. *Br. J. Psychiatry*, **158**, 200–204.

Kilbourne, A.M., Copeland, L.A., Zeber, J.E. *et al.* (2007) Determinants of complementary and alternative medicine use by patients with bipolar disorder. *Psychopharmacol. Bull.*, **40** (3), 104–115.

Linden, W. (2000) Psychological treatments in cardiac rehabilitation: review of rationales and outcomes. *J. Psychosom. Res.*, **48**, 443–454.

Miklowitz, D.J., Goldstein, M.J., Nuechterlein, K.H. *et al.* (1988) Family factors and the course of bipolar affective disorder. *Arch. Gen. Psychiatry*, **45**, 225–231.

Ng, F., Dodd, S. and Berk, M. (2007) The effects of physical activity in the acute treatment of bipolar disorder: A pilot study. *J. Affect. Disord.*, **101** (1–3), 259–262.

Olmsted, M.P., Daneman, D., Rydall, A.C. *et al.* (2002) The effects of psychoeducation on disturbed eating attitudes and behavior in young women with type 1 diabetes mellitus. *Int. J. Eat Disord.*, **32**, 230–239.

Peet, M. and Harvey, N.S. (1991) Lithium maintenance: I. A standard education program for patients. *Br. J. Psychiatry*, **158**, 197–200.

Perlis, R.H., Ostacher, M.J., Patel, J.K. *et al.* (2006) Predictors of recurrence in bipolar disorder: primary outcomes from the Systematic Treatment Enhancement Program for Bipolar Disorder (STEP-BD). *Am. J. Psychiatry*, **163** (2), 217–224.

Regier, D.A., Farmer, M.E., Rae, D.S. *et al.* (1990) Comorbidity of mental disorders with alcohol and other drug abuse. Results from the Epidemiologic Catchment Area (ECA) Study. *J. Am. Med. Assoc.*, **264** (19), 2511–2518.

Reinares, M., Colom, F., Martínez-Arán, A. *et al.* (2002) Therapeutic interventions focused on the family of bipolar patients. *Psychother. Psychosom.*, **71**, 2–10.

Reinares, M., Colom, F., Sánchez-Moreno, J. *et al.* (2008) Impact of caregiver group psychoeducation on the course and outcome of bipolar patients in remission: a randomized controlled trial. *Bipolar Disord.*, **10** (4), 511–519.

Scott, J., Colom, F., Popova, E. *et al.* (2009) Long-term mental health resource utilization and cost of care following group psychoeducation or unstructured group support for bipolar disorders: a cost-benefit analysis. *J. Clin. Psychiatry*, **70** (3), 378–386.

Simon, G.E., Ludman, E.J., Bauer, M.S. *et al.* (2006) Long-term effectiveness and cost of a systematic care program for bipolar disorder. *Arch. Gen. Psychiatry*, **63** (5), 500–508.

Simon, G.E., Ludman, E., Unützer, J., and Bauer, M.S. (2002) Design and implementation of a randomized trial evaluating systematic care for bipolar disorder. *Bipolar Disord.*, **4** (4), 226–236.

Simon, N.M., Otto, M.W., Weiss, R.D. *et al.* (2004) STEP-BD Investigators. Pharmacotherapy for bipolar disorder and comorbid conditions: baseline data from STEP-BD. *J. Clin. Psychopharmacol.*, **24** (5), 512–520.

Van Gent, E.M. (2000) Follow-up study of 3 years group therapy with lithium treatment. *Encephale*, **26**, 76–79.

Weiss, R.D., Griffin, M.L., Kolodziej, M.E. *et al.* (2007) A randomized trial of integrated group therapy versus group drug counseling for patients with bipolar disorder and substance dependence. *Am. J. Psychiatry*, **164** (1), 100–107.

23

The Role of Treatment Setting in the Pharmacotherapy of Bipolar Disorder

Jean-Michel Azorin

Department of Psychiatry, Ste Marguerite Hospital,
Marseille, France

Due to the increasing evidence that the costs of psychiatric hospitalization constitute the major component of treatment costs for bipolar patients (Keck *et al.*, 2000), it seems that nowadays third-party payers for psychiatric services have taken over from the civil rights upholders in challenging the justification for hospital treatment for such patients. As hospitalization appears to be inevitable in a vast majority of cases, as pharmacotherapy certainly is, there is an increased tendency to reduce the hospital length of stay of those patients during their manic and depressive phases, which go together with a dramatic reduction in hospital beds. The same trend towards managed care utilization as it was implemented in the U.S/ is now "threatening" European countries, one of the most refractory so far being France due to its public health maintenance organization system which provides inpatient as well as outpatient care, in accordance with its humanitarian and political tradition (since Pinel liberated the mentally ill from their chains).

As French clinicians are, in this regard, at a crossroads between tradition and modernism, it may be interesting to try to look at what we are about to lose but also acquire in changing their utilization of treatment settings for bipolar patients. These issues are in some ways generic to other countries as well.

23.1 IMPLEMENTATION OF DRUG TREATMENT ACCORDING TO PHASE AND SEVERITY OF ILLNESS

During manic and depressive phases of illness, hospitalization is often required for drug treatment. This is especially the case for severe, psychotic, and suicidal patients. For those refusing hospitalization, involuntary commitment may be necessary. Limited insight into illness, danger to self or others, significant impairment of daily activities, or uncontrollable behavior have to be considered for admission in "closed" units in the hospital. During the manic phase there is a need for a quiet and structured environment in so far as a high level of stimulation may drive and perpetuate the episode and lead to increased medication and dosage. This may be the reason why seclusion rooms are sometimes

Bipolar Psychopharmacotherapy: Caring for the patient, Second Edition. Edited by Hagop S. Akiskal and Mauricio Tohen.
© 2011 John Wiley & Sons, Ltd. Published 2011 by John Wiley & Sons, Ltd.

used. In any case, such an environment has to be provided during the hospitalization; mild and moderate patients too may benefit from it, when their home environment is a source of marked stress and high expressed emotion.

Open day hospital or outpatient treatments are alternatives in milder or moderately severe cases. When choosing to treat manic and depressive patients in these settings, clinicians need to carefully assess the quality and availability of family and social support which may take on some of the responsibility of the hospital staff, keeping in mind that mild and moderate episodes may progress to more severe forms unexpectedly.

The treatment setting can also influence the choice of drugs. The urge for rapid control of symptoms may have priority, especially in emergency rooms, leading to preferential use of intramuscular preparations, whereas in mood centers mood stabilizers tend to be preferentially prescribed as first line medications, even for acute episodes. Availability of drugs with mood stabilizing properties as intramuscular preparations may thereby facilitate and extend clinicians' compliance with current guidelines (Goodwin and Jamison, 2007; Menninger, 1995; American Psychiatric Association, 2002).

23.2 PRETREATMENT EVALUATION AND MONITORING OF PHARMACOTHERAPY

Prescribing a drug treatment, especially a mood stabilizer, in patients suffering from bipolar disorder, necessitates a careful pretreatment evaluation and further close monitoring. This is mainly due to the number of medical conditions contraindicating the use of mood stabilizers-above all lithium-likely to interfere with their use. Moreover the high frequency of side effects which can impinge on almost all body functions with this type of medication warrants a thorough assessment of baseline medical status. This is all the more true as nonadherence largely depends on the occurrence of side effects which has to be regularly monitored and which patients have to be informed of. Furthermore many of the available mood stabilizers necessitate blood levels monitoring. All the foregoing reasons explain why the pharmacotherapy of bipolar patients has to be conducted in a skilled medical environment. This is not the case for all settings, especially in some European countries where the therapeutic milieu, in either hospital or ambulatory centers, remains largely under the influence of psychodynamic practitioners. Such a milieu is typically associated with the tendency of bipolar disorder to be under-recognized and often misdiagnosed. It has been shown to be the case in France for both manic (Akiskal *et al.*, 1998) and depressive (Hantouche *et al.*, 1998) bipolar patients, however the same phenomenon has been observed in the U.S. too (Hirschfeld, Lewis, and Vornik, 2003). These patients are frequently receiving neuroleptics or antidepressants that may exacerbate their illness course and contribute to render it chronic. In France one may find a host of such patients in psychiatric hospitals or day care-centers with a diagnosis of "chronic psychotic" and a treatment based on neuroleptic depot preparations.

This emphasizes the need for mood centers, especially in European countries, as well as the usefulness of information and continuing medical education of clinicians on bipolar disorder. In addition to pharmacotherapy and medical expertise, these centers provide education of patient and significant others and psychotherapy (especially group psychotherapy) as adjunctive treatments (Colom *et al.*, 2003).

23.3   DRUG RESPONSE AND TREATMENT SETTING

Can the treatment setting influence the response to pharmacotherapy? It has been long known that hospitalization was likely to affect a patient's response to drugs. Inpatients were sometimes found to respond to drugs they has not responded to as outpatients (Kotin, Post, and Goodwin, 1973). Enhanced treatment adherence and influence of the therapeutic milieu have been evoked as explanations of this phenomenon. Controlled trials have demonstrated that monotherapy with a mood stabilizer could be effective in the short term; however it seems that maintenance treatment may often require more "aggressive" pharmacotherapy with a combination of drugs. In one study conducted in acute mania (Pope, McElroy, and Keck, 1991), of the 20 patients randomly assigned to divalproex, 9 responded with at least 50% improvement at the end of the 21-day study period; however after completion of the study when the investigators continued to follow the responders, they found that 1 patient discontinued divalproex due to side effects, 6 required the addition of antipsychotics or other mood stabilizers, and only 2 continued with monotherapy. In fact, combination treatment has been shown to be far more common than monotherapy among ambulatory bipolar patients (Solomon et al., 1997). Nearly 50% were found to receive three or more psychotropic agents, whereas only 18% received monotherapy, according to a survey conducted 10 years ago (Levine et al., 2000).

One reason which could explain those prescription patterns is the fact that bipolar patients are prematurely discharged, before they achieve full remission. Some studies (Cooke et al., 1996; Keitner et al., 1996) have found residual mania in about 70% of cases and residual depression in about 60%, which represent high rates of clinical symptomatology that have been demonstrated to increase the risk of relapse and recurrence (Keller et al., 1992).

In an NIMH study, *both* bipolar I and II patients spent nearly 50% of weeks – during an average of 13 years of naturalistic prospective follow-up – with some level of affective symptoms, mostly depressive in nature (Judd et al., 2002, 2003).

This gap between drug response and illness recovery may represent a serious challenge to our conception of modern pharmacotherapy. Short hospital stays thereby compromise patient welfare.

23.4   FROM EFFICACY TO EFFICIENCY OF PHARMACOTHERAPY IN BIPOLAR ILLNESS

One way to bridge this gap has been to emphasize the difference existing between the efficacy of a drug and its efficiency. The first concept refers to the pharmacological and symptomatic effect whereas the second stresses its consequences for the healing and easing of illness (Azorin, Naudin and Kaladjian, 2002). It is the first we are assessing when we measure a drug response with a rating scale, but we are referring to the second when we are speaking of quality of life and recovery. This difference is not without consequences on how we are taking care of our patients, even when we are prescribing a drug. If we are restricting ourselves to the concept of efficacy, we just expect from a medication a mere and direct physiological change, whereas referring to that of efficiency allows us to expect from the patient that he will be able to use the changes induced by the drug as a means to achieve recovery, that is an indirect effect. One could speak thereby of the antimanic or antidepressant effect of the drug which sets free the coping strategies the patient can use to recover. Mania or depression is certainly an illness, but from a psychodynamic and/or anthropological viewpoint it has also been considered as a crisis in identity, that is, temporary dissolution of a rigid, sclerotic identity, acquired through over-identification to social roles and value-fixation (Kraus, 1977). That means a particular way of being in relationship with oneself, the others and the world: in this context depression but also to some extent mania conveys the meaning of a threat to identity, and giving the patient a sick role has been deemed giving him a substitutive and protective identity, especially during the hospitalization phase. In certain cases premature discharge could thereby mean a new loss of identity and precipitate relapses. Offering patients a therapeutic milieu may be not just passively awaiting changes in rating scales using "magical" drugs, but trying, on the basis of these changes, to help them reconstitute a more flexible identity in an appropriate setting.

Traditional representations of the role of hospitalization in the treatment of mental disorders which still prevail in some European countries have been changing during the last decade. Progresses in pharmacotherapy and technical interventions may partly explain these changes, but economic pressure and the necessity of cost savings are certainly the main determinants.

Nevertheless, clinical experience suggests that bipolar patients characterized by their instability of mood may benefit from the highly structured setting offered by the psychiatric hospital. A mood episode is not only a phase in illness but also an identity crisis which necessitates a person-centered approach. The hospital represents a protected setting where the conflicts keeping this crisis going can be expressed and sometimes resolved (Goodwin and Jamison, 2007).

We still do not know what the consequences of losing benefit from such settings could be in the long run, in spite of the progress in modern treatments. Some of these consequences are, however, perceptible such as the "trans-institutionalization" phenomenon which has appeared in many countries, with an increasing number of bipolar patients found in prison populations (Goodwin and Jamison, 2007; London and Taylor, 1982). This is a grave problem facing Western psychiatry which, in its attempt to shorten acute psychiatric hospitalization for bipolar patients, is creating homelessness, with its resultant lack of family supervision, and the development of social marginalization of the mentally ill – and at worst leading to a criminal incarceration – instead of the more benign and humane psychiatric hospitalization when needed.

References

Akiskal, H.S., Hantouche, E.G., Bourgeois, M.L. *et al.* (1998) Gender, temperament, and the clinical picture in dysphoric mixed mania: Findings from a French national study (EPIMAN). *J. Affect. Disord.*, **50**, 175–186.

American Psychiatric Association (2002) *Guidelines for Bipolar Disorder. Practice Guidelines*, American Psychiatric Press, Washington, DC.

Azorin, J.M., Naudin, J., and Kaladjian, A. (2002) Efficacité et efficience des psychotropes. *Evol. Psychiatr.*, **67**, 170–183.

Colom, F., Vieta, E., Martinez-Aran, A. *et al.* (2003) A randomized trial on the efficacy of group psychoeducation in the prophylaxis of recurrences in bipolar patients whose disease is in remission. *Arch. Gen. Psychiatry*, **60**, 402–407.

Cooke, R.G., Robb, J.C., Young, L.T. *et al.* (1996) Well-being and functioning in patients with bipolar disorder assessed using the MOS 20-item short form (SF-20). *J. Affect. Disord.*, **39**, 93–97.

Goodwin, F.K. and Jamison, K.R. (2007) *Manic-Depressive Illness: Bipolar Disorders and Recurrent Depression*, Oxford University Press, Oxford.

Hantouche, E.G., Akiskal, H.S., Lancrenon, S. *et al.* (1998) Systematic clinical methodology for validating bipolar – II disorder: data in mid-stream from a French national multi-site study (EPIDEP). *J. Affect. Disord.*, **50**, 163–173.

Hirschfeld, R.M.A., Lewis, L., and Vornik, L.A. (2003) Perceptions and impact of bipolar disorder: how far have we really come? Results of the national depressive and manic-depressive association 2000 survey of individuals with bipolar disorder. *J. Clin. Psychiatry*, **64**, 161–174.

Judd, L.L., Akiskal, H.S., Schettler, P.J. *et al.* (2002) The long-term natural history of the weekly symptomatic status of bipolar I disorder. *Arch. Gen. Psychiatry*, **59**, 530–537.

Judd, L.L., Akiskal, H.S., Schettler, P.J. *et al.* (2003) A prospective investigation of the natural history of the long-term weekly symptomatic status of bipolar II disorder. *Arch. Gen. Psychiatry*, **60**, 261–269.

Keck, P.E., Mc Elroy, S.L., and Arnold, L.M. (2000) The costs of treatment of bipolar disorder, in *Bipolar Disorders: 100 Years After Manic-Depressive Insanity* (eds A. Marneros and J. Angst), Kluwer Academic Publishers, Dordrecht, pp. 437–448.

Keitner, G.I., Solomon, D.A., Ryan, C.E. *et al.* (1996) Prodromal and residual symptoms in bipolar I disorder. *Compr. Psychiatry*, **37**, 362–367.

Keller, M.B., Lavori, P.W., Kane, J.M. *et al.* (1992) Subsyndromal symptoms in bipolar patients. A comparison of standard and low serum levels of lithium. *Arch. Gen. Psychiatry*, **49**, 371–376.

Kotin, J., Post, R.M., and Goodwin, F.K. (1973) Drug treatment of depressed patients referred for hospitalization. *Am. J. Psychiatry*, **130**, 1139–1141.

Kraus, A (1977) *Sozialverhalten und Psychose Manisch-Depressiver*, Enke, Stuttgart.

Levine, J., Chengappa, K.N.R., Brar, J.S. *et al.* (2000) Psychotropic drug prescription patterns among patients with bipolar I disorder. *Bipolar Disord.*, **2**, 120–130.

London, W.P. and Taylor, B.M. (1982) Bipolar disorders in a forensic setting. *Compr. Psychiatry*, **23**, 33–37.

Menninger, W.W. (1995) Role of the psychiatric hospital in the treatment of mental illness, in *Comprehensive Textbook of Psychiatry/VI*, vol. **2** (eds H.I. Kaplan and B.J. Sadock), Williams and Wilkins, Baltimore, pp. 2690–2696.

Pope, H.G. Jr., Mc Elroy, S.L., and Keck, P.E. Jr. (1991) Valproate in the treatment of acute mania: a placebo-controlled study. *Arch. Gen. Psychiatry*, **48**, 62–68.

Solomon, D.A., Ryan, C.E., Keitner, G.I. *et al.* (1997) A pilot study of lithium carbonate plus divalproex sodium fort he continuation and maintenance treatment of patients with bipolar I disorder. *J. Clin. Psychiatry*, **58**, 95–99.

Pharmacological Prevention of Suicide in Bipolar Patients

Zoltán Rihmer

Department of Clinical and Theoretical Mental Health, and Department of Psychiatry and Psychotherapy, Semmelweis University, Faculty of Medicine, Budapest, Hungary

24.1 INTRODUCTION

The prediction and prevention of suicidal behavior among psychiatric patients is not only a great challenge for the psychiatrists, but could also be among the most reliable indicators of the efficacy of **clinicians**. Suicide behavior and particularly committed suicide, which is the most serious complication of untreated major psychiatric illness, is one of the most tragic events in human life. Although suicide is very complex, multi-causal behavior, involving several medical-biologic, psycho-social and cultural components, history of major mood disorders (particularly in the presence of previous suicide attempt) constitutes the most important risk factor. However, because the majority of mood disorder patients never commit (and up to 50% of them never attempt) suicide, other familial-genetic, clinical, and psychosocial risk factors also play a significant contributory role (Akiskal, 2007; Rihmer, 2005, 2007).

24.2 MOOD DISORDERS AND SUICIDAL BEHAVIOR

Psychological autopsy studies from several countries of the world consistently show that over 90% of consecutive suicide victims have one or more Axis I (mostly untreated) major psychiatric disorders at the time of their deaths, and major mood disorders (59–87%) schizophrenia/schizoaffective disorder (10–12%), and substance-use disorders (10–15%) are the most common principal diagnoses. Dysthymic disorder, anxiety disorders, person-ality disorders, or serious medical illness itself as the only diagnoses in suicide victims are quite rare, but they are commonly present as additional diagnoses (Cheng *et al.*, 2000; Goodwin and Jamison 1990; Hawton and van Heeringen 2000; Rihmer, Belső, and Kiss, 2002). Reviewing 17 follow-up studies on committed suicide in patients with primary affective disorders, Guze and Robins (1970) found that about 15% of formerly hospitalized depressed patients would die by suicide. Goodwin and Jamison (1990) also concluded that 19% of depressed patients (mainly inpatients) died by suicide. In their meta-analysis of studies on suicide risk in psychiatric disorders, Harris and Barraclough

Bipolar Psychopharmacotherapy: Caring for the patient, Second Edition. Edited by Hagop S. Akiskal and Mauricio Tohen.
© 2011 John Wiley & Sons, Ltd. Published 2011 by John Wiley & Sons, Ltd.

(1997) analyzed separately the risk of suicide in unipolar major depression and in bipolar disorder. They found that the risk of suicide was about 20-fold for patients with index diagnosis of unipolar major depression, and the same figure for bipolar disorder was 15. However, these three studies (Goodwin and Jamison, 1990; Guze and Robins, 1970; Harris and Barraclough, 1997) cannot provide a precise estimation of separate suicide risk in unipolar and bipolar disorder, that is, they overestimate the risk for unipolar depression and underestimate it for bipolar disorders. The main sources of these are that the index diagnosis frequently change during the follow-up from unipolar depression to bipolar disorder (Akiskal *et al.*, 1995; Goldberg, Harrow, and Whiteside, 2001; Akiskal *et al.*, 2003) and in the studies reviewed by the mentioned authors the diagnostic category of bipolar II depression (depression with hypomania but not with mania) which is the most common form of bipolar disorders has not been considered separately. It is very likely that the majority of bipolar II patients in these studies were included in the unipolar major depressive subgroup. In addition, recent results showed that about 50% of unipolar depressions were found to be bipolar depressions after careful and skillful probing for past hypomania or mania and when the bipolar spectrum disorders (that is, "unipolar" depression with bipolar family history, treatment-associated hypomania/mania in major depression, and depressive mixed state/agitation) were also considered (Akiskal *et al.*, 2005; Benazzi and Akiskal, 2003a; Ghaemi, Boima, and Goodwin, 2000).

24.3 RISK OF SUICIDAL BEHAVIOR IN BIPOLAR DISORDERS

Since specific diagnostic subtypes of major mood disorders (unipolar, bipolar I, and bipolar II) show several differences from both clinical and research perspective (Akiskal, 2002; Akiskal *et al.*, 1995; Goodwin and Jamison, 1990; Tondo *et al.*, 1999), it is logical to assume that each subgroup might have its own different suicide risk. Considering only the 10 studies, in which unipolar, bipolar I, and bipolar II patients were analyzed separately, and summarizing the data (Rihmer, 2005; Table 24.1), it can be seen that the rate of previous suicide attempts is the lowest in unipolar major depression (13%) and the rate of prior suicidal behavior in bipolar patients (types I and II combined) is much higher (28%) than that of unipolars. The lifetime rates of suicide attempts in both bipolar I and in bipolar II patients (26 and 33%, respectively) are also markedly elevated

Table 24.1 Lifetime prevalence of suicide attempt(s) in unipolar major depression, bipolar I and bipolar II disorder according to 10 independent studies, reviewed by Rihmer, 2005.

	Prior suicide attempt		Range
Diagnostic subtype	n	%	%
Unipolar major depression (n = 1328)	177	13	9–30
Bipolar disorder (I + II) (n = 1859)	525	28	10–61
Bipolar I (n = 1319)	349	26	10–50
Bipolar II (n = 540)	176	33	18–61

comparing to the same figure for unipolar patients. Re-analyzing the ECA database, Judd and Akiskal (2003) also reported that the rate of prior suicide attempt(s) was higher in bipolar II (34%) than in bipolar I (24%) patients, while the same figure for unipolar major depression was 16% (Chen and Dilsaver, 1996).

Investigating the clinical characteristics of 230 inpatients with recurrent major depression, Bulik et al. (1990) found that bipolar II diagnosis was significantly more frequent among the 67 patients who attempted suicide (19%) than in the 163 patients without suicide attempt (9%). Dunner, Gershon, and Goodwin (1976) reported that 3% of the 73 unipolar, 6% of the 68 bipolar I, and 18% of the 22 bipolar II patients died by suicide during their one to nine year follow-up study.

In contrast to the above-mentioned studies, Angst et al. (2002) found that during the 34–38-year follow-up study of hospitalized patients with major mood disorders (unipolar, n = 186, bipolar I and II combined, n = 220), a higher proportion of unipolar patients died by suicide than that of bipolar patients (14% vs. 8%). On the other hand, however, in their very recent long-term prospective follow up study (average 11 years) on 1983 unipolar major depressives and 843 bipolar (I + II) patients, Tondo, Lepri, and Baldessarini (2007) found five-times fold higher rate of completed suicide in bipolar I and II than in unipolar patients (0.25% of patients/year vs 0.05% of patients/year). This study also found that the ratio of attempted to completed suicide in bipolar II, bipolar I, and unipolar depression was 5, 11, and 10, respectively, indicating that the lethality of suicide attempts was far highest in bipolar II patients.

Although suicidal behavior is quite frequent among all patients with major mood disorders, the findings strongly suggest that bipolar II patients might be at particularly high risk (Akiskal, 2007). The two published reports where the prevalence of bipolar II, bipolar I, and unipolar depression have been analyzed separately among the suicide victims shows that among the 125 consecutive suicide victims with primary major depression at the time of suicide, 44% had bipolar II depression, 2% had bipolar I depression, and 54% had first episode or recurrent unipolar depression (Rihmer et al., 1990; Rihmer, Rutz, and Pihlgren, 1995; Table 24.2). Because the lifetime prevalence rates of DSM-III/IV bipolar II illness in the population are relatively low compared with unipolar major depression (2–5 and 15–17%, respectively) (Angst, 1998; Szádóczky et al., 1998), these results suggest that bipolar II disorder imparts a particularly high risk of committed suicide among the three different subgroups of major mood disorders.

Analyzing the specific diagnostic subtypes of 69 consecutive (nonviolent) suicide attempters with current DSM-IV major depression in Budapest, Hungary, it has been

Table 24.2 Diagnostic distribution of bipolar II, bipolar I and unipolar major depression among consecutive suicide victims with major depressive episode at the time of suicide.

Source	Bipolar II		Bipolar I		Unipolar	
	Rate	%	Rate	%	Rate	%
Rihmer et al. (1990)	46/100	46	1/100	1	53/100	53
Rihmer, Rutz, and Pihlgren (1995)	9/25	36	2/25	8	14/25	56
Total	55/125	44	3/125	2	67/125	54

found that 45 (65%) had unipolar major depression, 19 (28%) had bipolar II e depression, and 5 (7%) had bipolar I depression (Balázs *et al.*, 2003). Considering the fact that the lifetime prevalence rates of DSM-III-R unipolar major depression, bipolar II, and bipolar I disorder in the general population of Hungary are 15.1, 2.0, and 1.5% respectively (Szádóczky *et al.*, 1998), this study suggests that bipolar II patients are relatively overrepresented not only among depressed suicide victims (Rihmer *et al.*, 1990; Rihmer, Rutz, and Pihlgren, 1995), but also among depressed suicide attempters.

Bipolar patients with comorbid anxiety, substance-use, and personality disorders as well as bipolar depressives with DSM-IV atypical features are also at an increased risk of attempted or completed suicide (Chen and Dilsaver, 1996; Balázs *et al.*, 2003; Isometsä *et al.*, 1994; Sánchez-Gistau *et al.*, 2009; Tondo *et al.*, 1999; Vieta *et al.*, 1997). One of the major sources of the highest suicide risk in bipolar II patients may be the very high rate of atypical depression, comorbid anxiety disorders (Akiskal, 1981; Rihmer *et al.*, 2001, Sánchez-Gistau *et al.*, 2009), substance-use disorders (Akiskal, 1981; Vieta *et al.*, 1997; Brieger, 2000), and depressive mixed states, frequently called "agitated depression" (Akiskal *et al.*, 2005; Akiskal, 2007; Benazzi and Akiskal, 2003b; Koukopoulos and Koukopoulos 1999). The importance of depressive mixed states in predicting suicidal behavior is supported by several recent studies (Maser *et al.*, 2002; Akiskal *et al.*, 2005; Balázs *et al.*, 2006; Valtonen *et al.*, 2008) and current findings also show that cyclothymic/irritable affective temperaments, that are characteristic also mainly for bipolar II disorder, also increase the risk of suicidal behavior (Rihmer *et al.*, 2010). It should be noted, however, that in the majority of cases many suicide risk factors are present and they have an additive effect on the self-destructive behavior. (Maser *et al.*, 2002; Akiskal, 2007; Rihmer, 2005, 2007). Analyzing the clinical and demographic characteristics of more than 1000 bipolar I patients, admitted for an index manic episode, Azorin *et al.* (2009a, 2009b) found that the following risk factors were significantly associated with lifetime suicide attempts: multiple hospitalizations, depressive, or mixed polarity at first episode, cyclothymic temperament, lifetime anxiety disorder comorbidity, stressful life events before illness onset, younger age at onset, no free intervals between episodes, female sex, and higher number of prior episodes. Anxiety disorder comorbidity in bipolar patients is the rule rather than the exception (Chen and Dilsaver, 1996; Brieger, 2000; Rihmer *et al.*, 2001; Akiskal, 2002) and it is also true for juvenile patients with bipolar disorder (Dilsaver *et al.*, 2007). This study also found that in adolescent patients with bipolar disorder comorbid PTSD significantly increased the risk of prior suicide attempts even after controlling for the confounding effects of comorbid OCD, panic disorder, and social phobia.

Among bipolar patients, however, it is not the depressive episode, that is, the only risk period for suicide. In contrast to classical (that is, euphoric) mania, where suicidal tendency is extremely rare suicidal thoughts and attempts are relatively common in dysphoric (mixed) mania or hypomania (Isometsä *et al.*, 1994; Strakowski *et al.*, 1996; Tondo *et al.*, 1999).

Family history of suicide is a significant risk factor for suicide behavior, particularly in persons with bipolar disorder. Bipolar patients with positive family history of suicide in first-degree relatives were found to be significantly more likely to attempt suicide (38%) than those without (14%) (Roy, 1983), and it has been reported that 0.9% of unipolar depressives, 1.8% of bipolar I, and 2.9% of bipolar II patients had a family history of committed suicide (Dunner, Gershon, and Goodwin, 1976). Another study has found a 6.5-fold higher rate of suicide committed among the first-degree relatives of 129 bipolar II (3.9%) than that of the 188 bipolar I (0.6%) patients (Tondo et al., 1998).

Recent adverse life events, as well as permanent psychosocial stressors, have been shown to be also a risk factor for attempted or completed suicide, particularly in the frame of major depressive, mixed depressive, or dysphoric manic episodes (Cheng et al., 2000; Hawton and van Heeringen, 2000; Valtonen et al., 2008). However, it should be noted that these adverse life events are frequently the results of the patient's own (socially desinhibited) behavior during their manic of hypomanic episodes.

In spite of the fact that the lifetime prevalence of major mood disorders (unipolar and bipolar forms combined) in the population is about 20% (Angst, 1998; Szádóczky et al., 1998), they remain highly under-referred, underdiagnosed, and undertreated, and it is particularly true for bipolar II patients (Akiskal, 2007; Balázs et al., 2003; Isometsä et al., 1994; Goldberg, Harrow, and Whiteside, 2001; Rihmer et al., 1990; Rihmer, Belső, and Kiss, 2002). On the other hand, despite of the fact that up to 66% of suicide victims contact different levels of health care four weeks before suicide (Hawton and van Heeringen, 2000; Rihmer, Belső, and Kiss, 2002), the rate of adequate pharmacotherapy among depressed suicide victims is disturbingly low (Hawton and van Heeringen, 2000; Isacsson, 2000; Rihmer et al., 1990; Rihmer, Belső, and Kiss, 2002). Since successful acute and long-term pharmacotherapy of mood disorders relieves not only the clinical symptoms, but parallel with this also decreases or vanishes suicidality, appropriate acute, and long-term treatment of mood disorders can be declared as a key issue in suicide prevention (Baldessarini et al., 2006; Isacsson, 2000; Rihmer, Belső, and Kiss, 2002; Rihmer, 2007; Sondergard et al., 2008; Tondo and Baldessarini, 2000). Therefore, lacking treatment in patients with major mood (particularly bipolar) disorder as well as noncompliance with the treatment can also be considered as major suicide risk factors. Table 24.3 shows the clinically most important suicide risk factors in bipolar disorders.

24.4 SUICIDE PREVENTION IN BIPOLAR DISORDERS

Since suicidal behavior is a multicausal phenomenon with many biological, psychological, and cultural components, its prevention should also be complex, even in the case of bipolar disorder which is the "most biological" illness in the field of psychiatry and which requires long-term pharmacotherapy in the majority of the cases. Since bipolar disorders usually show a peak onset between 15 and 25 years of age, but there is 8–10 years of delay in correct diagnosis (Akiskal, 2002; Ghaemi, Boima, and Goodwin, 2000; Goodwin and Jamison, 1990; Szádóczky et al., 1998), early detection of bipolar the nature of the disorder, including the soft manifestations as well, is the first step in suicide prevention. Misdiagnosis of bipolar depression as unipolar depression results in treatment with antidepressants alone, and this can have negative effects on the course of the illness, because of inducing mixed depressive episodes, hypomanic or manic switches, rapid cycling, and therefore increasing the chance of suicidal behavior (Benazzi, 2003; Benazzi and Akiskal, 2003b; Ghaemi, Boima, and Goodwin, 2000; Henry et al., 2001; Koukopoulos et al., 1983; Rihmer and Akiskal, 2006).

Table 24.3 Clinically significant major suicide risk factors in bipolar disorders.

Diagnostic subtype
    Bipolar II > bipolar I
Previous suicide attempt
    Violent > non-violent
    High lethality > low lethality
Clinical features
    Severe depression, hopelessness, insomnia, guilt
    DSM-IV atypical features (hypersomnia, hyperphagia, mood-reactivity,
       rejection sensitivity, laden paraéysis, etc.)
    Mixed depressive episode/agitation
    Dysphoric (mixed) mania or hypomania
    Mixed affective episode
    Comorbid anxiety/anxiety disorders, substance-use, and personality disorders
    Cyclothymic/irritable affective temperament
Family history of suicide in first-and second degree relatives
Permanent adverse life situations, acute psychosocial stressors
Lacking adequate acute and long-term treatment/care
Noncompliance with the treatment

Table 24.4 Suicide prevention strategies in bipolar disorders. The role of health care.

  I. Elimination of acute suicide danger (emergency hospitalization, sedation, anxiolysis, crisis-intervention)
 II. Improving the diagnosis and treatment of bipolar disorders with particular regard to the soft clinical manifestations
     1. Education of health care workers, patients, and relatives
     2. Adequate acute and long-term treatment/aftercare (pharmacotherapy, non-pharmacological interventions such as psychoeducation, psychotherapy, cognitive therapy, family counselling/family therapy, etc.)
III. Improving the patients' compliance (psychoeducation, psychotherapy, cognitive therapy, etc.)
IV. Reducing the stigma against bipolar disorders via media

    The role of health care in the suicide prevention of bipolar patients is summarized in Table 24.4.

    As suicide behavior in bipolar patients occur mostly during severe pure or mixed depressive episodes and less frequently in the frame of dysphoric (mixed) mania, but practically never during euphoric mania and euthymia (that is, suicidal behavior in bipolar patients is state-and severity dependent phenomenon) (Isometsä *et al.*, 1994; Simpson and Jamison, 1999; Tondo *et al.*,1999; Rihmer, 2005, 2007), it is logical to assume that effective acute and long-term treatment has a strong protection against suicide, suicide attempts, and probably against other complications (secondary substance-use disorders, marital instability, loss of job, cardiovascular morbidity/mortality, violent behavior, and so on).

24.4.1   THE ROLE OF PSYCHOPHARMACONS IN SUICIDE PREVENTION OF BIPOLAR PATIENTS

While successful acute pharmacotherapy of depressive or mixed episodes can only prevent the risk of suicide connected with a given episode, it is only adequate prophylactic therapy that can provide long-term results in patients with bipolar illness.

24.4.1.1   Lithium and Antiepileptic Mood Stabilizers

The efficacy of lithium in the treatment of manic states and in prevention recurrences of bipolar patients is well documented (Goodwin and Jamison, 1990; Goodwin, 1999; Maj, Tortorella, and Bartoli, 2000; Bowden, 2002), and recent data indicate that combination of lithium (and other mood-stabilizers) with antidepressants reduces the chance of hypomanic or manic switching when bipolar depression is treated with antidepressants (Henry *et al.*, 2001; Mundo *et al.*, 2006). However, about 50% of bipolar patients do not show satisfactory prophylactic response to lithium; positive family history of bipolar illness, early onset, mania-depression-interval type of course predicts a good prophylactic response, while higher frequency of episodes, depression-mania-interval type of course, and comorbid substance-use disorders indicate poor response (Bowden, 2002; Goodwin and Jamison, 1990; Goodwin, 1999; Maj, Tortorella, and Bartoli, 2000). The place of antiepilectics (valproate, carbamazepine, lamotrigine) in the acute and long-term treatment of bipolar disorders is also well established. Predictors of better response to anticonvulsants than to lithium are mixed episodes, rapid cycling, comorbid substance-use disorders, and previous lithium nonresponse (Bowden, 2002; Goodwin and Jamison, 1990; Goodwin, 1999; Maj, Tortorella, and Bartoli, 2000).

In a recent, comprehensive review of 45 randomized, controlled, and open clinical studies (including 34 studies also providing data without lithium treatment) involving a total of 85 229 person-years of risk exposure. Baldessarini *et al.* (2006) reported about 80% risk reduction for attempted and completed suicides either in unipolar or in bipolar patients with long-term lithium treatment. The risk reduction was similar for suicide attempts and for completed suicides. The incidence-ratio of attempts-to-suicides increased 2.5 times with lithium treatment, indicating reduced lethality of suicuidal acts. The authors concluded that the robust reduction of suicidal behavior with lithium maintenance in bipolar and unipolar patients to overall levels was close to general population rates. This marked anti-suicidal potential of lithium seems to be more than the simple result of its episode-prophylactic effect, as it has been demonstrated that during the long term lithium prophylaxis of 167 recurrent bipolar or unipolar affective disorder patients with at least one prior suicide attempt, a significant reduction in the number of suicide attempts was found not only in the excellent responders (92%), but also in moderate responders (78%), and in poor responders (70%) (Ahrens and Müller-Oerlinghausen, 2001). The clinical importance of this finding is that in the case of lithium nonresponse, when the patient has one or more suicide risk factor, instead of switching lithium to another mood stabilizer, the clinician should retain lithium (even on a lower dose) and combine it with another mood stabilizer.

The marked anti-suicidal effect of lithium in bipolar and unipolar major mood disorder patients has also been supported recently from an epidemiological perspective: investigating the lithium levels in tap water in 18 municipalities in Japan in relation to the suicide mortality in each municipality, the authors found that lithium levels were significantly and negatively associated with suicide rate averages for 2002–2006 (Ohgami et al., 2009).

In a 34–38 year-long naturalistic follow-up study including 220 formerly hospitalized bipolar I and bipolar II patients, Angst et al. (2002) found that patients who received long-term pharmacotherapy (lithium, neuroleptics, antidepressants) tended to live longer and to have significantly (2.5-fold) lower suicide rate (13.1% vs. 5.2%) than untreated bipolars. Interestingly, they also found significantly lower rates from all natural deaths among treated vs. untreated bipolars.

In a randomized, open-label, perspective, 2.5-year-folow-up study Thies-Flechtner et al. (1996) investigated the number of suicide events in 175 bipolar, 110 schizoaffective, and 93 recurrent depressive patients. The patients were randomly assigned to lithium, carbamazepine, or amitriptyline. There were 14 serious suicide events (9 completed suicides and 5 serious attempts) during the study, and 7 out of the 14 events (6 suicides and 1 attempt) were among the bipolar patients. Most of the 14 suicide acts happened in the carbamazepine group (4 suicides and 5 attempts), and none of the 14 suicidal patients were taking lithium. These results also indicate that lithium has a strong antisuicidal effect which markedly exceeds its prophylactic efficacy. This effect may be related to the well-known antiaggressive and serotonin-agonistic activity of lithium (Ahrens and Müller-Oerlinghausen, 2001; Goodwin and Jamison, 1990).

On the other hand, however, in a retrospective chart review study of 140 out-patients with bipolar disorders treated continuously for a minimum of six months during a 23-year-period of private practice, Yerevanian, Koek, and Mintz (2003) found more than twofold reduction in nonlethal suicidal behavior during, compared with after, discontinuation of mood stabilizers (lithium, valproate, or carbamazepine). The frequency of nonlethal suicidal behavior was not different during treatment with lithium, compared with valproate or carbamazepine. It is also important to note that only one completed suicide (during a period off of lithium) occured in this sample.

In the most recent naturalistic, retrospective chart review study of 405 bipolar patients seen in a large US Veterans Administration health care system Yerevanian, Koek, and Mintz (2007a) analyzed the risk of suicidal behavior of the patients followed for a mean of three years. As there was only one completed suicide in this study the analysis was restricted only to suicide attempts and serious suicidal ideation resulting in hospital admission. The findings showed that mood stabilizer monotherapy (lithium, divalproex, carbamazepine) reduced the risk of suicidal behavior by more than 90%. Lithium and antiepileptic mood stabilizers showed similar benefits in this respect.

In a population-based retrospective "real word" cohort study on more than 20000 patients with bipolar I or bipolar II disorder Goodwin et al. (2003) compared the risk of suicide and suicide attempts during lithium treatment with that of during divalproex or carbamazepine treatment. There was no exposure to lithium, divalproex, or carbamazepine during 45% of all person-years of the follow-up (mean: 2.9 years). In this observational study, where milder or nonsuicidal cases were probably overrepresented among patients who had never been treated with any mood stabilizer, it has been found a 42% reduction in suicide death among patients taking lithium compared to those who were not treated with any mood stabilizers. After adjustment for age, sex, comorbid disorders, and concommittant use of other psychotropics, the authors found that the risk of suicide deaths and suicide attempts resulting in hospitalization were 2.7 and 1.8 times higher during treatment with divalproex and 1.5 and 2.9 times higher during treatment with carbamazepine than during treatment with lithium. These results are in good agreement with the findings of Thies-Flechtner et al. (1996), who reported that among patients treated for bipolar disorders the risk of suicidal behavior was lower during lithium treatment than during treatment with carbamazepine.

Using linkage of national registers, Sondergard et al. (2008) investigated the association between continued mood stabilizing treatment and suicide among all patients discharged nationwide from hospital psychiatry as an in- or outpatient during 1995 and 2000 in Denmark with an ICD-10 diagnosis of bipolar disorder (n = 5926). The results showed that patients who continued treatment with mood stabilizers (lithium, divalproex, lamotrigine, oxcarbazepine, and topiarmate) had a significantly decreased rate of suicide compared to patients who purchased mood stabilizers once only and the rate of suicide decreased consistently with the number of additional prescriptions. The authors also found that a switch to or augmentation with lithium to patients initiated on antiepileptic mood stabilizers was associated with a significantly reduced suicide rate whereas a switch to or augmentation with antiepileptics to patients first started on lithium showed no additional effect on suicide mortality. Although long-term treatment with lithium and antiepileptic mood stabilizers was associated with similar reduction in the suicide mortality, these results suggest that lithium may have some superiority in preventing suicide.

Analyzing the 12 662 Oregon Medicaid patients diagnosed with bipolar disorders and treated with mood stabilizers between 1998 and 2003 Collins and McFarland (2008) found that the adjusted hazard ratios (versus lithium) for suicide attempts were 2.7 for divalproex users (p = 0.001), 2.8 for carbamazepine users (not significant), and 1.6 for gabapentin users (not significant). For completed suicides the hazard ratios were 1.5 for divalproex users (not significant), 2.6 for gabapentin users (p = 0.001), and not available for carbamazepine users.

24.4.1.2 Antidepressants and Antipsychotics

The role of typical and atypical antipsychotics in the acute treatment of mania, mixed states, and psychotic depression is well considered (Bowden, 2002; Goodwin and Jamison, 1990; Maj, Tortorella, and Bartoli, 2000). Recent results suggest that some atypical antipsychotics (olanzapine quetiapine, and aripirazol) have long-term mood-stabilizing effect in patients with bipolar disorders (Keck and McElroy, 2003; Tohen et al., 2005; Young et al., 2008; Yatham et al., 2009), but their putative specific anti-suicidal effects need further studies.

Antidepressants have very limited value in the long-term treatment of bipolar disorders because of their mood-destabilizing effects (Benazzi, 2003; Bowden, 2002; Maj, Tortorella, and Bartoli, 2000; Rihmer and Akiskal, 2006). However, rates of hypomanic or manic switches during treatment with SSRIs are much lower than with TCAs, and mood stabilizers further reduce the risk of the mood switch (Bowden, 2002; Henry *et al.*, 2001). The study by Yerevanian and collegaues also showed that during the long-term pharmacotherapy of bipolar patients the risk of suicidal behavior is highest in patients with antidepressant and antipsychotic monotherapy (Yerevanian *et al.*, 2007b, Yerevanian, Koek, and Mintz, 2007c), lowest in patients with mood stabilizer monotherapy (Yerevanian, Koek, and Mintz, 2007a) and the risk of patients with combination therapy (mood stabilizers + antidepressants or antipsychotics) showed an intermediate position with similar risk of suicidal behavior to bipolar patients during the period "off" mood stabilizer (Yerevanian, Koek, and Mintz, 2007a, Yerevanian *et al.*, 2007b, Yerevanian, Koek, and Mintz, 2007c). This suggest that combination of antidepressants or antipsychotics with mood stabilizers substantially reduces (but does not eliminate) the elevated risk of suicide seen in patients on antidepressant or antipsychotic monotherapy, and only mood stabilizer monotherapy provides the best result in this respect. These findings have important clinical implications: clinicians who add antidepressants or antipsychotics to mood stabilizers to treat breakthrough depression or mania during the long-term treatment of their bipolar patients should consider that antidepressants and antipsychotics may increase the risk of suicidal behavior; therefore, they should keep their patients on these supplementary medications as short a time as possible and the main component of the long-term pharmacotherapy should be the mood stabilizer monotherapy.

24.4.2   THE ROLE OF PSYCHOSOCIAL INTERVENTIONS IN SUICIDE PREVENTION OF BIPOLAR PATIENTS

In the last decade more and more effective psychosocial interventions in the field of bipolar disorders were developed primarily for patients who show insufficient response to acute and long-term pharmacotherapy, who cannot tolerate drugs or who are noncompliant with the treatment (Bauer, 2002; Fountoulakis *et al.*, 2009). The main targets of these interventions are: preventing medication noncompliance with psychoeducation or with cognitive-behavioral therapy, lifestyle modification, teaching patients and relatives to identify early symptoms of relapse and obtain treatment as early as possible, and modification of family and other interpersonal conflicts (Bauer, 2002; Colom and Vieta, 2002; Lam *et al.*, 2003; Fava *et al.*, 2001). These psychosocial techniques specifically designed for relapse/recurrence prevention in bipolar patients are effective either alone, or mostly in conjunction with mood stabilizers, and they are discussed in detail elsewhere (Bauer, 2002; Colom and Vieta, 2002; Fountoulakis *et al.*, 2009; **Miklowitz in this book**). These psychosocial interventions, while reducing relapse/recurrence may indirectly reduce the risk of suicide. However, there is only one published study concerning the effect on suicidality of intensive psychosocial treatment that specifically targeted suicidality in bipolar disorder. Rucci *et al.* (2002) investigated the lifetime rates of suicide attempts among 175 bipolar I patients during a two-year-period of intensive pharmacotherapy (lithium, valproate, carmabazepine), and one of two adjunctive psychosocial interventions (psychotherapy specific to bipolar disorder or nonspecific intensive clinical management).

They found that the patients experienced 3-fold reduction in the rate of suicide attempts during the acute treatment phase and a 18-fold reduction during maintenance. There was no significant difference regarding suicide attempts between the two subgroups with different psychosocial interventions.

However, the interaction between pharmacotherapy and psychosocial interventions is quite complex. It has been reported that successful episode-preventive medication with mood stabilizers in bipolar patients counteracted dysfunctional cognitions (including lowered self-esteem), and adjunctive cognitive therapy could help to optimize the long-term course of bipolar illness (Wolf and Müller-Oerlinghausen, 2002).

Mental health professionals and physicians are, of course, unable to prevent all suicides. However, our present pharmacological and psychosocial intentions are effective enough to minimize the chance of suicide in patients with bipolar disorder that represents the highest risk of self-inflicted death.

References

Ahrens, B. and Müller-Oerlinghausen, B. (2001) Does lithium exert an independent antisuicidal effect? *Pharmacopsychiatry*, **34**, 132–136.

Akiskal, H.S. (1981) Subaffective disorders. Dysthymic, cylothymic and bipolar II disorders in the "borderline" realm. *Psychiatr. Clin. N. Am.*, **4**, 25–46.

Akiskal, H.S. (2002) Classification, diagnosis and boundaries of bipolar disorders: a review, in *Bipolar Disorder* (eds M. Maj, H.S. Akiskal, J.J. Lopez-Ibor, and N. Sartorius), John Wiley and Sons, Ltd., Chichester, pp. 1–52.

Akiskal, H.S. (2007) Targeting suicide prevention to modifiable risk factors: has bipolar II been overlooked? *Acta Psychiatri. Scand.*, **116**, 395–402.(Editorial).

Akiskal, H.S., Benazzi, F., Perugi, G. *et al.* (2005) Agitated "unipolar" depression re-conceptualized as a depressive mixed state: implications for the antidepressant-suicide controversy. *J. Affect. Disord.*, **85**, 245–258.

Akiskal, H.S., Hantouche, F.-G., Allilare, J.-F. *et al.* (2003) Validating antidepressant-associated hypomania (bipolar III): a systematic comparison with spontaneous hypomania (bipolar II). *J Affect. Disord.*, **50**, 143–151.

Akiskal, H.S., Maser, J.D., Zeller, P.J. *et al.* (1995) Switching form "unipolar" to bipolar II: n 11-year prospective study of clinical and temperamental predictors in 559 patients. *Arch. Gen. Psychiatry*, **52**, 114–123.

Angst, J. (1998) The emerging epidemiology of hypomania and bipolar II disorder. *J. Affect. Disord.*, **50**, 143–151.

Angst, F., Stassen, H.H., Clayton, P.J. *et al.* (2002) Mortality of patients with mood disorders: follow-up over 34–38 years. *J. Affect. Disord.*, **68**, 167–181.

Azorin, J.-M., Kaladjian, A., Adida, M. *et al.* (2009a) Risk factors associated with lifetime suicide attempts in bipolar I patients: findings from a French National cohort. *Compr. Psychiatry*, **50**, 115–120.

Azorin, J.-M., Kaladjian, A., Adida, M. *et al.* (2009b) Psychopathological correlates of lifetime anxiety comorbidity in bipolar I patients: findings from a French National cohort. *Psychopathology*, **42**, 380–386.

Balázs, J., Benazzi, F., Rihmer, Z. *et al.* (2006) The close link between suicide attempts and mixed (bipolar) depression: implications for suicide prevention. *J. Affect. Disord.*, **91**, 133–138.

Balázs, J., Lecrubier, Y., Csiszér, N. *et al.* (2003) Prevalence and comorbidity of affective disorders in persons making suicide attempts in Hungary: importance of the first depressive episodes and of bipolar II diagnoses. *J. Affect. Disord.*, **76**, 113–119.

Baldessarini, R.J., Tondo, L., Davis, P. *et al.* (2006) Decreased risk of suicides and attempts during long-term lithium treatment: a meta-analytic review. *Bipolar Disord.*, **8**, 625–639.

Bauer, M.S. (2002) Psychosocial interventions for bipolar disorder: a review, in *Bipolar Disorder* (eds M. Maj, H.S. Akiskal, J.J. Lopez-Ibor, N. Sartorius), John Wiley and Sons, Ltd., Chichester, pp. 281–313.

Benazzi, F. (2003) How could antidepressants worsen unipolar depression? *Pychother. Psychosom.*, **72**, 107–108 (ltr).

Benazzi, F. and Akiskal, H.S. (2003a) Refining the evaluation of bipolar II: beyond the SCID-IV guidelines for hypomania. *J. Affect. Disord.*, **73**, 33–38.

Benazzi, F. and Akiskal, H.S. (2003b) Clinical and factor-analytic validation of depressive mixed states: a report from the Ravenna-San Diego collaboration. *Curr. Opin. Psychiatry*, **16** (Suppl. 2), 70–78.

Brieger, P. (2000) Comorbidity in bipolar affective disorder, in *Bipolar Disorders. 100 Years After Manic Depressive Insanity* (eds A. Marneros and J. Angst), Kluwer Academic Publishers, Dordrecht, pp. 215–229.

Bowden, C.L. (2002) Pharmacological treatment of bipolar disorder: a review, in *Bipolar Disorder* (eds M. Maj, H.S. Akiskal, J.J. Lopez-Ibor, and N. Sartorius), John Wiley and Sons, Ltd., Chichester, pp. 191–221.

Bulik, C.M., Carpenter, L., Kupfer, S.J. *et al.* (1990) Features associated with suicide attempts in recurrent major depression. *J. Affect. Disord.*, **18**, 29–37.

Chen, Y.W. and Dilsaver, S.C. (1996) Lifetime rates of suicide attempts among subjects with bipolar and unipolar disorders relative to subjects with other axis I disorders. *Biol. Psychiatry*, **3**, 896–899.

Cheng, A.T.A., Chen, T.H.H., Chen, C.C. *et al.* (2000) Psychological and psychiatric risk factors for suicide. Case-control psychological autopsy study. *Br. J. Psychiatry*, **177**, 360–365.

Collins, J.C. and McFarland, B.H. (2008) Divalproex, lithium and suicide among medicaid patients with bipolar disorder. *J. Affect. Disord.*, **107**, 23–28.

Colom, F. and Vieta, E. (2002) Treatment adherence in bipolar patients. *Clin. Approaches Bipolar Disord.*, **1**, 49–56.

Dilsaver, S.C., Benazzi, F., Akiskal, H.S. *et al.* (2007) Post-traumatic stress disorder among adolescents with bipolar disorder and its relationship to suicidality. *Bipolar Disord.*, **9**, 649–655.

Dunner, D.L., Gershon, E.S., and Goodwin, F.K. (1976) Heritable factors in the severity of affective illness. *Biol. Psychiatry*, **11**, 31–42.

Fava, G.A., Bartolucci, G., Rafanelli, C. *et al.* (2001) Cognitive-behavioral management of patients with bipolar disorder who relapsed while on lithium prophylaxis. *J. Clin. Psychiatry*, **62**, 556–559.

Fountoulakis, K.N., Gonda, X., Siamouli, M. *et al.* (2009) Psychotherapeutic intervention and suicide risk reduction in bipolar disorder: a review of the evidence. *J. Affect. Disord.*, **113**, 21–29.

Ghaemi, S.N., Boima, E.E., and Goodwin, F.K. (2000) Diagnosing bipolar disorder and the effect of antidepressants: a naturalistic study. *J. Clin. Psychiatry*, **61**, 804–808.

Goodwin, F.K. (1999) Anticonvulsant therapy and suicide risk in affective disorders. *J. Clin. Psychiatry*, **60** (Suppl. 2), 89–93.

Goodwin, F.K., Fireman, B., Simon, G.E. *et al.* (2003) Suicide risk in bipolar disorder during treatment with lithium and divalproex. *J. Am. Med. Assoc.*, **290**, 1467–1473.

Goodwin, F.K. and Jamison, K.R. (1990) *Manic-Depressive Illness*, Oxford University Press, New York.

Goldberg, J.F., Harrow, M., and Whiteside, J.E. (2001) Risk for bipolar illness in patients initially hospitalized for unipolar depression. *Am. J. Psychiatry*, **158**, 1265–1270.

Guze, S.B. and Robins, E. (1970) Suicide and primary affective disorders. *Br. J. Psychiatry*, **117**, 437–438.

Harris, E.C. and Barraclough, B. (1997) Suicide as an outcome for mental disorders. *Br. J. Psychiatry*, **170**, 205–228.

Hawton, K. and van Heeringen, K. (eds.) (2000) *The International Handbook of Suicide and Attempted Suicide*. John Wiley and Sons, Ltd, Chichester.

Henry, C., Sorbara, F., Lacoste, J. *et al.* (2001) Antidepressant-induced mania in bipolar patients: identification of risk factors. *J. Clin. Psychiatry*, **62**, 249–255.

Isacsson, G. (2000) Suicide prevention – a medical breakthrough? *Acta Psychiatri. Scand.*, **102**, 113–117.

Isometsä, E.T., Henriksson, M.M., Aro, H.M. *et al.* (1994) Suicide in bipolar disorder in Finland. *Am. J. Psychiatry*, **151**, 1020–1024.

Judd, L.L. and Akiskal, H.S. (2003) The prevalence and disability of bipolar spectrum disorders in the US population: re-analysis of the ECA database taking into account subthreshold cases. *J. Affect. Disord.*, **73**, 123–131.

Keck, P.E. and McElroy, S. Jr. (2003) Redefining mood stabilization. *J. Affect. Disord.*, **73**, 163–169.

Koukopoulos, A., Caliari, B., Tundo, A. *et al.* (1983) Rapid cyclers, temperament and antidepressants. *Compr. Psychiatry*, **24**, 249–258.

Koukopoulos, A. and Koukopoulos, A. (1999) Agitated depressions as a mixed state and the problem of melancholia. *Psychiatr. Clin. N. Am.*, **22**, 547–563.

Lam, D.H., Watkins, E.R., Hayward, P. *et al.* (2003) A randomized controlled study of cognitive therapy for relapse prevention for bipolar affective disorder. *Arch. Gen. Psychiatry*, **60**, 145–152.

Maj, M., Tortorella, A., and Bartoli, L. (2000) Mood stabilizers in bipolar disorder, in *Bipolar Disorders. 100 Years After Manic Depressive Insanity* (eds A. Marneros and J. Angst), Kluwer Academic Publishers, Dordrecht, pp. 351–372.

Maser, J.D., Akiskal, H.S., Schettler, P. *et al.* (2002) Can temperament idedentify affectively ill patients who engage in lethal or non-lethal suicidal behavior? A 14-year prospective study. *Suicide Life Threat. Behav.*, **32**, 10–32.

Mundo, E., Cattaneo, E., Russo, M. *et al.* (2006) Clinical variables related to antidepressant-induced mania in bipolar disorder. *J. Affect. Disord.*, **92**, 227–230.

Ohgami H., Tearao T., Shiotsuki I. *et al.* (2009) Lithium in drinking water and risk of suicide. *Br. J. Psychiatry*, **194**, 464–465.

Rihmer, Z. (2005) Prediction and prevention of suicide in bipolar disorders. *Clin. Neuropsychiatry*, **2**, 48–54.

Rihmer, Z. (2007) Suicide risk in mood dsorders. *Curr. Opin. Psychiatry*, **20**, 17–22.

Rihmer, Z. and Akiskal, H.S. (2006) Do antidepressants t(h)reat(en) depressives? Toward a clinically judicious formulation of the antidepressant-suicidality FDA advisory in light of declining national suicide statistics from nay countries. *J. Affect. Disord.*, **94**, 3–13.

Rihmer, Z., Akiskal, K.K., Rihmer, A. *et al.* (2010) Current research on affective temperaments. *Curr. Opin. Psychiatry*, **23**, 12–18.

Rihmer, Z., Barsi, J., Arató, M. *et al.* (1990) Suicide in subtypes of primary major depression. *J. Affect. Disord.*, **18**, 221–225.

Rihmer, Z., Belső, N., and Kiss, K. (2002) Strategies for suicide prevention. *Curr. Opin. Psychiatry*, **15**, 83–87.

Rihmer, Z. and Kiss, K. (2002) Bipolar disorders and suicide risk. *Clin. Approaches Bipolar Disord.*, **1**, 15–21.

Rihmer, Z., Rutz, W., and Pihlgren, H. (1995) Depression and suicide on Gotland. an intensive study of all suicides before and after a depression-training programme for general practitioners. *J. Affect. Disord.*, **35**, 147–152.

Rihmer, Z., Szádóczky, E., Füredi, J. *et al.* (2001) Anxiety disorders comorbidity in bipolar I, bipolar II and unipolar major depression: results from a population-based study in Hungary. *J. Affect. Disord.*, **67**, 175–179.

Roy, A. (1983) Family history of suicide. *Arch. Gen. Psychiatry*, **40**, 971–974.

Rucci, P., Frank, E., Kostelnik, B. *et al.* (2002) Suicide attempts in patients with bipolar I disorder during acute and maintenance phases of intensive treatment with pharmacotherapy and adjunctive psychotherapy. *Am. J. Psychiatry*, **159**, 1160–1164.

Sánchez-Gistau, V., Colom, F., MAné, A. *et al.* (2009) A typical depression is associated with suicide attempt in bipolar disorder. *Acta Psychiatr. Scand.*, **120**, 30–36.

Simpson, S.G. and Jamison, K.R. (1999) The risk of suicide in patients with bipolar disorders. *J. Clin. Psychiatry*, **60** (Suppl. 2), 53–56.

Sondergard, L., Lopez, A.G., Andersen, P.K. *et al.* (2008) Mood stabilizing pharmacological treatment in bipolar disorders and risk of suicide. *Bipolar Disord.*, **10**, 87–94.

Strakowski, S.M., McElroy, S.L., Keck, P.E. Jr. *et al.* (1996) Suicidality among patients with mixed and manic bipolar disorder. *Am. J. Psychiatry*, **153**, 674–676.

Szádóczky, E., Papp, Zs., Vitrai, J. *et al.* (1998) The prevalence of major depressive and bipolar disorders in Hungary. *J. Affect. Disord.*, **50**, 153–162.

Thies-Flechtner, K., Müller-Oerlinghausen, B., Seibert, W. *et al.* (1996) Effect of prophylactic treatment on suicide risk in patients with major affective disorders. *Pharmacopsychiatry*, **29**, 103–107.

Tohen, M., Greil, W., Calabrese, J.R. *et al.* (2005) Olanzapine versus lithium in the maintenance treatment of bipolar disorder: a 12-month, randomized, double-blind, controlled clinical trial. *Am. J. Psychiatry*, **162**, 1281–1290.

Tondo, L., Baldessarini, R.J., Hennen, J. *et al.* (1998) Lithium maintenance treatment of depression and mania in bipolar I and bipolar II disorders. *Am. J. Psychiatry*, **155**, 638–645.

Tondo, L., Baldessarini, R.J., Hennen, J. *et al.* (1999) Suicide attempts in major affective disorder patients with comorbid substance use disorders. *J. Clin. Psychiatry*, **60** (Suppl. 2), 63–69.

Tondo, L. and Baldessarini, R.J. (2000) Reduced suicide risk during lithium maintenance treatment. *J. Clin. Psychiatry*, **61** (Suppl. 9), 97–104.

Tondo, L., Lepri, B., and Baldessarini, R. (2007) Suicidal risk among 2826 Sardinian major affective disorder patients. *Acta Psychiatr. Scand.*, **116**, 419–428.

Vieta, E., Benabarre, A., Colom, F. *et al.* (1997) Suicidal behavior in bipolar I and bipolar II disorder. *J. Nerv. Ment. Dis.*, **185**, 407–409.

Yatham, L.N., Kennedy, S.H., Schaffer, A. *et al.* (2009) Canadian Network for Mood and Anxiety Treatments (CANMAT) and International Society for Bipolar Disorders (ISBD) collaborative update of CANMAT guidelines for the management of patients with bipolar disorder: update 2009. *Bipolar Disord.*, **11**, 225–255.

Yerevanian, B.I., Koek, R.J., and Mintz, J. (2003) Lithium, anticonvulsants and suicidal behavior in bipolar disorder. *J. Affect. Disord.*, **73**, 223–228.

Yerevanian, B.I., Koek, R.J., and Mintz, J. (2007a) Bipolar pharmacotherapy and suicidal behaviour. Part 1: lithium, divalproex and carbamazepine. *J. Affect. Disord.*, **103**, 5–11.

Yerevanian, B.I., Koek, R.J., Mintz, J. *et al.* (2007b) Bipolar pharmacotherapy and suicidal behaviour. Part 2: the impact of antidepressants. *J. Affect. Disord.*, **103**, 13–21.

Yerevanian, B.I., Koek, R.J., and Mintz, J. (2007c) Bipolar pharmacotherapy and suicidal behaviour. Part 3: impact of antipsychotics. *J. Affect. Disord.*, **103**, 23–28.

Young, A., McElroy, S., Olausson, B. *et al.* (2008) Quetiapine monotherapy up to 52 weeks in patients with bipolar depression: continuation phase data from EMBOLDEN I and EMBOLDEN II. Poster presented at the 21st European College of Neuropsychopharmacology (ECNP) Conference, Barcelona, Spain, 2008 (Abstract).

Valtonen, H.M., Suominen, K., Haukka, J. *et al.* (2008) Differences in incidence of suicide attempts during phases of bipolar I and bipolar II disorders. *Bipolar Disord.*, **10**, 588–596.

Wolf, T. and Müller-Oerlinghausen, B. (2002) The influence of successful prophylactic drug treatment on cognitive dysfunction in bipolar disorders. *Bipolar Disord.*, **4**, 263–270.

25

Overview of Principles of Caring for Bipolar Patients

Hagop S. Akiskal[1] and Kareen K. Akiskal[1,2]

[1]International Mood Center, University of California at San Diego,
San Diego, CA, USA
[2]French Depressive and Manic-Depressive Association, Rennes, France

Il faut aimer les aliené*s* pour *ê*tre digne et capable de les server.'' ("The psychiatrist must have special love for the severely mentally ill, in order to deserve and be capable of serving them.").

Esquirol (1845)

25.1 INTRODUCTION

This overview chapter considers aspects of bipolar illness that have to do with its practical long-term clinical management on a day to day basis. In other words, we will cover what is generally considered the clinical art of how to care for these patients. This art, which obviously has to take into consideration the existing clinical science on bipolar disorder, nonetheless derives largely from the authors' intimate hands-on experience with patients and their families. It is based on the clinical experience of the first author (HSA) who has directed mood and/or bipolar clinics since 1973; as well as the patient advocacy experience of the second author (KKA), who responded to various crises telephone inquiries from families and patients. This dual experience of both authors spans more than the illness itself in that it involves, among others, familial, social, educational, financial, and legal aspects. The principles we enunciate herein are not meant to be an exhaustive discussion of these issues but instead focus on the main areas that need to be taken into consideration for optimal outcome.

Although formal "manualized" therapeutic programs for bipolar disorder exist, they derive from specific theoretical perspectives such as cognitive-behavior therapy and circadian rhythms, or their application in psycho-education. These are valuable contributions summarized in this book, but are limited to specific areas of dysfunction in bipolar illness. In this chapter, instead of applying particular theoretical perspectives in the treatment of

Bipolar Psychopharmacotherapy: Caring for the patient, Second Edition. Edited by Hagop S. Akiskal and Mauricio Tohen.
© 2011 John Wiley & Sons, Ltd. Published 2011 by John Wiley & Sons, Ltd.

bipolar disorder, we integrate therapeutic principles that we have learned from caring for bipolar patients and their families.

25.2 THE MAJOR PLAYERS IN BIPOLAR DISORDER

25.2.1 THE PATIENT

Although the depressive phase causes a great deal of suffering, both patient and family may initially ascribe it to misfortune, trauma, or love loss. Later they may invoke moral explanations such as "laziness." But ultimately when depression fully declares itself, recurring on a cyclical basis, especially in the face of observable dysfunction and disability and suicidal preoccupation or attempts, it becomes inescapable that both patient and significant others will understand that these manifestations constitute signs of a veritable illness. Patients and families are more likely to accept help for the depressive phase.

The manic phase with its poor judgment and lack of insight robs the patient of the capacity to understand the pathological nature of excited behavior. Significant others, too, may initially misunderstand manic signs and symptoms as indicative of misbehavior due to youthfulness, hardheadedness, or erotic excesses. Ultimately parents recognize the excited phases to be the hallmark of the illness, leading to grave dysfunction, but not so with the patient who continues to insist that they are feeling fit and well and that there is nothing wrong with their behavior. One of the tragedies of bipolar illness is that considerable destruction of the social fabric of the patient's life does occur as a result of numerous manic episodes (Krober, 1993) before they can be brought to accept treatment; some never do so.

Overall, the foregoing considerations suggest that if and when patients accept treatment it is likely to be for the depressive phase, that is, with anti-depressants which, in monotherapy, have the distinct disadvantage to switch the patient into the excited phase – or at least not to protect against it (Sachs *et al.*, 2007) – thereby leading to increased cycling (Kukopulos *et al.*, 1980) or mixed states (Akiskal and Mallya, 1987). Patients' motivation to continue with mood stabilizers, often given during crises against their will, is rarely adhered to beyond a short period. Because they do not feel ill in their excited phase, they can find a myriad of banal "rationales" to discontinue their mood stabilizing medication. Unfortunately there is a litany of side effects that they can invoke to stop their medication.

The main conclusion to be drawn from the foregoing statement is that the cognitive dysfunction of bipolar illness (Balanzá-Martínez *et al.*, 2010) – which unfortunately is not even in the criteria of DSM IV for bipolar disorder – represents the most handicapping aspect of the illness (Goldberg and Burdick, 2008). Such "illness agnosia" is the basis for the failure to understand the need for treatment, and is often associated with personal and social "deficits" (Akiskal, Azorin, and Hantouche, 2003a).

25.2.2 THE FAMILY

The cyclical recurrence of depressive and excited episodes is highly disruptive to family life. In addition, patients may use highly abusive language toward their loved ones.

Relationships with peers, especially of a romantic nature, are often strained, tempestuous and on a disaster path. Academic and professional promises are not fulfilled. The family is extremely frustrated and confused. Although they wish the best treatment for their bipolar member of the family, in the beginning years of the illness they may deny its presence because it is traumatic for the family to accept that yet another member of the family has come down with the illness. They hope and wish it will go away. Even if hospitalization is required, they may in the beginning opt against it to avert the stigma implied in psychiatric hospitalization for the affected member, as well as for the family at large.

Eventually the consequences of bipolar disorder become unbearable for the family – and *dire* for the patient. But the patient is typically unwilling to accept treatments involving restraints and imposition on their civil liberties. Such attitudes inaugurate the long phase of battles with family and significant others regarding the need for hospitalization and/or regular outpatient visits. These may eventually translate into legal conflicts between patients and the family. Not infrequently, these conflicts involve financial battles over inheritance, trust funds, and pensions. Under the worst scenario, adolescent and even older bipolar patients may accuse parents of inflicting trauma and emotional abuse – even sexual abuse (Akiskal, 2004). This is not to say that the latter never takes place. What is regrettable is that inexperienced or earnest mental health clinicians all too often take reports of "abuse" at their face value, instead of considering them as a reflection of the extreme emotional climate of a high expressed emotion (EE) family (Akiskal, 1996).

With chronically relapsing illness, it is often the mother who carries the brunt of the illness' burden. Such mothers themselves typically go through periods of despair, hope, and denial about their adult bipolar children. This is often a lonely despair, about which kin not living with the family are ignorant of or indifferent to; at worst, such kin may even display critical and angry attitudes toward the caregiving mother (i.e., "You are a bad mother" or "you are not taking care of your sick child"), or even worse ("Your child's illness is due to you having abandoned her"). Such criticism toward the mother is also routinely verbalized by the bipolar offspring, but unlike that of kin, may cycle into effusive expression of love and gratitude in a state-dependent fashion.

In the case of illness declaring itself in a marriage, separation or divorce is a common complication. Such individuals may return to their family of origin, where again the mother carries the burden of caring for an "adult child" – otherwise the patient may end up becoming institutionalized or homeless.

25.2.3 THE PSYCHIATRIST AND OTHER CLINICIANS

Nonpsychiatric physicians usually shun away from bipolar illness as a specialized area. Also many clinical psychologists consider bipolarity to represent the domain of psychiatry. This is fortunately gradually changing. Psychologists are increasingly assuming an important role on the therapeutic team in the long-term care of bipolar patients. The same is even truer for social workers, nurses, and doctors of pharmacy, who in today's mental health care system represent a cadre of valuable and essential members of bipolar or mood clinics.

Although psychiatrists during their training do gain experience in diagnosing and treating this illness, most university medical centers do not offer specialized training in bipolar disorder. As a consequence, unless a psychiatric trainee has a special interest in this area, his or her experiential base in this disorder is likely to be less than optimal, in particular, they gain little hands-on experience in the *long-term* care of bipolar patients.

Patients and their families are always seeking information to understand this illness and its frustratingly complex course. One of the most difficult problems for the patient and the family is to find the "right psychiatrist" who can manage bipolar disorder. That the number of such psychiatrists is relatively small, is not the fault of the psychiatrist, but rather the lack of vision in graduate medical education. Much of what most psychiatrists do in their clinical practice involves affective disorders in the broad sense, yet their formal educational curriculum does not reflect this. "Neurotic" and depressive disorders are relatively easy to comprehend and manage, and illnesses like schizophrenia and dementia have the veneer of organic disease, whereas bipolarity has such a complex interplay of social and occupational behavior that is less fathomable for the average psychiatric trainee. Their lack of exposure to phenomenology, psychology, pharmacology, and long-term course of bipolar disorder creates a major public health problem. So-called "classic bipolar" disorder is a platonic myth – from which most patients deviate in significant ways. An inexperienced clinician then will often misattribute bipolar disorder to other mental disorders such as schizophrenia, anxiety and unipolar disorders, or personality disorders (Akiskal and Puzantian, 1979; Hirschfeld, Lewis, and Vornik, 2003; Hantouche and Akiskal, 2004). Sadly, the cross-sectional erratic behavior of bipolar patients is often labeled "borderline" – if not frankly "psychopathic." Such labels alone will militate against any meaningful long-term alliance of patients with clinicians. Despite protests to the contrary, bipolar disorder remains under-diagnosed and under-treated (Albanese *et al.*, 2006; Zimmerman *et al.*, 2008; Smith and Ghaemi, 2010).

There are reasons to believe that continuing medical education programs focusing on bipolar disorder are beginning to positively impact the recognition and treatment of bipolarity in its broad expressions. There now exist pockets of clinical excellence in bipolar disorder and, refreshingly, many are in practice settings outside academia.

25.2.4   THE MOOD/BIPOLAR CLINIC

In part because of the reasons just discussed, there exist very few mood and or bipolar clinics in the world. Of the few existing ones, nearly all are located in the United States. They used to be called "lithium" clinics (Fieve, 1975), because rigorous use of lithium with due attention to medical aspects and blood levels was mandatory. This helped in the medicalization of bipolar disorders at a time when psychiatry was basking in psychodynamics. However, positive results with lithium were largely limited to bipolar patients who were willing to adhere to the relatively tight regimes required. These clinics were crucial for adherence to the prophylactic use of this agent (Akiskal, 1999) and suicide prevention (Muller-Oerlinghausen, Grof, and Schou, 1999).

Mood clinics had a broader agenda and emphasized integration of different therapeutic modalities. Although this was more congruent with the emergence of an "eclectic psychiatry," mood clinics did not become popular perhaps because they competed for the clientele of psychiatrists in both academia and general practice. In the process, what psychiatry missed was the opportunity for mood clinics to train residents and fellows to become specialists of mood disorders. In such clinics, routine prospective follow up revealed high rates of transformation of depression into bipolar disorder (Akiskal *et al.*, 1983), particularly bipolar II subtype (Akiskal *et al.*, 1978; Akiskal, 2005). This would have liberated psychiatrists from the rigidity in our formal diagnostic system for mood disorders where patients fall into the unipolar and bipolar molds. In clinical reality, most affectively ill patients fall in a spectrum between these extremes (see Chapter 2). But to properly appreciate this perspective, the clinician must experience over prospective follow-up, the gradual – though at times subtle – transformation of unipolar patients into soft bipolarity. Family history, especially when buttressed with family interviews, will further inform the psychiatrist where DSM-IV and ICD-10 fail abominably – as the proper diagnosis of bipolar disorder needs to be continuously revised by the evolving nature of affective and related disorders in family members. It is also important to appreciate that mood patients over prospective observation develop what otherwise might be regarded as "unusual" – namely, the common development, among others, of psychotic, panic, phobic, obsessive-compulsive, dysmorphic, bulimic, addictive, and impulse-control disorders (Perugi, Toni, and Akiskal, 1999). Such complexity is the rule, rather than the exception. Short of such an exposure to the familial and longitudinally evolving nature of affective illness, the psychiatrist in training could not gain optimal experience to the most common types of bipolar disorder. Furthermore, in such a setting a team of mental health professionals could bring their knowledge and experience to bear upon the treatment of these patients. Thereby, a therapeutic relationship would be forged between the patients, their families, and the clinic at large, including the trainees. This is a good scenario for treatment adherence – and makes caring possible.

The situation is different with the current bipolar programs in many academic centers which are primarily focused on industry supported pharmaceutical research and secondarily on research related to the psychobiology of the illness supported by National Health Institutes. Most of these programs are at the mercy of the vagaries of funding, which means that neither the staff nor the patients have long term continuity. This is a sad scenario, which does not take the lifelong nature of the illness into consideration. This is not to say that bipolar programs as they exist today do not advance knowledge. On the contrary, a great deal has been learned about the illness itself and its treatment – witness the large number of new treatments introduced over the last decade and a half, and which is the theme of this book. The problem is that most studies do not address the long term care of the patient. Even collaborative or cooperative programs from funding institutes – which have the luxury of longer follow up – do not primarily focus on the long term care of the patient, and sadly spend little funding to train specialists in bipolar disorder. Most research scientists who, by the very nature of their funding, train interviewers or raters of psychopathology rather than clinical practitioners. As a result, they produce research administrators who know more about methodology, institutional review boards and the art of "grantsmanship" than caring for bipolar patients.

Interestingly, there has been some interest to develop mood and bipolar clinics in private practice settings, including at least one in the setting of primary general medical care (Manning, Hyakal, and Akiskal, 1999). The primary care clinic in general medical settings provides an optimal opportunity for early detection of bipolar disorder. In this setting, Dr. Manning, in collaboration with the present authors' team, used the temperament evaluation of Memphis, Pisa, Paris, and San Diego (TEMPS) to detect subtle and early manifestations of bipolar disorder at the temperamental level (Akiskal *et al.*, 2005). In nonpsychiatric medical settings, it is more practical to use this instrument rather than instruments that detect hypomania, which require more formal psychometric understanding (Benazzi and Akiskal, 2009).

A pessimist might conclude that the gap between those who actually care for bipolar patients and those who do research on how to care for such patients is widening. An optimist might point out to a large volume of an increasingly sophisticated literature on caring for bipolar patients and their families, particularly from psychoeducational (Colom *et al.*, 2003) and collaborative care model (Bauer *et al.*, 2006) perspectives. The real question though is why psychiatry has not yet developed a sufficient number of mood or bipolar clinics to accommodate the somatic and psychosocial needs of these patients in an integrated fashion. That patients and families with bipolar illness have long been frustrated in this respect is perhaps the main driving force for the development of bipolar advocacy organizations.

25.2.5 MENTAL HEALTH ADVOCACY ORGANIZATIONS

The foregoing challenges, as well as the need for a long-term perspective led to the development of such organizations – several of which are devoted to depressive and bipolar disorders. They promised self-help support, education, destigmatization, advocacy for better services, advocacy for *relevant* research and administering research awards that are advancing knowledge about the needs of patients rather than mere theoretical or basic science developments. These lofty goals are obviously helpful for patients as well as for their families, and could impact public health (Lish *et al.*, 1994). Unlike the Alcoholics Anonymous model, these organizations typically endorse a spectrum of therapeutic modalities that span from the psychopharmacologic to the psychotherapeutic. Many members of these organizations also often seek the assistance of their local Alcoholics Anonymous chapters.

The major downside of these organizations is, because their main advisors, tend to be high level researchers rather than clinicians involved in the day to day care of patients. Optimally, both researchers and clinicians should be represented on these advisory boards. Advocacy organizations are vulnerable to the tensions and conflicts inherent to large organizations, including the inevitable clash of temperaments of its executive members. Nonetheless, these organizations have succeeded in bringing strong clout to the cause of de-stigmatization of bipolar disorder and the need for new research to both governmental and industry sources. In the United States, it has even become possible to have one rubric, the National Alliance of the Mentally Ill, to serve as a unifying voice for the mentally ill at large. Moreover, the National Alliance for Research in Schizophrenic and Affective Disorders (NARSAD) has sprung from the ranks of affluent families with offspring suffering from these disorders to become the world's leading charity dedicated to mental health research. It supports both established and promising investigators in their pursuit of innovative research leads in etiology, pathogenesis, and innovative treatments.

25.2.6 SOCIETY AND THE MEDIA

Bipolar patients are poorly understood by the public at large. This is generally true for all serious mental illness, but there are two aspects rather unique to bipolar disorder, and which often find resonance in the media. The first is that bipolar individuals are over-represented in the corporate world and in politics: scandals in the sexual and financial arena, so alluring to the media and to the public at large, tend to give a "bad name" to the illness. The other one is the tendency of some researchers and media to glamorize bipolarity as a "genius disease," especially in the artistic domain and theoretical science. This is problematic because such benefits characterize a minority of patients, usually at the soft end of the spectrum (Akiskal and Akiskal, 1988) or among the "unaffected" relatives of bipolar patients (Coryell *et al.*, 1989). Many patients are disappointed that their doctors are unable to help them reap the "benefits" of their illness. If not properly handled, this may create mistrust between the doctor and the patient. This could also generate conflict between bipolar patients, their employer and institutions in which they work. Patients may feel entitled to advantages and even tolerance for their outrageous behavior on the grounds that manic-depression confers creative spurts upon them. While greater understanding of bipolar disorder has occurred recently, this does not necessarily translate into greater tolerance of the irregular work habits of bipolar patients.

25.3 PRINCIPLES OF CARING

1. Bipolar illness is a disease with strong genetic determinants which is exacerbated and complicated by psychosocial factors. **Competent pharmacotherapy must be matched with sophisticated yet practical psychosocial interventions**. There is no longer such a philosophical divide between the two (Mundt, 2003; Fuchs, 2004). "Medication visits" are necessary but insufficient: Quality time is needed to explore and address psychotherapeutic issues (Table 25.1). However, such lofty goals are more easily articulated than carried out. In current practice, especially in public mental health settings, pharmacotherapy and psychotherapy are disassociated, thereby making their integration difficult. Combining them in one person, obligatorily a physician, has the disadvantage that psychiatrists may not have all the requisite skills for the newly developed unwieldy list of psychosocial interventions and, even if they did, it may be impractical for one person to administer them all. The so-called "team approach" is an optimal compromise, but has the danger of becoming administrative rhetoric rather than a genuine forum for integration. To

Table 25.1 Psychotherapeutic issues in bipolar disorder.

Denial of the illness
Developmental delays and emotional immaturity
Uneven careers, talent, and creativity
Financial extravagance
Burden on the family
Risky sexual behavior
Marriage, pregnancy, genetics
Tempestuous relationships, lovelife, divorce
Stigma about chronic illness
Effects of bipolar medications on temperament
Fears of return of illness episodes
Battle over control of the self
Self-regulation and regulation of self-esteem

Table 25.2 Factors in treatment non-adherence.

Cultural: stigma, anti-medication attitudes
Illness: no insight, mania, initial episodes
Comorbidity: alcohol/drug abuse
Medication: unacceptable side effects
Patient: young, low socio-economic status male, missing highs
Family: lack of supervision
Physician: inexperience, inconsistency, or hiding behind authoritarian attitudes
Health climate: undermining continuity of care

make things worse, patients and families may disrupt the precarious balance of integrated treatments. That's why treatments for bipolar patients must be administered by visionaries committed to practical tasks – a rare blend of talents.

2. **Availability of family members or significant others** who are willing to participate in the therapeutic process, who can monitor adherence to treatment, provide information about the course of illness under treatment and could be trusted during times of crisis. Such support and participation is crucial in bipolar disorder with its proverbially unpredictable exacerbations. Patients' denial of illness and reticence to seek help represent major factors in relapse, and the pivotal role of a caring family cannot be underestimated in this regard; adherence to treatment is a complex subject (Table 25.2); also see Jamison and Akiskal (1983). In the authors' experience, love and respect for or dependency upon a significant other or an authority figure in the family is crucial for treatment adherence.

3. The attitude of significant others which is of the greatest help is one of concern and **emotional warmth while maintaining objectivity**. Given the tempestuous interactions that occur in this illness, individuals close to the patient cannot avoid being – or coming across as – critical. While it is true that critical attitudes may

Table 25.3 Group therapy for bipolar patients.

To involve others (e.g., spouses) in the therapeutic process
To educate about the nature of the illness and its treatment
To challenge denial
To enhance compliance to prophylactic medication
To identify the impending signs of relapse
To impose external control over risk-taking
To explore new homeostatic strategies for the "stabilized" self

lead to further exacerbation of the illness – particularly depression – it would be unrealistic to think that they would not occur. It is warmth that counterbalances critical attitudes whether in bipolar disorder or schizophrenia (Okasha *et al.*, 1994), representing an important vehicle in facilitating caring.

4. Feedback by peers – meaning by other bipolar patients and other bipolar families – is often more effective than that given by professionals and the patient's immediate family. This means that exposure to peers in a format such as **group therapy** (Table 25.3) can play a fundamental role in combating denial (Graves, 1993).

5. **In mood charting** (which Kraepelin (1921) pioneered and in more recent times was introduced into clinical science by Robert Post [2008]), life events and prevalent mood on a daily basis can help the patient understand the connection of such moods to life events, for example, hypomania to sexual unfaithfulness, irritable mood to loss of job. However, unwieldy methods of charting deriving from research protocols are not of much use in routine practice. Mood charting is best individualized to make sure that it is patient-friendly.

6. **Limit setting** can be achieved through the group therapeutic process. However, in some instances, only a close family member can be trusted to place such limits. We are specifically referring to delegating financial control at critical junctures to a spouse, parent, or sibling. This pertains, among others, to checks, credit cards, and inheritance. As for the latter, lawyers may be necessary to protect the patient's and family's respective rights. In this endeavor, one must rely upon lawyers whose loyalty has been tested beforehand. Tragically, impulsive spending often leads to financial ruin before such measures are instituted. Mental health professionals regrettably have little or no training in such matters. The authors are familiar with cases where lawyers, instead of being patient advocates, further depleted the patients' financial means.

7. **Functioning is more important than mood stabilization.** While rapid control of mania in the acute phase is desirable, over-stabilizing patients with "aggressive" pharmacotherapy is unlikely to lead to treatment adherence in the long run. It is best if the psychiatrist "goes halfway" in meeting reasonable requests by the patient about dosage and the optimum mix of medications. Implicitly, the psychiatrist will still have the "upper hand" from a medical point of view, while permitting the patient some participation in the therapeutic choices. Once recovered from major episodes, permitting some degree of self-management is a valuable but difficult

goal to attain. Vigilance is necessary to make sure that the patient doesn't take this as a mandate to do as he or she pleases, while at the same time reassuring that the psychiatrist is aware of the difficulty the patient has in entirely surrendering the control of the self to some "ideal" of stabilization that is in a textbook's or guidelines' doses or blood levels. For instance, while it is true that better control of bipolar episodes is achieved with high lithium blood levels, most patients cannot tolerate such levels, hence they stop it (Gelenberg *et al.*, 1989). In summary, **the goal of treatment is *not* to aggressively overmedicate the patient to mediocrity;** the psychiatrist should endeavor to help patients attain their best functioning without risking relapse. This is a more delicate art than helping patients maintain optimum blood pressure or blood glucose. But the "battles" over chemistry and health between patients and doctors as to who controls or is in charge of the patient's temperament, life, and soul are analogous in principle in both internal medicine and psychiatry. The art of managing such matters, while fundamental in our teaching efforts, is difficult to transmit – yet they must be practiced. This is what makes being a doctor fundamentally different from being a scientist. It is amazing how the current craze for scientific medicine continues to obscure this difference. Our point is that the issues involved are not unique to psychiatry, and to express our reservation to the complacency of many in our field who feel that "evidence-based" guidelines represent a sufficient measure for practice.

8. It follows then that for the patient to trust a psychiatrist, he or she must **respect the patient's temperament** and individuality, that indeed his or her aim is to bring out the optimum of what is positive and desirable in patients' temperament in terms of interpersonal charm and professional achievement (Akiskal and Akiskal, 2005). Nonetheless, as alluded to earlier, it is generally best to downplay literature about bipolarity as a "genius disease." First of all, "genius" is multi-factorial and if it is associated with bipolarity, it is generally at the soft end of the bipolar spectrum and not at the psychotic end (Akiskal and Akiskal, 1988, 2007, 2010). While it is understandable that some literature advocates the idea that bipolar individuals are very successful individuals in the arts and other domains (Jamison, 1996; Arnold, 1995), the intent of this literature is best understood as an attempt to de-stigmatize the illness. The unfortunate fact is that despite many positive attributes, the majority of ill bipolar patients cannot be expected to be creative or eminent unless they are independently gifted – and the course of the illness permitting. In our report from a large urban mood clinic (Akiskal and Akiskal, 1988), "creativity" (which was liberally defined) was limited to basically 8% of bipolar II. Should too much be made of the prospects of eminence in bipolar disorder in a given patient, the patient may feel cheated that the psychiatrist and the team of mental health workers somehow failed in bringing the best in him or her.

9. **Comorbid personality disorder – particularly the "B label" – is best handled by not diagnosing it**, as more often than not, it is a reflection or complication of the illness (Akiskal, 2004). The emphasis must be on rigorous treatment of the bipolar illness itself. We have elsewhere shown that the use of temperament constructs is much more germane to understanding bipolar disorder, as they identify traits which

make individuals vulnerable to the illness, while at the same time fostering adaptive function (Akiskal, 1992; Akiskal *et al.*, 2005). Family members, like psychiatrists and psychologists, in their frustration often invoke characterologic factors to explain the unproductive or "bad" behavior of their bipolar kin. It is best to conceive of such behavior as "faulty habits" that maintain the illness or are developed to deal with it. Addressing such habits with behavioral interventions is more likely to lead to change in the desired direction than characterologic labels that fault the patient and exculpate the clinician. Social workers can play a vital role in this process as they are more likely to be Meyerian in philosophy.

10. Because psychiatric tragedies, including social scandals, often occur in the lives of bipolar patients, the psychiatrist must **be available at times of crisis**. A non-judgmental attitude by the psychiatrist when all others are "attacking" the patient would assure to enlist the patient's cooperation in solving the crisis with minimal consequences (Akiskal, 2000). Being nonjudgmental however does not mean that the psychiatrist is condoning the behavior that led to the crisis. Because such crises often stem from poor judgment due to (hypo)mania or depression (more often the former than the latter), the psychiatrist must attempt to steer the patient out of the crisis rather than wait for the patient to find his way out.

11. Related to the above, and given the fact that depression is more painful subjec-tively and less likely to impair insight than hypo-mania, outcome of prophylactic treatment is, in our experience, more likely to be associated with better adherence when initiated during the former. Despite one study favoring such a conclusion (Lenzi *et al.*, 1989), there is surprisingly little systematic data on this very critical subject. Thus, more attention needs to be paid to **phase-specific pharmacologic treatments**, such as Koukopoulos' notion, that "mania-depression-free interval" patients do better on lithium than those with "depression-mania-free intervals" (Koukopoulos *et al.*, 1995).

12. The most serious crisis in bipolar disorder is suicidality. The clinician should err on the safe side and consider admitting the patient to the hospital. Electrocon-vulsive therapy is an option which often proves to be life-saving. **Faced with a suicidal bipolar patient, half-baked theoretical or existential discussions must be avoided**. Although lithium is touted to be unique in its antisuicidal proper-ties (Goodwin *et al.*, 2003), probably most, if not all, approved agents for bipolar disorder are as effective (Angst *et al.*, 2002). Depressive mixed states (Benazzi and Akiskal, 2001), intrusion of hypomanic features into depressive episodes, is one of the most treacherous substrates for suicidality, because of the subtle nature of the mixed state. In our experience, such patients respond best to Ziprasidone, Olanzepine, or Divalproex.

13. **The psychiatrist should avoid taking a Calvinistic approach to alcohol and substance use**. Thus, one must not be unreasonable in prohibiting alcohol and/or marijuana which based on occasional use has not shown to have destabilized the patient. However, abstinence from stimulant agents, including caffeine, is mandatory. Opiate-dependent patients can be stabilized on methadone (Maremmani *et al.*, 2003).

14. Many bipolar patients, even in their trait condition are "activity junkies" (Akiskal, 2005). Unfortunately, most types of excessive activation – whether it is spending money, frequent travel, excessive risk-taking in sex, drugs of abuse, gambling, working two to three shifts – can destabilize them. The destabilizing effect of activation is also pertinent to therapeutic agents for depression – and we are specifically referring to antidepressants. They should be used sparingly, for rigorous indications (that is, severe or suicidal depression), and only for as long as needed. Thus, **antidepressants should almost always be administered along with mood-stabilizing or anti-manic medications**. "Bipolar-friendly" antidepressants (for example, bupropion) might be preferred, but even these are not entirely safe – from a switching standpoint – in monotherapy. Lamotrigine may prove to be a viable "antidepressant" for many *acute* bipolar depressions, and this may be particularly true for bipolar II.

15. **Sleep hygiene** is an important ingredient in the overall management of bipolar disorder. However, because yearning for freedom from time constraints (rhythmopathy) is part of the core pathology of the illness, it often remains an elusive goal. Pragmatic approaches are preferred over unwieldy protocols developed in chronobiology labs. Nonetheless, understanding of chronobiologic principles can help to develop individualized circadian approaches in situations of shift work and jet lag. Useful approaches to the rhythmopathy include total darkness which should enhance sedating pharmacotherapy to prevent sleep deprivation and maintain restorative sleep. Thus, given the anxious arousal and insomnia or decreased need for sleep in bipolar disorder, rather than solely depending on behavioral management, it is often desirable to use sedating properties of existing anti-bipolar agents to treat anxious arousal at night. By the same token, although it is best to treat bipolar patients combining approved medication for the bipolar indication – or those with evidence from controlled studies – an appropriate exception can be made for agents such as gabapentin or clonazepam, as possible augmentation agents for anxiolysis, or sleep restoration.

16. The same remarks apply to topiramate as an agent for weight reduction. **Weight management and associated metabolic issues** represent a relatively new challenge, and must be rigorously addressed. When weight is a major concern, although one must preferably use weight-neutral approved medications for bipolar disorder (for example,, Carbamazepine, Lamotrigene, Aripiprazole), this should not be at the expense of effectiveness. That is, if a bipolar patient responds best or exclusively to medication which leads to weight gain, it may sometimes be disastrous to substitute it with weight-neutral medication. Thus, rather than risking destabilization, the psychiatrist must consider concurrent weight management. This is obviously an art in which the field of medicine at large has yet to prove its worth in terms of long-term effectiveness. But one can learn something by trying different approaches which may fail in some, but work in others. In our experience, "diet" is a term that elicits frustration. Lifestyle changes, such as incorporating walking in one's daily routine, are more likely to be rewarding and effective.

17. Bipolar disorder is multidimensional and requires **rational polypharmacy** working on different substrates, which means that anti-psychotics, anti-convulsants, and

mood stabilizers are often to be combined. Because abrupt withdrawal of an agent from the medication regimen is likely to lead to premature or early relapse, it is generally best to augment rather than substitute agents in the medication regimen.

18. **It is generally futile to meddle with the patient's love life**, for this is hardwired! Nonetheless when the erotic life is tempestuous to such a degree it is causing extreme pain and suffering or it is hopelessly or delusionally fixated on unavailable love objects (erotomania), an open discussion can prepare the ground for exploratory psychotherapy. Regrettably, antipsychotics which reduce sexual desire may have to be used in some instances.

19. A great deal of research, covered in this book, supports the use of psycho-educational practices in treatment adherence and in reducing denial. What this literature does not sufficiently emphasize is that **psycho-education is a two-way street**. The doctor himself or herself must learn about the patient and his or her disease, not from textbooks, but from direct daily interactions with the patient and his or her family.

20. Side effects of medications are sometimes intolerable and may necessitate adjustment of dosage or even substitution with a better tolerated medication. However, **in a patient whose illness has been brought under reasonable remission, it is best not to make major adjustments in the medication regimen**. The risk of relapse is a more serious concern in this instance than the nuisance of certain side effects. This is a situation when the therapeutic relationship with the physician is extremely important for the patient to trust his or her judgment on this matter, namely that it is not always possible to eliminate all side effects, and once "good enough functioning" has been achieved, it is best not to risk destabilization. Nonetheless, all reasonable efforts must be made to make sure that all adjustments are made to assure that side-effects are tolerable enough to _not_ compromise adherence. The principle here is **meeting the patient half way**.

21. However, **periodic _minor_ adjustment of medication can be considered at times of expected major stress**, including circadian stress such as trans-meridian travel, or when past course has revealed seasonal exacerbation, or specific psychosocial situations leading to relapse, proper upward medication adjustment should be prescribed at the expected time of the occurrence of these stressful events.

22. **Supporting the family, the spouse, or other carers – and particularly the mother** – of bipolar patients is a cardinal principle that is often neglected in contemporary psychiatry. Not only is this necessary to make sure that the patient has an effective support in the family, but to prevent the family from breaking down. Family members of the patient often carry the same bipolar genes in dilute form, compared to that of the patient, and it is the stress of being exposed to an extremely ill offspring that for the first time brings about depression in the mother. Illness of one's offspring, from an evolutionary standpoint, represents an extreme stress for a woman. It is such stress operating on a modest genetic vulnerability that brings about a depressive outcome for the mother. Support to the family often requires individual or group therapy. Patient advocacy organizations can also play a vital role in this respect.

23. The value of **genetic counseling** is limited, because patients in our experience typically present after the fact (that is, when pregnant). The risks of bipolar medication for the fetus, especially that of lithium, in our experience are exaggerated. Nonetheless, pregnant bipolar patients may require careful assessment in consultation with gynecologists or specialized women's bipolar clinics which have experience in such matters. Prospectively identified patients, which can be accomplished in a mood clinic, can be provided with risk estimates for offspring, especially when family history is loaded with affective illness or has pedigrees with psychotic bipolar illness and/or suicide.

24. Bipolar patients are preferably treated in group practice. Such a setting will provide the opportunity for consultation from colleagues, or time limited appointments with other members of the team when the primary physician is on vacation or ill. This could help in diluting negative transference reactions, while at the same time giving the patient the benefit of a second or third opinion. Ideally however, and especially in the public domain where most bipolar patients are treated, a **mood or bipolar clinic** provides many advantages (Table 25.4). Such clinics provide an experienced, sophisticated multi-disciplinary team including psychiatrists, psychologists, social workers, nurses, and doctors of pharmacy. Not only does the team provide greater variety of treatments tailored to the different needs of the patient, but it is better able to assure adherence, longitudinal care, and prevention. It also provides a resource for other mental health professionals in the community. Thus a patient can have pharmacotherapy, psycho-education, individual psychotherapy, group therapy, behavioral therapy, and social interventions. Of all the psychosocial treatments, psycho-education has the best data-based status, and has been covered elsewhere in this volume. In the mood clinic setting it is also possible to provide support for the family care givers, making sure that they become acquainted with the psychological and social skills to monitor the patient's progress. Finally and most importantly, the setting of a mood clinic provides the opportunity to observe and diagnose illnesses in family members before they fully declare themselves. This could include spouses, siblings or children (Akiskal *et al.*, 1985a). This is of immense public health importance, yet it has been insufficiently capitalized in psychiatry (Berk *et al.*, 2010). This is regrettable given the inexorable course of the illness once it develops into full steam. Finally, secondary prevention can be achieved by family members identifying early signs of impending relapse. Patients

Table 25.4 The role of a mood or bipolar clinic.

Combines service, training, and research
Experienced multi-disciplinary staff
Focus on the family or couple
Sophisticated treatment
Better treatment adherence
Longitudinal care
Prevention
A resource for other mental health professionals

can also be taught to monitor their own behavior and mental state in achieving this goal. A combination of the two sources of information is needed, because in general caregivers might be oversensitive in identifying signs of a relapse, while patients often are less inclined to do so.

25. **Maximize treatment adherence**. The principles we have discussed will be defeated if reasonable treatment adherence is not achieved. Indeed, these principles should contribute significantly to such adherence. The following can help further maximize adherence: Educating both patient and family about early signs of relapse, monitoring adherence to medication, making sure appointments in the clinic are kept, minimize dosing frequency, tailoring medication side-effects to those which are least likely to interfere with a patient's functioning, medication support group therapy, and of course, psychoeducation.

25.4 SPECIAL CONSIDERATIONS FOR HYPOMANIC AND CYCLOTHYMIC PATIENTS

Much of the literature in the treatment of bipolar disorder is focused on bipolar I. In this section, we discuss adherence issues particularly relevant to hypomania, as well as special psychological problems posed by cyclothymic patients.

Bipolar patients are notoriously nonadherent with maintenance oral medication (Jamison and Akiskal, 1983). Many patients whose mood swings are attenuated by medication may complain of feeling "flat" (especially with lithium) because of a relative depression; others may describe memory problems, which are not easy to document. In such cases, it is necessary to rule out atypical relapses without vegetative signs or lithium-induced hypothyroidism (especially in women). The latter is best accomplished with the TRH stimulation test. Other patients complain that the loss of hypomanic drive and indefatigability adversely affects their work and relationships. Couples therapy may be indicated when treatment results in decreased assertiveness in a patient who previously took an active role in sexual and social activities. Other patients may complain of decreased productivity and creativity. However, a systematic survey conducted by Schou (1979) among artists showed actual decreases in creativity to be uncommon; indeed, more often than not, lithium offers the opportunity for more "even" periods devoted to interpersonal, scholastic, professional, and artistic pursuits. Recent data shows lithium-induced gray matter volume increases to underlie treatment response (Lyoo *et al.*, 2010).

Adherence can often be enhanced by using the lowest possible dose that is compatible with freedom from major episodes, without necessarily preventing all mood oscillations. Another strategy is to combine two medications with different mechanisms of action and side effect profiles, but administering each at "sub-therapeutic doses," which would be synergistic and therapeutic in combination. A trial-and-error period, during which the patient's mental status is closely followed, is necessary to establish such a balance. This approach is especially welcome by those bipolar patients who enjoy hypomanic moods.

Many bipolar patients have considerable psychological assets, such as personal charm, affective warmth, creative bent, and a high drive to fight for or advance various causes.

These assets can often be capitalized in attempts to reconstruct lives that have been shattered because of impulsiveness and poor social judgment. In general, depth interpretations are unlikely to change these impulsive excesses, and voluntary control of such behavior is desirable - for example, turning over the checkbook to the spouse (Akiskal, Khani, and Scott-Strauss, 1979).

The foregoing issues are particularly relevant in the treatment of the spectrum of bipolar II disorders. Because these conditions begin at an early age and pursue a periodic lifelong course, they may be mistaken for primary characterological disorders. These soft bipolar conditions are distinguished from the classical (or so-called major) mood disorders in that their baseline manifestations are subsyndromal, intermittent, and typically lifelong. That is, in the patient's *habitual* condition, the affective psychopathology does not necessarily crystallize into discrete episodes. However, clearcut and unmistakable syndromal episodes are not uncommonly superimposed on the lifelong course of these temperaments. It is this very intermittence that creates their resemblance to personality disorders. This is further reinforced by lifelong maladjustment in scholastic, occupational, and conjugal areas, secondary to chronically unstable and unpredictable moods. Finally, the mood change is often quite subtle, with behavioral and personal disturbances dominating the clinical presentation. For instance, in the University of Tennessee study of cyclothymic depressives (Akiskal *et al.*, 1977), affective manifestations were masked by interpersonal crises. Repeated marital failure or romantic breakups, episodic promiscuous behavior, alcohol and drug abuse, uneven work and school record, geographic instability, and dilettantism were the cardinal reasons for which these patients had come to clinical attention.

Unpredictability of moods is a major source of distress for cyclothymic individuals, who can't predict from one day to the next how they will feel. This undermines their sense of self and gives rise to apprehension, even during euthymic periods (Akiskal, Khani, and Scott-Strauss, 1979). Indeed, this temperamental propensity to change from one affective state to another with very little ego control over the change is one of the principal reasons why some psychodynamically oriented clinicians may consider cyclothymic and bipolar II disorders as an expression of "borderline" characterological psychopathology. Old and current data (Akiskal *et al.*, 1985b; Deltito *et al.*, 2001; Akiskal, 2004; Smith, Muir, and Blackwood, 2005) suggest that in many cases the direction of causality is in the opposite direction, that is, that borderline features arise from the affective instability. Mixed states of short duration with extreme irritability occur in all subtypes of cyclothymia and are often associated with sedative hypnotic and alcohol abuse. Borderline characterological psychopathology is usually most severe in cases in which such irritable periods predominate. These irritable cyclothymics (Akiskal and Mallya, 1987; Akiskal, Hantouche, and Lancrenon, 2003b) are habitually moody-irritable and choleric with infrequent euthymia; they tend to brood; are hypercritical, complaining, and obtrusive; and typically evidence dysphoric restlessness and impulsivity.

In view of their propensity to affective recurrences, cyclothymia and bipolar disorder NOS are at high risk for having stormy object relations, which often give rise to serious interpersonal disturbances. While these disturbances warrant considerable psychotherapeutic attention, such attention may prove futile in the absence of competent pharmacotherapy of the affective instability.

25.5 CONCLUSION

There has been a revolution in the epidemiology, clinical phenomenology, classification, pharmacological, psychotherapeutic, and public health aspects of bipolar disorder. Indeed, bipolar disorders can now be considered to constitute a **subspecialty in psychiatry**. This is particularly true given the lifelong nature of the illness, the unpredictable exacerbations, and the disruption in social, occupational, and conjugal life, substance and medical comorbidity, and the high risk of suicide. Such an illness requires a coordination of services involving psychiatrists, nurses, social workers, psychologists, and pharmacists. It is no longer possible to think of solo practice in the management of this illness. The spectrum aspects require attention to diagnostic sophistication, not only in the patient, but also in the family, serving the cause of early case detection. This would be a model of practice that is necessary to teach training psychiatrists and other mental health professionals. The substantial advances in science are unlikely to make any impact on prevention and public health without such clinical units.

Regrettably, some bipolar programs deliver research rather than care. It is the latter aspect that now needs to be instituted. For this to happen, there needs to be "political" change in the climate of academic psychiatry and public mental health. What we need is the proper structure of caring for the affectively ill, mood, or bipolar clinics – just as there exist diabetes clinics, glaucoma clinics, pain clinics – multidisciplinary clinics that conduct research, train specialists, while providing high quality care.

The worst scenario for bipolar patients is that the lack of structures for caring for them in the current shortage of psychiatric beds is creating a new asylum on the streets of "civilized nations," such as the United States, in the form of homelessness (Health Care for the Homeless Clinicians' Network, 2000) – or worse, turning the mentally ill into prison inmates, which is particularly a very serious problem for bipolar with polysubstance abuse in the states of Arizona and California. Such incarceration is contrary to the spirit of Pinel's (1809) humanitarian reforms which unchained the mentally ill and liberated them. Such liberation envisaged the right for hospital treatment when needed. It was not a blanket endorsement for keeping patients out of the hospital under any circumstances. Today the severely mentally ill are roaming in the streets and are liable to all the hazards and abuses of such an existence. Civilized nations must not tolerate such outcome for those unfortunate members of its society who are bipolar, **psychotically** ill and poor. There was a time when medical schools cared for the disadvantaged. Today, they erect proud institutes of molecular biology, cancer, and cardiovascular health. Modern psychiatry began two centuries ago with a humanitarian revolution, followed by one of understanding the mind, culminating in the psychopharmacological revolution. A major theme of this book is an eloquent example of the success of the latter paradigm as it pertains to bipolar disorder. Bipolar disease is a spectrum of genetically-based illnesses and, without competent modern pharmacotherapy, it is hopelessly impossible in most cases to attenuate its cyclic course and provide a life relatively free from major episodic eruptions, despair, and suicide. What we now need is a culture of caring within a broader social psychiatry. For psychiatry which does not safeguard the basic dignity of every man or woman with serious mental illness in not psychiatry at all.

Basic research is being pursued in bipolar disorder along many fronts. The most promising leads, in terms of understanding the causes and pathogenesis of bipolar disorder would probably come from genetics. Our team has identified genes for bipolar disorder, which pertain to their temperamental substrates (Greenwood *et al.*, 2009). Such leads might eventually facilitate early diagnosis and prevention.

Today, many young psychiatrists and psychologists, aspiring to emulate their academic seniors in universities and research hospitals, measure prestige and success in multimillion dollar grants, and/or the limelight in national and international congresses. Ultimately, what we lecture about ("teach"), write, and do, must be measured against a less "prestigious" but more humane goal of caring for patients on a daily basis. The names of such dedicated mental health professionals are typically absent from the list of lecturers in national and international symposia on bipolar disorder – and their names do not adorn the pages of this book. We dedicate this chapter to them.

References

Akiskal, H.S. (1992) Delineating irritable-choleric and hyperthymic temperaments as variants of cyclothymia. *J. Person. Disord.*, **6**, 326–342.

Akiskal, H.S. (1996) The prevalent clinical spectrum of bipolar disorders: beyond DSM-IV. *J. Clin. Psychopharmacol.*, **16** (Suppl. 1), 4s–14s.

Akiskal, HS (ed.) (1999) *Bipolarity: Beyond Classic Mania. Psychiatric Clinics of North America*, W.B. Saunders, London, September 1999.

Akiskal, H.S. (2000) Dysthymia, cyclothymia and related chronic subthreshold mood disorders, in *New Oxford Textbook of Psychiatry* (eds M. Gelder, J. Lopez-Ibor, and N. Andreasen), Oxford University Press, London, pp. 736–749.

Akiskal, H.S. (2004) Demystifying borderline personality: critique of the concept and unorthodox reflections on its natural kinship with the bipolar spectrum. *Acta Psychiatr. Scand.*, **110**, 401–407.

Akiskal, H.S. (2005) Searching for behavioral indicators of bipolar II in patients presenting with major depressive episodes: the "red sign", the "rule of three" and other biographic signs of temperamental extravagance, activation and hypomania. *J. Affect. Disord.*, **84**, 279–290.

Akiskal, H.S. and Akiskal, K. (1988) Re-assessing the prevalence of bipolar disorders: clinical significance and artistic creativity. *Psychiatr. Psychobiol.*, **3**, 29s–36s.

Akiskal, K. and Akiskal, H.S. (2005) The theoretical underpinnings of affective temperaments: implications for evolutionary foundations of bipolarity and human nature. *J. Affect. Disord.*, **85**, 231–239.

Akiskal, H.S. and Akiskal, K.K. (2007) In search of Aristotle: temperament, human nature, melancholia, creativity and eminence. *J. Affect. Disord.*, **100**, 1–6.

Akiskal, H.S. and Akiskal, K.K. (2010) The genius-insanity debate: focus on bipolarity, temperament, creativity and leadership. In Yatham, L. and Maj, M., *Bipolar Disorder: Clinical and Neurobiological Foundations*. pp. 83–89, John Wiley & Sons, Chichester, UK.

Akiskal, H.S., Akiskal, K.K., Haykal, R. *et al.* (2005) TEMPS-A: progress towards validation of a self-rated clinical version of the temperament evaluation of the Memphis, Pisa, Paris, and San Diego Autoquestionnaire. *J. Affect. Disord.*, **85**, 3–16.

Akiskal, H.S., Azorin, J.F., and Hantouche, E.G. (2003a) Proposed multidimensional structure of mania: beyond the euphoric-dysphoric dichotomy. *J. Affect. Disord.*, **73**, 7–18.

Akiskal, H.S., Hantouche, E.G., and Lancrenon, S. (2003b) Bipolar II with and without cyclothymic temperament: "dark" and "sunny" expressions of soft bipolarity. *J. Affect. Disord.*, **73**, 49–57.

Akiskal, H.S., Bitar, A.H., Puzantian, V.R. *et al.* (1978) The nosological status of neurotic depression: a prospective three-to-four year examination in light of the primary-secondary and unipolar-bipolar dichotomies. *Arch. Gen. Psychiatry*, **35**, 756–766.

Akiskal, H.S., Djenderedjian, A.H., Rosenthal, R.H. *et al.* (1977) Cyclothymic disorder: validating criteria for inclusion in the bipolar affective group. *Am. J. Psychiatry*, **134**, 1227–1233.

Akiskal, H.S., Downs, J., Jordan, P. *et al.* (1985a) Affective disorders in the referred children and younger siblings of manic-depressives: mode of onset and prospective course. *Arch. Gen. Psychiatry*, **42**, 996–1003.

Akiskal, H.S., Chen, S.E., Davis, G.C. *et al.* (1985b) Borderline: an adjective in search of a noun. *J. Clin. Psychiatry*, **46**, 41–48.

Akiskal, H.S., Khani, M.K., and Scott-Strauss, A. (1979) Cyclothymic temperamental disorders. *Psychiatr. Clin. N. Am.*, **2**, 527–554.

Akiskal, H.S. and Mallya, G. (1987) Criteria for the "soft" bipolar spectrum: treatment implications. *Psychopharmacol. Bull.*, **23**, 68–73.

Akiskal, H.S. and Puzantian, V.R. (1979) Psychotic forms of depression and mania. *Psychiatr. Clin. N. Am.*, **2**, 419–439.

Akiskal, H.S., Walker, P.W., Puzantian, V.R. *et al.* (1983) Bipolar outcome in the course of depressive illness: phenomenologic, familial, and pharmacologic predictors. *J. Affect. Disord.*, **5**, 115–128.

Albanese, M.J., Clodfelter, R.C., Jr., Pardo, T.B. *et al.* (2006) Underdiagnosis of bipolar disorder in men with substance use disorder. *J. Psychiatr. Pract.*, **12**, 124–127.

Angst, F., Stassen, H.H., Clayton, P.J. *et al.* (2002) Mortality of patients with mood disorders: follow-up over 34–38 years. *J. Affect. Disord.*, **68**, 167–181.

Arnold, L. (1995) *The Price of Greatness*, Guilford, New York.

Balanzá-Martínez, V., Selva, G., Martínez-Arán, A. *et al.* (2010) Neurocognition in bipolar disorders- a closer look at comorbidities and medications. *Eur. J. Pharmacol.*, **626**, 87–96.

Bauer, M.S., McBride, L., Williford, W.O., Glick, H. *et al.* (2006) Collaborative care for bipolar disorder: Part II impact on clinical outcome, function, and costs. *Psychiatr. Serv.*, **57**, 937–945.

Benazzi, F. and Akiskal, H.S. (2001) Delineating bipolar II in the Ravenna-San Diego collaborative study: the relative prevalence and diagnostic significance of hypomanic features during major depressive episodes. *J. Affect. Disord.*, **67**, 115–122.

Benazzi, F. and Akiskal, H.S. (2009) The modified SCID Hypomania module (SCID-Hba): a detailed systematic phenomenological probing. *J. Affect. Discord.*, **117**, 131–136.

Berk, M., Hallam, K., Malhi, G.S. *et al.* (2010) Evidence and implications for early intervention in bipolar disorder. *J. Ment. Health.*, **19**, 113–126.

Colom, F., Vieta, E., Martinez-Aran, A. *et al.* (2003) A randomized trial on the efficacy of group psychoeducation in the prophylaxis of recurrences in bipolar patients whose disease is in remission. *Arch. Gen. Psychiatry*, **60**, 402–407.

Coryell, W., Endicott, J., Keller, M. *et al.* (1989) Bipolar affective disorder and high achievement: a familial association. *Am. J. Psychiatry*, **146**, 983–988.

Deltito, J., Martin, L., Riefkohl, J. *et al.* (2001) Do patients with borderline personality disorder belong to the bipolar spectrum? *J. Affect. Disord.*, **67**, 221–228.

Esquirol, J.E.D. (1983 *Des Maladies Mentales*, Balliere, Paris. (Translated by E.K. Hunt as mental maladies: a treatise on insanity. Philadelphia: Les and Blanchard, 1845).

Fieve, R.R. (1975) The lithium clinic: a new model for the delivery of psychiatric services. *Am. J. Psychiatry*, **132**, 1018–1022.

Fuchs, T. (2004) Neurobiology and psychotherapy: an emerging dialogue. *Curr. Opin. Psychiatry*, **17**, 479–485.

Gelenberg, A.J., Kane, J.M., Keller, M.B. *et al.* (1989) Comparison of standard and low serum levels of lithium for maintenance treatment of bipolar disorder. *N. Engl. J. Med.*, **321**, 1489–1493.

Goldberg, Joseph. and Burdick, K. (2008) *Cognitive Dysfunction in Bipolar Disorder: A Guide for Clinicians*, American Psychiatric Publishing, Inc., Arlington.

Goodwin, F.K., Fireman, B., Simon, G.E. *et al.* (2003) Suicide risk in bipolar disorder during treatment with lithium and divalproex. *J. Am. Med. Assoc.*, **290**, 1467–1473.

Graves, J.S. (1993) Living with mania: a study of outpatient group psychotherapy for bipolar patients. *Am. J. Psychother.*, **47**, 113–126.

Greenwood, T.A., Akiskal, H.S., Akiskal, K.K. *et al.* (2009) *Genome-wide Association Study of Temperament as an Intermediate Phenotype for Bipolar Disorder Reveals Significant Associations to Three Novel Loci*. Paper presented at the World Congress of Psychiatric Genetics, Nov 4–8, 2009, San Diego, CA, USA.

Hantouche, E.G. and Akiskal, H.S. (2004) Traiter le patient bipolaire. *Ann. Méd. Psychol.*, **162**, 164–168.

Health Care for the Homeless Clinicians' Network (2000) Mental illness, chronic homelessness: an american disgrace. *Heal. Hand.*, **4**, 1–5.

Hirschfeld, R.M., Lewis, L., and Vornik, L.A. (2003) Perceptions and impact of bipolar disorder: how far have we really come? Results of the national depressive and manic-depressive association 2000 survey of individuals with bipolar disorder. *J. Clin. Psychiatry.*, **64**, 161–174.

Jamison, K.R. (1996) *Touched with Fire: Manic Depressive Illness and the Artistic Temperament*, Free Press, New York.

Jamison, K.R. and Akiskal, H.S. (1983) Medication compliance in patients with bipolar disorders. *Psychiatr. Clin. N. Am.*, **6**, 175–192.

Koukopoulos, A., Reginaldi, D., Minnai, G., Serra, G., Pani, L., and Johnson, F.N. (1995) The long-term prophylaxis of affective disorders. *Adv. Biochem. Psychopharmacol.*, **49**, 127–147.

Kraepelin, E. (1921) Manic Depressive Insanity and Paranoia. Edinburgh.

Krober, H.L. (1993) Illness perception and coping with illness of bipolar manic-depressive patients. *Fortschr. Neurol. Psychiatr.*, **61**, 267–273.

Kukopulos, A., Reginaldi, D., Laddomada, P. *et al.* (1980) Course of the manic-depressive cycle and changes caused by treatment. *Pharmakopsychiatr. Neuropsychopharmakol.*, **13**, 156–167.

Lenzi, A., Lazzerini, F., Placidi, G.F. *et al.* (1989) Predictors of compliance with lithium and carbamazepine regimens in the long-term treatment of recurrent mood and related psychotic disorders. *Pharmacopsychiatry*, **22**, 34–37.

Lish, J.D., Dime-Meenan, S., Whybrow, P.C. *et al.* (1994) The National Depressive and Manic-depressive Association (DMDA) survey of bipolar members. *J. Affect. Disord.*, **31**, 281–294.

Lyoo, K., Dager Stephen, R., Kim Jieun, E. *et al.* (2010) Lithium-induced gray matter volume increase as a neural correlate of treatment response in bipolar disorder: a longitudinal brain imaging study. *Neuropsychopharmacology*, **25**, 1743–1750.

Manning, J.S., Hyakal, R.F., and Akiskal, H.S. (1999) The role of bipolarity in depression in the family practice setting. *Psychiatr. Clin. N. Am.*, **22**, 689–673.

Maremmani, I., Pacini, M., Lubrano, S. *et al.* (2003) Dual diagnosis heroin addicts. The clinical and therapeutic aspects. *Heroin. Add. Rel. Clin. Probl.*, **5**, 7–98.

Muller-Oerlinghausen, B., Grof, P., and Schou, M. (1999) Lithium and suicide prevention. *Br. J. Psychiatry*, **175**, 90–91.

Mundt, C. (2003) Psychotherapy and the novel biological paradigms – how do they relate? *Seishin. Shinkeigaku. Zasshi.*, **105**, 171–184.

Okasha, A., El Akabawi, A.S., Snyder, K.S. *et al.* (1994) Expressed emotion, perceived criticism, and relapse in depression: a replication in an Egyptian community. *Am. J. Psychiatry*, **151**, 1001–1005.

Perugi, G., Toni, C., and Akiskal, H.S. (1999) Anxious-bipolar comorbidity: Diagnostic and treatment challenges. *Psychiatr Clin North Am*, **22**, 565–583.

Pinel, P. (1809) *Traite medico-philosophique sur l'alienation mentale* [Medico-philosophical treatise on mental alienation], Paris, Brosson, 1809. Reprint fascimile, Paris, Clin Comar Byla, 1975.

Post, R.M. and Leverich, G.S. (2008) *Treatment of Bipolar Illness*, WW Norton & Co, New York.

Sachs, G.S., Nierenberg, A.A., Calabrese, J.R. *et al.* (2007) Effectiveness of adjunctive antidepressant treatment for bipolar depression. *N. Engl. J. Med.*, **356**, 1711–1722.

Schou, M. (1979) Artistic productivity and lithium prophylaxis in manic-depressive illness. *Br. J. Psychiatry*, **135**, 97–103.

Smith, D.J. and Ghaemi, N. (2010) Is underdiagnosis the main pitfall when diagnosing bipolar disorder? Yes. *Br. Med. J.*, **340**, c854.

Smith, D.J., Muir, W.J., and Blackwood, D.H. (2005) Borderline personality disorder characteristics in young adults with recurrent mood disorders: a comparison of bipolar and unipolar depression. *J. Affect. Disord.*, **87**, 17–23.

Zimmerman, M., Ruggero, C.J., Chelminski, I. *et al.* (2008) Is bipolar disorder overdiagnosed? *J. Clin. Psychiatry*, **69**, 935–940.

Index

abuse, childhood 323
N-acetylcysteine (NAC) 291, 293, 294, 434
activation, excessive 498
addictions 294
   see also substance use disorders
adenosine 425, 426
ADHD *see* attention deficit hyperactivity disorder
adherence to treatment
   caring principles 494, 499, 501
   older bipolar patients 382
   psychoeducation 451–3
   risperidone LAI 170
adolescence, abuse in 323
adolescent bipolar disorder *see* pediatric bipolar
   disorder
advocacy organizations 492–3
agitated depression 394, 474
   see also mixed states
agomelatine 427
agranulocytosis 134–5
alcohol use
   caring principles 497
   combination therapy 287, 290, 291, 293
   gender differences 322–3
   psychoeducation 453–4
   valproate 33, 291
allopurinol 426
alopecia 36
alternative therapies 453
American Psychiatric Association (APA)
   DSM-IV 2–3, 392, 393, 411
   treatment guidelines 225–7
AMPA receptors 428, 429
antiarrhythmic drugs 239
anticonvulsants 61–71
   complex combination therapy 290, 291, 292,
     293
   mixed states 25, 28–29, 32, 50–51, 55,
     61–62, 86–7, 356, 358, 401, 402,
     404
   older patients 375, 377

pediatric patients 32, 33–34, 36–37, 53, 64,
   182, 355–9
rapid cyclers 31, 51, 63, 417
suicide prevention 477–479, 480–1
treatment guidelines 226
women 37, 38, 46–47, 53, 56, 290, 327–332,
   333–4, 335, 336
see also carbamazepine; lamotrigine; valproate
antidepressants 299–307
   breastfeeding 335
   bupropion 291, 295, 306, 401, 455
   caring principles 498
   clinical guidelines 306–7
   complex combination therapy 292, 498
   future research 306
   gender differences 329
   MAO inhibitors 300, 303, 307
   mixed states 401, 402, 404, 405
   mood stabilizers as 299–300
   older patients 379, 380–1
   in pregnancy 332–3
   rapid cyclers 305–306, 309, 329, 413–414,
     416, 417, 418–9
   self-prescription and 456
   SNRIs 300, 309
   SSRIs 300, 303, 304–309, 329, 332–3
     see also fluoxetine; paroxetine
   suicidality 300, 302–303, 306–309, 306, 475,
     479–80
   treatment guidelines 226, 227, 299
   tricyclics 300, 301–303, 307, 329, 332–3, 413
   see also depression, novel therapeutic
     approaches
antiepileptics *see* anticonvulsants
antipsychotics
   first generation (typical; classical) 109–126,
     132–3, 140
     gender differences in responses to 327
     nursing mothers 335
     second generation's efficacy compared *see*
       below

Bipolar Psychopharmacotherapy: Caring for the patient, Second Edition. Edited by Hagop S. Akiskal and Mauricio Tohen.
© 2011 John Wiley & Sons, Ltd. Published 2011 by John Wiley & Sons, Ltd.